Communications in Computer and Information Science   1211

Commenced Publication in 2007
Founding and Former Series Editors:
Simone Diniz Junqueira Barbosa, Phoebe Chen, Alfredo Cuzzocrea,
Xiaoyong Du, Orhun Kara, Ting Liu, Krishna M. Sivalingam,
Dominik Ślęzak, Takashi Washio, Xiaokang Yang, and Junsong Yuan

More information about this series at http://www.springer.com/series/7899

Ana Roque · Arkadiusz Tomczyk ·
Elisabetta De Maria · Felix Putze ·
Roman Moucek · Ana Fred ·
Hugo Gamboa (Eds.)

Biomedical Engineering Systems and Technologies

12th International Joint Conference, BIOSTEC 2019
Prague, Czech Republic, February 22–24, 2019
Revised Selected Papers

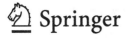 Springer

Editors
Ana Roque
Universidade Nova de Lisboa
Caparica, Portugal

Elisabetta De Maria
Nice Sophia Antipolis University
Nice Cedex 2, France

Roman Moucek
University of West Bohemia
Pilsen, Czech Republic

Hugo Gamboa
Universidade Nova de Lisboa
Caparica, Portugal

Arkadiusz Tomczyk🆔
Lodz University of Technology
Łódź, Poland

Felix Putze
University of Bremen
Bremen, Germany

Ana Fred
Instituto de Telecomunicações
University of Lisbon
Lisbon, Portugal

ISSN 1865-0929   ISSN 1865-0937 (electronic)
Communications in Computer and Information Science
ISBN 978-3-030-46969-6   ISBN 978-3-030-46970-2 (eBook)
https://doi.org/10.1007/978-3-030-46970-2

This Springer imprint is published by the registered company Springer Nature Switzerland AG
The registered company address is: Gewerbestrasse 11, 6330 Cham, Switzerland

Preface

The present book includes extended and revised versions of a set of selected papers from the 12th International Joint Conference on Biomedical Engineering Systems and Technologies (BIOSTEC 2019), held in Prague, Czech Republic, during February 22–24, 2019. BIOSTEC is composed of five colocated conferences, each specialized in a different knowledge area, namely BIODEVICES, BIOIMAGING, BIOINFORMATICS, BIOSIGNALS, and HEALTHINF.

BIOSTEC 2019 received 271 paper submissions from 47 countries, of which only 8% are included in this book. This reflects our care in selecting those contributions. These papers were selected by the conference chairs and their selection was based on a number of criteria that included the classifications and comments provided by the Program Committee members, the session chairs' assessment, and the program chairs' meta review of the papers that were included in the technical program. The authors of selected papers were invited to submit a revised, extended, and improved version of their conference paper, including at least 30% new material.

The purpose of the BIOSTEC joint conferences is to bring together researchers and practitioners, including engineers, biologists, health professionals, and informatics/computer scientists. Research presented at BIOSTEC included both theoretical advances and applications of information systems, artificial intelligence, signal processing, electronics, and other engineering tools in areas related to advancing biomedical research and improving healthcare.

The papers selected to be included in this book contribute to the understanding of relevant trends of current research on the biomedical engineering field. In particular, the book contains chapters describing novel trends in biodevices, namely the potential to apply microfluidic platforms to analyze cell deformability in biological fluids, the development of algorithms to compare electrical impedance diagnostics, the simulation of the magnetic navigation of micro robots in the body, or even a new platform for the robotic rehabilitation of balance impairment. This book also includes papers on machine learning – and specifically deep learning – for biosignal processing in medical contexts. This includes the classification of cardiac arrhythmias, stress, or non-stationarity of heart rate. Another trend is the focus on applicable sensor setups with high mobility and low degree of intrusiveness, such as commercially available wearables. Another set of papers included in this book contribute to the understanding of relevant trends of current research on medical image analysis. This includes both classic methods like active contours and modern deep learning techniques like convolutional neural networks. In both cases the crucial element is domain knowledge provided by the experts. It can be expressed either in natural language, which need to be transformed into semantic constraints applied while contour evolution, or as an annotated set of data, which is directly used for neural network training. Another group of papers presents novel algorithms to deal with involved research problems in structural bioinformatics, genomics and proteomics, model design and evaluation, and drug discovery. Finally, some papers describing the role and acceptance of socially assistive robots in rehabilitation, detection of cognitive impairments and early Alzheimer's dementia, GDPR compliance of mHealth, and improvement of data management in healthcare by adopting FAIR principles and standardizing clinical caremaps were also included.

We would like to thank all the authors for their contributions and also to the reviewers who helped to ensure the quality of this publication.

February 2019

Ana Roque
Arkadiusz Tomczyk
Elisabetta De Maria
Felix Putze
Roman Moucek
Ana Fred
Hugo Gamboa

Organization

Conference Co-chairs

Ana Fred   Instituto de Telecomunicações and University
of Lisbon, Portugal

Hugo Gamboa   LIBPhys, Universidade Nova de Libsboa, Portugal

Program Co-chairs

BIODEVICES

Ana Roque   UCIBIO, Universidade Nova de Lisboa, Portugal

BIOIMAGING

Arkadiusz Tomczyk   Lodz University of Technology, Poland

BIOINFORMATICS

Elisabetta De Maria   Université Côte d'Azur, CNRS, I3S, France

BIOSIGNALS

Felix Putze   Universität Bremen, Germany

HEALTHINF

Roman Moucek   University of West Bohemia, Czech Republic

BIODEVICES Program Committee

Andreas Bahr	University of Kiel, Germany
Mohammed Bakr	CCIT-AASTMT, Egypt
Steve Beeby	University of Southampton, UK
Jan Cabri	Luxembourg Institute of Research in Orthopedics, Sports Medicine and Science (LIROMS), Luxembourg
Carlo Capelli	University of Verona, Italy
Vítor Carvalho	IPCA-EST, Algoritmi Research Centre, UM, Portugal
Hamid Charkhkar	Case Western Reserve University, USA
Youngjae Chun	University of Pittsburgh, USA
Alberto Cliquet Jr.	University of São Paulo and University of Campinas, Brazil
Pedro Estrela	University of Bath, UK
Maria Evelina Fantacci	University of Pisa, INFN, Italy

Renato Varoto	University of Campinas, Brazil
Pedro Vieira	Universidade Nova de Lisboa, Portugal
Bruno Wacogne	FEMTO-ST, UMR CNRS 6174, France
Richard Willson	University of Houston, USA
Hakan Yavuz	Çukurova Üniversity, Turkey
Alberto Yufera	Universidad de Sevilla, Spain

BIODEVICES Additional Reviewers

Mattia Dimitri	University of Florence, Italy

BIOIMAGING Program Committee

Jesús B. Alonso	Universidad de Las Palmas de Gran Canaria, Spain
Peter Balazs	University of Szeged, Hungary
Richard Bayford	Middlesex University, UK
Alpan Bek	Middle East Technical University, Turkey
Obara Boguslaw	University of Durham, UK
Alberto Bravin	European Synchrotron Radiation Facility, France
Alexander Bykov	University of Oulu, Optoelectronics and Measurement Techniques Laboratory, Finland
Rita Casadio	University of Bologna, Italy
Alessia Cedola	CNR, Institute of Nanotechnology, Italy
Heang-Ping Chan	University of Michigan, USA
Paola Coan	LMU Munich, Germany
Miguel Coimbra	University of Porto, Portugal
Christos Constantinou	Stanford University, USA
Giacomo Cuttone	Laboratori Nazionali del Sud Catania (INFN), Italy
Alexandre Douplik	Ryerson University, Canada
Edite Figueiras	Champalimaud Foundation, Portugal
P. Gopinath	Indian Institute of Technology Roorkee, India
Dimitris Gorpas	Technical University of Munich, Germany
Tzung-Pei Hong	National University of Kaohsiung, Taiwan, China
Jae Youn Hwang	DGIST, South Korea
Kazuyuki Hyodo	High Energy Accelerator Research Organization, Japan
Xiaoyi Jiang	University of Münster, Germany
Patrice Koehl	University of California, USA
Algimantas Krisciukaitis	Lithuanian University of Health Sciences, Lithuania
Pavel Kříž	University of Chemistry and Technology Prague, Czech Republic
Adriaan Lammertsma	VU University Medical Center Amsterdam, The Netherlands
Sang-Won Lee	Korea Research Institute of Standards and Science, South Korea
Ivan Lima Jr.	North Dakota State University, USA

Hua Lin	Shanghai Institute of Optics and Fine Mechanics, Chinese Academy of Sciences, China
Honghai Liu	Children's Hospital of Pittsburgh of UPMC, USA
Siyu Ma	Massachusetts General Hospital, USA
Joanna Isabelle Olszewska	University of West Scotland, UK
Kalman Palagyi	University of Szeged, Hungary
George Panoutsos	University of Sheffield, UK
Tae Jung Park	Chung-Ang University, South Korea
Gennaro Percannella	University of Salerno, Italy
Gabriele Piantadosi	Università Federico II di Napoli, Italy
Ales Prochazka	University of Chemistry and Technology, Czech Republic
Wan Qin	University of Washington, USA
Alessandra Retico	Istituto Nazionale di Fisica Nucleare, Italy
Benjamin Risse	University of Münster, Germany
Bart Romeny	Eindhoven University of Technology (TU/e), The Netherlands
Sherif S. Sherif	University of Manitoba, Canada
Olivier Salvado	CSIRO, Australia
Ravi Samala	University of Michigan, USA
K. C. Santosh	The University of South Dakota, USA
Emanuele Schiavi	Universidad Rey Juan Carlos, Spain
Jan Schier	The Institute of Information Theory and Automation, Czech Academy of Sciences, Czech Republic
Mário Secca	CEFITEC, Universidade Nova de Libsboa, Portugal
Gregory Sharp	Massachusetts General Hospital, USA
Leonid Shvartsman	Hebrew University, Israel
Vijay Singh	Massachusetts Institute of Technology, USA
Milan Sonka	University of Iowa, USA
Chikayoshi Sumi	Sophia University, Japan
Chi-Kuang Sun	National Taiwan University, Taiwan, China
Piotr Szczepaniak	Lodz University of Technology, Poland
Pablo Taboada	University of Santiago de Compostela, Spain
Arkadiusz Tomczyk	Lodz University of Technology, Poland
Carlos Travieso-González	Universidad de Las Palmas de Gran Canaria, Spain
Benjamin Tsui	Johns Hopkins University, USA
Vladimír Ulman	Masaryk University, Czech Republic
Sandra Ventura	Escola Superior de Saúde do Politécnico do Porto, Portugal
Irina Voiculescu	University of Oxford, UK
Yuanyuan Wang	Fudan University, China
Quan Wen	University of Electronic Science and Technology of China, China
Hedi Yazid	LATIS, National School of Engineering of Sousse, Tunisia
Hongki Yoo	Hanyang University, South Korea

Zeyun Yu   University of Wisconsin at Milwaukee, USA
Habib Zaidi   Geneva University Hospital, Switzerland

BIOIMAGING Additional Reviewers

Wei Wei   University of Washington, USA
Xin Xie   Becton Dickinson and Company, USA

BIOINFORMATICS Program Committee

Tatsuya Akutsu   Kyoto University, Japan
Hesham Ali   University of Nebraska at Omaha, USA
Jens Allmer   Hochschule Ruhr West University of Applied Sciences,
                                 Germany
Francois Andry   Philips, France
Joel Arrais   Universidade de Coimbra, Portugal
Zafer Aydin   Abdullah Gul University, Turkey
Emiliano   Universidad Nacional de Colombia, Colombia
  Barreto-Hernandez
Payam Behzadi   Shahr-e-Qods Branch, Islamic Azad University, Iran
Judith Blake   Jackson Laboratory, USA
Leonardo Bocchi   Università di Firenze, Italy
Luca Bortolussi   University of Trieste, Italy
José Cerón Carrasco   Universidad Católica San Antonio de Murcia, Spain
Young-Rae Cho   Baylor University, USA
Mark Clement   Brigham Young University, USA
Federica Conte   National Research Council of Rome, Italy
Antoine Danchin   Institut Cochin INSERM U1016, CNRS UMR 8104,
                                 Université Paris Descartes, France
Thomas Dandekar   University of Würzburg, Germany
Sérgio Deusdado   Instituto Politecnico de Bragança, Portugal
Santa Di Cataldo   Politecnico di Torino, Italy
Eytan Domany   Weizmann Institute of Science, Israel
Richard Edwards   University of Southampton, UK
François Fages   Inria, France
Maria Evelina Fantacci   University of Pisa, INFN, Italy
António Ferreira   Universidade de Lisboa, Portugal
Giulia Fiscon   National Research Council of Rome (CNR), Italy
Liliana Florea   Johns Hopkins University, USA
Alexandre Francisco   Universidade de Lisboa, Portugal
Bruno Gaeta   University of New South Wales, Australia
Max Garzon   The University of Memphis, USA
Igor Goryanin   University of Edinburgh, UK
Christopher Hann   University of Canterbury, New Zealand
Ronaldo Hashimoto   University of São Paulo, Brazil
Volkhard Helms   Universität des Saarlandes, Germany

Seiya Imoto	University of Tokyo, Japan
Sohei Ito	National Fisheries University, Japan
Bo Jin	MilliporeSigma, Merck KGaA, USA
Giuseppe Jurman	Fondazione Bruno Kessler, Italy
Yannis Kalaidzidis	Max Planck Institute Molecular Cell Biology and Genetic, Germany
Natalia Khuri	Wake Forest University, USA
Inyoung Kim	Virginia Tech, USA
Toralf Kirsten	University of Leipzig, Germany
Jirí Kléma	Czech Technical University in Prague, Czech Republic
Ivan Kulakovskiy	Russia
Yinglei Lai	George Washington University, USA
Carlile Lavor	University of Campinas, Brazil
Matej Lexa	Masaryk University, Czech Republic
Pawel Mackiewicz	Wroclaw University, Poland
Prashanti Manda	The University of North Carolina at Greensboro, USA
Elena Marchiori	Radboud University, The Netherlands
Andrea Marin	University of Venice, Italy
Majid Masso	George Mason University, USA
Petr Matula	Masaryk University, Czech Republic
Giancarlo Mauri	Università di Milano Bicocca, Italy
Paolo Milazzo	Università di Pisa, Italy
Vincent Moulton	University of East Anglia, UK
Chad Myers	University of Minnesota, USA
Helder Nakaya	University of São Paulo, Brazil
David Naranjo-Hernández	University of Seville, Spain
Jean-Christophe Nebel	Kingston University, UK
José Oliveira	University of Aveiro, DETI/IEETA, Portugal
Oscar Pastor	Universidad Politécnica de Valencia, Spain
Marco Pellegrini	Consiglio Nazionale delle Ricerche, Italy
Matteo Pellegrini	University of California, Los Angeles, USA
Horacio Pérez-Sánchez	Catholic University of Murcia, Spain
Nadia Pisanti	Università di Pisa, Italy
Olivier Poch	ICube UMR7357, CNRS, Université de Strasbourg, France
Alberto Policriti	Università degli Studi di Udine, Italy
Gianfranco Politano	Politecnico di Torino, Italy
Junfeng Qu	Clayton State University, USA
Javier Reina-Tosina	University of Seville, Spain
Laura Roa	University of Seville, Spain
Simona Rombo	Università degli Studi di Palermo, Italy
Eric Rouchka	University of Louisville, USA
Olivier Roux	École Centrale de Nantes, France
Claudia Rubiano Castellanos	Universidad Nacional de Colombia, Colombia
Carolina Ruiz	WPI, USA

J. Salgado	University of Chile, Chile
Alessandro Savino	Politecnico di Torino, Italy
Jaime Seguel	University of Puerto Rico at Mayaguez, USA
Noor Akhmad Setiawan	Universitas Gadjah Mada, Indonesia
João Setubal	Universidade de São Paulo, Brazil
Hamid Shahbazkia	University of Central Asia, Kyrgyzstan
Anne Siegel	CNRS, France
Christine Sinoquet	University of Nantes, France
Pavel Smrz	Brno University of Technology, Czech Republic
Gordon Smyth	Walter and Eliza Hall Institute of Medical Research, Australia
Yinglei Song	Jiansu University of Science and Technology, China
Peter Stadler	Universität Leipzig, IZBI, Germany
David Svoboda	Masaryk University, Czech Republic
Peter Sykacek	University of Natural Resources and Life Sciences, Austria
Takashi Tomita	Japan Advanced Institute of Science and Technology, Japan
Alexander Tsouknidas	Aristotle University of Thessaloniki, Greece
Juris Viksna	University of Latvia, Latvia
Thomas Werner	University of Michigan, Germany
Malik Yousef	Zefat Academic College, Israel
Alexander Zelikovsky	Georgia State University, USA
Wen Zhang	Icahn School of Medicine at Mount Sinai, USA
Zhongming Zhao	University of Texas, USA
Leming Zhou	University of Pittsburgh, USA
Jiali Zhuang	Molecular Stethoscope Inc., USA

BIOINFORMATICS Additional Reviewers

Eugene Baulin	Institute of Mathematical Problems of Biology, Russian Academy of Sciences, Russia
Giovanna Broccia	University of Pisa, Italy
Artem Kasianov	VIGG, Russia
Jakob Ruess	Inria Paris, France
Cátia Vaz	INESC-ID, Portugal

BIOSIGNALS Program Committee

Bruce Denby	Sorbonne Université, France
Jean-Marie Aerts	M3-BIORES, Katholieke Universitëit Leuven, Belgium
Eda Akman Aydin	Gazi University, Turkey
Raul Alcaraz	Biomedical Engineering Research Group, University of Castilla-La Mancha, Spain
Robert Allen	University of Southampton, UK
Jesús B. Alonso	Universidad de Las Palmas de Gran Canaria, Spain

Carlos Thomaz	Centro Universitário FEI, Brazil
Ana Tomé	University of Aveiro, Portugal
Carlos Travieso-González	Universidad de Las Palmas de Gran Canaria, Spain
Ahsan Ursani	Mehran University of Engineering and Technology, Pakistan
Egon L. van den Broek	Utrecht University, The Netherlands
Bart Vanrumste	Katholieke Universiteit Leuven, Belgium
Michal Vavrecka	Czech Technical University, Czech Republic
Pedro Vaz	University of Coimbra, Portugal
Fernando Velez	Universidade da Beira Interior, Portugal
R. Vinothkanna	Koneru Lakshmaiah Education Foundation, India
Yuanyuan Wang	Fudan University, China
Quan Wen	University of Electronic Science and Technology of China, China
Didier Wolf	CRAN, UMR CNRS 7039, Université de Lorraine, France
Chia-Hung Yeh	National Sun Yat-sen University, Taiwan, China
Rafal Zdunek	Politechnika Wroclawska, Poland

BIOSIGNALS Additional Reviewers

Karl Daher	University of Applied Sciences and Arts Western Switzerland, Switzerland
Laercio Silva Junior	Centro Universitário da FEI, Brazil
Emanuel Teixeira	Unversidade da Beira interior, Portugal

HEALTHINF Program Committee

Francois Andry	Philips, France
Wassim Ayadi	LERIA, University of Angers, France, and LaTICE, University of Tunis, Tunisia
Omar Badreddin	University of Texas El Paso, USA
Payam Behzadi	Shahr-e-Qods Branch, Islamic Azad University, Iran
Sorana Bolboaca	Iuliu Hatieganu University of Medicine and Pharmacy, Romania
Alessio Bottrighi	Università del Piemonte Orientale, Italy
Andrew Boyd	University of Illinois at Chicago, USA
Klaus Brinker	Hamm-Lippstadt University of Applied Sciences, Germany
Federico Cabitza	Università degli Studi di Milano-Bicocca, Italy
Eric Campo	LAAS CNRS, France
Guilherme Campos	IEETA, Portugal
Manuel Campos-Martinez	University of Murcia, Spain
Marc Cavazza	University of Greenwich, UK
Sergio Cerutti	Polytechnic University of Milan, Italy
James Cimino	UAB School of Medicine, USA

Mihail Cocosila	Athabasca University, Canada
Miguel Coimbra	University of Porto, Portugal
Emmanuel Conchon	XLIM, France
Carlos Costa	Universidade de Aveiro, Portugal
Liliana Dobrica	University Politehnica of Bucharest, Romania
Stephan Dreiseitl	Upper Austria University of Applied Sciences at Hagenberg, Austria
George Drosatos	Democritus University of Thrace, Greece
Martin Duneld	Stockholm University, Sweden
Farshideh Einsele	Berne University of Applied Sciences, Switzerland
Christo El Morr	York University, Canada
José Fonseca	UNINOVA, Portugal
Christoph Friedrich	University of Applied Sciences and Arts Dortmund, Germany
Ioannis Fudos	University of Ioannina, Greece
Henry Gabb	University of Illinois at Urbana-Champaign, USA
Angelo Gargantini	University of Bergamo, Italy
James Geller	New Jersey Institute of Technology, USA
Laura Giarré	Università degli Studi di Palermo, Italy
Juan Miguel Gómez	Carlos III University of Madrid, Spain
Yves Gourinat	ISAE-SUPAERO, France
Alexandra Grancharova	University of Chemical Technology and Metallurgy, Bulgaria
David Greenhalgh	University of Strathclyde, UK
Tahir Hameed	Merrimack College, USA
Vitaly Herasevich	Mayo Clinic, USA
Cirano Iochpe	Universidade Federal Do Rio Grande Do Sul, Brazil
Dragan Jankovic	University of Nis, Serbia
Petr Ježek	University of West Bohemia, Czech Republic
Eleni Kaldoudi	Democritus University of Thrace, Greece
Noreen Kamal	University of Calgary, Canada
Finn Kensing	University of Copenhagen, Denmark
Josef Kohout	University of West Bohemia, Czech Republic
Eduan Kotze	University of the Free State, South Africa
Tomohiro Kuroda	Kyoto University Hospital, Japan
Craig Kuziemsky	MacEwan University, Canada
Sofia Kyratzi	University of the Aegean, Greece
Elyes Lamine	University of Toulouse, IMT Mines Albi, CGI, France
Nekane Larburu Rubio	Vicomtech, Spain
Giuseppe Liotta	University of Perugia, Italy
Nicolas Loménie	Université Paris Descartes, France
Guillaume Lopez	Aoyama Gakuin University, Japan
Martin Lopez-Nores	University of Vigo, Spain
Jose Alberto Maldonado	Universitat Politècnica de València, Spain
Alda Marques	University of Aveiro, Portugal
Ken Masters	Sultan Qaboos University, Oman

James McGlothlin	Fusion Consulting Inc., USA
Rebecca Meehan	Kent State University, USA
Lourdes Moreno	Universidad Carlos III De Madrid, Spain
Roman Moucek	University of West Bohemia, Czech Republic
Hammadi Nait-Charif	Bournemouth University, UK
Binh Nguyen	Victoria University of Wellington, New Zealand
Heinrich Niemann	University of Erlangen-Nuernberg, Germany
José Oliveira	University of Aveiro, DETI/IEETA, Portugal
Agnieszka Onisko	Bialystok University of Technology, Poland
Thomas Ostermann	Witten/Herdecke University, Germany
Nelson Pacheco da Rocha	University of Aveiro, Portugal
Rui Pedro Paiva	University of Coimbra, Portugal
Vimla Patel	The New York Academy of Medicine, USA
Sotiris Pavlopoulos	ICCS, Greece
Fabrizio Pecoraro	National Research Council, Italy
Carlos Pereira	Federal University of Rio Grande Do Sul (UFRGS), Brazil
Liam Peyton	University of Ottawa, Canada
Enrico Piras	Fondazione Bruno Kessler, Italy
Josiah Poon	The University of Sydney, Australia
Arkalgud Ramaprasad	University of Illinois at Chicago, USA
Grzegorz Redlarski	Gdansk University of Technology, Poland
Ita Richardson	University of Limerick, Ireland
Marcos Rodrigues	Sheffield Hallam University, UK
Alejandro Rodríguez González	Centro de Tecnología Biomédica, Spain
Valter Roesler	Federal University of Rio Grande do Sul, Brazil
Elisabetta Ronchieri	INFN, Italy
Carolina Ruiz	WPI, USA
George Sakellaropoulos	University of Patras, Greece
Ovidio Salvetti	National Research Council of Italy (CNR), Italy
Akio Sashima	AIST, Japan
Jacob Scharcanski	Universidade Federal do Rio Grande do Sul (UFRGS), Brazil
Bettina Schnor	Potsdam University, Germany
Jan Sliwa	Bern University of Applied Sciences, Switzerland
Berglind Smaradottir	University of Agder, Norway
Åsa Smedberg	Stockholm University, Sweden
Jan Stage	Aalborg University, Denmark
Jiangwen Sun	Old Dominion University, USA
Chia-Chi Teng	Brigham Young University, USA
Francesco Tiezzi	University of Camerino, Italy
Markos Tsipouras	Technological Educational Institute of Epirus, Greece
Lauri Tuovinen	Dublin City University, Ireland
Mohy Uddin	King Abdullah International Medical Research Center (KAIMRC), Saudi Arabia

Gary Ushaw   Newcastle University, UK
Aristides Vagelatos   CTI, Greece
Egon L. van den Broek   Utrecht University, The Netherlands
Sitalakshmi Venkatraman   Melbourne Polytechnic, Australia
Francisco Veredas   Universidad de Málaga, Spain
Justin Wan   University of Waterloo, Canada
Szymon Wilk   Poznan University of Technology, Poland
Xuezhong Zhou   Beijing Jiaotong University, China
André Zúquete   IEETA, Universidade de Aveiro, Portugal

HEALTHINF Additional Reviewers

José Alberto   Universidad de León, Spain
  Benítez-Andrades
Katarzyna Borgiel   Ecole d'ingénieurs ISIS, France
Rejane Dalcé   Ecole d'ingénieurs ISIS, France
Gerardo Lagunes García   Universidad Politécnica de Madrid, Spain
Lucia Prieto Santamaria   Universidad Politécnica de Madrid, Spain

Invited Speakers

Hossam Haick   Israel Institute of Technology, Israel
Andres Diaz Lantada   Universidad Politecnica de Madrid, Spain
Henrique Martins   Universidade da Beira Interior, Portugal

Contents

Health Informatics

Biomedical Electronics and Devices

Design and Evaluation of the Platform
for Weight-Shifting Exercises
with Compensatory Forces Monitoring

Wiktor Sieklicki[1]([☒]) [iD], Robert Barański[2] [iD], Szymon Grocholski[1], Patrycja Matejek[1], and Mateusz Dyrda[1]

[1] Gdańsk University of Technology, Gdańsk, Poland
wiktor.sieklicki@pg.edu.pl
[2] AGH University of Science and Technology, Kraków, Poland
robertb@agh.edu.pl

Abstract. Details of a platform for the rehabilitation of people with severe balance impairment are discussed in the paper. Based upon a commercially available static parapodium, modified to fit force sensors, this device is designed to give a new, safe tool to physiotherapists. It is designed for the patients who cannot maintain equilibrium during a bipedal stance and need to hold to or lean on something during the rehabilitation. Visual, real-time information about weight distribution between left and right leg as well as the information about the force applied to the pillows supporting the patient's body is provided to the patient with help of a LED display. The control system allows registering forces applied by the patient to the device and analyze them after the therapy. The results of a preliminary evaluation of the device are presented in the paper with four healthy and one Cerebral Palsy ataxic participants. Two exercise scenarios are tested showing significant dependence between balance impairment and compensatory forces measured by the device, as well as a notable difference in how the subject strives for better results if the visual feedback is provided.

Keywords: Robotic rehabilitation · Balance training · Visual biofeedback · Biomedical electronics · Balance impairment

1 Introduction

Free body movements, walking and finally, locomotion gives the feeling of independence and personal safety. Diminished ability to achieve or maintain standing posture has a direct impact on general Activities of Daily Living (ADL) [1, 2] and increase the risk of falling [3–6]. It has also significant developmental and sociological consequences to an impaired person as well as to the family [1, 7, 8].

Cooperation of nervous, muscular, skeletal and fascia systems together with developed integrity of reactions, reflexes, tonus, acquired sensory system information as well as the intellectual, emotional and social capacity, determines the ability to execute free body movements and maintain equilibrium [9, 10]. Impaired balance is thus common

A. Roque et al. (Eds.): BIOSTEC 2019, CCIS 1211, pp. 3–28, 2020.
https://doi.org/10.1007/978-3-030-46970-2_1

among patients with neurological damage like Cerebrovascular Accidents (stroke) [8, 11–13], Traumatic Brain Injuries (TBI) [14], Spinal Cord Injuries (SCI) [15], Cerebral Palsy (CP) [7, 8], Parkinson's Disease (PD) [4, 16] and Multiple Sclerosis (MS) [3].

In many cases, the necessity to use rehabilitation aids emerge. Moreover, assistance from a third-person often becomes inevitable when dealing with everyday tasks as well as during the therapy sessions. Physical therapists working with balance impaired individuals have a highly demanding job being physically involved in exercises. Their goal is usually, to assist the patient in achieving a vertical position. This necessity comes from many advantages of keeping the upright body position [17, 18]. Training sessions can include extensive physical exercises during which a patient may burden their weight onto an assisting person at any moment. The intensity and duration of training sessions, therefore, have to consider the physical strength and endurance of a therapist. This limitation applies to any person assisting the patient. During everyday tasks, those are often parents, who are not necessarily trained nor physically prepared to bear the weight of their child as it gets older. As a result, people with severe balance deficits often end up in a wheelchair. The willingness to exercise in the standing position thus may fade as the main short term goal of locomotion is achieved. Ultimately, almost 40% of the untreated Dystonia patients and 24% of the injured spinal cord patients use a wheelchair [8]. In the case of Cerebral Palsy, it is reported that 29% and 41% of patients use a wheelchair indoors and outdoors respectively [19]. As much as 90% of patients using a wheelchair are classified at level IV-V of the Gross Motor Function Classification System (GMFCS) [19, 20].

Verticalization exercises are beneficial if a standing posture is maintained for 30 min to 4 h a day [17, 21]. Martinsson and Himmelmann ([22]) reported positive physical outcomes when patients maintained the standing posture for 60 up to 90 min a day. They also found no positive effects of staying in a vertical position for less than 30 min a day. In another study, standing for not less than 7.5 h a week was beneficial for the patients' health [14].

For a mildly affected patient this amount of time is achievable, but to lessen the boredom of repetitive, long-lasting exercises numerous rehabilitation aids targeting balance disorders have been developed. Interactive devices challenge patients with various means and are meant to diversify training sessions [23–25]. Often force platforms are introduced to make rehabilitation exercises more attractive to patients, thus maximize the time spent in training sessions [26, 27]. Recently a Nintendo Wii Fit has been widely offered as a low budget, weight-bearing assessment and exercise tool [28]. It provides a balance performance monitoring with visual and auditory feedback. Low cost and high availability of the platform makes it an interesting choice for therapists but some studies show, that not all patients can profit from this system [29, 30].

The free-standing exercises are not suitable if the patient is reluctant to an activity that exerts a risk of falling or an injury. Patients with severe balance disorders (GMFCS III-IV) and those who cannot keep an erect posture at all (GMFCS V) may need constant support of their trunk. For those patients, weight-relieving or side-supporting frames and harness-like systems (parapodium, walkers) are available. Parapodium is usually a modular frame with a wide base. Its function is to support a patient in an upright position by various elements of the device. The parapodia can be of two kinds: static parapodium, which stabilizes the body of the patient in an upright position, and can provide support in the chest, hip, lumbar and knee areas, or a dynamic parapodium, which stabilizes a patient's body while allowing one to move around. This device is not suitable for gait training though, because the movement of the device is achieved through a side to side rocking movement, which does correspond to a correct walking pattern. Active forms of work with a patient held upright in a parapodium usually focus on activating patients' manual and cognitive skills. It is possible because a parapodium allows the patient to free their arms from supporting the body, while in most cases, simultaneously blocking their legs. A similar device is a walker. The patient strapped into the walker may move around on his feet being held upright. Unfortunately, there are no strong arguments to back the thesis, that exercising with the use of walkers allows to minimize coordination dysfunction, which in turn would allow the patient to be able to retain their balance without the help of assisting devices [31, 32].

The fact, that losing equilibrium may happen at any moment during training sessions or any other activity often narrows the rehabilitation to passively standing in parapodium. Quickly it becomes boring and annoying, especially if the patient has to keep the stance every day for over 30 min. There are only a few rehabilitation tools for stability assessment and enhancement available for the patients who need assisting devices to maintain an upright position.

An example of a commercially available device answering this need is a static-dynamic parapodium BalanceReTrainer [13]. It keeps the patient in an upright position while allowing them for an inclination in coronal and sagittal planes for up to 10 degrees. Passive springs act against the frame's inclination. The feet of the patient remain attached to the floor. The device uses visual feedback that shows the patient the current inclination of their upper body. Measurements of the inclination are registered via accelerometers. The patient is requested to control the inclination of the body and follow instructions shown on a screen in front of him. The assessment of the patient's stability is based upon the concordance of the directions and amounts of inclination requested by the program and executed by the patient. Michalska and colleagues reported that training with BalanceReTrainer showed some improvements in weight-bearing abilities in CP patients, although mainly for patients classified at the level I and II of the GMFCS [33]. The limitation of this device is that the patient's Centre of Pressure (CoP) is significantly affected by a possible leaning on the device. Identification of the CoP during an unperturbed stance has become a well-established static posturography technique for the standing balance assessment. Displacement of the CoP is considered a representation of the equilibrium control to keep the Center of the body Mass (CoM) within the area of support [34]. In the case where the base of support is not only the two platforms beneath the patient, but also side pillows or additional handles, balance control extends beyond ankle/hip strategies ([35]) and the CoM displacement cannot be interpreted as CoP displacements acquired by force platforms only. There is no information gathered about the pressure applied by the patient to various parts of the Balance ReTrainer. Therefore, the device does not allow to properly assess the patient's CoP. Moreover, because the spring mechanism is the resistor for patient movements, the force required to perform an inclination rises, as the inclination gets greater.

Another device developed to facilitate therapy of balance impaired individuals, providing firm support to the patient's body is KineAssist [1]. Initially designed as a portable system providing the patient with the possibility to walk while actively supporting their trunk in a vertical position. The device is also actively following the patient's steps, which makes KineAssist a more robust walker with wider functionality. There is no information about the patient's CoP position and displacement though. KineAssist recently changed the design and it became a stationary system with a treadmill beneath it. This made the device potentially suitable for exercises in stance and stability assessment.

Lokomat [36, 37] is probably the most commercially successful device designed for balance impaired individuals. In basic form is has 4 Degrees of Freedom (DoF) - left and right knee and hip joints. This way it can assist and guide the hip and the knee movements while the ankle joint is moved passively with a spring system. The patient is held uprights by the set of suspenders. Additional feature includes a waist connection providing hips side movements and prevents backward movement. Lokomat is a gait training device though, and balance exercises in static stance cannot be executed nor it can help in the assessment of stability.

All of the mentioned devices are commercially available. KineAssist being a HDT Global product is sold by Woodway, Inc. Balance ReTrainer, under the name Thera-Trainer Balo, is a product of Thera Trainer. Lokomat is a product of Hocoma. One of the major drawbacks of mentioned rehabilitation robots is their cost ranging from $6.500 (Thera-Trainer Balo), $140.000 (KineAssist), up to $330.000 (Lokomat).

Measurements of the weight distribution between left and right leg, together with the visual feedback, can be successfully done with the use of force platforms as it was proposed by various authors [10, 28]. It is a cheap and widely available solution. This device though is not suitable for people compelled to use a parapodium in order to maintain a standing position. If force platforms were to be used together with a parapodium, patients could act upon the supports exerting compensatory forces. This could lead to the consolidation of improper muscle tonus in bipedal stance, making patients even less able to maintain a standing position without being supported by the parapodium. The compensatory forces applied to the parapodium, necessary to compensate disturbances of stability, influence pressure distribution on the patients' base of support. Proper assessment of stability based on CoP displacement analysis in such setup is thus difficult and does not provide correct results [38]. The visual systems designed to assess the stability neither can be used in such case, because there is no information about direction/amount of compensatory forces exerted by the patient to the parapodium.

Those observations led the authors to develop JStep. A suitable device for patients, who are not able to maintain an upright position without the aid of a physiotherapist and orthopedic aids. It is designed for training and assessment of the weight-shifting asymmetry as well as compensatory strategies of balance impaired individuals within a fall-safe environment. JSetp was initially described in [39], where authors briefly described its features and construction. A single case of use was there presented. The purpose of this study is to provide the proper background information and precise design criteria for this rehabilitation device, complete calibration procedures, as well as the mechanical and electrical features not described in the previous paper. This includes the compensatory forces identification and analysis. Moreover, in this study authors wish to present results of testing the device with five healthy and one CP patients with the aim to indicate balance-shifting variations and accompanying compensatory forces.

We focused on the condition affecting a particular patient, so the objective was to design a device that meets the requirements of an Ataxic Cerebral Palsy patient rehabilitation. In general, this covers requirements of the individuals classified at level I-IV of the GMFCS. Some dysfunctions are not framed by the GMFCS though. Eligibility criteria for the patients who can use the device, are listed: a) the individual has enough muscle strength to operate his limbs, trunk and head, b) individual has only mildly affected sight (LogMAR visual acuity ≤ 0.45, Snellen: $\leq 20/56$ or $\leq 6/17$, decimal ≤ 0.35) [40, 41], c) individual is communicative and understands verbal commands.

Criteria for the development of the device are presented in Sect. 2 of this paper; the device structure, sensory system, visual feedback are described in Sect. 3; in Sect. 4 the evaluation of the device, participants description, exercises' scenarios and tests results are presented; conclusions and discussion are presented in Sect. 5.

2   Design Criteria

A compulsory feature of a rehabilitation system targeting balance impairment of patients classified at level IV-V of the GMFCS would be a fall-safe environment. Lifting the threat of falling should give patients the possibility to comply more closely with the exercise protocol [42, 43]. This is particularly difficult for the device which purpose is to exercise balance [4]. It requires that the device is either following movements of the patient (e.g., powered walker, exoskeleton), or allows him to move within (e.g., parapodium, harness-like support system) with a possibility to hold/lean on.

An important aspect of the rehabilitation is that it refers to an impaired person who needs a therapy, not just the impairments that are to be cured. Physiotherapists' task is therefore not only to administer the physical exercises but also to find the most attractive way to work with the specific patient [44]. On the other hand, repetition strategy is considered strongly influential for maintaining brain changes acquired during the rehabilitation [45]. This requires consistent practice with repetitive movements. It is not necessarily interesting nor meaningful for the patient though, what in turn may reduce their willingness to participate in rehabilitation. Some patients may not recover or gain standard mobility at all. Even though, for the sake of their health it is crucial to proceed with balance exercises and motivate them to keep the bipedal stance during the day [17, 18]. The Rehabilitation device should therefore provide possibilities to engage patients more in exercises and give them enjoyable, task-based training protocol [13, 46].

Visual feedback may encourage patients to persist in their efforts and create positive reinforcement [29, 47]. To achieve this, a close interaction between the subject's actual equilibrium management and the outcomes of a single task should be evident for the patient. Since cognitive and cognitive-motor based training are reported effective to improve standing balance [48] both actual weight-bearing as well as forces exerted onto the fall-preventing structure displayed in front of the patient could enhance this improvement. Minimizing the compensatory forces exerted onto the fall-preventing structure might become a new goal for the training. The capability of the on-demand weight-shifting as well as the values of the compensatory forces during the task should be monitored to provide a track record of the patient's performance.

If keeping the balance during the rehabilitation is an issue, the therapeutic techniques presume that the patient may use their arms to hold to e.g., parallel bars, thus retain the equilibrium during exercises. Patients' stance model becomes quadrupedal this way, making it impossible to properly assess the CoP. To address this problem, the device should identify the forces transferred to the handles, harnesses, parallel bars or side pillows by the patient while one compensates for imbalance. As the result, an objective measure of compensation necessary to avoid losing the equilibrium could be: a) the amount of time the patient availed the support while executing a specific task [49], b) the amount and direction of force applied to the support while executing the task.

An adequate method of visualization should be provided to properly inform the patient about actual readings of the system. The minimal distance between the patient and the visualization panel, with respect to the minimal dimension of letters/controls lights displayed on the visualization panel, is calculated for the visual acuity $n = 0.35$ (in Snellen decimal scale). The letters height $h[m]$ is obtained from the visual angle formula (1), where Θ (equals 5 min of arc for letters [50] and has to be converted to degrees), $d[m]$ is the distance between the eye and the letter, and n is the Snellen visual acuity decimal representation. This means the visualization panel installed 2 m away from the patient's head should have letters taller than 8.31 mm. The control lights diameter should be greater than 1 min arc what results in 1.6 mm of diameter on a distance of 2 m according to (1) if theta equals 1 min of arc [50]. For the lights to be distinguishable, the distance between them should also be 1.6 mm.

$$h = 1/n \cdot 2 \cdot d \cdot \tan(\Theta/2) \tag{1}$$

The ability to shift the body weight onto a single leg plays a significant role in walking. Weight transfer between right and left legs should be considered one of the tasks practicable with the use of the rehabilitation device. Another widely accepted condition is for the subject to stand still in bipedal stance and to distribute weight equally on both legs. With this setup, a weight-bearing capacity assessment is usually linked [51, 52]. The rehabilitation device should, therefore, enable to assign both exercises scenarios [53, 54]. As reported by Goldie and coll. ([53]), the therapeutic approach should focus on improving weight-shifting to both legs, independently which is the affected one. The differences in the patient's capacity to transfer the correct amount of weight onto a selected leg can be considered a weight-shifting asymmetry [55]. The amount of time the demanded weight distribution should be maintained during tests is usually considered when functional balance tests are conducted [9]. Based on the testing procedures of weight-bearing capacity assessment, 5 s should be enough ([53]).

Since the interaction between the patient and the device is based upon the forces exerted to the device, the patient's performance can be considered a quantitative assessment of the balance. According to Mancini and Horak ([49]), automatic algorithms for quantifying balance control during prescribed tasks are necessary to make the quantitative measures of balance feasible for clinical practice. Moreover, they conclude that the user-friendly interfaces and convenient data storage as an electronic medical records are important.

3   JStep Rehabilitation Platform

The device is built on the foundation of a static, standing frame PJMS 180 (Fig. 1, left). It is a commercially available parapodium. This ensures that the patient is safely held upright in the bipedal stance. The patient stands in the parapodium with his feet on two independently mounted platforms (Fig. 1, right). The distance between the platforms is adjustable in the coronal plane. The patient is kept in the vertical, bipedal stance by a set of pillows on the sides, as well as on the front and in the rear of the parapodium. Adjustment of the pillows position can be done matching height of the hips of the patient and keeping desired distance between left and right pillows. The patient can lift his legs and bend the knees on demand. If the patient has little control over the extensor muscles of legs, a rubber-like horizontal bar on the height of the tibia may be installed limiting the forward movement of the knees. The device provides real-time visualization of the body weight distribution between the left and the right leg. Weight shifting is visualized on a panel installed in front of the patient (Fig. 1d). It also provides information about leaning of the patient on pillows of the parapodium.

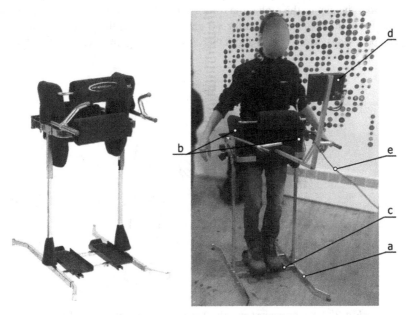

Fig. 1. Unmodified parapodium (left), and JStep during testing (right): a) mechanical structure, b) sensorized pillows, c) sensorized feet platforms, d) visualization panel, e) USB cable to PC.

3.1   Sensory Layer

Two sets of sensors are embedded in the structure. One set is implemented for measurements of weight applied to the platforms on which the patient stands. This solution assimilates JStep to a standard, static force platform. For this task, four YZC-161 load cells are placed beneath each platform. The advantage of those sensors is that they have a very low profile (12 mm) while being able to measure and withstand significant loads (up to 40 kg each). Additionally, they are extremely cheap ($10 for a pack of four sensors). The second set of sensors is responsible for the measurement of compensatory forces applied to the pillows. Those load cells are mounted in between the parapodium frame and the pillows. Each pillow is capable of sensing the force acting perpendicularly to its surface. Load cells used in the pillows are beam type load cells NA27-005, which are also quite inexpensive sensors costing approx. $10 apiece.

Weight shifting from one leg to another implies movements of the hips to the sides. Preliminary tests showed, that approx. 3 cm of space between the pillows and the patient's hips is enough to shift the body weight completely to one leg while keeping a vertical posture. Because the pillows provide a constant feeling of support to the patient though, this gap should be kept minimal. Based on the preliminary tests, a 90 kg and 155–185 cm tall individual leaning against the side pillow (the setup presented in Fig. 2, left) produces max. $F_{side} = 41$ N of force. Similar results were obtained for the individual leaning against the rear pillow (the setup presented in Fig. 2, right) with max. force $F_{rear} = 38$ N registered. Those values are dependent on how wide is previously discussed gap. The wider the gap is, the higher the forces applied to the pillows due to leaning are. The forces listed above are acquired for a 3 cm gap between the patient's hips and the pillows on both sides. More details about the sensors' arrangement can be found in [39].

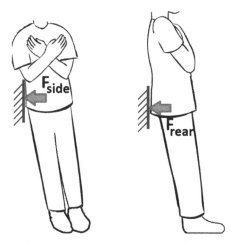

Fig. 2. Leaning against side (left) and rear (right) pillows model.

Verification of the stability and the reliability of both NA27-005 and YZC-161 was done after mounting them into the device. Sensors of this type have a close correlation between signal output level and the supply voltage. For example, the NA27 sensors, according to the technical specification, have a sensitivity of 1 mV/V. In practice, this means that the sensitivity increases with the rise of the supplying voltage. In our design, a 5 V supplying voltage was chosen. This is because the ATmega 328P, used as a central unit, powered from a 9 V battery, provides enough power to obtain a stable 5 V using the TL78L05 voltage stabilizer. The stability of the voltage supplying the sensor is of utmost importance because any change (even momentary) in the input of the transducer instantly changes the sensitivity and thus, the level of the output signal.

The supply voltage stability tests were carried out with the assumption, that the expected time of a single training session with the use of the device shall be less than an hour. Various loads were applied to the sensor during the supply voltage stability test. The mean value of the supply voltage reached 5.02 V with a standard deviation of 1 mV (representing 0.2% of the supply voltage). The percent coefficient of variation of the supply voltage is calculated to be 0.002%. It is considered that such small changes in the supply voltage should not have a significant effect on the output signal.

An analog-to-digital converter (A/D) incorporated into the ATmeg328P system is a 10-bit converter operating in the standard voltage range of 0 V to 5 V. As a result, its quantization step is approx. 4.88 mV. Since the expected voltage level measured directly from the force sensor is several to several dozen mV, the signal fed directly to the input of the A/D converter without any conditioning system would be burdened with a very large quantization error. For this reason, an implemented signal conditioning is composed of a low-pass filter, an amplifier and the A/D converter (Fig. 3).

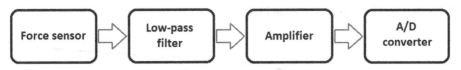

Fig. 3. Signal conditioning diagram.

It is assumed that significant signal variations during the measurement will not take place more often than several times per second. Therefore, a passive filter with a cut-off frequency of 10 Hz is used. The scheme of the filtration system is shown in Fig. 4, left. To achieve the assumed cut-off frequency, parameters with values of R = 166 kOhm, and C = 1 μF are chosen.

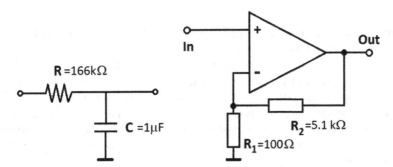

Fig. 4. Low-pass filter (left), and a general diagram of an operational amplifier in a non-inverting configuration (right).

An amplifier has a role of sensing the difference between the voltage signals that are applied to its inputs and multiply it by a gain A. For our application, a standard, inexpensive (less than $1 apiece) operational amplifier TL084 is used in a non-inverting configuration (Fig. 4, right). The gain A is determined by an Eq. (2). The values of the R1 and R2 resistors are chosen to be R1 = 100 O and R2 = 5.1 kOhm giving a gain of A = 52.

$$A = 1 + (R_2/R_1) \tag{2}$$

An important aspect of the strain gauge based force sensors is that the temperature variations may strongly influence the sensor's readouts. This effect can be minimized if the measurements are done in stable conditions (e.g. laboratory). However, independently from the environment influence, the excitation voltage increases the stain gauge's temperature creating a temperature drift.

To determine the characteristics of the NA27-005 temperature drift due to excitation voltage, a single sensor was tested in a room with a constant temperature of 24 °C ± 1 °C. Readouts were acquired from the moment the voltage was applied to the sensor till 60 min after. No mechanical load was applied to the sensor during the tests. The resulting characteristics conditioned with a low-pass filter and converted with use mentioned earlier A/D converter is presented in Fig. 5.

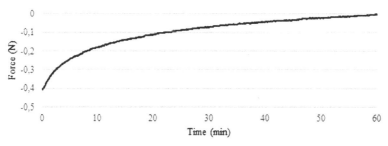

Fig. 5. NA27-005 force sensor temperature drift due to excitation voltage characteristics under the constant environment temperature conditions (24 °C ± 1 °C).

Tests revealed, that in a period of 60 min the readings increased of 0.4 N, which is approximately 1% of the measurement range (50 N). The change was most evident (50% of the total change) during the first 8 min of the test (0.2 N). Subsequent 0.1 N of the change was noticed after 21 min and finally after 60 min from the beginning of the test. The readings change rate can be defined as 0.007 N/min after 10 min from applying the excitation voltage. To solve this issue it is recommended to start the system 10 min before the measurements are taken. Another solution is to use larger gages and higher resistance gages. This would decrease the power necessary to be dissipated per unit area of a strain gauge.

The parameters of linear regression $(ax + b)$ determining the dependence of the load applied to the sensor and the sensor's output voltage were also calculated. For this reason, tests were carried out in a room with a constant temperature of 24 °C ± 1 °C within 3days. 90 subsequent measurements with the use of 1, 2, and 3 kg load were done. The coefficients a and b were calculated and for all of the regression equations, the R^2 was not lower than 0.9999996, showing a linear relationship between the load and the output voltage signal.

All the above tests were carried out to check the reliability of signals from chosen force sensors. It should be noted that at the current stage of the project, the exact values of the force applied to the pillows are not of utmost importance. Rather the information about forces' variation is utilized in proposed training algorithms. Nevertheless, the knowledge about the sensors' stability rises the credibility of the system and opens up the possibility of using those sensors in the future if such functionality will be desired.

3.2 Visual Feedback Layer

Literature research [29, 47, 48], as well as the authors' observation of ataxic CP individuals, proved that the information about the weight-bearing and compensatory forces applied to the device has to be shown in a simple and informative way. Significant difficulties in reading and understanding complex information by patients with vestibular system damage do not allow the use of any numerical display with digits changing as, for example, patients shift their weight.

Our proposition for visual feedback is a Light Emitting Diode (LED) display incorporating five bars, each representing one sensing surface of the parapodium – left and right feet platform, left, right and back pillows ([39]). Each bar is composed of several LED lights placed in a row. Two yellow-red tapering bars in the center of the display are used for displaying the information about shifting the body weight between the left and right leg. When the force is equally distributed between left and right leg, yellow LEDs are illuminated (four of them on each side). Changing the body weight distribution to one of the legs results in illuminating more of the LED lights on this side. In other words, the more weight is on the side, the more LEDs are illuminated. Each LED corresponds to an amount of weight normalized as a percentage of body weight (%BW) shifted to the particular leg (Table 1). In this way, if the patient keeps the equilibrium or the weight-bearing is within a 56% threshold of the body weight, four yellow LEDs on both sides are illuminated. A shift of the body weight on an e.g. left leg so that 70% of body weight is kept on this leg results in six LEDs illuminated on the left bar. It does not necessarily mean though, that on the right bar there will be two LEDs illuminated. This number is influenced by the amount of force the patient exerts on the pillows of the parapodium to compensate for the loss of the equilibrium.

Leaning against the side pillows is represented by two LED bars placed on the sides of the display. Each bar is composed of 7 green LED lights placed in a row. Leaning against the back pillow is represented by a single LED bar on the bottom of the display. This bar is also composed of 7 green LED lights placed in a row. We noticed during the initial trials, that the patient was more enthusiastic and content with his actions when the successful movements resulted in as many illuminated LEDs as possible. Switching the LEDs off was associated for the patient with doing something wrong. Because of that switching-off, rather than illuminating LEDs was chosen as the measure of applied compensatory forces. When there are no forces applied to the pillows, all LEDs are thus illuminated. During the calibration process (discussed in subsequent Subsection) a maximum force (R_{max}^n, where n = {LP, RP, BP}, which stands for Left Pillow, Right

Pillow and Back Pillow respectively) applicable by a patient to each pillow is registered. As soon as a force of more than 15% of R_{max}^n is applied, a pair of utmost LED light on both ends of a corresponding LED bar is switched-off, resulting in 5 LEDs left illuminated. With a force of 30% of R_{max}^n applied to a particular pillow, only three LEDs are left illuminated. Applying more than 40% of the R_{max}^n force to a pillow results in only one LED left illuminated. This feature is organized differently to how the leaning on the device is managed in previous paper ([39]).

Table 1. The amount of LEDs illuminated for a respective load applied to a corresponding leg.

Amount of weight in % of total body weight (%BW) shifted to one leg	Amount of LED lights illuminated for a respective load
90–100%	8
79–89%	7
68–78%	6
57–67%	5
44–56%	4
32–43%	3
20–31%	2
9–19%	1
0–8%	0

Such a display arrangement allows understanding the body weight distribution at a glimpse of an eye. Therefore, it is easy to set a goal of the exercise as the patient can easily observe his weight shifts and possible leaning. It should also let the patient put more attention to execute the task, rather than focusing on reading the information from the display. The simplicity of the display is achieved at the expense of the resolution of the readings. Independent of what is shown to the patient on the LED display though, raw data is sent directly to the PC (Personal Computer) for further analysis.

The hardware layer of the LED display includes five SN74HC595 8-bit shift registers. This solution minimizes necessary analog outputs from a control unit to operate that many LED lights. Each LED bar is operated by one shift register. The operational frequency of the shift registries is approx. 25 MHz. Considering a 16 MHz clock frequency of the ATmega328P, the refresh rate of LEDs when all of the LEDs were illuminated was achieved approx. 15 Hz. This is considered enough to interpret LEDs as constantly illuminated.

3.3   Sensors' Calibration

The spasticity of some muscle groups in CP can cause the inability to equalize the body weight between the left and right leg. It does not, however, conclude for the inability of maintaining stability. The device allows calibrating the force range for each of the surfaces with force sensors so that it is tailored to the patient's capabilities and needs. Adjustment of the device performance to the patients of various weight is done thanks to the calibration of sensors.

The calibration is based on measuring the maximum force applied by the patient to the specific sensing surface and scaling the range of the readings accordingly. As discussed in the previous Subsection, maximum force applicable to the sensors is R_{max}^n, where $n = \{LP, RP, BP, LL, RL\}$ which stands for Left Pillow, Right Pillow, Back Pillow, Left Leg and Right Leg respectively. The result is, that the first LED and all LEDs up to the last one of a selected bar on the display are illuminated when minimum and maximum force is applied to a particular sensor respectively. The JStep functioning algorithm with a calibration loop is presented in Fig. 6.

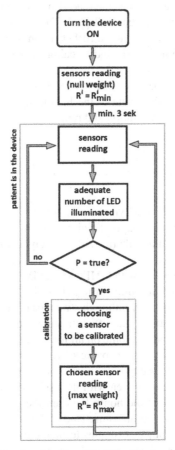

Fig. 6. An algorithm of the JStep functioning, with calibration loop included in which R represents current readouts, R_{max} stands for maximum readouts obtainable for a particular sensor and n is a sensor index {left pillow, right pillow, back pillow, left leg or right leg}. "P" is an action of pressing the button on a top of the LED display box.

Each time the device is switched on, the first three seconds average reading is considered a null level for a sensor. During that time the patient cannot be in the device. The system enters the operational mode after three seconds after which the patient may enter the device. As long as the button "P" on a top of the LED display box is not pressed, the device shows current sensors' readings in a form of the illuminated LED bars. It also sends numerical data to the computer. If the button "P" is pressed, the device enters calibration mode and one single light of a LED bar corresponding to the left foot platform starts flashing. Each push of the button "P" shifts the illuminated LED to a subsequent LED bar representing the left leg platform, right leg platform, left pillow, right pillow, and rear pillow. After five seconds, while the LED of the desired sensor is flashing, it enters a state in which readings from this sensor are being gathered for two seconds. At this point, the patient is asked to apply as much force to this sensing surface as he is capable. The system picks maximum value read (Rn) during that time and sets it as the maximum value readable for this sensor (R_{max}^n). This information is mapped to eight levels (in case of leg platforms) so that the LED bar can be lit properly. Afterward, the system goes back to operational mode and to calibrate another sensor, this procedure has to be repeated.

The presented procedure does not influence readouts sent to PC via USB. The user cannot change the raw data values sent to the PC during the process. The calibration refers only to the LED display resolution and range.

4 Evaluation

4.1 Participants

Three healthy males (age: 25.7 ± 3.2yrs, height: 169.2 ± 12.8 cm, body mass: 66.9 ± 8.5 kg), one healthy female (age: 32yrs, height: 166 cm, body mass: 58 kg), and one Cerebral Palsy in the cerebellum male (age: 18yrs, height: 175 cm, body mass: 61 kg) volunteered for the evaluation study.

The CP participant is classified with GMFCS level IV. His motor abilities allow him to sit and keep the torso upright while sitting. He's also capable of keeping his head upright and execute reaching tasks although dysmetria, tremor, and dyssynergia are evident. He has strong astigmatism and difficulties in controlling eye movements when tired. The subject moves around his home on all fours. He is unable to keep the bipedal stance without any support but he is capable of rising to the stance and keeping the upright standing posture if allowed to hold to stable support (e.g. furniture). Making the steps is challenging for the subject even with the use of external support. An assistant is necessary to walk him around the house but then the patient leans on the assistant giving him full control over the equilibrium. Due to the legs' spasticity, plantar flexion is present permanently. The subject struggles to maintain an upright standing position because he has to flex the knees, keep his weight on the toes and rotate his hips backward achieving anterior pelvic tilt. The result of such a posture is that the subject does not bring his hips into contact with the front pillow of a parapodium at all.

The one female participated in the study is a health professional who is knowledgeable about youth with CP and the GMFCS. All the participants provided informed consent prior to data collection.

4.2 Exercises Scenarios

Most of the design criteria discussed in Sect. 2 are addressed through the sole concept of the device as a static frame, supporting the patient on-demand, as well as the sensory system with proper visualization of the forces the patient may exert to the supporting surfaces. A task-based approach with an embedded engagement mechanism needs more explanation though.

There are many exercise scenarios possible to realize with the use of a discussed device. In this paper, we would like to focus on exercises aiming to:

- increase the capability for on-demand weight-shifting and control over the amount of weight transferred onto a particular leg,
- decrease the amount of force exerted on the support surfaces, necessary to compensate for temporary loss of equilibrium while shifting the body weight.

The two objectives can be addressed with similar exercises scenarios. Given the possibilities provided by the LED display, two exercises are further described:

- Exercise 1: Illuminate a given amount of LED lights related to the body weight distribution.

The goal is to shift the body weight between the left and right leg to illuminate a given number of LEDs chosen from two tapering LED bars (described in Subsect. 3.2). To complete the assignment, the given LED has to be kept illuminated for five consecutive seconds. Thus, the subject has to achieve and maintain a demanded weight distribution for 5 consecutive seconds. The subject has 120 s to succeed. Otherwise, the system automatically ends the assessment. In practice, one chosen LED light (from a set of 4 through 8) representing the left leg load is switched on at the LED display and starts blinking. It's a signal for the subject to shift his weight until this particular LED is illuminated and keep it illuminated for five consecutive seconds. The following round is similar but this time another light (from a set of 4 through 8) representing second leg is blinking.

- Exercise 2: Illuminate a given amount of LED lights related to the body weight distribution while refraining from switching-off any LED lights related to the forces applied to the pillows.

Here, the subject has to execute the same algorithm as in the first exercise but this time leaning on the device results in switching-off the LED lights on the display. Applying too much force to the pillows makes it impossible to accomplish the task. In practice, the weight-shifting assignment is managed alike the first exercise, but the subject has to pay attention not to lean against the pillows. Applying the force to the pillows results in switching-off the green LED lights and as soon as there is only one green LED light left illuminated (at any of the green LED bars), the whole task is suspended. Up until the subject stops leaning on the device, LED bars related to the body weight distribution are switched off.

For the sake of completing this exercise, a feasible threshold of force applicable to the pillows has to be set, otherwise, an individual with stability deficits will not be able to finalize this task at all. After some trial tests, the threshold value was set to 40% of the maximum force applicable to this particular pillow by this particular patient, as discussed in Subsect. 3.2. This is in line with a very important aspect of gamification, which is the win-loss ratio. To keep the patient actively involved in the game, hence in the rehabilitation process, a game designer has to maintain the game challenging for the patient but at the same time plausible to succeed.

An algorithm responsible for selecting a task (LED light number) for consecutive rounds in both of the exercises is alike. To provide an equal distribution of tasks, each subsequent assignment is different from the previous one for this particular leg. Such a feature has been achieved by removing a LED light number that was chosen the last round from a set of LED lights numbers that are considered for the current round.

The subjects were asked not to grasp the parapodium frame with their hands. To facilitate that, they were given two small cylindrical objects to hold with their hands.

For the evaluation purposes, the device was located in a room with a constant temperature of 24 °C ± 1 °C. Tests were carried out during day time, assuring a similar light intensity in the room between the subsequent trials and for all the subjects.

Each healthy subject performed both the exercises scenarios for about half an hour resulting in approx. 70 assignments. Assessment of their capabilities is done based on those assignments and is further discussed in Subsect. 4.3. In the case of the CP subject, the device was provided solely for him for the duration of six weeks. During this time the subject was asked to work with the assignments and complete each of them twice, every day. If the subject was sick or unable to perform his duty that day he was asked to complete his task the other day additionally to the scheduled exercises for that day. He was also asked to carry out the calibration procedure for the null weight and maximum weight for all the sensors each day before he did the assignments.

4.3 Data Aggregation

All the results gathered include: date and time; current number of exercise (1 or 2); current round number r, where $r = \{1,..10\}$; LED number k selected as a target for the exercise, which refers to the requested body weight distribution ($k = \{4,5,6,7,8\}$); amount of time spent on completing the exercise (T_a); amount of time spent with a correct body weight distribution (T_s); and for the second exercise, the amount of time the patient applied the force to the pillows higher than a threshold (T_p).

After each round the system sends an update to the PC with new information about the current training. At this stage of the project saving the results for each participant is done manually. This refers also to post-processing of the data, which is currently done in MS Excel 2010 environment. A script written in the Visual Basic is run for each spreadsheet with collected data. Following steps in order to obtain results are: removing null results, aggregation of the results for each exercise scenario, each task and each leg separately, building the charts and calculation of the linear regression function.

4.4 Results

During six week time period the CP patient performed the first exercise scenario 154 times and the second exercise scenario 113 times. It took him 23 days to complete all these exercises.

The amount of time necessary for the patient to achieve and maintain the desired body weight distribution for five consecutive seconds (T_a) is the first quality criteria. For the CP patient, the exemplary results of T_a gathered in a time span of 42 days while executing the exercise 1 are shown in Fig. 7, left. Here the task was to keep the body weight evenly distributed between left and right leg with a maximum 56% of the weight on the one leg (fourth LED illuminated on the display for one leg). A trend function: $y = -1.08t + 72$ with a coefficient of determination $R^2 = 0.11$ are obtained. The plot show very similar results to one presented as an example in [39] with some of the data points excluded though. This is because the normalization of the body weight is done with a different percentage levels used for illuminating particular LEDs what allowed to better distribute the body weight representation between consecutive LEDs.

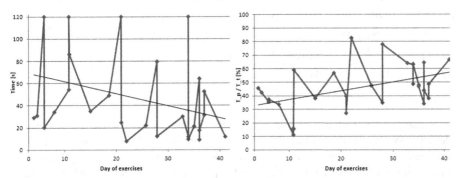

Fig. 7. Results obtained for CP participant: on the left - time necessary to complete the task in exercise 1 - T_a; on the right - percentage of time necessary to complete the exercise during which patient achieved desired body weight distribution but not necessarily maintained it for consecutive 5 s - $T_{s\%}$. Data presented for case where the patient's weight had to be distributed evenly with up to 56% of weight on left leg.

The T_a linear trend function for all the body weight transfer cases, calculated for the six weeks training time of a CP patient is presented in Table 2. Presented in Fig. 7, left case corresponds to the trend function listed in Table 2, third row, last column. Here, the activity which initially required approximately 70 s to complete (compound b of the $y = ax + b$ function) after 6 weeks of training was more often achieved in only 25 s. A decrease in time necessary to succeed in exercise 1 as the training proceeded can be noticed for all the body weight transfer cases except 90–100% of the body weight transferred on one leg case. Here the time required to complete the exercise extended throughout the training period for both left and right leg. Based on a trend function, the time necessary to complete the exercise for both legs combined is presented also as a percentage value (ΔT_a) of the initial result. From those numbers it can be concluded, that the calculated time necessary to complete exercise 1 was decreased 63% in the case where the task was to keep the equilibrium. Best results were obtained for the case where the task was to minimally (57–67% of the body weight) transfer the body weight to one leg. Here the improvement was calculated 88%.

Table 2. Linear trend function $y = ax + b$ of T_a and $T_{s\%}$ in function of days (t) the exercises were performed for subsequent body weight distribution cases. LL stands for the left leg, RL - right leg, and TO – combined results from both legs. Additionally, ΔT_a is a percentage change of time necessary to complete the exercise for both legs combined based on a trend function T_a (TO).

	100–90% of body weight on one leg	89–79% of body weight on one leg	78–68% of body weight on one leg	67–77% of body weight on one leg	Up to 56% of body weight on one leg
T_a (LL)	$1.09t + 36$	$-0.82t + 86$	$-0.77t + 58$	$-1.45t + 65$	–
T_a (RL)	$0.87t + 84$	$-1.77t + 110$	$-0.57t + 58$	$-1.56t + 76$	–
T_a (TO)	$0.32t + 74$	$-1.31t + 100$	$-0.66t + 59$	$-1.5t + 71$	$-1.08t + 72$
$T_{s\%}$ (LL)	$-0.63t + 61$	$0.69t + 25$	$0.3t + 40$	$0.64t + 33$	–
$T_{s\%}$ (RL)	$-0.28t + 15$	$1.12t + 8$	$0.6t + 33$	$0.83t + 28$	–
$T_{s\%}$ (TO)	$0.13t + 25$	$1.01t + 13$	$0.44t + 37$	$0.75t + 31$	$0.64t + 30$
ΔT_a [%]	-16	53	46	88	63

To compare the results with healthy participants the exemplary results showing T_a calculated as a mean value of all the healthy participants is shown in Fig. 8, left. The participants had to accomplish the task at least 12 times, not necessarily during an extended training period like in the case of CP patient. Here, in the case where the task

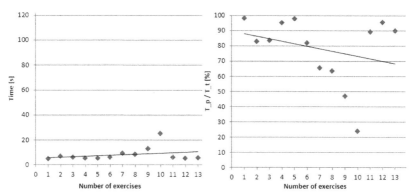

Fig. 8. Healthy participants' results: on the left – mean time required to complete the task in exercise 1 (T_a); on the right - percentage of mean time necessary to complete the exercise during which patient achieved desired body weight distribution but not necessarily maintained it for consecutive 5 s ($T_{s\%}$). Data presented for the case where the patients' weight had to be distributed evenly with up to 56% of weight on one leg.

was to keep the body weight evenly distributed with a maximum 56% of the body weight transferred on one leg, the calculated trend function is: $y = 0.02t + 2$ with a coefficient of determination $R^2 = 0.76$.

Mean values of time ($\overline{T_a}$) required to complete the task in exercise 1 together with standard deviation for both CP patient and healthy patients are presented in Table 3. For the CP patient the most time was required to complete the task of putting the whole body weight on one leg (80 s on average). This result was mainly due to high results for loading the right leg (97 s on average). The tendency was maintained as for the time required to complete the task in case of transferring the body weight to the left and right leg across all the load cases. This result clearly shows the weight-shifting asymmetry in CP patient's behavior. Healthy patients did not show such a tendency. Moreover, much lower standard deviations were calculated for the healthy patients suggesting that this might be a proper indicator of the balance impairments.

Table 3. Data referring mean time $\overline{T_a}$ necessary to complete the task in exercise 1 calculated as combined results from both legs (total) as well as for the left and right leg separately in all five body weight distribution cases. LL stands for the left leg and RL stands for the right leg.

	Percentage of body weight on one leg:	100–90%	89–79%	78–68%	67–57%	Up to 56%
CP patient (mean)	$\overline{T_a}$ total [s]	80, SD = 46	73, SD = 40	45, SD = 30	37, SD = 34	47, SD = 39
	$\overline{T_a}$ (LL) [s]	60, SD = 51	67, SD = 43	43, SD = 28	33, SD = 30	–
	$\overline{T_a}$ (RL) [s]	97, SD = 35	79, SD = 39	46, SD = 33	41, SD = 37	–
Healthy patients (mean)	$\overline{T_a}$ total [s]	16, SD = 10	12, SD = 2	16, SD = 7	14, SD = 2	12, SD = 2
	$\overline{T_a}$ (LL) [s]	13, SD = 3	13, SD = 4	22, SD = 13	15, SD = 9	–
	$\overline{T_a}$ (RL) [s]	14, SD = 3	15, SD = 3	11, SD = 2	12 SD = 1	–

The second quality criterion for both of the exercises is $T_s\%$ which is the amount of time during which the desired body weight distribution was achieved but not necessarily maintained for consecutive five seconds. The T_s in its nominal value is highly dependent upon the overall time of completing the task. It has to be therefore further discussed as:

$$T_s\% = T_s/T_a \cdot 100\% \tag{3}$$

The exemplary results for $T_s\%$ are presented in Fig. 7, right. In this case, the task was to distribute the body weight evenly between left and right leg with a maximum 56% of the body weight on one leg. Exercises were done in a timespan of 42 days. A complete list of $T_s\%$ results obtained for the CP patient is presented in 4th to 6th row of Table 2. For the case where the task was to distribute the body weight evenly between left and right leg the $T_s\%$ trend function $y = 0.64t + 30$ with a coefficient of determination $R^2 = 0.2$ was obtained. Similarly to the T_a results, $T_s\%$ show improvement across all the cases but one - 100–90% of the body weight transferred to one leg. Although it is not completely true, because even though the result obtained for the left leg show worsening (a compound of the $y = ax + b$ function is -0.63), b compound is very high (=61) showing high success ratio from the beginning. Again, worst results are thus for the right leg with trend function calculated to be y = −0.28t + 15. In all load cases, the *b* compound of the trend function for the right leg was the lowest. Mean results for healthy participants are presented for comparison in Fig. 8, right, showing significant spread.

A dataset from Table 3 referring mean time $\overline{T_a}$ for CP patient is presented in Fig. 9. It provides a quick information about posture dissymmetry. It is instantly notable, that tasks involving shifting body weight to the right leg require more time to accomplish. It may be assumed, that those tasks are more difficult for the patient to execute. Also, the more weight is to be transferred to the right leg, the more difficult the task becomes. In the task of transferring body weight onto the left leg, the patient did not succeed only twice (for 87 times the task was assigned) whereas in the case of transferring body weight onto the right leg it happened 11 times throughout all 67 times the task was assigned. This also indicates problems with the weight-shifting abilities.

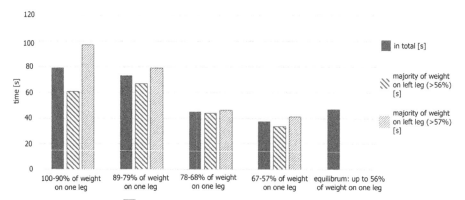

Fig. 9. Mean time value $\overline{T_a}$ necessary to complete a task in exercise 1 for CP subject- data divided for five levels of body weight distribution and presented for each leg separately as well as for both legs combined (total).

Personal observations of the patient, while he was in training, revealed that most of the time he did not succeed happened when he was distracted by a nearby discussion or was anxious to do something else in the time he was exercising. It is disputable therefore if a drop-out ratio should be considered as an important parameter for determining weight-shifting abilities.

Results referring second goal of exercises, that is to estimate and possibly decrease the amount of force exerted on the support surfaces (necessary to compensate for a temporary loss of equilibrium while shifting the body weight) are shown in Fig. 10, left. Those results are obtained for a CP subject, whereas the mean results for the healthy participants are shown in Fig. 10, right. The CP subject tends to lean on the parapodium especially when the information about applied force was not provided to the patient at the time. The best results for this scenario subject achieved for the case, where the task was to shift the body weight of 68–78% to the left leg. The patient leaned on the parapodium for half the time required to succeed in the task ($T_p = 50\%$). Most leaning occurred when the task was to transfer more than 79% of the body weight to one of the legs ($T_p \cong 80\%$). Mean value across all the cases for the CP patient was calculated to be $\overline{T_p} = 69\%$.

When the information about the force was displayed to the subject (exercise 2), he achieved best results for the left leg ($T_p = 16\%$ for the 79–89% loading case) and the mean $\overline{T_p}$ time was calculated to be 30% of the task realization time, what is a far better result than in exercise 1.

For comparison of results between CP and healthy subjects, the mean $\overline{T_p}$ time for all the healthy subjects is presented in Fig. 10, right. It is evident, that healthy subjects did not need support in order to finish the task. The worst results here were obtained for the 90–100% task scoring $T_p = 12\%$. This may suggest, that 3 cm of clearance between hips and pillows might not be enough for shifting the weight without touching the pillows.

Restriction inflicted in the second exercise by the presence of side and rear pillows extended the time necessary for the CP patient to achieve and maintain the desired body weight distribution for five consecutive seconds (T_a). Mean value $\overline{T_a}$ was calculated for 100–90%, 89–79%, 78–68%, 67–57% and for the equilibrium with up to 56% of the weight on one leg cases to be 61, 75, 62, 81 and 71 s respectively. Here the differences in shifting body weight over left or right leg are not so obvious: $\overline{T_a}$ (LL): 20, 81, 56, 99 s, whereas $\overline{T_a}$ (RL): 82, 58, 73, and 64 s for each mentioned above weight cases.

The task of transferring the body weight properly to the left and right leg in the second exercise was assigned 57 and 56 times respectively. In the case of the left leg, the patient did not manage to achieve success in the 120 s time limit six times and for the right leg, it was eight times. This resulted in standard deviations of T_a SD = 38 for the left leg and SD = 66 for the right leg results. Again, the drop-out cases were mostly inflicted by external disturbances.

The results in the case of the second exercise are much more consistent and show very similar T_a values for all four cases where the weight had to be shifted onto the left

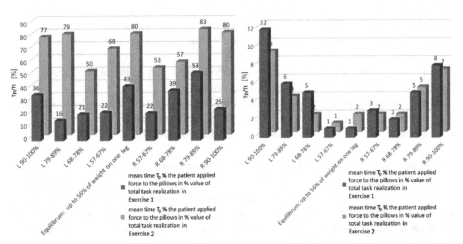

Fig. 10. Mean time value $\overline{T_p}$ the force was applied to the pillows during the realization of the task. Results presented for exercise 1 and exercise 2: results obtained for a CP subject (left), and results obtained for healthy participants (right).

leg. We noticed very little improvement of T_a and $T_s\%$ parameters over the six-weeks training time in case of the second exercise. This is probably due to a very high difficulty the patient had with completing the task of shifting the body weight while simultaneously caring not to lean on the device.

5 Conclusions and Discussion

In the paper, authors have presented a device for training and assessment of the weight-shifting asymmetry and compensatory forces monitoring within a fall-safe environment. The discussed assisting device is suitable for patients, who are not able to maintain an upright position without the aid of a physiotherapist and orthopedic aids. It enables training of weight-shifting in the coronal plane and provides visual feedback informing about the patient's current body weight distribution as well as the forces inflicted on the pillows while leaning on the device.

Our concept fits the needs of the individuals classified at level I-IV of the GMFCS and who has enough muscle strength to operate the limbs, trunk, and head. In order to utilize the visual feedback function, the patient may have only mildly affected sight, has to be communicative and understand verbal commands.

The body weight distribution, as well as the compensatory forces inflicted on the device, necessary to minimize the disturbances of stability, are presented in the form of illuminated LED lights at the front of the patient. Such functionality gives the patient and the physiotherapists real-time information about body weight distribution. Furthermore, it provides a wider knowledge about the compensation the patient may need to keep the upright standing position.

Two exercises are proposed to train stability with the use of the device. Both involve shifting the patient's body weight in the coronal plane so that it matches requested body weight distribution. The second though requires the patient to avoid leaning on the side and rear pillows of the parapodium. Performing proposed exercises allows for the estimation of the capabilities of the patient. As an outcome of executing the exercises, a set of parameters measured and calculated during the training session is achieved:

- the amount of time necessary for the patient to achieve and maintain the desired body weight distribution for five consecutive seconds (T_a),
- the amount of time during which the desired body weight distribution was achieved but not necessarily maintained for consecutive five seconds (T_s),
- the amount of time the patient leaned on the parapodium (T_p).

The device was tested with four healthy and one ataxic Cerebral Palsy subjects. CP subject was training for 6 weeks period. During this time the patient performed 267 times the exercises described. It means the patient spent approximately 30 h in the device safely standing and performing exercises, which is already a great success. Some of the results are already presented in [39], others include an analysis of forces applied to the side pillows for both the exercises and the comparison of the CP patients results to the healthy subjects' results. Moreover, current results had been normalized with different percentage levels of body weight used for illuminating particular LEDs, which allowed to better distribute the body weight representation between the consecutive LEDs.

Very high readouts were collected for the T_p in case of a CP subject (leaning on the device for up to 83% of the time required to complete the exercise) in comparison to the healthy subjects (up to 12%). For this reason, the device might be considered suitable for an assessment of the compensatory forces applied to the parapodium. Moreover, a significant improvement in T_p was observed for the case when the currently inflicted compensatory forces were shown to the patient in respect to the case when this information was hidden. This was not observed in the case of healthy patients. Furthermore, high values of T_p, for exercise 1 in comparison to exercise 2 suggest, that informing the patient verbally, that he should not lean on the device does little in comparison to the patient's self-awareness if he is restricted from winning a game unless he does not stand correctly. This particular result is of great significance, because it suggests, that gamification has the ability to further increase patient's efforts in order to pursue rehabilitation goals. This may be achieved if the game mechanics is carefully adjusted to match the physical rehabilitation requirements.

Another indicator of the possible issues with maintaining the balance is that the mean time necessary to complete the task $\overline{T_a}$, while executing exercise 1, was lower ($\overline{T_a} = 57$ s) than in the case of executing exercise 2 ($\overline{T_a} = 67$ s). This means that the restriction inflicted in the second exercise by the presence of side and rear pillows does require from the patient more attention to the compensatory forces inflicted to the device. This result can be further exploit in order to create training scenarios for the weight-shifting asymmetry with necessary compensatory forces minimization.

Further works include the development of a more sophisticated environment, where the patient is motivated to pursue the best results based on the gratification system embedded in a computer game. Moreover, the game scenarios should include increasing difficulty of the tasks required from the patient. This includes an initial level of repetitive movements, intermediate level of some movements variability and finally an advanced level of random body weight distribution requests.

References

1. Patton, J., et al.: KineAssist: design and development of a robotic overground gait and balance therapy device. Top. Stroke Rehabil. **15**, 131–139 (2008). https://doi.org/10.1310/tsr1502-131
2. Harun, A., Semenov, Y.R., Agrawal, Y.: Vestibular function and activities of daily living. Gerontol. Geriatr. Med. **1**, 233372141560712 (2015). https://doi.org/10.1177/2333721415607124
3. Cattaneo, D., De Nuzzo, C., Fascia, T., Macalli, M., Pisoni, I., Cardini, R.: Risks of falls in subjects with multiple sclerosis. Arch. Phys. Med. Rehabil. **83**, 864–867 (2002). https://doi.org/10.1053/apmr.2002.32825
4. Allen, N.E., Sherrington, C., Paul, S.S., Canning, C.G.: Balance and falls in parkinson's disease: a meta-analysis of the effect of exercise and motor training. Mov. Disord. **26**, 1605–1615 (2011). https://doi.org/10.1002/mds.23790
5. Geurts, A.C.H., de Haart, M., van Nes, I.J.W., Duysens, J.: A review of standing balance recovery from stroke. Gait Posture **22**, 267–281 (2005). https://doi.org/10.1016/j.gaitpost.2004.10.002
6. Horak, F.B.: Postural orientation and equilibrium: what do we need to know about neural control of balance to prevent falls? Age Ageing **35**(Suppl 2), ii7–ii11 (2006). https://doi.org/10.1093/ageing/afl077

7. Batra, M., Sharma, V.P., Batra, V., Malik, G.K., Pandey, R.M.: Postural reactions: an elementary unit for development of motor control. Disabil. CBR Incl. Dev. **22**, 134–137 (2011). https://doi.org/10.5463/dcid.v22i2.30

8. Bronstein, A.M.: Clinical disorders of balance, posture and gait. Arnold (2004)

9. Horak, F.B.: Clinical assessment of balance disorders. Gait Posture **6**, 76–84 (1997). https://doi.org/10.1016/s0966-6362(97)00018-0

10. Winter, D.A., Patla, A.E., Frank, J.S.: Assessment of balance control in humans. Med. Prog. Technol. **16**, 31–51 (1990)

11. Roerdink, M., Geurts, A.C.H., de Haart, M., Beek, P.J.: On the relative contribution of the paretic leg to the control of posture after stroke. Neurorehabil. Neural Repair. **23**, 267–274 (2009). https://doi.org/10.1177/1545968308323928

12. Drużbicki, M., Przysada, G., Rykała, J., Podgórska, J., Guzik, A., Kołodziej, K.: Ocena przydatności wybranych skal i metod stosowanych w ocenie chodu i równowagi osób po udarze mózgu Evaluation of the effectiveness of selected scales and methods used in the assessment of gait and balance after a cerebral stroke. Przegląd Med. Uniw. Rzesz. 21–31 (2013). https://doi.org/10.15584/ejcem

13. Matjacić, Z., Hesse, S., Sinkjaer, T.: BalanceReTrainer: a new standing-balance training apparatus and methods applied to a chronic hemiparetic subject with a neglect syndrome. NeuroRehabilitation. **18**, 251–259 (2003)

14. Katz, D.I., White, D.K., Alexander, M.P., Klein, R.B.: Recovery of ambulation after traumatic brain injury. Arch. Phys. Med. Rehabil. **85**, 865–869 (2004). https://doi.org/10.1016/j.apmr.2003.11.020

15. Dietz, V., Fouad, K.: Restoration of sensorimotor functions after spinal cord injury. Brain **137**, 654–667 (2014). https://doi.org/10.1093/brain/awt262

16. Ferrazzoli, D., et al.: Balance dysfunction in Parkinson's disease: the role of posturography in developing a rehabilitation program. Parkinsons Dis. **2015**, 1–10 (2015). https://doi.org/10.1155/2015/520128

17. Walter, S.J., Sola, G.P., Sacks, J., Lucero, Y., Langbein, E., Weaver, F.: Indications for a home standing program for individuals with spinal cord injury. J. Spinal Cord Med. **22**, 152–158 (1999). https://doi.org/10.1080/10790268.1999.11719564

18. Verschuren, O., Peterson, M.D., Balemans, A.C.J., Hurvitz, E.A.: Exercise and physical activity recommendations for people with cerebral palsy. Dev. Med. Child Neurol. **58**, 798–808 (2016). https://doi.org/10.1111/dmcn.13053

19. Rodby-Bousquet, E., Hägglund, G.: Use of manual and powered wheelchair in children with cerebral palsy: a cross-sectional study. BMC Pediatr. **10**, 59 (2010). https://doi.org/10.1186/1471-2431-10-59

20. Palisano, R.J., Rosenbaum, P., Bartlett, D., Livingston, M.H.: Content validity of the expanded and revised gross motor function classification system. Dev. Med. Child Neurol. **50**, 744–750 (2008). https://doi.org/10.1111/j.1469-8749.2008.03089.x

21. Tardieu, C., de la Tour, E.H., Bret, M.D., Tardieu, G.: Muscle hypoextensibility in children with cerebral palsy: I. Clinical and experimental observations. Arch. Phys. Med. Rehabil. **63**, 97–102 (1982)

22. Martinsson, C., Himmelmann, K.: Effect of weight-bearing in abduction and extension on hip stability in children with cerebral palsy. Pediatr. Phys. Ther. **23**, 150–157 (2011). https://doi.org/10.1097/pep.0b013e318218efc3

23. Shumway-Cook, A., Hutchinson, S., Kartin, D., Price, R., Woollacott, M.: Effect of balance training on recovery of stability in children with cerebral palsy. Dev. Med. Child Neurol. **45**, 591–602 (2003)

24. Shirota, C., et al.: Robot-supported assessment of balance in standing and walking. J. Neuroeng. Rehabil. **14**, 80 (2017). https://doi.org/10.1186/s12984-017-0273-7

25. Shanahan, C.J., et al.: Technologies for advanced gait and balance assessments in people with multiple sclerosis. Front. Neurol. **8**, 708 (2018). https://doi.org/10.3389/fneur.2017.00708
26. Park, D.-S., Lee, G.: Validity and reliability of balance assessment software using the Nintendo Wii balance board: usability and validation. J. Neuroeng. Rehabil. **11**, 99 (2014). https://doi.org/10.1186/1743-0003-11-99
27. Clark, R.A., McGough, R., Paterson, K.: Reliability of an inexpensive and portable dynamic weight bearing asymmetry assessment system incorporating dual Nintendo Wii Balance Boards. Gait Posture **34**, 288–291 (2011). https://doi.org/10.1016/j.gaitpost.2011.04.010
28. Goble, D.J., Cone, B.L., Fling, B.W.: Using the Wii Fit as a tool for balance assessment and neurorehabilitation: the first half decade of "Wii-search". J. Neuroeng. Rehabil. **11**, 12 (2014). https://doi.org/10.1186/1743-0003-11-12
29. Liuzzo, D.M., et al.: Measurements of weight bearing asymmetry using the Nintendo Wii fit balance board are not reliable for older adults and individuals with stroke. J. Geriatr. Phys. Ther. **40**, 37–41 (2017). https://doi.org/10.1519/jpt.0000000000000065
30. Reed-Jones, R.J., Dorgo, S., Hitchings, M.K., Bader, J.O.: WiiFit^{TM} Plus balance test scores for the assessment of balance and mobility in older adults. Gait Posture **36**, 430–433 (2012). https://doi.org/10.1016/j.gaitpost.2012.03.027
31. Livingstone, R., Paleg, G.: Measuring outcomes for children with cerebral palsy who use gait trainers. Technologies **4**, 22 (2016). https://doi.org/10.3390/technologies4030022
32. Paleg, G., Livingstone, R.: Outcomes of gait trainer use in home and school settings for children with motor impairments: a systematic review. Clin. Rehabil. **29**, 1077–1091 (2015). https://doi.org/10.1177/0269215514565947
33. Michalska, A., Dudek, J., Bieniek, M., Tarasow-Zych, A., Zawadzka, K.: The application of the balance trainer parapodium in the therapy of children with cerebral palsy. Fizjoterapia Pol. **11**, 273–285 (2011)
34. Winter, D.A., Patla, A.E., Ishac, M., Gage, W.H.: Motor mechanisms of balance during quiet standing. J. Electromyogr. Kinesiol. **13**, 49–56 (2003). https://doi.org/10.1016/s1050-6411(02)00085-8
35. Winter, D.A., Prince, F., Frank, J.S., Powell, C., Zabjek, K.F.: Unified theory regarding A/P and M/L balance in quiet stance. J. Neurophysiol. **75**, 2334–2343 (1996). https://doi.org/10.1152/jn.1996.75.6.2334
36. Colombo, G., Joerg, M., Schreier, R., Dietz, V.: Treadmill training of paraplegic patients using a robotic orthosis. J. Rehabil. Res. Dev. **37**, 693–700 (2000)
37. Jezernik, S., Colombo, G., Keller, T., Frueh, H., Morari, M.: Robotic orthosis lokomat: a rehabilitation and research tool. Neuromodulation Technol. Neural Interface **6**, 108–115 (2003). https://doi.org/10.1046/j.1525-1403.2003.03017.x
38. Noé, F., Quaine, F.: Insertion of the force applied to handles into centre of pressure calculation modifies the amplitude of centre of pressure shifts. Gait Posture **24**, 382–385 (2006). https://doi.org/10.1016/j.gaitpost.2005.10.001
39. Sieklicki, W., Barański, R., Grocholski, S., Matejek, P., Dyrda, M., Klepacki, K.: A new rehabilitation device for balance impaired individuals. In: BIODEVICES 2019 - 12th International Conference on Biomedical Electronics and Devices, Proceedings; Part of 12th International Joint Conference on Biomedical Engineering Systems and Technologies, BIOSTEC 2019 (2019)
40. Elliott, D.B., Flanagan, J.: Assessment of visual function. In: Elliott, D.B. (ed.) Clinical Procedures in Primary Eye Care, pp. 29–81. Elsevier, Amsterdam (2007)
41. Ghasia, F., Brunstom, J., Tychsen, L.: Visual acuity and visually evoked responses in children with cerebral palsy: gross motor function classification scale. Br. J. Ophthalmol. **93**, 1068–1072 (2009). https://doi.org/10.1136/bjo.2008.156372

42. Jacobson, B.H., Thompson, B., Wallace, T., Brown, L., Rial, C.: Independent static balance training contributes to increased stability and functional capacity in community-dwelling elderly people: a randomized controlled trial. Clin. Rehabil. **25**, 549–556 (2011). https://doi.org/10.1177/0269215510392390

43. Veneman, J.F., et al.: Design and evaluation of the LOPES exoskeleton robot for interactive gait rehabilitation. IEEE Trans. Neural Syst. Rehabil. Eng. **15**, 379–386 (2007). https://doi.org/10.1109/tnsre.2003.818185

44. Bayona, N.A., Bitensky, J., Salter, K., Teasell, R.: The role of task-specific training in rehabilitation therapies. Top. Stroke Rehabil. **12**, 58–65 (2005). https://doi.org/10.1310/bqm5-6ygb-mvj5-wvcr

45. Kilgard, M.P.: Cortical map reorganization enabled by nucleus basalis activity. Science **279**, 1714–1718 (1998). https://doi.org/10.1126/science.279.5357.1714

46. Matjacić, Z., Johannesen, I.L., Sinkjaer, T.: A multi-purpose rehabilitation frame: a novel apparatus for balance training during standing of neurologically impaired individuals. J. Rehabil. Res. Dev. **37**, 681–691 (2000)

47. Catherine, W., Brenda, B.J., Elsie, C.G.: Use of visual feedback in retraining balance following acute stroke. Phys. Ther. **80**, 886–895 (2000). https://doi.org/10.1093/ptj/80.9.886

48. Pasma, J.H., Engelhart, D., Schouten, A.C., van der Kooij, H., Maier, A.B., Meskers, C.G.M.: Impaired standing balance: the clinical need for closing the loop. Neuroscience **267**, 157–165 (2014). https://doi.org/10.1016/j.neuroscience.2014.02.030

49. Mancini, M., Horak, F.B.: The relevance of clinical balance assessment tools to differentiate balance deficits. Eur. J. Phys. Rehabil. Med. **46**, 239–248 (2010)

50. Bailey, I.L., Lovie, J.E.: New design principles for visual acuity letter charts. Am. J. Optom. Physiol. Opt. **53**, 740–745 (1976)

51. Stoller, O., et al.: Short-time weight-bearing capacity assessment for non-ambulatory patients with subacute stroke: reliability and discriminative power. BMC Res. Notes **8**, 723 (2015). https://doi.org/10.1186/s13104-015-1722-7

52. Rogers, M.W., Martinez, K.M., Waller, S.M., Gray, V.L.: Recovery and rehabilitation of standing balance after stroke. In: Stroke Recovery and Rehabilitation, pp. 343–374 (2009)

53. Goldie, P.A., Matyas, T.A., Evans, O.M., Galea, M.P., Bach, T.M.: Maximum voluntary weight-bearing by the affected and unaffected legs in standing following stroke. Clin. Biomech. (Bristol, Avon) **11**, 333–342 (1996)

54. Rougier, P.R., Genthon, N.: Dynamical assessment of weight-bearing asymmetry during upright quiet stance in humans. Gait Posture **29**, 437–443 (2009). https://doi.org/10.1016/j.gaitpost.2008.11.001

55. Kamphuis, J.F., de Kam, D., Geurts, A.C.H., Weerdesteyn, V.: Is weight-bearing asymmetry associated with postural instability after stroke? A systematic review. Stroke Res. Treat **2013**, 1–13 (2013). https://doi.org/10.1155/2013/692137

Reinventing Biomedical Engineering Education Working Towards the 2030 Agenda for Sustainable Development

Andrés Díaz Lantada$^{(\boxtimes)}$

Mechanical Engineering Department, ETSI Industriales, Universidad Politécnica de Madrid,
c/José Gutiérrez Abascal, 2, 28006 Madrid, Spain
andres.diaz@upm.es

Abstract. The engineering design of successful medical devices relies on several key factors, including: orientation to patients' needs, collaboration with healthcare professionals throughout the whole development process and the compromise of multi-disciplinary research and development (R&D) teams formed by well-trained professionals, especially biomedical engineers, capable of understanding the connections between science, technology and health and guiding such developments. Preparing engineers in general and biomedical engineers in particular to work in the medical industry, in connection with the development of medical devices, is a challenging process, through which the trainee should acquire a broad overview of the biomedical field and industry, a well-balanced combination of general and specific knowledge, according to the chosen specialization, several technical abilities linked to modern engineering tools and professional skills. Besides, understanding that biomedical engineering (BME), may constitute a fundamental resource to achieve global health coverage, biomedical engineers trainees should be made aware of their social responsibility and ethical issues should be always considered in the BME field and in BME education. Ideally, fulfilling the 2030 Agenda, especially as regards the Sustainable Development Goals (SDGs) on "Good Health and Well Being" & "Quality Education", should become the driving context for the biomedical engineers and the biomedical engineering educators of the future. Among the existing teaching-learning methodologies that can be employed for providing such holistic training, project-based learning is presented here and illustrated by means of successful experiences connected to the mentioned SDGs. The great potential of PBL to transform, not only courses on BME, but also complete programmes of studies in BME, and the strategies to connect BME education with the SDGs, are analyzed and discussed in depth. Emerging trends in the field of collaboratively developed open source medical devices (OSMDs) are presented in connection with the concept of "BME education for all".

Keywords: Project-Based Learning (PBL) · Engineering education · Biomedical Engineering (BME) · Sustainable development · Open Source Medical Devices (OSMD) · Service learning · Collaborative design · Co-creation

© Springer Nature Switzerland AG 2020
A. Roque et al. (Eds.): BIOSTEC 2019, CCIS 1211, pp. 29–54, 2020.
https://doi.org/10.1007/978-3-030-46970-2_2

1 Introduction

The engineering design of successful medical devices relies on several key factors, including: orientation to patients' needs, collaboration with healthcare professionals throughout the whole development process and the compromise of multi-disciplinary research and development (R&D) teams formed by well-trained professionals, especially biomedical engineers, capable of understanding the connections between science, technology and health and guiding such developments. Preparing engineers in general and biomedical engineers in particular to work in the medical industry, in connection with the engineering of medical devices, is a challenging process, through which the trainee should acquire a broad overview of the biomedical field and industry, a well-balanced combination of general and specific knowledge, according to the chosen specialization, several technical abilities linked to modern engineering tools and professional skills. Understanding that biomedical engineering (BME), if adequately applied to the development of equitable healthcare technologies, may constitute a fundamental resource to achieve global health coverage [1] is a fundamental question. Besides, biomedical engineers trainees should be aware of their social responsibility and ethical issues should be always considered in the BME field and its education. Ideally, fulfilling the 2030 Agenda for Sustainable Development [2], especially as regards the Sustainable Development Goals (SDGs) numbers 3 & 4 on "Good Health and Well Being" & "Quality Education", should become the driving context for the biomedical engineers and the BME educators of the future.

Problem-based learning, project-based learning, experiential learning, game-based learning, learning in collaborative project and environments, among others, are just different versions of highly formative and integrative learning experiences that place students in the center of the teaching-learning process, in accordance with a desire for a more holistic training for the 21st Century, especially in engineering education [3]. In all these project-related teaching-learning methodologies, student teams face a real life (typically engineering) problem, more or less simplified, and perform the specification, design, prototyping and testing of a product, a process, an event or, generally speaking, a system. In some cases prototyping and testing is achieved just virtually, but there is a critical analysis of results and a public exposition and subsequent debate for increased learning throughout the groups of students taking part in the course(s). In addition, creativity, decision making and critical thinking are fostered and professional tools for engineering practice (i.e. design and simulation software, prototyping tools…) are applied, so as to prepare students, as globally as possible, for their professional and personal lives. Knowledge acquisition is necessary, but the development of specific professional skills and transversal abilities, for more adequately applying the acquired knowledge to solve real challenges, is fundamental in modern education [4]. All this is in connection to what accreditation agencies, i.e. ABET and ENAEE, have been proposing in the last decades. This education based on learning objectives and professional outcomes is also essential for the recently implemented European Area of Higher Education and aligned with the UNESCO's World Declaration on Higher Education for the 21st Century [5].

The varied types of PBL experiences mainly differ in the level of depth, to which the project, product, process or system is specified, designed, implemented and managed or operated, and in the proposed context and desired level of realism, which depends also on the time and resources available for students living through the formative experience [6–8].

The "conceive – design – implement – operate" or "CDIO" approach to project-based learning, in a way, encompasses all the aforementioned types of active learning experiences [9]. In fact, the complete CDIO cycle involves the whole life-cycle of any engineering project or system, from specification and planning, through the design, engineering and construction, towards full operation, maintenance and end of life. Furthermore, the CDIO educational model goes beyond traditional project-based learning, as it involves also actuations, within the institutions and the professionals committed to "rethinking engineering education", aimed at continuous quality improvements in all engineering education-related processes. To this end, the support of a set of CDIO standards (see: http://www.cdio.org [10]), together with the sharing of good practices in the CDIO events, is fundamental. Among the characteristics of these CDIO educational experiences, is the permanent search for educational contexts with an increased level of realism (when compared to more classic project- and problem-based learning experiences) and, therefore, with a higher potential social impact. In many cases the CDIO projects are linked to real research and innovation projects or to industrial, entrepreneurial and social activities, in which highly transformative objectives are settled down and relevant human needs are addressed [11–13]. Clearly, the CDIO approach to reformulating engineering education is already having a worldwide transformative impact, with more than 150 higher education institutions worldwide having adopted its model and standards.

All this also links with service learning, defined by Jacobi as "a form of experiential education, in which students engage in activities that address human and community needs together with structured opportunities for reflection designed to achieve desired learning outcomes" [14]. Ideally, the solutions developed in these learning experiences reach society and transform it. This project-based service learning model adds to the previously listed types of active and integrative learning experiences and is clearly within the scope of CDIO. This hybridization between service learning and project-based learning can have additional impact if open source and collaborative approaches to engineering and its education are also involved and promoted, as recent international "express CDIO" learning experiences have put forward [15], in connection with the "UBORA educational model", described further on in this study as paradigmatic example in BME.

Finally, among the more recent project-based and active learning educational models in engineering education [16], it is also important to note the MIT's "NEET" or "New Engineering Education Transformation model", whose main elements are its project-centric curriculum and its organization in "threads" around a series of projects focused on new machines and systems. In fact, the NEET model is similar to CDIO but focuses on highly innovative fields: digital cities, autonomous machines, living machines, advanced materials or renewable energies.

Considering all the above, this study analyzes and discusses the - project-based learning - future of biomedical engineering education on the basis of inspiring references, motivating discussions with colleagues and students and personal experiences (ranging 10 years, including some 100 medical devices completely developed and 100 more concepts designed and with around 1000 students involved). Some aspects of the study have been recently presented by the author in a "keynote speech" in the 2019 Biodevices Conference (12th International Conference on Biomedical Electronics and Devices) and published in the related proceedings [17]. This expanded version better connects with the 2030 Agenda and may provide an innovative CDIO-related approach to BME education, in which the SDGs play a more relevant role, connected to specific topics of courses and projects. Along the study, the great potential of PBL to transform, not only single or scattered courses on BME, but also complete programmes of studies in BME, and the strategies to connect BME education with the SDGs, are analyzed and discussed in depth. Emerging trends in the field of collaboratively developed open source medical devices (OSMDs) [18–20] are presented in connection with the concept of "BME education for all".

To illustrate the OSMD field, the "UBORA" project is put forward as a recent paradigmatic example (UBORA means "excellence" in Swahili). This initially Euro-African (and now already global) initiative is focused on the promotion of OSMDs by means of innovation through education, by the creation of a "Wikipedia" of medical devices, the "UBORA e-infrastructure", which also guides designers in the systematic engineering design process and supports online collaboration through the process, and by the constitution of a truly international community of developers devoted to OSMDs. The varied project-based learning activities performed within the first couple of years of UBORA project's endeavors are also briefly discussed and some results illustrated. Besides, the "UBORA e-infrastructure" and the more than 100 open source biodevices concepts and prototypes developed in collaboration by a global community of around 400 users, and shared through such online infrastructure, are also analyzed, focusing on advances since its official presentation [1, 15, 20]. Finally, some potentials and challenges in the OSMD field are discussed, in connection with the "BME education for all" concept.

2 Project-Based Learning and Biomedical Devices

2.1 Introduction

Biomedical engineering (BME) has been since its origins a truly transformative field of engineering, which may even lead to equitable access to healthcare technologies and universal health care in the future, as previously introduced, according to World Health Organization's objectives [21]. However, this field and related transformations rely on the collaboration of engineers from all areas, whose training should make them successful developers of effective, efficient, ergonomic, user-oriented, in some cases even hedonomic, safe, replicable, cost competitive, ethically and socially responsible, sustainable and regulation compliant medical devices.

Project-based learning, connected to the development of real medical devices, is arguably the best strategy for training engineers, from a wide set of environments, towards successful professional practice in the medical industry, as happens with engineering education in general. In fact, PBL and challenge-based instruction prove very appropriate in BME, not just for organizing single courses and providing an introduction to the medical industry and to medical technology, but also for adequately implementing and being the backbone of whole programmes of studies and for career development, as presented and discussed in an excellent review [22]. Hybridizing PBL with service learning and connecting it with the needs of the developing world, may enhance the learning outcomes and better connect students with a more guided transition to professional practice, especially if the results are shared [1, 15, 23]. In terms of impact, it is also interesting to mention the process for developing medical technologies proposed by Stanford's Biodesign initiative, both for education and innovation [24]. Their proposed "identify – invent – implement" cycle is quite similar to the CDIO cycle and approach used here as reference and inspiring conception of modern engineering education.

The following subsections provide some guidelines, proposals and ideas for the straightforward and successful design, implementation and operation of PBL experiences in the biomedical engineering field. The proposed teaching-learning activities are focused on the design, manufacturing and testing of biodevices, and the indications are based on recommendations from key references [22–29] and on author's experience [30–32]. An emphasis on how to connect BME with the SDGs and with global health concerns is provided and illustrated with real cases of study in Sects. 3 to 6.

2.2 Planning the Learning Objectives

When planning project-based teaching-learning experiences, it is interesting to start by analyzing the global purpose and by listing down the learning objectives envisioned for the concrete course or programme of studies. Asking ourselves how our students may be involved in the medical industry in their future career paths and what we would like them to master, as regards the development life cycle of innovative medical devices, seems a good start option. A set of high-level learning objectives for any bioengineering design course focused on training students through the complete development process of medical technologies may include the following:

O.1. Ability to conceive, design, produce and operate innovative medical devices by applying systematic engineering-design methodologies for improved results when addressing global health concerns.

O.2. Ability to promote research and innovation strategies in biomedical engineering and in the medical device industry, so as to better take into consideration the voice of patients, associations and healthcare professionals.

O.3. Understanding the fundamental relevance of standardization and the need for considering existing regulatory paths, so as to achieve safe and compliant prototypes of medical devices ready for production.

O.4. Capability to create value proposals linked to innovative medical devices or technologies and to generate viable entrepreneurial activities within the biomedical industry.

O.5. Capability to learn for researching and developing innovative technologies and to mentor their application to innovative medical devices with improved performance, usability and societal impact, as compared with current gold standards

Once the learning objectives are defined, the context and boundaries need to be established, in accordance with the temporal framework and available resources for our course and considering the overall objectives and desired outcomes of the complete engineering programme.

2.3 Establishing the Context: PBL and Service Learning

Student and professor motivation are the keys of success in engineering education and establishing a motivating context of shared dreams is essential, towards truly successful and career inspiring PBL experiences, especially in such a transformative field as BME: Our students should always understand that engineering must aim at improving the world and our global society. Medical technologies are part of this process of change, in connection with the UN Global Goal number 3 on "Good health and well-being", but also linked to numbers 8 on "Decent work and economic growth" and 9 on "Industry, innovation and infrastructure", among others.

In consequence, PBL experiences in the BME field, if possible, should be contextualized in connection with relevant health concerns and should try to respond to the needs of patients and healthcare professionals. Ideally, when external advisors from hospitals, associations, companies or NGOs working in low-resource settings are involved, the context and ideas for the projects, to be developed by student groups within the PBL experience, can be linked to real specific needs or concrete challenges, hence transforming the PBL experience into a service learning challenge, in which ethical issues can be additionally developed in class.

Evidently the context is marked also by the background of our students and by the global objectives and outcomes of the whole programme: A medical device engineering design course within a robotics engineering programme may concentrate on medical robotics projects (i.e. design of surgical manipulators or artificial hands); while student projects in a mechanical engineering programme may focus on the design and manufacturing of implants (i.e. prostheses for articular repair or artificial valves).

At the same time, biomedical PBL experiences in materials science programmes may even connect with the field of biofabrication, through the design of scaffolding materials and other artificial constructs (at least conceptually); while PBL tasks in industrial organization engineering may tackle supply chain problems or focus on quality and risk management, as related with real production processes, to cite some examples. Student background should be also considered, perhaps leaving more conceptual projects to the first engineering courses and those requiring more technical design, manufacturing and experimental skills to the final year of the Bachelor's degrees or to the Master's and even PhD levels.

2.4 Defining Contents and Boundaries

With the previously listed high-level learning objectives in mind (O.1-O.5), for any bioengineering design course focused on training students through the complete development process of medical technologies or devices, the following basic contents are proposed. They can serve as topics for lessons or modules depending on the available time and temporal framework of the concrete course. They can also act as structuring elements for PBL experiences, which can range from just one week to even a whole academic year, as previous examples have shown [15, 33, 34]. The proposed basic contents include:

- Engineering design methodologies for biomedical devices.
- Conceptual design and creativity promotion tools.
- Design for usability and risk mitigation.
- Design considering standards and regulations.
- Prototyping and testing of biodevices.
- Mass-personalization and mass-production options.
- Commercialization paths and supply chain issues.
- Sustainable development of biodevices and ethical issues in BME.

These basic contents can be completed with specific modules for adapting a generic or sort of "universal" bioengineering design course to the specific needs of completely varied engineering programmes. For instance, a module on "biosignals" may adapt and reinforce these contents for an electronic engineering programme, while a module on "biomechanics and biomaterials" may be adequate for completing a course for a materials science or mechanical engineering programme. In some cases, specific training for transversal skills may be provided, including seminars on teamwork abilities, project and time management skills, and communication techniques, among others. Regarding the scope and boundaries of the PBL experience, depending also on the available time and resources, the projects may focus just on the specification and conceptual stages, or reach up to the design, prototyping and testing phases.

2.5 Implementing and Assessing

A good definition of objectives, context and contents typically leads to straightforwardly implementable PBL experiences, although some unforeseen events may always take place. Counting with well-maintained manufacturing resources, with rapid responding suppliers and with software licenses, renewed with enough time before the start of the courses, are among the good practices we can cite. Promotion of communication between professors and students, with at least monthly face-to-face meetings and tutorials and with intermediate presentation of results and through a consistent plan of distributed deliverables, is also advisable. Regarding evaluation, involving students in their own assessment, especially through peer-review activities within the working groups, may be considered as an additional control tool for PBL. In addition, the promotion of positive interdependence, by making students work in complex enough projects, and some degree of individual assessment, i.e. through specific questions in oral presentations or by means of additional deliverables or evaluation tasks, are the more basic options for achieving a good ambience of collaboration within the teams, without losing individual control upon students that may fade away in teamwork activities [8].

3 BME Courses Focused on Engineering Medical Devices

Along the last decade, at Universidad Politécnica de Madrid (UPM), our team has applied the previously explained considerations, regarding learning objectives, context, boundaries, contents, communication and evaluation, to the creation of four CDIO-oriented courses on BME for different programmes of study. The four courses are: "Design of Medical Devices", "Biomedical Engineering", "Bioengineering Design" and "MedTech", respectively belonging to: the "Bachelor's Degree in Biomedical Engineering", the Master's Degree in Mechanical Engineering", the "Master's Degree in Industrial Engineering" and the "Master's Degree in Organizational Engineering". In all of them, students, working in groups, live through the complete engineering-design cycle of innovative medical devices connected to global health concerns or to emergent health issues. As shown in Table 1, which presents a versatile structure of modules and contents for BME education through CDIO courses focused on medical device design, all these courses share a block of common fundamentals. These fundamentals introduce students to systematic engineering design methodologies, adequately adapted to the medical industry, and to key aspects on design for usability, standards, regulations, safety, ethics, sustainability, specification and planning, creativity promotion and conceptualization, design, prototyping and testing. These fundamentals have proven also of great value in the implementation of one-week "express CDIO" experiences, such as the UBORA Design Schools, in which our team takes part and which are also included in Table 1 for comparative purposes as a relevant and inspiring scalable example (see Sect. 6 and [18]).

Apart from the common learning module focused on the fundamentals, necessary because all students of these courses face for the first time the complete development of a medical device, there are additional learning modules, which can be combined depending on the actual programme of study, the specialization or background of students and the temporal framework (one year, one semester or even one week).

Regarding students' evaluation, it is important to highlight that the proposed topics and medical devices developed are complex enough to encourage positive interdependence between members of the teams, so that each member of a team is needed for achieving the overall success. The experiences and level of exigency are planned, so that there may be enough workload to let all students work hard and enjoy the experience, thanks to learning by doing in a challenging environment. In addition, we are encouraging individual assessment, complementing the teamwork activities with individual deliveries, through personal interviews and during the public presentations of their final results with individualized questions (which account for a 25% to a 30% of the global qualification). The evaluation of professional skills counts with the help of ad hoc designed assessment sheets or rubrics, as part of an integral framework for the promotion of engineering education beyond technical skills, consequence of recent educational innovation projects [32]. We are also considering the introduction of peer-evaluation techniques to some extent, although our main concern with this relies on the potential harm that the good ambience of collaboration within the teams might suffer.

Table 1. Versatile structure of modules and contents for BME education and CDIO initiatives focused on medical device design.

Module	Course: Name of Engineering Programme (*at UPM, **developed by the UBORA team); Level (& year); Course duration (& ECTS equivalent):	Design of Med. Devices — BSc in Biomedical Eng.* — 4th year — 1 semester (4 ECTS)	Bioengineering — MSc in Mechanical Eng.* — 1st (Master's level) — 1 semester (3 ECTS)	Bioengineering Design — MSc in Industrial Eng.* — 1st (Master's level) — 2 semesters (12 ECTS)	MedTech — MSc in Org. Eng.* — 1st (Master's level) — 2 semesters (12 ECTS)	UBORA Design Schools — Intl. events-hackathons** — Varied — 1 intense week (3 ECTS)
FUNDAMENTALS	Introduction to biomedical engineering and medical devices	x	x	x	x	x
FUNDAMENTALS	Sustainability and ethical aspects in biomedical engineering	x	x	x	x	x
FUNDAMENTALS	Product planning: The relevance of a medical need	x	x	x	x	x
FUNDAMENTALS	Conceptual design and creativity promotion: Design for-with users	x	x	x	x	x
FUNDAMENTALS	Basic engineering I: From the concept to the design	x	x	x	x	x
FUNDAMENTALS	Basic engineering II: From the design to the prototype	x	x	x	x	x
FUNDAMENTALS	Basic engineering III: Testing and validation of medical devices	x	x	x	x	x
FUNDAMENTALS	Detailed engineering: Standardization and safety issues	x	x	x	x	x
BASIC MECH. ISSUES	Overview on human biomechanics	x	x	x	x	x
BASIC MECH. ISSUES	Overview on biomaterials for biodevices	x	x	x	x	x
BASIC MECH. ISSUES	Basic computer-aided design seminar	x			x	x
BASIC MECH. ISSUES	Basic FEM-based modeling seminar	x			x	x
ADVANCED MECHANICAL & MANUFACTURING ISSUES	Key aspects in human biomechanics			x	x	
ADVANCED MECHANICAL & MANUFACTURING ISSUES	Key aspects in human fluid mechanics			x		
ADVANCED MECHANICAL & MANUFACTURING ISSUES	Advanced computer-aided design seminar		x	x		
ADVANCED MECHANICAL & MANUFACTURING ISSUES	Advanced FEM-based modeling seminar		x	x		
ADVANCED MECHANICAL & MANUFACTURING ISSUES	Special technologies for mass-personalization and mass-production	x	x	x		
ADVANCED MECHANICAL & MANUFACTURING ISSUES	Micro- and nano-fabrication of biomedical micro- and nano-systems	x	x	x	x	x
COMMERCIALIZ. OF MEDICAL TECHNOLOGY	Lean entrepreneurship methods	x			x	
COMMERCIALIZ. OF MEDICAL TECHNOLOGY	Key aspects for project and team management				x	
COMMERCIALIZ. OF MEDICAL TECHNOLOGY	Quality control and standards in the biomedical sector				x	
COMMERCIALIZ. OF MEDICAL TECHNOLOGY	Open innovation, collaborative design and blue economy	x	x	x	x	x
COMMERCIALIZ. OF MEDICAL TECHNOLOGY	Evaluation of technical and economical sustainability				x	
COMMERCIALIZ. OF MEDICAL TECHNOLOGY	Approaching the clients and users				x	
SPECIALIZED WORKSHOPS	Medical signals with open source electronics and sensors					x
SPECIALIZED WORKSHOPS	Medical imaging, movement tracking and image processing					x
SPECIALIZED WORKSHOPS	Electronic rapid prototyping and paper-based medical devices					x
SPECIALIZED WORKSHOPS	3D scanning combined with 3D printing for personalized devices					x
SPECIALIZED WORKSHOPS	Conflict management in teamwork and promotion of personal skills	x	x			x
CASES & TRENDS	Cases of study: Real medical device development projects	x	x		x	x
CASES & TRENDS	Future trends: Tissue engineering and biofabrication	x	x	x		x
CASES & TRENDS	Future Trends: Labs- and organs-on-chips	x	x	x		x
CASES & TRENDS	Future trends: Towards equitable healthcare through OSMDs	x	x	x	x	x

In all these experiences summarized in Table 1, living through a complete CDIO cycle is proposed, although in some particular situations it is only possible to cover in depth the conceptual and design phases, normally due to time restrictions or to the complexity of a selected device or challenge. In the UPM courses, the conceptual stages are supported by creativity-promotion tools and methods such as TRIZ, use of morphological boxes and systematic procedures for promoting the generation, association and selection of ideas. The design stages count with industrial state-of-the-art modeling and simulation software of main engineering disciplines. In addition, the UPM courses count with the support of well-equipped industrial manufacturing labs, where several design and simulation software, testing facilities, rapid prototyping technologies, usually by means of additive manufacturing and rapid form copying and pre-production tools, are available. In any case, more affordable fab labs are also perfect for educational purposes. Prototyping facilities are very relevant for letting students live trough the complete development process of innovative medical devices, from the conceptual and design phases, to the implementation and operation stages, which are normally more difficult to achieve [8]. Arduino and Bitalino kits and libraries of sensors and actuators are also available, as well as biomechanical models for performance evaluation.

To illustrate the potential of this approach and its relevant educational and societal impact Figs. 1, 2 and 3 present selected examples from medical devices engineered by UPM students. These results or selected cases of study also show the importance of counting with a versatile structure of contents and modules, which can be combined, to easily implement new courses for different programmes. As can be appreciated, the medical devices from Fig. 1, corresponding to the "Design of Medical Devices" course (one semester) from the UPM BSc in Biomedical Engineering, deal with biomedical signals and incorporate electronic components and sensors, topics in which students are well prepared. On the other hand, the medical devices from Fig. 2 focus on more mechanical devices, as they correspond to the "Bioengineering" course (one semester) from the UPM MSc in Mechanical Engineering. Results from Fig. 3 correspond to the "Bioengineering Design" and "MedTech" courses, performed in collaboration between the UPM MSc in Industrial Engineering and the UPM MSc in Organizational Engineering [33]. These selected cases from Fig. 3 show a higher level of development and complexity, as they are carried out along a whole academic year with students from different backgrounds collaborating, which leads to very remarkable results. In these cases, an additional degree of interaction with healthcare professionals, which act as external advisors, is encouraged.

In order to maintain these experiences alive, to continuously motivate both students and professors, to avoid repetition of devices and even eventual bad practices (i.e. students copying from projects developed in previous years), it is important to find new topics for the medical devices to be developed. To this end, thematic years can be proposed, in which the medical devices to be developed are proposed by students, but within a specific context (i.e. ageing society, maternal health, devices for mental health, solutions for tissue engineering and biofabrication, devices for sport practice, among others). Furthermore, this thematic/monographic experiences help to better connect the courses with the 2030 Agenda, as discussed in Sect. 5.

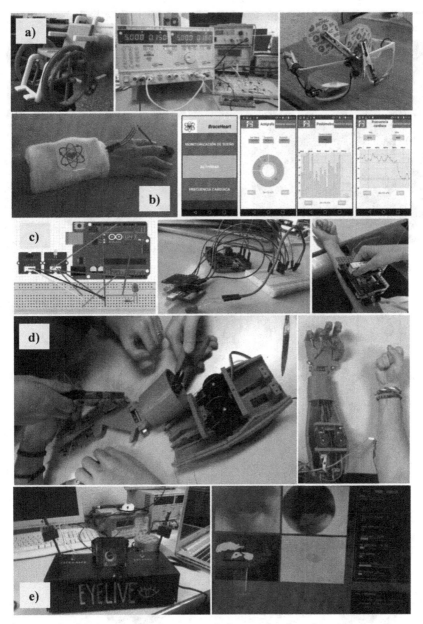

Fig. 1. Examples from medical devices, as result from project-based teaching-learning experiences developed in the "Design of Medical Devices" course in the BSc in Biomedical Engineering at UPM. a) Device for ocular control of wheel-chair. b) Device for activity monitoring with associated app. c) Hedonomic LEGO-based system for infrared vein detection in children. d) Prototype of myoelectric prosthetic arm. e) Device for mouse pointer control by eye movement tracking for patients with ALS.

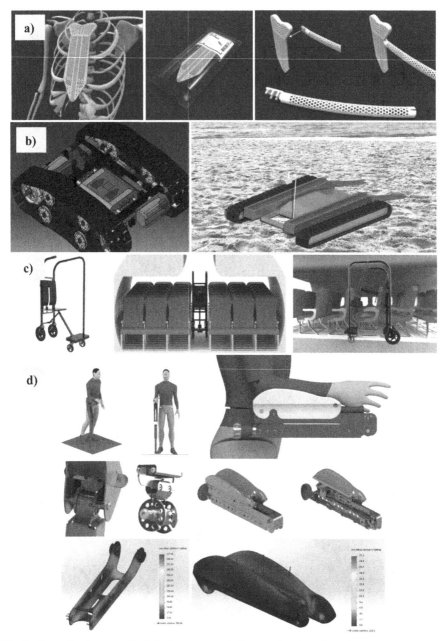

Fig. 2. Examples from medical devices, as result from project-based teaching-learning experiences developed in the "Bioengineering" course in the MSc in Mechanical Engineering at UPM. a) Lightweight sternum and rib prostheses. b) Crawler track undercarriage system for adapting wheelchairs to different environments (i.e. beach). c) System for helping disabled persons enter a plane. d) Foldable ergonomic crutch: Design and dummy, detailed components and mechanical evaluation.

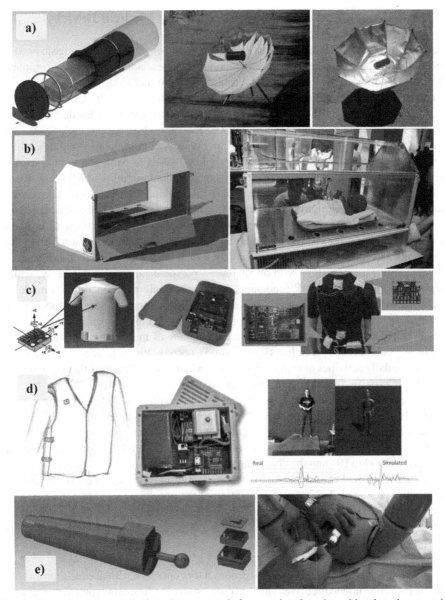

Fig. 3. Examples from medical devices, as result from project-based teaching-learning experiences developed in the "Bioengineering Design" and "MedTech" courses, performed in collaboration between the MSc in Industrial Engineering and the MSc in Organizational Engineering, both at UPM. a) Concept, prototype and experimental validation for a solar powered autoclave for remote settings. b) Low-cost do-it-yourself cradle with autonomous temperature and airflow control. c) System for wrong back posture detection and correction. d) System for detecting falls with wearable sensors driven by artificial intelligence trained with the support of a video game. e) Amnioscope for examining the amniotic cavity tested in delivery simulator.

4 BME Programmes Based on Engineering Medical Devices

The same versatile structure applied to PBL/CDIO courses in BME, with a basic or fundamentals module and some specialization moduli, can be adapted to construct complete BME programmes, in which the engineering of medical technology is the fundamental element of the curricular structure. This clearly connects with the CDIO approach and with the MIT-NEET model. However this study – see Fig. 4 – considers up to the doctoral level, in line with the seven EURAXESS doctoral training principles [34], and possibly aims at a higher level of versatility, modularity, interoperability and flexibility. In fact, higher engineering education in general and BME in particular should evolve towards more flexible programmes of study, capable of maintaining a high level of rigour and exigency in necessary scientific-technological fundamentals, but also of providing students with more opportunities for personalized paths and career development plans.

Modular structures, as the one proposed in Fig. 4 for BME education, are very adequate for setting international standards, for promoting the international mobility of students and for the establishment of international degrees, by collaboration among different universities, in line with an increased personalization and flexibility, while keeping a stable core of BME fundamentals, as previously mentioned. Such modular structures also help to renew engineering education by updating the more advanced modules, in many cases according to the more recent trends and in connection with research and development projects, while leaving the fundamentals more stable. In this way, the demanding bureaucratic procedures (verifications, accreditations, re-accreditations) that collapse the daily activities of many centers, even when minor changes to the programmes of study are proposed, could be also minimized.

Consequently, Fig. 4 presents a structure with modules including: "Science fundamentals", "Ethics and sustainability", "Biotechnology fundamentals", "Culture and multidisciplinary issues", "Advanced science", "Advanced biotechnology", "Contemporary issues", "Professional practice" and several modules devoted to engineering medical devices: "CDIO I to III" and the "Final degree theses". With such a structure, up to a 20–25% of activities deal with project-based or challenge-based experiences, around a 30% of activities are devoted to the personalization of the programme and to constructing a singular career path for each student, and around a 50% of the degrees deal with science and technology, with some compulsory courses and some eligible ones. Table 2 presents such learning modules, ordered in accordance with the structure of Fig. 4, together with possible courses examples.

Such a modular structure, the related proposal for contents for BME education and the holistic focus on knowledge dissemination, promotion of technical outcomes and training of professional and personal skills is aligned with the principles of the UNESCO's World Declaration on Higher Education for the 21st Century [5]. It would be also compliant with the guides from relevant accreditation bodies (i.e. ABEC and ENAEE) and would help to systematically integrate the 2030 Agenda and the SDGs as drivers of engineering education and practice, as analyzed and discussed in the following section.

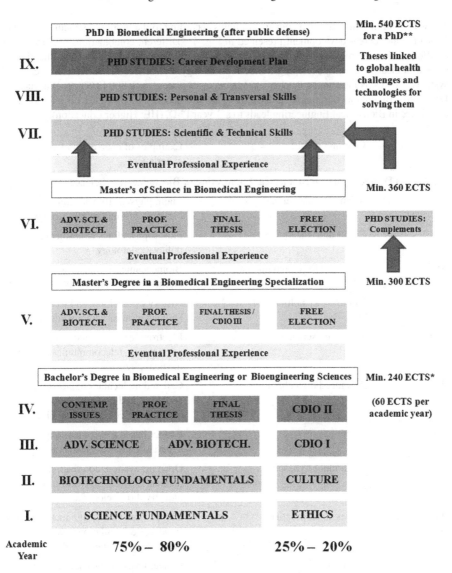

Fig. 4. Versatile, modular, interoperable and flexible structure for programmes of study in biomedical engineering education and career development in connection with the engineering of medical devices for global health concerns.

Table 2. Learning modules and courses examples according to the proposed structure for BME Education and career development presented in Fig. 4. *Different combinations lead to majors in: Biomaterials, biomechanics and biodevices, health informatics, biosignals and bioimaging…, all with a clear focus on developing medical technology. **MEMS: Micro-electro-mechanical systems, NEMS: Nano-electro-mechanical systems. ***Access with 300 ECTS from a Master's Degree in a Bioengineering major leads to a 4-year PhD, access with 360 ECTS from a Master's of Science in Biomedical Engineering leads to a 3-year PhD. (HE: Higher Education).

Academic year	Learning modules	Examples of courses and learning experiences
Bachelor's Degree studies in Biomedical Engineering or Bioengineering Sciences		
I	Science fundamentals	Math, physics, (bio-)chemistry, biology, informatics, physiology
I	Ethics and sustainability	Philosophy, ethics & aesthetics, policy, deontology
II	Biotechnology fundamentals	Biomechanics, biomaterials, bioinformatics, bio-signals
II	Culture and multidiscipl.	History of medicine and technology, languages, anthropology, nutrition
III*	Advanced science	Electromagnetism, electronics, energy engineering, telecommunications, medical physics
III*	Advanced biotechnology	Cell and molecular engineering, genomics and proteomics, bioimaging, computational biology
III	CDIO I	Project-based service learning experiences for low resource settings
IV	Contemporary issues	Open innovation, co-creation of medical devices, blue economy, industry 4.0, society 5.0
IV	Professional practice	Co-op, biodevice design methodology, standards & regulations, work in hospital, humanitarian aid
IV	CDIO II	Project-based service learning experiences for a set of selected clinical needs
IV	Final degree thesis	Complete development cycle of innovative medical devices or technologies
Master's Degree studies in Biomedical Engineering (start after completing 240 ECTS in HE)		
V & VI*	Advanced science and biotechnology	Tissue engineering, biofabrication, genomics, bio-MEMS-NEMS**
V & VI	Professional practice	Co-op, commercialization of medical technologies, management, work in hospital, humanitarian aid

(continued)

Table 2. (*continued*)

Academic year	Learning modules	Examples of courses and learning experiences
V & VI	Personal configuration	Design and simulation workshops, teamwork skills, leadership
V & VI	Final degree thesis-CDIO III	Complete development cycle of innovative medical devices or technologies
PhD studies in Biomedical Engineering (start after completing a min. of 300 ECTS in HE***)		
VI/VII–IX	Scientific & technical skills	Scientific methods, laboratory practice, software and hardware
VI/VII–IX	Personal and transversal skills	Communication, teamwork skills, leadership, policy making
VI/VII–IX	Career development planning	Personal branding and networking, value creation, entrepreneurship

5   Connecting BME Courses and Programmes with the SDGs

To systematically connect BME courses and programmes of study with the SDGs, especially with SDG3 on "Good Health and Well Being" and SDG4 on "Quality Education", which are those more linked to BME and its education, it is interesting to map the goals and their specific targets and to search for associations with teaching learning initiatives and topics for courses and CDIO-PBL tasks. The results for these analyses are presented in Table 3, which shows connections between "Good Health and Well Being" and BME education, and in Table 4, which focuses on the relationships between "Quality Education" and BME.

At UPM our team is already applying some of these proposed courses, teaching-learning initiatives and activities, so as to synergize BME with the SDGs. As can be seen from the cases of study included in Figs. 1, 2 and 3, several medical devices developed by our groups of students focus on maternal health and infants, aim at promoting the well-being of disabled people or have been designed considering usability conditions in low resource settings and remote rural areas. In some cases, these devices derive from project-based service learning initiatives, in which students have collaborated with patients associations and in some cases they have participated with their ideas (and with success) in start-up creation programmes or in international medical device design competitions, including the UBORA design competitions. Co-creation and open source strategies are also applied in the mentioned courses and many of the medical devices developed are shared through the UBORA e-infrastructure, presented in detail in the following section. The effort of mapping the SDGs with the activities in our BME course has helped our team to reinvent them.

Table 3. Connection of courses, teaching-learning activities and initiatives in BME education with some selected targets of the SDGs: 3. "Good Health and Well Being".

Selected targets of the goals, for which biomedical engineering is essential (summarized versions)	Proposed courses, teaching-learning activities and initiatives to synergize biomedical engineering education with the SDGs on "Good Health and Well Being"
3.1. Reduce the global maternal mortality ratio to less than 70 per 100,000 live births	– Topics for courses: devices for maternal health as cases of study. Debates in ethics lessons – CDIO-PBL tasks on medical devices for: monitoring pregnancy, apps supporting timely advices
3.2. End preventable deaths of newborns and children under 5 years (to at least as low as 12 per 1,000 live births and under-5 mortality to at least as low as 25 per 1,000 live births)	– Topics for courses: devices for infant health as cases of study. Debates in ethics lessons – CDIO-PBL tasks on medical devices for: monitoring health state of newborns and children, harm-less point-of-care diagnosis and vaccination, supporting healthy musculoskeletal development, detection of allergens
3.4. Reduce by one third premature mortality from non-communicable diseases through prevention and treatment and promote mental health and well-being	– Topics for courses: point-of-care testing and diagnoses as topic for bio-MEMS-NEMS courses – CDIO-PBL tasks on medical devices for: point-of-care testing in low resource settings, monitoring of mental health & well being in urban, sub-urban and rural areas
3.8. Achieve universal health coverage, including financial risk protection, access to quality essential health-care services and to safe, effective, quality & affordable essential medicines and vaccines for all	– Topics for courses: debates in ethics lessons and courses on open-innovation and blue economy – CDIO-PBL tasks on medical devices for: performing safe surgeries, updating donated equipments, improving and controlling the immunization supply chain
3.C. Substantially increase health financing and the recruitment, development, training and retention of the health workforce in developing countries	– Topics for courses: debates on universal health coverage and its possible sustainability – Develop educational initiatives including: stays in hospitals as BME trainees, cooperation between universities and hospitals for capacity building
3.D. Strengthen the capacity of all countries, in particular developing countries, for early warning, risk reduction and management of national and global health risks	– Topics for courses: debates on global health concerns – CDIO-PBL tasks on medical devices for: enhancing smartphones for supporting health management, helping with the implementation of e-health systems
In all selected targets, which may benefit from the development of medical devices in connection with biomedical engineering educational tasks	Promote co-creation of open source medical devices, whose development and usability information is freely shared, for the benefit of society, through online tools: (i.e. https://platform.ubora-biomedical.org/)

Table 4. Connection of courses, teaching-learning activities and initiatives in BME education with some selected targets of the SDGs: 4. "Quality Education".

Selected targets of the goals, for which biomedical engineering is essential (summarized versions)	Proposed courses, teaching-learning activities and initiatives to synergize biomedical engineering education with the SDGs on "Quality Education"
4.3. Ensure equal access for all women and men to quality vocational, tertiary and technical education, including university	– Topics for courses: debates on gender issues – Develop educational initiatives including: development of medical devices, in which gender may play a relevant role, i.e. due to special prevalence, ergonomic aspects...
4.4. Increase the number of youth and adults who have relevant skills, including technical and vocational skills, for employment, decent jobs and entrepreneurship	– Topics for courses: Lean start-up models, management, value creation, career path planning – Develop educational initiatives including: Spin-off/start-up creation challenges based on PBL activities
4.7. Ensure that all learners acquire the knowledge and skills needed to promote sustainable development	– Topics for courses: Debates on sustainable industries – Develop educational initiatives including: PBL-CDIO activities, in which analyzing the life-cycle is essential
4.A. Build and upgrade education facilities that are child, disability and gender sensitive and provide safe, nonviolent, inclusive and effective learning environments for all	– CDIO-PBL tasks on medical devices for: supporting people with disabilities to perform their daily activities – Develop educational initiatives including: cooperation with patient association for service learning approaches
4.B. Expand globally the number of scholarships available to developing countries, for enrollment in higher education	– Develop educational initiatives including: global classrooms and innovative mobility programmes thanks to the versatile, modular and flexible structure proposed. Promote sponsorship programmes connected to mobility and project-based service learning activities
4.C. Increase the supply of qualified teachers for developing countries and promote international cooperation for teacher training	– Topics for courses: at PhD level, involve early stage researchers as mentors in learning activities – Develop educational initiatives as in 4.B. Share teaching resources online (see UBORA platform below)
In all selected targets, which may benefit from the development of medical devices in connection with biomedical engineering educational tasks	Promote co-creation of open source medical devices, whose development and usability information is freely shared, for the benefit of society, through online tools: (i.e. https://platform.ubora-biomedical.org/)

6   Towards "BME education for all" in Connection with the SDGs: The UBORA Open Source & Collaborative Model

6.1   The UBORA Project, e-Infrastructure and Community and the SDGs

The UBORA research, development and training model for transforming the biomedical industry towards equitable healthcare technologies derives from experiences conceived, designed, performed and validated within the H2020 "UBORA: Euro-African Open Biomedical Engineering e-Platform for Innovation through Education" project (GA-731053) during years 2017 and 2018. These experiences have counted with the fundamental support of the UBORA e-infrastructure, an open-access design environment envisioned for the co-creation of open source medical technologies according to real needs, which has been also developed in the UBORA project, as detailed below.

6.2   Open Source Medical Devices

UBORA focuses on the promotion of research and training activities in BME pursuing the collaborative development of open source medical devices (OSMDs). These devices are developed by sharing concepts, design files, documentation, source-code, blueprints and prototypes, testing results and all collected data, with other professional medical device designers. These interactions should benefit the whole life cycle of the devices or products under development and ideally lead to safer performance, thanks to increased peer-review through the co-creation process [18–20, 35]. The open source approach is clearly connected to the SDGs on "Healthcare and Well Being" and "Quality Education" and also to their specific targets. Besides, the "UBORA educational model" derives from CDIO, in some cases hybridized with service learning, and works with some recommendations from the previously presented mapping of teaching-learning activities with the SDGs of interest, aiming at free quality education worldwide in the BME field.

6.3   UBORA: Much More Than a "Wikipedia" of Biodevices

The UBORA e-infrastructure, implemented for supporting the nascent OSMD community in both research, co-creation/-design and teaching-learning or educational tasks (see: https://platform.ubora-biomedical.org/) includes features such as: a) a section for specifying medical needs, through which patients and healthcare professionals can ask for technological solutions; b) a section for sharing technological solutions, through which engineers can showcase their proposals for the future of medical care; c) a meta-structure for supporting biomedical engineers, engineering students and professors in the field to guide the development of innovative medical technologies, in a step-by-step process following systematic engineering-design processes, answering and filling in the questions and sections provided by the e-infrastructure; d) a community with already more than 400 co-creators; and e) a section for sharing open teaching materials for free, in connection with the "BME education for all" concept.

6.4 Arranging and Training a Global Community Focused on OSMDs

When planning to arrange and train a global community of designers and developers of OSMDs, in which international collaboration should play a central role for the near future, it became clear for the UBORA consortium, led by Prof. Arti Ahluwalia from the University of Pisa, that PBL should be used as overall teaching-learning strategy. Consequently, different types and formats of PBL experiences have been conceived and carried out in the last two years, which have involved around 30 mentors and well-beyond 300 students (now engineers), leading to a collaborative community of more than 400 members from some 30 countries distributed through Africa, America, Asia and Europe and interacting through the UBORA e-infrastructure.

UBORA PBL experiences include: thematic medical device design competitions, one-week medical device design schools and final degree theses linked to biodevice development. In 2017 the UBORA Design Competition (online, February–June) and Design School (Nairobi, December) focused on child and maternal health, while in 2018 the UBORA Design Competition (online, January–May) and Design School (Pisa, September) focused on ageing-related issues. More than 100 participants have taken part in each of the competitions, while 40 students have participated in each design school, which follow an *"express PBL approach, from concept to prototype in 5 days"* [15]. These PBL activities are now performed on an annual basis and additional ones (mainly UBORA competitions and UBORA design schools) can be *ad hoc* conceived and implemented for focusing on more specific topics, health issues, contexts or locations, for colleagues and institutions interested in exploring open source approaches to the development of medical technology. Besides, the UBORA e-infrastructure is already supporting the development of different medical technology design courses, within different engineering programmes at the universities involved in the UBORA project consortium. Its use as teaching-learning environment for fostering PBL methodologies in bioengineering programmes is open to all colleagues interested in *learning-by-doing* with their students.

6.5 Some Cases of Success

When exploring the OSMDs developed within the UBORA e-infrastructure it is possible to find technological concepts and prototype solutions for most medical technology missions, including: prevention, diagnosis, surgery, therapy and monitoring. Besides, most medical areas are already being covered, from pediatrics to geriatrics, from internal medicine, through general surgery, to traumatology and orthopedics. All these devices can be also used for teaching-learning purposes as cases of study to analyze and illustrate all possible aspects involved in the co-creation of novel medical technologies. Here, by means of example, we present some selected cases of study mentored by the author and developed together with his students at UPM, either during their final degree projects, or along their participation in the different courses detailed in Sect. 3, in which PBL is used as driving methodology for teaching medical technology development and for promoting BME in Spain. The selected cases of study have been developed with the support of the UBORA e-infrastructure and their complete information, from documentation, to design files for manufacturing, is freely shared, thanks to the design of the

UBORA e-infrastructure following FAIR (findable, accessible, interoperable, reusable) data principles.

Figure 5 illustrates the personalized design and the 3D printed prototype of a shoulder splint for injured joint immobilization, as example of several ergonomic aids and splints developed within UBORA by UPM. Computer-aided design is performed, after optical scanning of the healthy volunteer, by using surface based design operation with Siemens NX-11 design software and final meshing with Autodesk Meshmixer. 3D printing for ergonomic validation is accomplished using a BCN-Sigma 3D printer and white poly(lactic acid) (PLA) filament. Figure 6 schematically presents the development of a portable cooler for vaccines based on the use of Peltier cells, in line with one of the targets of SDG3 (target 3.8), in which maintaining the cold chain of vaccines is described as a global health concern. The circuit design, based on the use of open source electronics (Arduino control board) and the preliminary 3D printed prototype, with the Peltier cell and refrigerator mounted upon the cooler top and isolating panels placed inside the printed cage, are shown. Additional information on these devices, which are now cases of study for several courses, is shared through the UBORA online research and innovation infrastructure (see: https://platform.ubora-biomedical.org/).

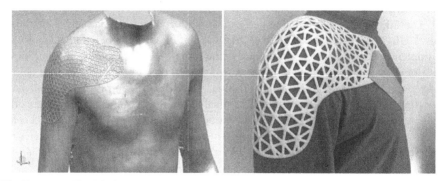

Fig. 5. Personalized design and 3D printed prototype of a shoulder splint for injured joint immobilization. Designer: Eduardo Martínez. Collaborator: Marina Maestro. Mentor: Andrés Díaz Lantada.

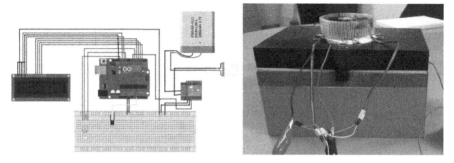

Fig. 6. Circuit design and preliminary prototype of a portable cooler for vaccines using Peltier cells. Designers: Isabel Álvarez and Elena Crespo. Mentor: Andrés Díaz Lantada.

7 Future Perspectives

7.1 Main Potentials

Innovation in BME education leads also to new approaches for developing medical technology, which is evolving at a rapid pace thanks to emergent trends including: affordable rapid prototyping tools, 3D printers and the "maker" movement; co-creation and collective intelligence strategies for developing medical technology; artificial intelligence and novel human-device biointerfaces; artificial fabrication of tissues and organs; and open source approaches for reshaping the medical industry, among others. OSMDs are here to stay as a changing force, towards a more equitable medical industry and accessible medical technologies, but also as shared cases of study to transform the future of BME education, which will be project-based, challenge-based and oriented to providing real solutions and services to healthcare professionals, patients and society. The benefits of OSMDs for the democratization of these solutions and for rethinking BME towards the 2030 Agenda in mind, aiming at global health coverage in the near future, can be understood, if we consider examples from other industries (i.e. electronics and software), which have been already transformed through open source software and hardware and through educational innovation.

The co-creation processes, in which these OSMDs rely, also turn out to be very positive for patients and healthcare professionals, due to the promotion of bottom-up innovation, and for educators and students, due to improved training of personal and professional skills. All these beneficial aspects of open source biodevices can be multiplied by means of adequate training strategies, aimed at the creation of a cohort of designers and developers, capable of mentoring this emergent area of open source medical technologies and focused on international, intersectoral and interdisciplinary collaboration throughout the whole innovation chain. In turn, this can lead to worldwide achieving the "BME education for all" concept, a scenario, in which access to engineering education, especially in the BME field, will be on the basis of motivation and merit and will not be hindered by social, economic, religious, cultural or gender discriminations.

7.2 Key Challenges

Possibly the more relevant challenges to tackle in this novel "BME education for all" scenario, so as to promote the democratization of medical technology by adequately training the BME engineers of the future, deal with making OSMDs have a truly transformative impact. For this open source medical technology co-creation paradigm to succeed, it is important to highlight: i) the need for solutions to guarantee the traceability of materials, design files and manufactured components in open design and production lines; ii) the need for resources to systematically and safely track design changes in collaborative design environments and e-infrastructures; iii) the need for changes in existing regulations and for new standards adequately considering and guiding developers, within these collaborative and open design and manufacturing approaches to medical device innovation; and, above all, iv) the need for BME training programmes, in which open source co-creation approaches play a central role, as part of the PBL activities that should vertebrate the programmes of study.

Capacity building in low-resource settings, by creating a workforce of rule-changing biomedical engineers and BME professors, in places where access to medical technology is more urgent and where the co-creation with healthcare professionals and patients can be of special relevance, is another fundamental issue. We expect that all these challenges will be solved in the near future, essentially through international collaboration using online co-creation environments, such as the UBORA e-infrastructure, which is open to all medical technology developers and users, as well as to educators, for constructive interactions.

8   Conclusions

Innovation through education (one of the mottos of the UBORA project and community) is an excellent, sustainable and responsible strategy for transforming any industry and for walking towards the fulfillment of the United Nations Global Goals for Sustainable Development. Within BME, training engineers for working in international teams and for collaborating in the development of open source medical technologies can constitute a very relevant driver of change in years to come. To this end, BME education should be also continuously updated, not only to incorporate the more advanced technological trends, but also as regards teaching-learning methodologies and activities capable of engaging students, of constructing international research communities and of providing the holistic training needed for innovating in such a complex field as BME. The presented PBL courses and the analyzed structure for PBL-supported programmes of study put the 2030 Agenda and the SDGs in the foreground of BME education and innovation. The proposed modularity applied both to courses and complete programmes is interesting in terms of scalability and internationalization of the proposed approaches to the future of BME education. The highlighted UBORA e-infrastructure, a recently established collaborative environment for the co-creation of medical devices, and related UBORA teaching-learning experiences provide pioneering examples of collaborative research and education in BME, as a way for setting the foundations of the OSMD field.

Acknowledgements. This document expands the Biodevices 2019 keynote speech presented by Prof. Dr. Andrés Díaz Lantada, who acknowledges the consideration of the Conference Chairs for their kind invitation. Besides, the author acknowledges the UBORA "*Euro-African Open Biomedical Engineering e-Platform for Innovation through Education*" project, funded by the European Union's "Horizon 2020" research and innovation programme, under grant agreement No. 731053, and all colleagues from the UBORA consortium, inspiringly led by Prof. Arti Ahluwalia from the University of Pisa.

References

1. Ahluwalia, A., De Maria, C., Díaz Lantada, A.: The Kahawa Declaration: a manifesto for the democratization of medical technology. Global Health Innov. **1**(1), 1–4 (2018)
2. United Nations General Assembly: Transforming our World: the 2030 Agenda for Sustainable Development, on 21 October 2015, A/RES/70/1 (2015)

3. Larmer, J.: Project-based Learning vs. Problem-Based Learning vs. X-BL. Edutopia, San Rafael (2014)
4. Shuman, L.J., Besterfield-Sacre, M., Mc Gourty, J.: The ABET professional skills, can they be taught? Can they be assessed? J. Eng. Educ. **94**, 41–55 (2005)
5. UNESCO: World Declaration on Higher Education for the Twenty-First Century: Vision and Action, Adopted by UNESCO's World Conference on Higher Education, 9 October 1998 (1998)
6. De Graaf, E., Kolmos, A.: Characteristics of problem-based learning. Int. J. Eng. Educ. **19**(5), 657–662 (2003)
7. Larmer, J., Mengeldoller, J., Boss, S.: Setting the standard for project based learning: a proven approach to rigorous classroom instruction. ASCD & Buck Institute for Education (2015)
8. Díaz Lantada, A., et al.: Towards successful project-based learning experiences in engineering education. Int. J. Eng. Educ. **29**(2), 476–490 (2013)
9. Crawley, E.F., Malmqvist, J., Östlund, S., Brodeur, D.R.: Rethinking Engineering Education: The CDIO Approach, pp. 1–286. Springer, Cham (2007). https://doi.org/10.1007/978-3-319-05561-9
10. CDIO Standards 2.0. http://www.cdio.org/implementing-cdio/standards/12-cdio-standards
11. Kontio, J.: Inspiring the inner entrepreneur in students: a case study of entrepreneurship studies in TUAS. In: 6th International CDIO Conference, Montréal, Canada (2010)
12. Cea, P., Cepeda, M., Gutiérrez, M., Muñoz, M.: Addressing academic and community needs via a service-learning center. In: 10th International CDIO Conference, Barcelona, Spain (2014)
13. Norrman, C., Bienkowska, D., Moberg, M., Frankelius, P.: Innovative methods for entrepreneurship and leadership teaching in CDIO-based engineering education. In: 10th International CDIO Conference, Barcelona, Spain (2014)
14. Jacoby, B.: Service-Learning in Higher Education: Concepts and Practices. Jossey-Bass, San Francisco (1996)
15. Ahluwalia, A., et al.: Biomedical engineering project based learning: Euro-African design school focused on medical devices. Int. J. Eng. Educ. **34**(5), 1709–1722 (2018)
16. Graham, R.: The Global State of the Art in Engineering Education. MIT Press, Cambridge (2018)
17. Díaz Lantada, A.: Project based learning and biomedical devices: the UBORA approach towards an international community of developers focused on open source medical devices. In: Proceedings of the 12th International Joint Conference on Biomedical Engineering Systems and Technologies, BIOSTEC 2019 – Vol. 1: Biodevices, pp. 7–13 (2019)
18. De Maria, C., Mazzei, D., Ahluwalia, A.: Open source biomedical engineering for sustainability in African healthcare: combining academic excellence with innovation. In: ICDS 2014, The Eight International Conference on Digital Society, pp. 45–53 (2014)
19. De Maria, C., Mazzei, D., Ahluwalia, A.: Improving African healthcare through open source biomedical engineering. Int. J. Adv. Life Sci. **7**(1 & 2), 10–19 (2015)
20. Ahluwalia, A., et al.: Towards open source medical devices: challenges and advances. In: Biodevices 2008, Madeira, Portugal, 19–21 January 2018 (2018)
21. United Nations General Assembly: Global health and foreign policy, Resolution A/67/81, 12 December 2012
22. Abu-Faraj, Z.O.: Bioengineering/ biomedical engineering education and career development: literature review, definitions and constructive recommendations. Int. J. Eng. Educ. **24**(5), 990–1011 (2008)
23. Sienko, K.H., Sarvestani, A.S., Grafman, L.: Medical device compendium for the developing world: a new approach in project and service-based learning for engineering graduate students. Global J. Eng. Educ. **15**(1), 13–20 (2013)

24. Yock, P.G., et al.: Biodesign: The Process of Innovating Medical Technology, 2nd edn., pp. 1–952. Cambridge University Press, Cambridge (2015)
25. King, P.H., Fries, R.: Designing biomedical engineering design courses. Int. J. Eng. Educ. **19**(2), 346–353 (2003)
26. King, P.H., Collins, J.C.: Ethical and professional training of biomedical engineers. Int. J. Eng. Educ. **22**(6), 1173–1181 (2006)
27. King, P.H.: Design and biomedical engineering. Int. J. Eng. Educ. **15**(4), 282–287 (1999)
28. Krishnan, S.: Project-based learning with international collaboration for training biomedical engineers. In: Proceedings of the IEEE Engineering in Medicine and Biology Society, pp. 6518–6521 (2011)
29. Morss Clyne, A., Billiar, K.L.: Problem-based learning in biomechanics: advantages, challenges and implementation strategies. J. Biomech. Eng. **138**(7), 070804 (2016)
30. Díaz Lantada, A., Ros Felip, A., Jiménez Fernández, J., Muñoz García, J., Claramunt Alonso, R., Carpio Huertas, J.: Integrating biomedical engineering design into engineering curricula: benefits and challenges of the CDIO approach. In: 11th International CDIO Conference, Cheng-Du, China (2015)
31. Díaz Lantada, A., et al.: CDIO experiences in Biomedical Engineering: preparing Spanish students for the future of biomedical technology. In: 12th International CDIO Conference, Turku, Finland (2016)
32. Hernandez Bayo, A., et al.: Integral framework to drive engineering education beyond technical skills. Int. J. Eng. Educ. **30**(6B), 1697–1707 (2014)
33. Díaz Lantada, A., et al.: Coordinated design and implementation of Bioengineering Design and MedTECH courses by means of CDIO projects linked to medical devices. In: 14th International CDIO Conference, Kanazawa, Japan (2018)
34. European Commission, EURAXESS: Doctoral training principles (web visited in May 2019). https://euraxess.ec.europa.eu/belgium/jobs-funding/doctoral-training-principles
35. Ravizza, A., et al.: Collaborative open design for safer biomedical devices. In: Third WHO Global Forum on Medical Devices, Geneva, Switzerland (2017)

Magnetic Three-Dimensional Control System for Micro Robots

Gaby Isabel Manzo Pantoja$^{(\boxtimes)}$ (ID), Martín Alonso Muñoz Medina$^{(\boxtimes)}$ (ID), and OscarAndrés Vivas Albán$^{(\boxtimes)}$ (ID)

FIET, University of Cauca, Calle 5 No. 4-70, Popayán, Colombia
{mgaby,maamunoz,avivas}@unicauca.edu.co
http://www.unicauca.edu.co

Abstract. The microrobots are devices that in recent years have had a great development and that hope to revolutionize the area of medicine. In this area, they are designed in order to study difficult access spaces in the human body without the use of cables or external power. One of the great unknowns for modern researchers is to know in advance how the operation of these platforms will be so the development of specialized simulations becomes mandatory, in this case a particular arrangement of Helmholtz and Maxwell coils is proposed where it is allowed analyze the current consumption of these by moving the microbot all this through a simulation in two particular parts of the human body.

Keywords: Magnetic navigation systems · Micro robot · Human body

1 Introduction

The technological advance in the area of medical robotics has contributed greatly in the improvement of surgical procedures, positioning particularly minimally invasive surgery as one of the greatest advances in technology in recent years due to the enormous improvement that this represents in the condition of patients and in the rehabilitation process [15], reinforcing the concept of high quality in surgical procedures, which among other things represents prevention rather than attention, precision, repeatability and decrease in the intrución to the body of the patient [7].

In recent years the use of microrobots has been proposed as an aid to various surgical procedures, taking advantage of the large size of some organs in the human body, all under the supervision of a physician specialized in this type of procedure; all this waiting for future improvements in microrobots, allow them to reach even smaller places [7]. It can be said that the inclusion of microrobots within medicine, opens a wide range of benefits to patients, such as product

Supported by University of Cauca.

A. Roque et al. (Eds.): BIOSTEC 2019, CCIS 1211, pp. 55–79, 2020.
https://doi.org/10.1007/978-3-030-46970-2_3

of the convergence between these areas of knowledge, such as the mobility of automatas through certain cavities in the human body in order to perform operations without transcendental lacerations and with a minimum trauma [16]. Another example of this type of procedure are those made with micro robots that use fiber optic cables under the continuous surveillance of a surgeon who is in charge of observing and directing the progress [10], concluding in this way that the operations to beings humans with microrobots will be the next tangible breakthrough in science [15].

The intrusion of endoscopic capsules and micro robots that navigate the fluids of the spine are clear examples of the mix between the field of robotics and medicine. In both cases, the replacement of conventional mechanisms with smaller ones, as is the case with pills with tiny cameras, causes a considerable reduction in the trauma patients face after these procedures, including even complex surgeries such as biopsies [18].

The appearance of microrobots has made it possible to reach remote areas within the human body, this has led to foresee that in the coming years medical robots will have one of their biggest challenges: to further modify the size of microrobots, this due to the continuous desire of scientists entering and studying new parts of the human body, which are currently not viable due to factors such as the size of the devices, the surface where they are immersed is not uniform, and the cavities where they enter are highly sensitive. To achieve a better study and analysis of some diseases, a microrobot should be able to navigate through the human body, reach a region of interest and once there, develop the desired task. Therefore, it is important that the type of locomotion is adapted to the medium in question and the activation is at the time and place required [13].

For this investigation, two different sections of the human body have been chosen to simulate the movement of a microbot in the three possible axes of movement: the pancreas and the subarachnoid region. This selection was made due to the large number of postoperative complications that complicate conventional laparoscopies in the pancreas that could be diminished by minimally invasive procedures such as the one that will be presented next; On the other hand the subarachnoid region is one of the parts of the human being less studied this due to its small size and the great difficulty of accessing this region, for this reason a large part of the surgeries that are posed in this area are not satisfactory In this case, just as in the pancreas, minimally invasive surgeries could be the solution.

2   Working Area for the Simulation

2.1   Subarachnoid Region of the Human Head

As mentioned above, the study of microrobots has had a broad growth, it could be said that nowadays the possibility of using them in a great variety of medical procedures, such as the transport of drugs in different parts of the human body, complex procedures such as Brachytherapy and hyperthermia, the transport of stem cells that reconstruct damaged tissues in different parts of the human body and the thermoablation, is a future that is closer and more tangible [21]. In some particular cases, there are micro robots with the ability to enhance the treatment of cancer in the central nervous system or move in areas of the digestive tract quickly and safely [21].

Many promising applications have been studied in the area of the nervous system, among which the use of neuronal prostheses and deep brain stimulation are highlighted. These applications are developed with the help of wirelessly guided microrobots, the main advantage being the fact that can be kept in the human body as implants; it is assured that the number of surgical procedures that have been performed with robotic assistance tripled from 80,000 to 250,000 between 2007 and 2010, all thanks to the inclusion of this type of surgeries [6].

One of the areas of the body with greater coextensiveness at the time of a surgical intervention is the human brain, despite many efforts made in recent years [20], the administration of drugs remains a challenge, mainly because the brain has a natural barrier formed by endothelial cells which are closely connected to each other covering the inside of the walls of the cerebral vessel and which serve as protection for the brain from external threats, in a large percentage it is impossible to overcome this barrier so many drugs [26], more exactly the 98% of them fail to pass to the central nervous system to fight cases of urgent treatment such as brain tumors and even cancer [24]. For the most part, this type of systematic medical procedures seek to enter the brain through surgeries such as craniotomy, although in many other cases of great innovation it has been sought that by means of lumbar punctures, microrobots enter the human body through the opening of the vertebrae L3 and L4 (third and fourth vertebra respectively) thus achieving to leave the skull intact and also be able to manipulate the device externally by means of catheters or magnetic systems [25], due to the above described, the subarachnoid region of the human brain was selected to study the movement of the microbot using the proposed coil array.

Figure 1 shows a representation of the measurement of the subarachnoid region in an average adult [11].

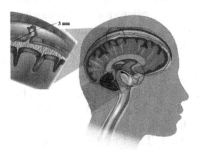

Fig. 1. Measurement of the subarachnoid region in an average adult.

2.2 Pancreas Region of the Human Body

Minimally invasive surgery has reached many sectors of medicine and the pancreas has not been an area outside of this advance, in fact laparoscopic surgery of the pancreas can be considered as a breakthrough procedure and should be performed exclusively by the exhaustive pancreatic experience. Initially, laparoscopic procedures involving the pancreas included only the staging of tumors in patients receptive to open resection. In this order of ideas, it is affirmed that unlike other abdominal surgeries, the laparoscopic approach in the pancreas has not been developed to a great extent, either due to technical reasons or due to the large number of postoperative complications that occur in receiving patients of this type of procedures.

Even so, the advance in technology has meant that the instruments with which this type of surgery is performed have improved greatly, leading a large number of surgeons and engineers to consider again pancreatic laparoscopy, including the use of micro robots in this type of such minor procedures [9].

In other cases, the barriers of this type of procedures include even the retroperitoneal location of the pancreas, the proximity to large vascular structures and the threat of an inadequate elimination of the disease to be attacked. For example, in the case of laparoscopies, laparoscopic distal pancreotomy is safe and feasible in comparison with common and traditional procedures [19]. The laparoscopic distal pancreotomy reduces the length of hospital stay, the blood loss and reduces the recovery time. This is where medical robotics is presented as the solution to the limitations of the same as those practiced to the three-dimensional visualization of great scope and this added to the skill of the surgeon that results in the ability to reduce the factors associates [6]. Currently, the control of sugar levels in the blood (especially for diabetics) is a very important issue, which is why this area was chosen for the analysis of the mobility of the microbot using the proposed coil array, as this way, in a future could be reached to measure glucose levels or even the injection of drugs that help counteract side effects of this disease in the bloodstream.

In the present investigation, the simulation of a Maxwell and Helmholtz coil array was used to magnetize the micro robot and move it along the subarachnoid region of the human head and pancreas. This arrangement consists of a pair of Maxwell coils and two pairs of stationary Helmholtz coils.

In this particular case, it has been decided to study the human pancreas, for this we must bear in mind that the pancreas contains a main duct which has a series of branches that extend along the organ. Said cavities have a diameter variation between 2 and 3 mm in all their extension. It is very important to model these pipelines with fidelity, because in this way you are not altering the results obtained in simulation. The Fig. 2 shown the anterior description.

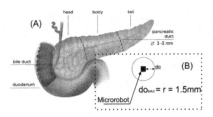

Fig. 2. View of the pancreas [17].

3   Brief Description of the Magnetic Navigation

One of the disadvantages translates into small scales, it is microrobot of the energy necessary to move, until now magnetic systems are presented as one of the solutions more in line with the needs of contemporary systems, these are also given as the set of software and hardware used in the work areas in the same way that a microrobot is oriented and directed by means of the magnets, generally, there is a main magnet in the project of a frontal field that is in the entire operating region [5]. In other cases, two magnets are used, a support for them and a positioner that selectively changes the location of the magnets helping the movement of them [28].

On the other hand, [4] designed a magnetic navigation system that had two pairs of helmholtz and maxwell coils that generated a uniform magnetic flux in order to obtain a static system that could displace an object in the x and y axes. Over the years, this system was improved and reduced in size due to the elimination of a pair of Maxwell coils, which makes the transportation of the mechanism easier and consumes less power [4]. Similarly, [12] analyzed and proposed a magnetic propulsion system consisting of three Helmholtz coils and one Maxwell coil, which added details of mobile enhancement not seen in earlier models.

In this order of ideas it can be stated that the use of electromagnets, has as its main advantage the direct control of the magnetic fields and gradients generated which leads to better control the device while it is in motion, on the other hand generates considerable energy consumption in some cases, so the designed combination of coils between Helmholtz and Maxwell must be carefully analyzed.

The currents necessary for the operation of magnetic navigation systems are an important factor to take into account when studying electromagnetic propulsion systems.

For the previously described case (3D locomotion system) it is stated that for the generation of uniform magnetic fields in the three pairs of Helmholtz and Maxwell coils, the number of turns of the winding is fundamental, since the size of the winding is directly proportional to the magnetic field that the entire system may have, it can be concluded that handling these magnetic fields is not complicated [29].

When working with microrobots, the tencological problems are usually normal, inconveniences such as lack of innovation and progress in the creation of motors and cables are common. It is very difficult to find solenoids smaller than $1\,mm^3$, this also because the maximum current density is limited by the dissipation of energy, which means that it is directly related to the size of the microbot [8].

4 Description of the Coils Used in Current Analysis

4.1 Description of Maxwell Coils

The Maxwell coils consist of two coils side by side that generate a certain amount of current which goes in opposite directions to drive the objects determined by the user. They are used to a large extent when working on magnetic propulsion projects, since they generate constant magnetic gradients to produce uniform propulsion forces at the center of the coil [2].

The magnetic flux density and its gradient, associated with the arrangement of Helmholtz and Maxwell coils along the main axis, can be approximated to a constant value. Therefore, said quantities will depend directly on the current applied to the system, by the following equations:

$$B = \frac{8}{5\sqrt{5}} \frac{\mu_0 N_H}{R_H} \overrightarrow{I} = k * I_H, \tag{1}$$

$$\nabla * B = \frac{48\sqrt{3}}{49\sqrt{7}} \frac{\mu_o * N_M}{R_M^2} \overrightarrow{I} = g * I_M, \tag{2}$$

where:

- N_H: number of laps of the pair of Helmholtz coils.
- R_H: radius of the Helmholtz coil pair.
- I_H: current obtained in the pair of Helmholtz coils.
- k: constant value.
- ∇: magnetization gradient.
- B: magnetic field.
- μ_0: constant value.
- N_M: number of turns of the Maxwell coil pair.
- R_M: radius of the Maxwell coil pair.
- $\overrightarrow{I}$: current vector obtained.
- I_M: current obtained in the pair

Where k and g are proportional coefficients, which depend on the radius of the coils and the number of turns for Helmholtz and Maxwell respectively. In order to simplify the model, it is assumed that the robot is a solid disk, immersed in a liquid with a small Reynolds number (the Reynolds number is a dimensionless quantity that has the same value in any coherent system of units and allows to determine if a fluid is laminar or turbulent), perpendicular to its axis. With that consideration, the drag force in a closed space can be approximated by:

$$\overrightarrow{F_D} = \frac{4\pi\mu_d v}{log\frac{2d_0}{r} - \frac{1}{4}\frac{r}{d_0}^2} \times h, \tag{3}$$

where:

- $\overrightarrow{F_D}$: drag force vector.
- μ_d: dynamic viscosity of the fluid.
- v: speed handled by the micro robot.
- r: robot radio.
- d_0: distance from the center of the micro robot to the space where it is confined
- h: thickness of the micro robot.

On the plane, the forces present are summarized below:

$$\overrightarrow{F_{mag}} + \overrightarrow{F_D} = m\overrightarrow{a}, \tag{4}$$

where:

- F_{mag}: magnetization force.
- $\overrightarrow{F_D}$: drag force vector.
- m: mass of the micro robot.
- $\overrightarrow{a}$: acceleration of the microrobot in the XYZ plane.

4.2 Description of Helmholtz Coils

Helmholtz coils are a particular type of pairs of coils mounted on a common axis at a fixed distance and whose spacing is equal to the common radius. In essence, by passing a certain amount of equal currents through them, a highly uniform magnetic field is generated within a limited space on the centroid between the coils. Thus, Helmholtz coils are ideal for use in the magnetic fields of a device when it is tested, and in this way produce precise and repeatable results [27]. Currently, a large number of studies have been carried out on the Helmholtz coils, and from these it has been concluded that the results which these coils offer are accurate and repeatable only while the location and orientation of the device under test can be maintained and repeated within a portion of the magnetic field. It is important to take into account that the magnetic field used must be uniform throughout the device under test (so the center of this must always be in the center of the coils). In other words, for maximum accuracy and repeatability of the test, the position and orientation of the device must be the same for the duration of the [27] test.

The magnetic navigation of a microbot can be expressed as shown in Eq. 5. The torque obtained when flowing an electric current through the coils is proportional to the magnetic field that is generated and is responsible for giving direction to the microbot, making it align with the generated magnetic field.

In the other hand, the magnetic force is proportional to the gradient of the magnetic field and is responsible for giving an impulse to the microbot, which takes it from one place to another, it can be concluded that all objects within a magnetic field will develop a pair and a force. In the following equation, the magnetic pair (which aligns the microrobot with the lines of the magnetic field) will be calculated in Eq. 6.

$$\overrightarrow{F} = V.(\overrightarrow{M}.\bigtriangledown)\overrightarrow{B} \tag{5}$$

$$\overrightarrow{\tau} = V\overrightarrow{M}x\overrightarrow{B} \tag{6}$$

In this:

- $\overrightarrow{F}$: vector of the general strength of the robot.
- V: volume of the robot.
- $\overrightarrow{M}$: robot magnetization vector.
- $\bigtriangledown$: magnetization gradient.
- τ: torque needed by the micro robot.
- $\overrightarrow{B}$: magnetic field vector.

Equation 6 can be expressed in a more intuitive way as shown above, here, the microrobot autoagulation vector is displayed in the three possible axes of movement, in this way it is much simpler to analyze some of the axes of be necessary.

$$\overrightarrow{\tau} = V(M_yB_z - M_zB_y)\overrightarrow{i}$$
$$+ V(M_zB_x - M_xB_z)\overrightarrow{j} + V(M_xB_y - M_yB_x)\overrightarrow{k} \tag{7}$$

Where M_x, M_y and M_z denote the magnetization value of each axis and B_x, B_y and B_z the magnetic field vector in each axis [2].

The objective of the use of the combinations of the Maxwell - Helmholtz pairs, is to drive a microbot on the x, y, z axis and also on more than one axis. For this reason, the two Helmholtz coils are placed perpendicularly to generate a vector sum of the uniform magnetic fields, and the two Maxwell coils are positioned perpendicularly to generate a vector sum of the magnetic fields of the gradient.

Helmholtz coils combined with Maxwell coils can be used to generate a certain magnetic force to navigate in a desired direction. To manipulate the microrobot correctly, two points must be taken into account:

- High uniformity in the magnetic field of the Helmholtz coils and uniform magnetic field of the Maxwell coils.
- There must be a high magnetic force with less current to reduce the heating of the coils and the energy consumption of the coils.

For conventional Helmholtz and Maxwell coils, the coil width and height parameters must be less than the coil radius. This type of coils are not suitable for use in magnetic navigation systems whose magnetic fields require high electric currents, since they will require a greater magnetic force and this causes the coils to become very hot. Thick coils with multiple turns could be a good option to design coils of greater magnetic force that consume the same amount of current.

5   Mathematical Model Used to Calculate Currents

For this project, the designed system was taken from [23] where it is initially considered as a black box, where there are a series of inputs and outputs as will be described below.

The system entries are:

- θ y ϕ: position angle of the micro robot with respect to the Maxwell and Helmholtz coils.
- M: magnetization of the micro robot.
- F: force with which the micro robot moves.
- B_M, B_Hx, B_Hy, B_Hz: parameters of the Maxwell and Helmholtz coils as the number of laps they carry and the radius of these.

The outputs of the system are:

- I_{Hx}: current of the Helmholtz coils on their x axis.
- I_{Hy}: current of the Helmholtz coils on their y axis.
- I_{Hz}: current of the Helmholtz coils on their z axis.
- I_M: current of the Maxwell coils.
- τ: torque needed by the micro robot.
- V: speed that the micro robot carries when moving.

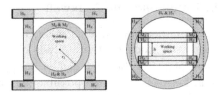

Fig. 3. Representation in blocks of the proposed system, taken from [3].

The arrangement of the coils to be used is the one proposed by [3] is shown in Fig. 3 consist in a Helmholtz type configuration that is located along an axis, separated by a distance d_h that is equal to its radius r_h. There is also a pair of Maxwell coils whose separation in their electromagnets d_m is $\sqrt{3}rm$, being r_m the radius of the coils, with the flow of the currents in opposite directions.

The magnetic field produced by a pair of Helmholtz coils of the x axis can be determined by the law of Biot-Savart, this is supported by [14] for the mathematical design of the coils that will be used, is described below:

$$H_{HX} = \left[k.\frac{ix.nx}{rx}, 0, 0 \right]^T \tag{8}$$

$$H_{HY} = \left[0, k.\frac{iy.ny}{ry}, 0 \right]^T \tag{9}$$

$$H_{HZ} = \left[0, 0, k.\frac{iz.nz}{rz}\right]^{T} \tag{10}$$

The following is the value of the constant k, [14]:

$$k = \left(\frac{4^{\frac{3}{2}}}{5}\right) \tag{11}$$

In next equations was shown that the total magnetic field is compounded by the sum of the partial magnetic fields, that is, those related to the axes x, y and z. It is obtained that:

$$H_H = H_{HX} + H_{HY} + H_{HZ} \tag{12}$$

From where it can be calculated that:

$$\overrightarrow{H_H} = k\left[\frac{ix.nx}{rx}, \frac{iy.ny}{ry}, \frac{iz.nz}{rz}\right]^{T} \tag{13}$$

$$\left[\frac{A}{m}\right]$$

5.1 Explanation of the Mathematical Method Used to Calculate the Currents in Helmholtz and Maxwell

In the study by [23], the mathematics that is going to be shown below was proposed in order to focus the study on the analysis of the currents required by the system. A cartesian plane can be imagined whose vector will be $\overrightarrow{H_H}$ and which will be represented between the three possible axes of movement which will be x, y z and where the relations between the vector and the axes will be given by the angles θ and ϕ then, 14, 15 and 16 are obtained:

$$x = H_H sen\theta cos\theta \tag{14}$$

$$y = H_H sin\theta sin\phi \tag{15}$$

$$z = H_H cos\theta \tag{16}$$

Reorganizing get that:

$$k\frac{ix.nx}{rx} = H_H sen\theta cos\phi \tag{17}$$

$$k\frac{iy.ny}{ry} = H_H sen\theta sen\phi \tag{18}$$

$$k\frac{iz.nz}{rz} = cos\theta \tag{19}$$

In this way we proceed to calculate the probable current necessary for the Helmholtz coils. The Eqs. 20, 21 and 22 were used for this calculation.

$$ix = \frac{H_H rx}{knx} sen\theta cos\phi \tag{20}$$

$$iy = \frac{H_H ry}{kny} sen\theta sen\phi \tag{21}$$

$$iz = \frac{H_H rz}{knz} cos\theta \tag{22}$$

The next step in the research already mentioned was calculate the torque generated by the Helmholtz coils that is essential for the current analysis, which is represented in the following equation:

$$\vec{\tau} = V[M \times B] \tag{23}$$

In this, V is the volume of the micro robot, μ_0 is the permeability of the medium and M is the magnetization constant.

Once the current in the Helmholtz coils was calculated, the next step was calculate the characteristic equation of the current used in the Maxwell coil and that will be explained below: First, the magnetic field generated in the Maxwell coils was calculated and explained in the following way:

$$H_m = \left[\frac{-1}{2} gmx, \frac{-1}{2} gmy, gmz \right] \tag{24}$$

Where gm is a constant expressed by:

$$gm = k \frac{nm.Im}{rm^2} \tag{25}$$

From where it can be seen that:

$$k = \frac{16}{3} \left(\frac{3}{7} \right)^{\frac{5}{2}} \tag{26}$$

Now, it is necessary to calculate the force with which the micro robot goes to a place:

$$F = \mu.V.|M|.|\nabla H| \tag{27}$$

Then it get:

$$F = \mu V |M| \frac{nmImK}{rm^2} \tag{28}$$

Finally it proceed to clear Im, to obtain the current of the Maxwell coils:

$$Im = \frac{Frm^2}{\mu V |M| nmK} \tag{29}$$

This concludes the calculation of the equations that would describe the currents needed in Maxwell and Helmholtz, and that will be analyzed later in the two proposed work areas: subarachnoid region of the head and human pancreas.

6   Anthropometry Related to the Project

To perform this type of simulations it is necessary to define the area where the micro robot will be mobilized, in this case two different studies will be used to determine the exact measurements of said space, since it is known that in the human body, that in many natural phenomena, the measures are governed by the Gaussian distribution [1]. Frequently when a homogeneous population is presented, the distribution of the anthropometric distributions is considered normal, and therefore the calculations made with them and in general all the statistical procedures are carried out through the properties of the distribution, which is very convenient given the ease of processing data of this type.

To develop the simulations of the project, two studies were considered that pretended to measure the anthropometry of the chosen parts of the human body; the anthropometry analyzed by [1] from which the case study of people between 18 and 65 years was taken, where the anthropometry of the workers was analyzed, was in charge of giving the values used for the human head. From this study we obtain the Table 1:

Table 1. Anthropometry table of the human head [1].

Length (mm)	Width (mm)	Height (mm)
150	176	281

Subsequently, we took the data obtained in the study of [22] where the standard measure of the pancreas was analyzed. From these we analyzed what would be the ideal measurements for the simulation of this corporeal space, from here we conclude the Table 2 that describes the distance between the coils, given that priority was given to the external space that covers the abdomen. From this study we obtain the Table 2:

Table 2. Anthropometry table of the human abdomen [22].

Coil type	Axis	Distance	Radio (cm)
Maxwell	x	40.00	23.09
	y	31.17	18.00
	z	10.34	11.00
Helmholtz	x	38.00	38.00
	y	20.00	20.00
	z	13.20	13.20

Once the measurements of the parts of the human body were made, we used Blender software to create two different figures of the human body (since both surgeries could be in two different ways, placing the patient in different positions). In order to simulate a functional human head, a not so deep cavity was made in the center of a previously modeled skull, in order to have a working area as real as possible to a physical one. Later a second model was made, inspired by the research carried out by [17], which was proposed, it became a second model, it was inspired by research, work, in the pancreas with a microrobot, but only in the x and y axes, this model was preserved in the user interface but internally it is exactly the same mathematic description above, this in order to guarantee an adequate comparison between the currents and the two parts of the human body which of course are different in size. Figure 4 shows the measures that human head usually has.

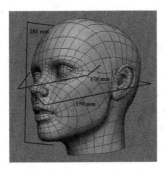

Fig. 4. Measurement of the regular human head [23].

Figure 5 shows the measures that the human pancreas can have, being the subarachnoid area little studied, it has not been possible to have a model like the one shown below, although it is presumed that a normal measurement in the subarachnoid space in adults it should not be less than 3 mm, as it was said was a previous section.

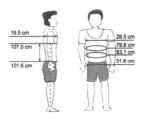

Fig. 5. Measurement of the average adult human abdomen [17].

As mentioned earlier, the development tool that was used was Unity3D, which is a development engine for the creation of games and interactive and didactic 3D content, which is fully integrated and offers many features to facilitate the development of video games and other platforms. It is available as a development platform for Microsoft Windows, OS X, Linux.

The main purpose of this experiment is to take a micro robot, and place it in a specific area of the human body, where it will later be given a direction (taking into account the direction of the existing magnetic field) to later apply a force and analyze which is the result of the currents obtained, taking into account these parameters. Both parts: the subarachnoid and pancreas regions, are small areas of the human body and also require a lot of study, so this type of procedure is of great importance to expand the medical barrier and achieve, in the future, enormous advances in the area of bioengineering

7   Results

In preliminary studies a simulation of the human head was performed in its subarachnoid section in the Unity3D software where the coil mathematics was governed by the equations previously explained, as a great innovation for this research, a new scene was develop in which the movement of the micro robot in the pancreas is analyzed. In this way, a second innovation is added since a more detailed movement in the vessels of the region of the human body studied as seen in Fig. 9 is now proposed, this adds a completely new level of detail that will allow the surgeon to have a better visibility of what his device is doing and greatly minimize human-machine errors.

The parameters that are used to model the microbot and also the coils are shown below in Table 3 both in the pancreas and in the subarachnoid area of the head. It is important to clarify, that the coils used in both areas are different, since the size of these is different and therefore have different requirements.

Where:

- Hx: Helmholtz coil in x.
- Hy: Helmholtz coil in y.
- Hz: Helmholtz coil in z.
- M: Maxwell coil.
- Mr: micro robot.
- Mag: magnetization.

Table 3. Table of environment parameters and proposed micro robot in the subarachnoid and pancreas area.

	Subarachnoid region	Pancreas region
Strength magnetic field	0.01 N 3183 A/m	0.05 N 3193 A/m
N Laps Hx	340	380
N spins Hy	110	3900
N turns Hz	340	370
Radio Hx	0.09 m	38 cm
Radio Hy	9 m	38 cm
Radio Hz	8.5 m	38 cm
N spins M	6000	3800
Radio M	14.5 m	0.214 m
Mag Mr	3000	3000
Radio Mr	500	500

Subsequently, the parameters taken into account for the modeling of the coils that were used in the abdomen are described,

In the proposed interface in Fig. 6 the arrangement of coils to be used for the subarachnoid area is shown, the yellow coils are the Helmholtz coils and the blue coils are the Maxwell coils. On the left side, there is a small panel that, when pressed, returns the values that will be of interest to the user, such as current, speed, and angles.

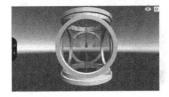

Fig. 6. Initial scene in subarachnoid simulation [23].

Figure 7 represents the model created in Unity for modeling the human pancreas, as can be seen the position in which the patient is going to intervene is different than the one proposed in the project based on the subarachnoid region of the human head and the modeling of the coils also, since the pancreas is immersed in the human abdomen, it is not possible to carry the coils inside this cavity, these must be large enough to surround the torso and create the current that the micro robot needs for its operation.

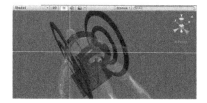

Fig. 7. Initial scene in pancreas simulation.

Next, the representation of the lines of the magnetic field in the subarachnoid region of the human head and also in pancreas will be shown. Basically the operation of these is similar in both areas, since in both the field lines are initially without lines as shown in Fig. 8, this in order that the user aligns them with his keyboard so that the micro robot rotates in this position, the microbot in both cases is represented by a small point and its direction is characterized by a red line, it is important to add that the size of the microbot is variable and the user is the one who decides the size of it. Once the micro robot has been aligned to the magnetic field, a force must be applied from the keyboard so that the microbot moves in this direction, which can be on the x and z axis. Figure 8 also shows the interior of the proposed human head, which, as mentioned above, has at its center the brain and a space between it and the walls that represent the arachnoid section. At this point, only current on the "z" axis is evident since the magnetic field lines are only directed on this axis.

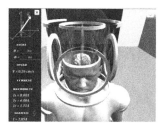

Fig. 8. View of the brain inside the skull [23]. (Color figure online)

Figure 9 shows the inside of the simulation that was used for the analysis of the movement and later study of the currents in the human pancreas, this in the investigation of [17] and later analysis and modification made in this investigation.

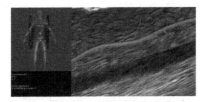

Fig. 9. View of the interior of the pancreas.

In this research we propose a new view of the microrobot used as can be seen in Fig. 10, initially it indicates where the movement of the microrobot starts and it travels to its final point, the human pancreas, the visibility has changed completely from the [23] study where you had a more rustic view and the main objective was to show the magnetic field lines, in this opportunity has been validated the correct use of these lines, so it has been given a broader approach to visualization that the doctor has at the time of performing the surgery, so additionally have simulated the microelements that would navigate along with the microrobot (platelets, red blood cells, etcetera).

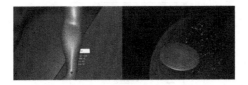

Fig. 10. Main escene in pancreas simulation. (Color figure online)

When the user has done the necessary tests in both proposed areas, the data must be analyzed in MATLAB mathematical software. This is a mathematical software tool that offers an integrated development environment (IDE) with a programming language of its own (M language), allows the analysis of results to subsequently graph them, in this way it can see in a three-dimensional image the results that are obtained.

Figures 11, 12 and 13 represent the comparison of the results of the currents obtained in the x, y and z axes between the sections studied taking into account the parameters mentioned above

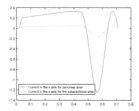

Fig. 11. Current obtained in the Helmholtz coils for subarachnoid and pancreas area, x-axis.

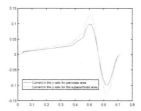

Fig. 12. Current obtained in the Helmholtz coils for subarachnoid and pancreas area, y-axis.

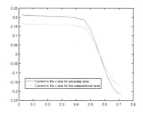

Fig. 13. Current obtained in the Helmholtz coils for subarachnoid and pancreas area, z-axis.

The currents obtained for the subarachnoid and the pancreas area for the characteristics of the micro robot are the following:

The currents obtained in this system and for both regions are not large compared to those recorded by other studies where they also use sets of coils, for example the one made by [14] where currents of 100 A, 85.1 A and 68.8 A are reached, although considering that the coils were not designed in the same way as in the study mentioned above. It is important to clarify that the results obtained refer to what the user entered in the simulation system, taking into account the previous knowledge that this could have of the area where he was going to work. It is difficult to make a real comparison of the amount of current that can be implemented since this system has not been built in a real space and therefore has not been tested in a subarachnoid area or physical pancreas. It is expected that in later studies these data can be obtained to compare them with those obtained in these simulations (Table 4).

Table 4. Currents obtained for subarachnoid and pancreas region.

	Pancreas	Subarachnoid area
Hx	1.1 A	1.3 A
Hy	1.1 A	0.2 A
Hz	1.1 A	1.1 A
M	1.8 A	2 A

8 Analysis of the Responses of the Currents to the Change in the Magnetic Field

In order to determine the limits of movement of the micro robot related to the current consumption of the electromagnets that move it, four tests per organ were made with different magnetic fields, since it is well known that by changing this value the consumption of energy by of the system also changes. For this, the respective calculations were made taking into account the angles θ and ϕ previously mentioned in which the micro robot could possibly move, and in this way obtain the answers of the Figs. 14, 15, 16 and 17.

Initially a test was made to the system using a magnetic field equal to $1\,\mathrm{T/A}$ in the subarachnoid area of the human head, to later graph the response of the current I (A) with respect to the time T (ms). In Fig. 14 the responses for the x axis are shown in red, and in green and z in blue. For the first axis, a current is obtained that does not vary beyond 0.05 A and then drops to −0.015 A and finally stabilizes again at a value close to 0.05 A. For the second axis a current that increases its value can be seen slowly until you have a sharp change to 0.5 ms and get to 0.17 A and go down quickly to −0.125 A and go back up to 0 A.

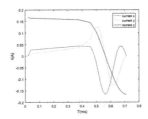

Fig. 14. Response with magnetic field $1\,\mathrm{T/A}$ in subarachnoid region. (Color figure online)

Next, the system was tested using a magnetic field equal to $10\,\mathrm{T/A}$, to later plot the response of the current I (A) with respect to the time T (ms). Figure 15 shows the answers for the x axis in red, and in green and z in blue. For the first axis a current is obtained with a very similar response in all its axes, this time changes the current range that can reach; for example, 0.05 A was the limit in the first experiment and 0.5 A the limit in the second. This same logic is applied for the other results: this time the current peaks are 0.5 A and -1.6 A for the x axis, 1.4 A and -1.4 A for the y axis, and 1.6 A and -1.6 A for the z axis.

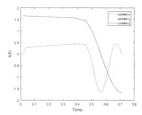

Fig. 15. Response with magnetic field $10\,\mathrm{T/A}$ in subarachnoid region. (Color figure online)

Next, the system was tested using a magnetic field equal to $12\,\mathrm{T/A}$, to later graph the response of the current I (A) with respect to the time T (ms). Figure 16 shows the answers for the x axis in red, and in green and z in blue. It was decided to make a test with a value close to the previous one since from this point the limit established in the previous study to this made in the Biorobotics Institute of the Scuola Superiore Sant Anna is reached, which is 2 A. In Fig. 16 shows that the established limit is reached on the z-axis as soon as the simulation starts and on the x-axis that limit is reached halfway through the simulation process, being 1.5 A and -1.5 A the top of the y-axis.

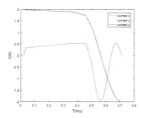

Fig. 16. Response with magnetic field $12\,\mathrm{T/A}$ in subarachnoid region. (Color figure online)

Subsequently the system was tested using a magnetic field equal to $20\,\mathrm{T/A}$, to later appreciate the responses for the x axis in red, and in green and z in blue. Once this value has been reached in the evaluated magnetic field, the current obtained has already exceeded the limit established by the Institution named above; as you can see, the limit of the x-axis and the z-axis pass the 3 A and -3 A, while the y-axis almost reaches 2.5 A and -2.5 A.

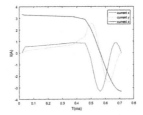

Fig. 17. Response with magnetic field 20 T/A in subarachnoid region.

The same number of tests was then made in the model created for the pancreas with the same values as those tested in the subarachnoid area in order to compare both behaviors. Initially a simulation was made with a magnetic field equal to 1 T/A. In Fig. 18 the responses for the x axis are shown in red, and in green and z in blue. For the first axis, a current is obtained that does not vary beyond 0.03 A and then drops to −0.016 A and finally stabilizes again at a value close to 0.05 A. For the second axis there is a current that starts at approximately 0.03 A and remains stable to descend abruptly to almost −0.03 A, finally on the third axis it can see a current that starts at 0 A and rises gently until a small peak of 0.02 A to go down to −0.02 A and climb again slowly.

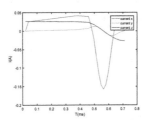

Fig. 18. Response with magnetic field 1 T/A in pancreas. (Color figure online)

In Fig. 19 the responses for the x axis are shown in red, and in green and z in blue. For the first axis, it gets a current that starts at 0 A and has an abrupt rise to 0.25 A and slowly rises to 0.4 A to drop quickly to a little beyond −1.5 A to rise again with the same speed. In the second axis, a current is observed that stays smooth until it rises after a while and goes down again. In the third axis, the current starts its course with approximately 0.25 A, it remains stable and decreases sharply until −0.25 A

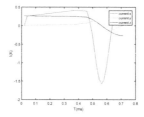

Fig. 19. Response with magnetic field 10 T/A in pancreas. (Color figure online)

In Fig. 20 the responses for the x axis are shown in red, and in green and z in blue. For the first axis, it gets a current that starts at approximately 0 A and rapidly rises to 0.5 A to fall dramatically to almost −2 A which, as previously stated, would be the proposed limit. The second axis shows a current that, as in the previous cases, does not show a great change in its beginnings, later it decreases until reaching a neutral point. In the third axis it see something similar to the previously described, the current remains stable to grow and decrease rapidly until neutralized again.

In Fig. 21 the responses for the x axis are shown in red, and in green and z in blue. For the first axis,a current is observed that rises rapidly to have then an exponential growth and a dramatic fall that removes this current from the established parameters as it takes it beyond 3 A. The remaining currents in the axes present a similar behavior as in the previous tests as they grow slowly and then decrease to stabilize at a neutral point.

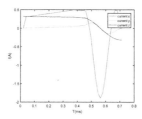

Fig. 20. Response with magnetic field 12 T/A in pancreas. (Color figure online)

It can be concluded that, as in the first tests, the currents did not change their response form but their values due to the change in the magnetic field.

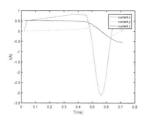

Fig. 21. Response with magnetic field 20 T/A in pancreas. (Color figure online)

9 Conclusions

This article shows the analysis of currents in two different regions of the human body with a magnetic system, getting a user to align the magnetic field lines at will to later apply a force and be able to move the microrobot in the area described: subarachnoid and pancreas region, subsequently, the behavior of the currents obtained at the change in the applied magnetic field is analyzed.

The system in which the areas of the chosen human body were immersed, consists of an arrangement of three Helmholtz coils and a pair of stationary Maxwell coils. Two areas of the human body completely different from each other were selected, in size and location obtaining different currents values. The aforementioned was modeled in the Blender software having previously analyzed investigations wich conclude on the regular measures so that they may have.

Initially an analysis was made of the currents that could be used in the subarachnoid area of the head and later in the human pancreas. For this, the user must have previously configured the software with the parameters that he considers that define the work area, in this way when the microbot is going to move, it will do so in the closest possible way to reality, since its environment external resembles the real one and can also move in three dimensions and through certain types of cavities as shown in previous sections of this article.

In addition, an analysis was made of the currents in both parts of the body when the magnetic field in which they are submerged changes, with this it has been concluded that the current in the z-axis is the one that suffers the most abrupt changes in its form in comparison with both cases of study, this due to the change of the windings and of the measures that these will have since as it was said before, a new region of the human body also implies a change in the design of the coils; similarly it is concluded that for both cases, the maximum magnetic field (ideal) in which the experimentation can be developed would be $12\,T/A$ since at this point the limit proposed in past investigations is crossed.

It also proposes the idea of build the real prototype of the proposed coils and make tests in a living area in order to have a real comparison of the data obtained in simulation and those that can be reached get in a real physical environment.

References

1. Ávila, R., Prado, L., González, E.: Dimensiones antropométricas de la población latinoamericana. Universidad de Guadalajara, Centro Universitario de Arte, Arquitectura y Diseño, División de Tecnología y Procesos, Departamento de Producción y Desarrollo, Centro de Investigaciones en Ergonomía, México (2007)
2. Cao, Q., Han, X., Zhang, B., Li, L.: Analysis and optimal design of magnetic navigation system using Helmholtz and Maxwell coils. IEEE Trans. Appl. Supercond. **22**(3), 4401504–4401504 (2012)
3. Choi, H., Cha, K., Jeong, S., Park, J.O., Park, S.: 3-D locomotive and drilling microrobot using novel stationary EMA system. IEEE/ASME Trans. Mechatron. **18**(3), 1221–1225 (2013)

4. Choi, H., Choi, J., Jeong, S., Yu, C., Park, J.O., Park, S.: Two dimensional loco-motion of a microrobot with a novel stationary electromagnetic actuation system. Smart Mater. Struct. **18**(11), 11–17 (2009)
5. Creighton, F.M., Burgett, S.: Magnetic navigation system, US Patent 7.019.610, 28 March 2006
6. Daouadi, M., et al.: Robot-assisted minimally invasive distal pancreatectomy is superior to the laparoscopic technique. Ann. Surg. **257**(1), 128–132 (2013)
7. Dario, P., Carrozza, M.C., Benvenuto, A., Menciassi, A.: Micro-systems in biomed-ical applications. J. Micromech. Microeng. **10**(2), 235 (2000)
8. Elwenspoek, M., Wiegerink, R.: Mechanical Microsensors. Springer, Heidelberg (2012)
9. Fernández-Cruz, L., Cesar-Borges, G., López-Boado, M.A., Orduña, D., Navarro, S.: Minimally invasive surgery of the pancreas in progress. Langenbeck's Arch. Surg. **390**(4), 342–354 (2005). https://doi.org/10.1007/s00423-005-0556-5
10. Flynn, A.M., Udayakumar, K., Barrett, D.S., McLurkin, J.D., Franck, D.L., Shect-man, A.: Tomorrow's surgery: micromotors and microrobots for minimally invasive procedures. Minim. Invasive Ther. Allied Technol. **7**(4), 343–352 (1998)
11. Frydrychowski, A.F., Szarmach, A., Czaplewski, B., Winklewski, P.J.: Subarach-noid space: new tricks by an old dog. PLoS ONE **7**(5), e37529 (2012)
12. Ha, Y.H., Han, B.H., Lee, S.Y.: Magnetic propulsion of a magnetic device using three square-Helmholtz coils and a square-Maxwell coil. Med. Biol. Eng. Comput. **48**(2), 139–145 (2010). https://doi.org/10.1007/s11517-009-0574-5
13. Haga, Y., Esashi, M.: Biomedical microsystems for minimally invasive diagnosis and treatment. Proc. IEEE **92**(1), 98–114 (2004)
14. Jeon, S., Jang, G., Choi, H., Park, S.: Magnetic navigation system with gradient and uniform saddle coils for the wireless manipulation of micro-robots in human blood vessels. IEEE Trans. Magn. **46**(6), 1943–1946 (2010)
15. Joseph, J.V., Arya, M., Patel, H.R.: Robotic surgery: the coming of a new era in surgical innovation. Expert Rev. Anticancer Ther. **5**(1), 7–9 (2005)
16. Mack, M.J.: Minimally invasive and robotic surgery. JAMA **285**(5), 568–572 (2001)
17. Medina, M.A.M., Vivas, O.A., Riccotti, L.: Herramienta para la simulación del movimiento de un micro robot para aplicaciones médicas a partir de un arreglo de bobinas basadas en Maxwell-Helmholtz. (herramienta de simulación para nave-gación de microrobots). Rev. EIA **15**(30), 151–160 (2018)
18. Menciassi, A., Quirini, M., Dario, P.: Microrobotics for future gastrointestinal endoscopy. Minim. Invasive Ther. Allied Technol. **16**(2), 91–100 (2007)
19. Merchant, N.B., Parikh, A.A., Kooby, D.A.: Should all distal pancreatectomies be performed laparoscopically? Adv. Surg. **43**(1), 283–300 (2009)
20. Murphy, W., Black, J., Hastings, G.W.: Handbook of Biomaterial Properties. Springer, New York (2016). https://doi.org/10.1007/978-1-4939-3305-1
21. Nelson, B.J., Kaliakatsos, I.K., Abbott, J.J.: Microrobots for minimally invasive medicine. Annu. Rev. Biomed. Eng. **12**, 55–85 (2010)
22. Panero, J., Zelnik, M.: Las dimensiones humanas en los espacios interiores: estándares antropométricos (1984)
23. Pantoja., G.I.M., Medina., M.A.M., Albán., O.A.V.: Magnetic three-dimensional pose control system for micro robots in the human head. In: Proceedings of the 12th International Joint Conference on Biomedical Engineering Systems and Technolo-gies - Volume 1: BIODEVICES, pp. 65–74. INSTICC, SciTePress (2019). https://doi.org/10.5220/0007483400650074
24. Pardridge, W.M.: Blood-brain barrier drug targeting: the future of brain drug development. Mol. Interventions **3**(2), 90 (2003)

25. Purdy, P.D., Fujimoto, T., Replogle, R.E., Giles, B.P., Fujimoto, H., Miller, S.L.: Percutaneous intraspinal navigation for access to the subarachnoid space: use of another natural conduit for neurosurgical procedures. Neurosurg. Focus **19**(1), 1–5 (2005)
26. Thijssen, H., Keyser, A., Horstink, M., Meijer, E.: Morphology of the cervical spinal cord on computed myelography. Neuroradiology **18**(2), 57–62 (1979). https://doi.org/10.1007/BF00344822
27. Webb, W., Penny, E., Sundstrom, L., Shappell, R.: Helmholtz coil system, US Patent App. 11/263,332, 3 May 2007
28. Werp, P.R., Creighton, F.M.: Magnetic navigation system, US Patent 7.774.046, 10 August 2010
29. Yu, C., et al.: Novel electromagnetic actuation system for three-dimensional locomotion and drilling of intravascular microrobot. Sens. Actuators A Phys. **161**(1–2), 297–304 (2010)

Features of Using Nonlinear Dynamics Method in Electrical Impedance Signals Analysis of the Ocular Blood Flow

A. A. Kiseleva[1], P. V. Luzhnov[1]([⊠]), and E. N. Iomdina[2]

[1] Bauman Moscow State Technical University, 2-nd Baumanskaya 5, 105005 Moscow, Russia
peterl@hotmail.ru
[2] Helmholtz National Medical Research Center of Eye Diseases,
Sadovaya-Chernogryazskaya 14/19, 105062 Moscow, Russia

Abstract. The article describes an approach to constructing an algorithm for qualitative and quantitative comparison of electrical impedance diagnostics signals using the nonlinear dynamics method. The biophysical factors for the electrical impedance diagnostics signal formation and their relationship with a variety of the developed algorithm parameters are presented. The method with the transpalpebral rheoophthalmography signal attractor reconstruction is considered. The optimal reconstruction parameters have been chosen to construct an attractor in the given coordinates space. It has been carried out the analysis of the reconstructed attractors mass centers position for the transpalpebral rheoophthalmography signals, on the basis of which the decision rule has been formulated for comparing and dividing the signals into groups. The results have been verified on electrical impedance signals of the eye blood flow. The application of the developed technique is shown on the example of transpalpebral rheoophthalmography signal analysis in patients with primary open-angle glaucoma.

Keywords: Nonlinear dynamics · Transpalpebral rheoophthalmography · Blood flow · Eye · Glaucoma

1 Introduction

The normal eye function is determined by its high-grade tissue blood flow level. The hemodynamic eye studies provide the ophthalmologist an additional information about the pathogenesis in case of such ocular pathologies as myopia, diabetic retinopathy, glaucoma. The main points are the possibility of early diagnosis and evaluation of the disease treatment in the future. The urgency of research in this area is due to the prevalence of ophthalmic diseases data.

Electrical impedance diagnostics allows non-invasive assessment of the blood flow state in various human body segments. It generates diagnostic information about the pulse volume in the tested segment. In addition, with the help of electrical impedance diagnostics, it is possible to obtain additional information about the biomechanical properties of blood vessels and the level of blood flow in them. The electrical impedance

A. Roque et al. (Eds.): BIOSTEC 2019, CCIS 1211, pp. 80–89, 2020.
https://doi.org/10.1007/978-3-030-46970-2_4

method principle is based on recording the changes in the total resistance (the impedance) when a high-frequency, low-amplitude probing current passes through the tissue.

There is a technique for the eye study, called rheoophthalmography [1, 2]. In [3, 4] the transpalpebral rheoophthalmography (TP ROG) technique is described, in which electrodes are superimposed on a closed eyelid [5]. The results of mathematical modeling were used during the development of this technique considering the particular anatomical structure of the vascular bed of the eyeball, which helps to increase the measurement accuracy [6]. Studies of the eye blood flow during the progression of myopia have been conducted, and the possibility of using this technique for the early myopia diagnosis in children [3] has been shown. A feature of signal analysis in the myopia diagnosis is mainly the study of the anterior part of the eye (see the Fig. 1).

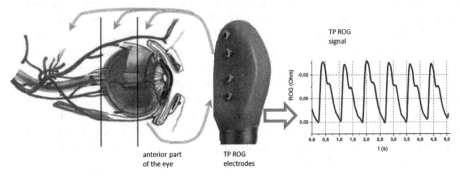

Fig. 1. The main technique and research areas for analysis TP ROG diagnostic signals.

In the case of glaucoma, the changes in blood flow are observed in all eye parts. Moreover, in the structure of ophthalmopathology, primary open-angle glaucoma (POAG) occupies one of the first places among eye diseases. Currently, the pathogenesis of the development and progression of POAG is associated with increased intraocular pressure (IOP). Increased IOP damages the nerve cells of the retina, from which the optic nerve is formed, which is manifested by a gradual loss of vision. However, other factors can lead to the progression of POAG. One of the risk factors for the POAG progression and progressive deterioration of vision in this disease is a decrease in the level of blood circulation in the brain and eye vessels. The study of hemodynamics with POAG eyes will give the necessary information about the clinical progression.

A number of studies described in [7, 8] have been conducted to analyze the TP ROG signals in patients with POAG. It is shown that the amplitude parameters estimation becomes more informative using waveform analysis. Thus, the TP ROG signals analysis includes a qualitative and quantitative analysis. Qualitative signal analysis involves determining the type of pulse wave. It is influenced by biophysical, biomechanical and hydrodynamic factors. In the aggregate, they influence on the type of the pulse wave and further determine the result of diagnosis in the qualitative signals analysis. At this moment, the method of analyzing the TP ROG signals pulse waveform hasn't been developed.

This type of waveform analysis is possible in two ways: with the help of amplitude graphic methods, and with the help of non-linear dynamics methods [8, 9]. Using the nonlinear properties of the system, it is possible to describe a combination of these factors and their mutual influence on each other.

An important role in the formation and manifestation of system nonlinear properties is played by dynamic processes, in particular, the dynamic chaos. First of all, the chaos is characterized by internal self-sustaining fractal fluctuations [10]. This effect is found in the analysis of many biological signals – studies of the heart electrical activity [11], brain neural activity [12], respiration [13], and blood supply of the various organs. It becomes possible to carry out signals qualitative and quantitative comparison using the phase-spatial representation of signals, so called attractors [14].

TP ROG signals studies using the attractors have been carried out [7, 8], but the question of choosing the most appropriate parameters of the algorithm remains open. On the other hand, the biophysical principles of TP ROG signals forming carry information about the functioning of the ocular blood circulatory system. The analysis of biophysical principles in conjunction with the form of recorded signals allows to generate the necessary parameters of the algorithm. They can be applicable to the development of diagnostic algorithms based on nonlinear dynamics methods. It is very important in the POAG early diagnosis and separation of the POAG stages [15, 16].

Thus, the main goal of this work is to analyze the biophysical principles of TP ROG signals formation and the subsequent selection of the most optimal parameters for constructing attractors using the nonlinear dynamics method for TP ROG signals analysis in patients with POAG.

2 Materials and Methods

The biophysical factors of the TP ROG signals formation are as follows: the features of the heart, the tone, the innervation of the blood vessels and the vessels walls state in the examined diagnosis area.

It is distinguished the electrical impedance signal structure of the pulse component during the cardiac intervals analysis. The TP ROG signal cardiointerval starts with a "steep climb" that goes to the top of the systolic wave. After that, there is a decrease in the signal level until the beginning of the next cardiointerval. The slope is not the same during the signal increasing, it is divided into two parts. The first part is the period of quick blood circulation, which lasts until the maximum derivative of the signal is reached (see the Fig. 2). The second part is the period of slow blood filling which lasts until the signal systolic peak signal [7]. The systolic apex determines the rheographic signal amplitude and generates a systolic wave. The systolic wave is followed by a local signal minimum called an incisura. Following the incisura, a diastolic wave is recorded.

The amplitude and shape of the rheographic signal are influenced by the blood flow nature and the visco-elastic properties of the blood vessels walls, both directly in the study area and in the adjacent sections of the vessels bed at various levels. The period of quick blood filling is considered, firstly, as a manifestation of the physiological heterogeneity of the left ventricle expulsion period, and secondly, as a reflection of the hemodynamic properties of large-caliber arterial vessels. The period of slow blood filling falls on the

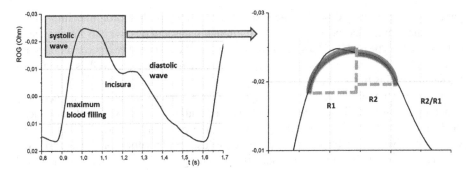

Fig. 2. The structure of TP ROG signal cardiointerval and parameters of the systolic wave.

phase of reduced expulsion in the left ventricle. The diastolic wave is determined by the blood flow speed through arterioles and precapillaries into the capillary system, by blood pressure, as well as by the visco-elastic characteristics of the investigated area vessels and distal located vessels.

All these factors together affect the pulse wave form and determine the result during the TP ROG signals waveform analysis.

The tasks of analyzing the pulse waveform includes:

– determination of the beginning and end of the TP ROG signals cardiointervals;
– determination of the top systolic wave type;
– determination of the systolic and diastolic waves ratio and the subsequent TP ROG signals classification.

For each type of the signal contour analysis, it is necessary to select the boundaries of cardiointervals in time. Selection boundaries methods can be divided into three groups: threshold methods, methods for comparing with patterns and spectral methods. In real-time working conditions, preference is given to threshold methods. During the TP ROG signals analysis, the algorithm with the threshold method of finding boundaries will determine the systolic component of the cardio interval, as well as the duration of the quick blood filling phases and diastole. Thus, it is necessary to use one amplitude parameter and one-time parameter.

For solving the second problem of determining the systolic wave type, the methods of comparison with templates can be used. The choice of the pattern type is determined by the main hemodynamic factors affecting the TP ROG signals. With low peripheral resistance, it is minimal contribution to the formation of a reflected systolic wave from the distal regions. The return effect weakens, and the signal has a high amplitude, a pointed apex and a short period of quick blood filling. With high peripheral resistance, the influence of reflection is more stable, and as a result, during the period of slow blood filling, the systolic part of the signal becomes flatter. The apex of the TP ROG signals is also flattened.

As a template for analysis, it is possible to use a triangular pattern, a semicircular pattern or a bell-shaped pattern. The triangular pattern contains the least number of parameters, but it also describes the systolic apex least accurately. The bell-shaped pattern most accurately describes the systolic apex, but it also has a complex implementation. Therefore, it has been chosen a semicircular pattern in this work to automatically determine the type of TP ROG signals systolic wave. It consists of two parts: an increase and a decline. It is characterized by two radiuses (see the Fig. 2), as well as the ratio of the second radius to the first.

In solving the third task of classifying the TP ROG signals waveform, it is necessary to define a diastolic wave in order to develop an algorithm. It can be a difficult task due to the fact that the diastolic wave of the TP ROG signals may not be expressed. In previous works, to solve this problem, it was proposed to use an algorithm for constructing the signal attractor with its subsequent analysis. According to the characteristic of the blood vessels tonus [17, 18], it makes possible to divide the TP ROG signals into three main types: the hypotonic type, the normotonic type and the hypertonic type.

To construct the TP ROG signals attractor, the analysis of phase – spatial portraits is used. It allows to classify the signals not only by their quantitative characteristics (the value of wave amplitudes, the duration), but also with the help of pulse filling waveform analysis. This analysis consists of the following steps:

– selection of the attractor parameters;
– reconstruction of the attractor with the selected parameters;
– analysis of the obtained attractor form;
– classification of the pulse blood filling waveform at TP ROG signals.

The signal attractor or phase portrait can be constructed in two ways. The first method uses the time delay method. It includes the reconstruction of pseudo-phase portraits using the values of the signal samples $x(t)$ on the subspace with the coordinates $x(t + d)$, where d is the time delay. The second method is based on displaying the phase portrait on a subspace with coordinates $x(t)$ and $x'(t + d)$, where $x'(t + d)$ is the first derivative of the signal $x(t)$ [8].

Both of these methods involve the selection of parameters for constructing an attractor. The process of attractor reconstruction is based on building a new or reconstructed attractor by the sequence of samples of the signal $x(t)$ under consideration. The new attractor has the same properties as the original one. For this purpose, m-dimensional vectors are constructed, and for sufficiently large m, the parameters of the reconstructed attractor in the m-dimensional space coincide with the parameters of the original attractor.

The key role for calculating all parameters of the obtained attractor belongs to the correct selection of the displacement d. Typically the offset is selected so that each reconstructed next vector adds the most informative data about the attractor or less can be correlated with the previous one. This can be achieved by using a priori knowledge of the TP ROG waveform. During the analysis of the pulse blood filling signals, the following components should be distinguished: the period of quick blood filling, the systolic wave and the diastolic wave. Based on their duration analysis, the values of 0.08 s and 0.22 s have been chosen.

The Fig. 3 shows an example of the resulting attractor on the model signal of the pulse. The type of signal and the resulting signal attractor are shown.

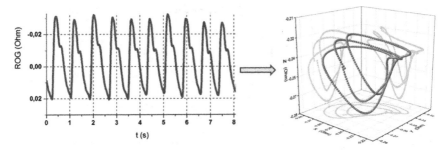

Fig. 3. The example of TP ROG signal and the resulting signal attractor.

Further, it is analyzed the obtained form of the attractor. Projections onto three sub-space (XY, YZ, XZ) are considered. The attractor shape and its projections are approximated by simple geometric shapes to carry out the classification of the pulse filling waveforms. These can be done with the help of the following figures: a sphere, an ellipsoid, a pyramid with a triangular base, a parallelepiped. The corresponding projections for them are as follows: a circle, an ellipse, a triangle, a rectangle. More complex geometric shapes in our work have not been considered due to the difficulty of using them in the algorithm for waveform automatic classification.

In the tasks of analyzing the pulse wave shape, it becomes possible to determine the correlation of systolic and diastolic waves. At the same time other tasks require additional iterations of the algorithm. In order to minimize them, it has been proposed to modify the algorithm and consider not the signal attractors, but its derivatives. Since both the task of determining the beginning and the end of the TP ROG signals cardiointervals and the task of determining the type of the systolic wave apex are biophysically determined by the periods of quick and slow blood filling during the systole phase, these processes will be reflected in the construction of the derived signal attractor.

The advantage of this algorithm is a more accurate separation of the cardiocycle signal into systolic and diastolic components, as well as the ability to determine the beginning of the cardiointerval. The Fig. 4 show the derivative of the pulse blood filling signal and its reconstructed attractor. The selected areas correspond to the systolic and diastolic components of the original signal.

When analyzing the shape of the attractor (see the Fig. 4), it is used the approximation by the rotation ellipsoid. The projections of the obtained attractor are optimally determined using two ellipses. The first ellipse describes the systolic part, and the second describes the diastolic part of the pulse blood filling signal.

The introduction of two geometric figures approximating the projection of the attractor allows us to formulate another classification algorithm parameter for the TP ROG signals form. Considering the positions of the two ellipses mass centers, it becomes possible to calculate the distance parameter between their mass centers. It is proposed to use this distance to analyze the shape of the obtained attractor projections. When constructing an algorithm for automatic classification of the TP ROG signals wave shape, the separation has been carried out according to three main types: a hypotonic type, a normotonic type and a hypertonic type.

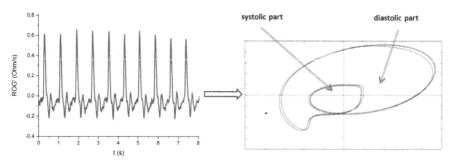

Fig. 4. The derivative of the TP ROG signal and its reconstructed attractor.

The model signals of each type have been considered: a normotonic type, a hypotonic type, a hypertonic type. Based on the analysis of the calculated parameters, it has been formulated the requirements for the mass centers location for each signal type. It has been determined that the mass center coordinates of the systolic component are identical for signals of all types. Therefore, it has been proposed to use a combination of the two approaches described above to construct TP ROG signals attractors.

For combining all three analysis tasks (the determination of the beginning and the end of the cardiointervals, the determination of the systolic wave apex type, the determination of the systolic and diastolic waves ratio) in this paper, an algorithm for constructing an attractor is proposed. In this algorithm the first two axes of the phase space have the dimension of the signal and the third is the derived signal. In this case, the first two parameters of displacement are associated with the biophysical processes of the two waves formation on the signal – systolic and diastolic. These displacements also reflect the refractory interval between consecutive cardiointervals. The third parameter, given by the signal derivative, is associated with the biophysical principles of forming a quick blood filling region. In addition, it is associated with the moments of the beginning and the end of the cardiointerval on the signal of the pulse volume.

To these parameters it is necessary to add the distance parameter between the mass centers of two ellipses approximating the attractor projection (see the Fig. 5). With the help of this algorithm, it becomes possible to conduct an automatic analysis of the recorded TP ROG signals shape, their subsequent classification and further diagnosis.

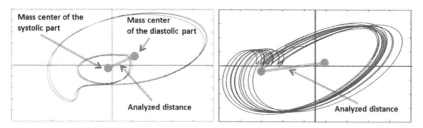

Fig. 5. The mass centers of the approximating ellipses in previous coordinates (left) and in developed phase space.

The developed algorithm works in the phase space of three coordinates (XYZ), in which the construction of the TP ROG signals attractor is carried out. The first and second axes have the signal dimension. The displacement parameter for the second axis is 0.08 s, the displacement parameter for the third axis is 0.22 s. The third axis has the dimension of the first signal derivative.

In the selected coordinates space, it is constructed a signal attractor with a duration of at least 10 s. In this case duration makes it possible to take into account at least one complete respiration cycle during the analysis. Then, on the projections, two approximating ellipses are constructed, each pair describes systolic and diastolic TP ROG signals waves. The mass centers of the approximating ellipses are calculated, and the distance between them is calculated (see the Fig. 5). Then the decision rule is introduced for TP ROG signals classification. The decision rule includes the coordinates of the mass centers of the systolic and diastolic signal components, the distance between them. The threshold values of all parameters depend on the projection subspace. In the Fig. 5 it is shown an example of the decision rule formation for model signals of electrical impedance diagnostics normalized to the maximum amplitude. The separation of the electrical impedance diagnostics signal can be carried out in this way according to three vascular types: a hypotonic type, a normotonic type and a hypertonic type. Carrying out this TP ROG signals separation into the types in patients with POAG, it is quite informative, since it represents an additional opportunity to study the relationship between the stage of POAG, arterial pressure and IOP. As a result, an ophthalmologist has an algorithm for automatically classification of the TP ROG signals waveform, both according to the disease stages, and according to the vascular tone types in POAG.

3 Compliance with Ethical Requirements

This study was performed in accordance with the Declaration of Helsinki and was approved by the Local Committee of Biomedical Ethics of the Moscow Helmholtz Research Institute of Eye Diseases. A written informed consent was obtained from all participants.

4 Results

A study has been conducted on the TP ROG signals in patients with different stages of POAG. Four groups of patients have been considered: healthy subjects, patients with the first POAG stage of glaucoma, patients with the second POAG stage of glaucoma, and patients with the third stage of glaucoma. Each group consisted of 8 signals of each type. The duration of all signals was 10 s.

The following Table 1 shows the distance between mass centers for each type of the signal.

Comparing the obtained values, it can be concluded that the algorithm developed for analyzing the pulse waveform makes it possible to determine the beginning and the end of the TP ROG signals cardiointervals, determine the systolic wave apex type and also allows to determine the correlation of systolic and diastolic waves with the subsequent classification of the TP ROG signals.

Table 1. The distance between mass centers of TP ROG signals.

Type signal	Distance between centers
Healthy subjects	0.2 ± 0.18
POAG I stage	0.3 ± 0.26
POAG II stage	0.6 ± 0.25
POAG III stage	0.6 ± 0.33

5   Conclusions

As a result of this work, it has been developed an algorithm for TP ROG signals classification based on nonlinear dynamics methods. For this purpose, the attractor parameters have been justified, the parameters have been selected, and the attractor has been reconstructed with the selected parameters on the model signals and the TP ROG signals of patients with POAG. The analysis of the obtained attractor form has been carried out, and the possibility of classifying the pulse waveform in the TP ROG signals has been shown.

In the future, it is planned to conduct a study of the algorithm in the separation TP ROG signals in real time. It is also possible to use the developed algorithm for the study at an early stage of the disease of the relationship between changes in the ocular hemodynamics, blood pressure and biomechanical properties of eye tissue.

Conflict of Interest. The authors declare that they have no conflict of interest. The paper was supported by a grant from RFBR (No. 18-08-01192).

References

1. Lazarenko, V.I., Kornilovsky, I.M., Ilenkov, S.S., et al.: Our method of functional heography of eye. Vestn. oftalmol. **115**(4), 33–37 (1999)
2. Lazarenko, V.I., Komarovskikh, E.N.: Results of the examination of hemodynamics of the eye and brain in patients with primary open-angle glaucoma. Vestn. oftalmol. **120**(1), 32–36 (2004). https://doi.org/10.21687/0233-528X-2017-51-3-22-30
3. Luzhnov, P.V., Shamaev, D.M., Iomdina, E.N., et al.: Transpalpebral tetrapolar reoophtalmography in the assessment of parameters of the eye blood circulatory system. Vestn. Ross. Akad. Med. Nauk **70**(3), 372–377 (2015). https://doi.org/10.15690/vramn.v70i3.1336
4. Luzhnov, P.V., Shamaev, D.M., Iomdina, E.N., et al.: Using quantitative parameters of ocular blood filling with transpalpebral rheoophthalmography. IFMBE Proc. **65**, 37–40 (2017). https://doi.org/10.1007/978-981-10-5122-7_10
5. Shamaev, D.M., Luzhnov, P.V., Iomdina, E.N.: Modeling of ocular and eyelid pulse blood filling in diagnosing using transpalpebral rheoophthalmography. IFMBE Proc. **65**, 1000–1003 (2017). https://doi.org/10.1007/978-981-10-5122-7_250
6. Shamaev, D.M., Luzhnov, P.V., Iomdina, E.N.: Mathematical modeling of ocular pulse blood filling in rheoophthalmography. IFMBE Proc. **68**(1), 495–498 (2018). https://doi.org/10.1007/978-981-10-9035-6_91

7. Luzhnov, P.V., Shamaev, D.M., Kiseleva, A.A., et al.: Using nonlinear dynamics for signal analysis in transpalpebral rheoophthalmography. Sovremennye tehnologii v medicine **10**(3), 160–167 (2018). https://doi.org/10.17691/stm2018.10.3.20

8. Kiseleva, A.A., Luzhnov, P.V., Nikolaev, A.P., Iomdina, E.N., Kiseleva, O.A.: Nonlinear dynamics method in the impedance signals analysis of the eye blood flow of patients with glaucoma. In: Proceedings of 12th International Joint Conference on Biomedical Engineering Systems and Technologies BIODEVICES, vol. 1, pp. 75–80 (2019). https://doi.org/10.5220/0007554800750080

9. Kiseleva, A., Luzhnov, P., Dyachenko, A., Semenov, Y.: Rheography and spirography signal analysis by method of nonlinear dynamics. In: Proceedings of the 11th International Joint Conference on Biomedical Engineering Systems and Technologies BIODEVICES, vol. 1, pp. 136–140 (2018). https://doi.org/10.5220/0006579301360140

10. Betelin, V.B., Eskov, V.M., Galkin, V.A., et al.: Stochastic volatility in the dynamics of complex homeostatic systems. Dokl. Math. **95**, 92 (2017). https://doi.org/10.1134/S1064562417010240

11. Elhaj, F., Salim, N., Harris, A., Swee, T., Ahmed, T.: Arrhythmia recognition and classification using combined linear and nonlinear features of ECG signals. Comput. Methods Programs Biomed. **127**, 52–63 (2016). https://doi.org/10.1016/j.cmpb.2015.12.024

12. Akar, S.A., Kara, S., Agambayev, S., Bilgic, V.: Nonlinear analysis of EEG in major depression with fractal dimensions. In: 37th Annual International Conference of the IEEE on Engineering in Medicine and Biology Society, pp. 7410–7413 (2015). https://doi.org/10.1109/embc.2015.7320104

13. Gracia, J., et al.: Nonlinear local projection filter for impedance pneumography. EMBEC/NBC -2017. IP, vol. 65, pp. 306–309. Springer, Singapore (2018). https://doi.org/10.1007/978-981-10-5122-7_77

14. Takens, F.: Detecting strange attractors in turbulence. In: Rand, D., Young, L.-S. (eds.) Dynamical Systems and Turbulence, Warwick 1980. LNM, vol. 898, pp. 366–381. Springer, Heidelberg (1981). https://doi.org/10.1007/BFb0091924

15. Flammer, J., Orgul, S., Costa, V.P., et al.: The impact of ocular blood flow in glaucoma. Prog. Retin. Eye Res. **21**, 359–393 (2002)

16. Kurysheva, N.I., Parshunina, O.A., Shatalova, E.O., et al.: Value of structural and hemodynamic parameters for the early detection of primary open-angle glaucoma. Curr. Eye Res. **42**(3), 411–417 (2017)

17. Schmetterer, L.: Ocular perfusion abnormalities in glaucoma. Russian Ophthalmol. J. **4**, 100–109 (2015)

18. Siesky, B., Harris, A., Ehrlich, R., Kheradiya, N., Lopez, C.R.: Glaucoma risk factors: ocular blood flow. In: Schacknow, P., Samples, J. (eds.) The Glaucoma Book, pp. 111–134. Springer, New York (2010). https://doi.org/10.1007/978-0-387-76700-0_11

Analogue Fluids for Cell Deformability Studies in Microfluidic Devices

A. S. Moita[1]([⊠]) [iD], C. Caldeira[1], I. Gonçalves[1,2], R. Lima[2,3], E. J. Vega[4],
and A. L. N. Moreira[1]

[1] IN+ - Center for Innovation, Technology and Policy Research, Instituto Superior Técnico,
Universidade de Lisboa, Av. Rovisco Pais, 1049-001 Lisbon, Portugal
anamoita@tecnico.ulisboa.pt

[2] Metrics, Mechanical Engineering Department, University of Minho, Campus de Azurém,
4800-058 Guimarães, Portugal

[3] CEFT, Faculdade de Engenharia da Universidade do Porto (FEUP), R. Dr. Roberto Frias,
4200-465 Porto, Portugal

[4] Área de Mecánica de Fluidos, Dpto. de Ingeniería Mecánica, Energética y de los Materiales,
Escuela de Ingenierias Industriales, Universidade de Extremadura, Campus Universitario,
Av. de Elvas, s/n, 06006 Badajoz, Spain

Abstract. This study concerns the development and test of analogue fluids which can be used in tests focused on cell deformability studies. The analogue fluids were characterized in terms of their main physico-chemical properties, the size distribution of the particles (mimicking the cells) and on their deformability. From the various approaches tested here, a solution of water DD with a surfactant (Brij40), giving rise to semi-rigid particles, has shown the greatest potential to be used as an analogue fluid. This analogue fluid depicts a particle size distribution that is representative of the biosamples to be studied in our future work. Furthermore, simple filtering processes allow to narrow the particle size distribution, giving rise to a homogeneous solution with particles depicting sizes and deformability ratios that are compatible with red blood cell preparations. The flow and velocity behaviours of this analogue fluid inside a microchannel also support the potential to use it also as an analogue blood fluid for hemodynamic studies.

Keywords: Analogue fluids · Microfluidic devices · Cell deformability · Clinical diagnostics · Lab-on-a-chip

1 Introduction

Microfluidic devices are pointed as high potential diagnostic tools, capable of providing cost effective diagnostics in harsh environments, such as those found in developing countries [1]. Furthermore, they can potentially perform several sample manipulation operations and biochemical analysis [2–5], allowing a significant reduction of samples and reagents, a better control of the reactions (due to the short characteristic length scales) and a marginal manual handling, thus minimizing contamination issues [6]. Despite of these advantages and of the extensive research that has been performed towards the

© Springer Nature Switzerland AG 2020
A. Roque et al. (Eds.): BIOSTEC 2019, CCIS 1211, pp. 90–101, 2020.
https://doi.org/10.1007/978-3-030-46970-2_5

development of these devices within the last decade, there are still several obstacles to overcome, particularly when using droplet based microfluidic devices [7]. Hence, lab-on-chip operational systems for clinical diagnostics are just now maturing at real application levels, e.g. [8].

Microfluidic devices are also particularly suitable to explore specific biosamples properties, in the context of label free diagnostics. For instance, cell deformability and especially large deformability regimes have been recently reported to provide useful information on the process of metastasis [9]. These recent findings agree with previous studies, scarcely reported in the literature, which suggest correlations between the deformability ratio of the cells and the stage of malignancy [10]. Such correlations require a deeper study but are worth to be explored. In fact, there are several pathologies which are related with cell deformability and stiffness modifications that can be explored in custom made microfluidic devices. For instance, hyperglycemia in diabetes mellitus is reported in several studies to reduce the deformability of red blood cells, among other rheological modifications [11–13]. In this context, microfluidic devices are also privileged means to study and simulate specific *in vivo* cell behaviours and mechanisms, such as those observed in microcirculation e.g. [13, 14]. Hence, in line with the development of microfluidic devices for clinical diagnostics, it is vital to devise biofluid analogues which can mimic the properties not only of healthy, but also of the pathological behavior. This is important not only to understand the pathophysiological behavior of the cells and of the biofluids but also to allow a better design of the devices without the need to use real biofluids, which are difficult to obtain, due to medical, ethical, economical and safety issues.

Following this line of thought and subsequently to our previous work, which was mainly focused on the development of a microfluidic device for cancer diagnostics based on cell deformability [15–18], this part of the work is now focused on the development of analogue fluids that can be tested in the previously devised microfluid chips. Different solutions were considered to produce the analogue fluids, namely, using xanthan gum solutions and suspensions of polymers and surfactants solved in water, the latter resulting on the precipitation of small semi-rigid particles. The analogue fluids are then characterized in terms of their main physical properties, of the resulting particle size distribution and on the evaluation of particles behavior and deformability. Although the main objective is to develop a lab-on-a-chip for cancer diagnostics, at this preliminary stage, the analogue fluids devised here are supposed to mimic the behavior of red blood cells preparations, given the previous experience of the working group in this issue e.g. [13, 15–19] and to facilitate the comparison with values (e.g. deformability ratios) already reported in the literature.

2   Experimental Procedure

As aforementioned, the present work proposes different strategies to develop biomimetic (blood) fluids which are then tested and characterized. The testing procedure that is proposed here comprises the characterization of the physico-chemical properties of the analogues, a full characterization of the resulting particle size distribution (to see if it matches with the characteristic sizes of the cells) and a detailed characterization of their deformability behaviour to be compared with that of real cells. Since the microfluidic system that is being devised under the scope of the global project concerns the use of electrowetting as external actuation, the fluids are also tested to check on their response to electrostatic actuation. The procedures followed in each of these stages are described in the following subsections.

2.1 Preparation and Characterization of the Analogue Fluids

The various analogue fluids to be characterized and tested are water DD based solutions with xanthan gum, polymeric particles and a surfactant which results in the precipitation of semi-rigid surfactant particles.

The xanthan gum solutions were prepared with the concentrations of 0.05wt% and 0.35wt%. Xanthan gum was used to mimic the shear thinning behavior of blood. The rheological data was obtained under temperature-controlled conditions, with an accuracy of ±5%. The measurements were performed ATS RheoSystems (a division of CANNON® Instruments, Co). The viscosity vs shear rate curves were fitted using the Cross model [20], as described in [21].

The suspensions with polymeric particles were prepared with PMMA - Poly(methyl methacrylate) using a concentration of 1wt%. Different particle sizes were tested, namely 5 μm, 10 μm and 20 μm, to fit the correct range of sizes corresponding to characteristic cells sizes (including the red blood cells). Finally, the third approach considered was adding to the water small amounts of Brij40, a nonionic polyoxyethylene surfactant from Thermo Fisher. This procedure resulted in the precipitation of semi-rigid microparticles which remained suspended in the water in a stable manner. Except for the xanthan gum solutions, all the other analogues depicted viscosities close to those of water, at room temperature (20 ± 3 °C). Besides viscosity, surface tension and density were the main evaluated physico-chemical properties. Surface tension σ_{lv} was measured using the optical tensiometer (THETA from Attention). The final surface tension values were averaged from 15 measurements taken at room temperature. Measurements have standard mean errors always lower than 0.35. Density ρ was evaluated from basic concentration calculations. The measured values for the various solutions are summarized in Table 1.

Table 1. Density and surface tension (measured at room temperature 20 ± 3 °C) of the analogue fluids tested in the present work [18].

Solution	Density ρ [kg/m^3]	Surface tension σ_{lv} [mN/m]
Xanthan gum 0.05wt%	997	72.0
Xanthan gum 0.35wt%	997	72.95
Water DD + PMMA particles (1wt%)	999	58.65
Water DD + Brij40	999	21.10

2.2 Characterization of Particles Sizes Distribution Using Laser Scanning Fluorescent Confocal Microscopy

PMMA and surfactant solutions were further analyzed to characterize the size distribution of the particles suspended in the solutions, based on extensive post-processing of images taken with a Laser Scanning Confocal Microscope (SP8 from Leica), using an in-house code developed in MATLAB. Rhodamine B (Sigma Aldrich) was used as fluorophore, with a concentration of 3.968×10^{-6} g/ml, which does not alter the physico-chemical properties of the analogue fluids [16]. The solutions were excited using a 552 nm wavelength laser, fixing the laser power to 10.50 mW (3.00% of its maximum power). The gain of the microscope photomultiplier was fixed at 550 V. These values were chosen after a sensitivity analysis on the contrast of the image (before the post-processing) and on the Signal to Noise Ratio (SNR). The images were recorded in the format 1024×1024 pixels^2 and the scanning frequency was set to 400 Hz. For the optical arrangement used, the lateral and axial resolutions for most of the measurements are $R_l = 0.375$ μm and $R_a = 1.4$ μm. The optical slice thickness was 2.2 μm.

2.3 Characterization of Particles Deformability and Flow Dynamic Behaviour of the Analogue Fluids

To study the flow dynamic behavior and deformability of the particles of the analogue fluids, the fluids flow in a PDMS – Polydimethylsiloxane channel with the geometry represented in Fig. 1. For this part of the study, very dispersed solutions were considered, with only 1% of particles, to avoid clogging issues, which were recurrent with larger concentrations, particularly for the analogue solutions with the PMMA particles.

The flow was constant pressure driven using a (KD Scientific, USA). Particles sizes and velocities were taken from image post-processing procedures using ImageJ. Images were taken using a high-speed camera (Phantom v7.1; Vision Research, USA), with a resolution of 640×640 px^2 or 512×768 px^2 and with a frame rate of 4000 fps. The lens used had a 20X magnification and the pixel size was 1.185 px/μm.

The flow was accelerated in the contraction section which promotes the deformation of the particles. Particles velocity was evaluated by tracking their displacement between consecutive images. The deformability ratio was accessed by quantifying the

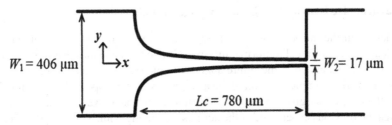

Fig. 1. Schematic with the geometry and main dimensions of the microchannel used to study the flow behavior and deformability of the particles formed in the analogue fluids tested in the present work.

deformation index, DI, as defined in [22]:

$$DI = \frac{L_{major} - L_{minor}}{L_{major} + L_{minor}} \tag{1}$$

where, L_{major} and L_{minor} represent the major and minor axis lengths of the particle.

2.4 Evaluation of the Response of the Analogue Fluids to Electrostatic Actuation

The response of the analogue fluids was evaluated based on the measurement of the contact angles variation, for subsequent values of an applied tension. The contact angles (angles formed between the solid surface and the tangent to the droplet profile under equilibrium conditions of the liquid-solid-vapor interfacial tensions) were measured with an optical tensiometer (THETA from Attention) using the sessile drop method. The measurements were performed inside a Perspex chamber with quartz windows, to avoid optical distortion, under continuously controlled temperature and relative humidity conditions, assured with a DHT 22 Humidity & Temperature Sensor connected to an Arduino. Temperature measurements were acquired with a sample rate of 0.5 Hz and an accuracy of ±0.5 °C. Relative humidity measurements were taken at a sample rate of 0.5 Hz, with an accuracy of 2–5%.

A 25 μm diameter tungsten wire (Goodfellow Cambridge Ltd), acting as an electrode, was dipped inside the droplets to be tested. The counter electrode on which the droplets were deposited was a copper cylinder with 19 mm of diameter and 20 mm height. A 10 μm Teflon film (Goodfellow Cambridge Ltd) was used as the dielectric layer. A very thin film of sodium chloride was placed between the counter electrode and the dielectric to avoid the presence of an air gap [23]. Both electrodes were connected to a Sorensen DCR600-.75B power supply and DC voltage was applied, for a range between 0–230 V in 25 V increments. The final curves were averaged from at least six assays, obtained under similar experimental conditions. Droplet volume was kept constant and equal to 3 μl.

The set-up and experimental procedures are extensively described in [24].

3   Results

3.1 Particle Size Distribution in the Analogue Fluids

As explained in the introduction, the analogue fluids to be developed are intended to mimic real biofluids for cell deformability-based cancer diagnostics. More specifically the main project is aimed at the future analysis of pleural effusions. However, for this stage of the work, a simpler version of the analogues was developed, mainly mimicking blood cell preparations, given the wider collection of data that is available in the literature and given the previous experience of the authors in hemodynamic studies. However, one will broad the analysis of the particle size distribution and of the particles deformability to evaluate the potential to adapt these analogues to mimic different types of biofluids.

Concerning their rheological properties, the xanthan gum solutions depict a shear thinning behaviour, close to that of blood. Nevertheless, these solutions cannot mimic the potential rheological modifications caused by cells deformation as they do not contain solid particles. In this context the polymeric suspensions and the surfactant solutions provide a much more realistic approach. In line with this, the first step was to characterize the particles size distribution of the polymeric and of the surfactant solutions.

Qualitatively, looking at the images taken with the confocal microscope to the PMMA and to the surfactant solutions, they suggest a strong trend for the PMMA particles to agglomerate and form large rigid clusters with irregular shapes, as illustrated in Fig. 2.

A completely different behavior is depicted by the semi-rigid particles which precipitate as the surfactant is added to water DD. Hence, Fig. 3a) shows a homogeneous distribution of spherical particles without any visible agglomeration. The particle size distribution obtained for unfiltered solutions is relatively wide, as confirmed in Fig. 3b).

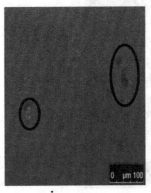

Fig. 2. Illustrative image of a PMMA solution (characteristic size of the particles is 5.46 ± 0.38 μm taken with the Laser Scanning Confocal Microscope - Leica SP8). The images were taken with an objective with 20X magnification and a numerical aperture of 0.75 [18].

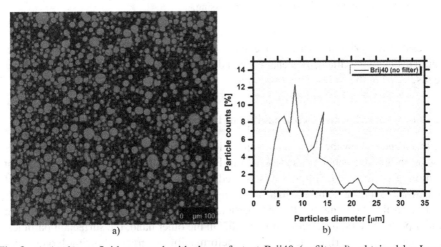

Fig. 3. a) Analogue fluid prepared with the surfactant Brij40 (unfiltered), obtained by Laser Scanning Fluorescent Confocal Microscopy (objective of 20x magnification and 0.75× numerical aperture) [18]. b) Size distribution of the semi-rigid particles obtained by image post-processing.

It is worth mentioning that having a particle size distribution more heterogeneous is in fact an advantage for the current study, since the pleural fluid (and other biofluids) samples may have different cells, with different morphologies, being the size distribution obtained here, similar to that reported by [10] using pleural effusions.

These solutions can, however, be easily uniformized in terms of particles size distributions by simply filtering the solutions. Indeed, Fig. 4a) clearly shows a more homogeneous solution, that is confirmed by the narrower particles size distribution shown in Fig. 4b). Hence, the surfactant solutions seem to be a flexible solution to mimic different biofluid flows, within a variety of characteristic sizes of the cells.

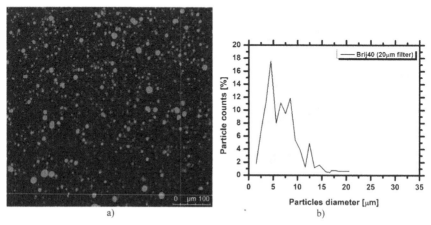

Fig. 4. a) Analogue fluid prepared with the surfactant, obtained by Laser Scanning Fluorescent Confocal Microscopy (objective of 20x magnification and $0.75\times$ numerical aperture) after filtering the solution with a 20 μm filter [18]. b) Respective size distribution of the semi-rigid particles of the filtered solution obtained by image post-processing.

Besides analyzing the particle size distribution in the analogue fluids, it is also relevant to evaluate the fluid flow behavior and deformability of the particles. These issues are discussed in the following sub-section.

3.2   Flow Behavior and Deformability of the Particles in the Analogue Fluids

Figures 5 and 6 show the deformation and velocity of the particles in the analogue fluids flowing in the microchannel represented in Fig. 1, as a function of their displacement position. The surfactant solution was filtered with a 20 μm filter to control the size of the particles keeping them within a size compatible with that of cells.

The results show that the PMMA particles depict smaller deformation indexes, for similar particle velocities, being more rigid. On the other hand, the surfactant particles, being naturally semi-rigid, depict higher deformability degrees, showing larger flexibility, as they allow for a wider range of deformability ratios. Thus, these semi-rigid particles are also more appropriate to microcirculation studies, being less prone for aggregation and consequently will trend to clog less.

Largest deformations naturally occur at the position within the channel where the particles attain a maximum velocity, as the particles are deformed under hydrodynamic effects. However, while the PMMA particles, being rigid, have a very low restitution ability, keeping a constant deformation along the microchannel, the surfactant particles suffer a strong deformation at the maximum velocity position, depicting a continuously lower deformation as the velocity and consequently the hydrodynamic forces promoting their deformation decrease. This behavior is much closer to that of a real cell, when compared to the deformation behavior obtained with the PMMA particles.

The DI values presented in Fig. 5 are averaged from at least three particle tracking tests. However, maximum deformation values could be quite higher. Hence, maximum deformation index DI that was obtained for the PMMA and Brij40 particles is represented in Fig. 7, together with real deformation values reported for human red blood cells in [22].

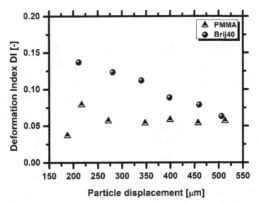

Fig. 5. Deformation of PMMA and surfactant particles in the analogue fluids flowing in a microchannel, as a function of their displacement position in the channel.

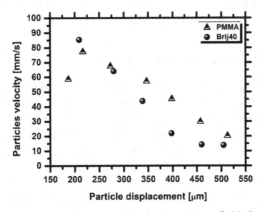

Fig. 6. Velocity of PMMA and surfactant particles in the analogue fluids flowing in a microchannel, as a function of their displacement position in the channel.

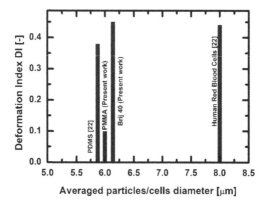

Fig. 7. Deformation index DI as a function of the initial (averaged) particles diameter for the particles used in different analogue fluids, compared with the deformation index of red blood cells, taken from [22].

This confirms the trend reported in Figs. 5 and 6 of the PMMA particles to present a more rigid behavior, being able to deform less than the Brij40 particles and less than the real red blood cells. Furthermore, looking at wider scenario, Brij40 particles are closer to replicate a wider range of deformability ratios of cells. Indeed, although the methodology reported by [10] for malignant diagnostics is quite complex and requires a more complete treatment of the data, [10] defined different profiles, associated to different stages of malignancy, which were mainly defined by distributions of the deformability (which [10] defined as the ratio L_{major}/L_{minor}). These deformability distributions were represented as a function of the initial diameter of the cells. Overall, considering that cell diameters in [10] ranged between 1 and 25 μm, this range of diameters is covered by the particle sizer distributions obtained with the Brij40 analogue, which show deformability ranges of the order of 1.25 or higher, in agreement with those reported in [10]. This analysis must be adapted for our case study and for the various strategies that will be used to deform the cells, but these preliminary results suggest a good potential of the Brij40 solution to be used in our deformability studies.

3.3 Electrostatic Response of the Analogue Fluids

Finally, given that the analogue fluids devised here are planned to be tested with droplet based microfluidic devices working with electrostatic actuation, it is relevant to evaluate the electrostatic response of the analogue fluids. For that purpose, millimetric droplets of each of the analogue fluids were tested as described in Subsect. 2.4. The results of these tests are depicted in Fig. 8, which shows the variation of the equilibrium contact angle under actuation, as a function of the applied voltage.

All the analogue fluids respond well to an electrostatic actuation, as confirmed by the decrease of the contact angle with the applied voltage, according to Young-Lippmann equation. The curves obtained here do not follow exactly Young-Lippmann equation since this classic theory does not account for various phenomena such as energy dissipation and contact line saturation. These curves are in good qualitative agreement with

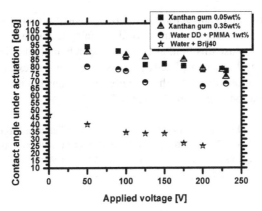

Fig. 8. Electrostatic response of the analogue fluids: contact angle of an actuated droplet (3 μl of volume) deposited on a Teflon substrate, as a function of the applied voltage [18].

those reported in [24]. Nevertheless, it must be mentioned that, in this case, the Brij40 solution has a reduced surface tension, due to the addition of the surfactant (see Table 1), which limits its response to the electrostatic actuation. This is clear, given the smaller range of contact angles variation that is obtained with this solution, as a function of the applied voltage, when compared to other water-based solutions. Such reduced response may be even more limited when analyzing the dynamic response of the fluids, thus affecting the handling of the samples. To overcome this issue, it is recommended to customize the surface properties of the microfluidic devices, to turn the contact surfaces more repellent to the samples. This is in fact in line with recommendations given in previous studies where we reported the progress in the development of the microfluidic devices [15–18].

4 Final Remarks

The present work addresses the development and characterization of analogue fluids to be used in the test of microfluidic devices to be used in the future, for cancer diagnostics, based on cell deformability. At this earlier stage of the work, the fluids devised here are closer to blood analogues, as there is more data available for comparison in the literature and due to previous working experience of the research group. Different approaches were followed, namely using xanthan gum to mimic non-Newtonian characteristics that are depicted in blood, polymer (PMMA) particles suspended in water DD solutions and an alternative original approach consisting in adding a surfactant (Brij40) to water DD, which led to the precipitation of semi-rigid particles. The analogue fluids were characterized in terms of their main physico-chemical properties, the size distribution of the particles (mimicking the cells) and on their deformability.

Results sustain a high potential of the solution with the surfactant to be used as an analogue fluid to mimic different types of biofluids. Hence, the particles size distribution spontaneously obtained in the unfiltered solution is representative of the biosamples to be studied in our future work, namely in pleural effusions. Furthermore, simple filtering processes allow to narrow the particle size distribution, giving rise to a homogeneous solution with particles depicting sizes and deformability ratios that are compatible with red blood cell preparations. The fluid flow dynamics of this analogue inside a microchannel also supports the potential to use this fluid as an analogue in hemodynamic studies.

All the analogues tested here depicted a positive response to an external (electrostatic) actuation, which also allows the use of these analogues in many lab-on-chips, which often use electrostatic actuation in the sample manipulation.

Acknowledgements. Authors are grateful to Fundação para a Ciência e a Tecnologia (FCT) for financing the contract of A.S. Moita through the IF 2015 recruitment program (IF 00810-2015) and for partially financing this research through the exploratory project associated to this contract.

References

1. Yager, P., et al.: Microfluidic diagnostic technologies for global public health. Nature **442**(7101), 412–418 (2006)
2. Takahashi, K., Hattori, A., Suzuki, I., Ichiki, T.: Non-destructive on-chip cell sorting system with real-time microscopic image processing. J. Nanobiotechnol. **2**, 1–8 (2014)
3. Gossett, D., et al.: Label-free cell separation and sorting in microfluidic systems. Anal. Bioanal. Chem. **397**, 3249–3267 (2010). https://doi.org/10.1007/s00216-010-3721-9
4. Shields, I.V., Reyes, C.D., López, G.P.: Microfluidic cell sorting: a review of the advances in the separation of cells from debulking to rare cell isolation. Lab Chip **16**, 1230–1249 (2010)
5. Chim, J.C.R.M.: Capillary biochip for point of use biomedical application, M.Sc. thesis, Instituto Superior Técnico, Universidade de Lisboa (2015)
6. Lin, C.C., Wang, J.H., Wu, H.W., Lee, G.B.: Microfluidic immunoassays. JALA - J. Assoc. Lab. Autom. **15**(3), 253–274 (2010)
7. Geng, H., Feng, J., Stabryl, L.M., Cho, S.K.: Dielectroetting manipulation for digital microfluidics: creating, transporting, splitting, and merging droplets. Lab-on-Chip **17**, 1060–1068 (2017)
8. Dance, A.: The making of a medical microchip. Nature **545**, 512–514 (2017)
9. Hu, S., Wang, R., Tsang, C.M., Tsao, S.W., Sun, D., Lam, H.W.: Revealing elasticity of largely deformed cells flowing along confining microchannels. RSC Adv. **8**, 1030–1038 (2018)
10. Gossett, D.R., et al.: Quantitative diagnosis of malignant pleural effusions by single-cell mechanophenotyping. Sci. Transl. Med. **5**(212), 212ra163 (2013)
11. Zhang, J., Johnson, P.C., Popel, A.S.: Effects of erythrocyte deformability and aggregation on the cell free layer and apparent viscosity of microscopic blood flows. Microvasc. Res. **77**(3), 265–272 (2009)
12. Ong, P.K., Kim, S.: Effect of erythrocyte aggregation on spatiotemporal variations in cell-free layer formation near on arteriolar bifurcation. Microcirculation **20**(5), 440–453 (2013)
13. Pinho, D., Campo-Deaño, L., Lima, R., Pinho, F.T.: In vitro particulate analogue fluids for experimental studies of rheological and hemorheological behavior of glucose-rich RBCs suspensions. Biomicrofluidics **11**, 054105 (2017)
14. Rodrigues, R.O., et al.: In vitro blood flow and cell-free layer in hyperbolic microchannels: visualizations and measurements. BioChip J. **10**(1), 9–15 (2016)
15. Vieira, D., Mata, F., Moita, A.S., Moreira, A.L.N.: Microfluidic prototype of a lab-on-chip device for lung cancer diagnostics. In: Proceedings of the 10th International Joint Conference on Biomedical Engineering Systems and Technologies - Volume 1: BIODEVICES, Porto, Portugal, 21–23 February 2017, pp. 63–68 (2017)

16. Moita, A.S., Vieira, D., Mata, F., Pereira, J., Moreira, A.L.N.: Microfluidic devices integrating clinical alternative diagnostic techniques based on cell mechanical properties. In: Peixoto, N., Silveira, M., Ali, H.H., Maciel, C., van den Broek, Egon L. (eds.) BIOSTEC 2017. CCIS, vol. 881, pp. 74–93. Springer, Cham (2018). https://doi.org/10.1007/978-3-319-94806-5_4

17. Moita, A.S., Jacinto, F., Mata, F., Moreira, A.L.N.: Design and optimization of an open configuration microfluidic device for clinical diagnostics. In: Cliquet Jr., A., et al. (eds.) BIOSTEC 2018. CCIS, vol. 1024, pp. 49–64. Springer, Cham (2019). https://doi.org/10.1007/978-3-030-29196-9_3

18. Moita, A.S., Caldeira, C., Jacinto, F., Lima, R., Vega, E.J., Moreira, A.L.N.: Cell deformability studies for clinical diagnostics: tests with blood analogue fluids using a drop based microfluidic device. In: 12th International Conference on Biomedical Electronics and Devices – Volume 1: BIODEVICES 2019, 22–24 February 2019, Prague, Czech Republic, pp. 99–107 (2019). ISBN 978-989-758-353-7

19. Rodrigues, R.O., Pinho, D., Faustino, V., Lima, R.: A simple microfluidic device for the deformability assessment of blood cells in a continuous flow. Biomed. Microdevice 17(6), 108 (2015). https://doi.org/10.1007/s10544-015-0014-2

20. Cross, M.M.: Rheology of non-Newtonian fluids: a new flow equation for pseudoplastic systems. J. Colloid Sci. 20, 417–437 (1965)

21. Moita, A.S., Herrmann, D., Moreira, A.L.N.: Fluid dynamic and heat transfer processes between solid surfaces and non-Newtonian liquid droplets. Appl. Therm. Eng. 88, 33–46 (2015)

22. Pinho, D.M.D.: Blood rheology and red blood cell migration in microchannel flow. Ph.D. thesis. Faculdade de Engenharia da Universidade do Porto (2018)

23. Restolho, J., Mata, J.L., Saramago, B.: Electrowetting of ionic liquids: contact angle saturation and irreversibility. J. Phys. Chem. C 113, 9321–9327 (2009)

24. Moita, A.S., Laurência, C., Ramos, J.A., Prazeres, D.M.F., Moreira, A.L.N.: Dynamics of droplets of biological fluids on smooth superhydrophobic surfaces under electrostatic actuation. J. Bionic Eng. 13, 220–234 (2016)

Bioimaging

Stepwise Transfer of Domain Knowledge for Computer-Aided Diagnosis in Pathology Using Deep Neural Networks

Jia Qu[1,4]([✉]), Nobuyuki Hiruta[2], Kensuke Terai[2], Hirokazu Nosato[3], Masahiro Murakawa[1,3], and Hidenori Sakanashi[1,3]

[1] University of Tsukuba, Tsukuba 305-8573, Japan
[2] Toho University Sakura Medical Center, Sakura 285-8741, Japan
[3] National Institute of Advanced Industrial Science and Technology (AIST), Tsukuba 305-8560, Japan
[4] Mitsubishi Electric Corporation, Tokyo, Japan
Kyoku.Ka@dc.MitsubishiElectric.co.jp

Abstract. Deep learning using deep convolutional neural networks (DCNNs) has demonstrated unprecedented power in image classification. Subsequently, computer-aided diagnosis (CAD) for pathology imaging has been largely facilitated by DCNN approaches. However, because DCNNs require massive amounts of labeled data, the lack of availability of such pathology image data as well as the high cost of labeling new data is currently a major problem. To avoid expensive data labeling efforts, transfer learning is a concept intended to overcome training data shortages by passing knowledge from the source domain to the target domain. However, weak relevance between the source and target domains generally leads to less effective transfers. Therefore, following the natural step-by-step process by which humans learn and make inferences, a stepwise fine-tuning scheme is proposed by introducing intermediate domains to bridge the source and target domains. The DCNNs are expected to acquire general object classification knowledge from a source domain dataset such as ImageNet and pathology-related knowledge from intermediate domain data, which serve as fundamental and specific knowledge, respectively, for the final benign/malignant classification task. To realize this, we introduce several ways to provide pathology-related knowledge by generating an intermediate dataset classified into various corresponding pathology features. In experiments, the proposed scheme has demonstrated good performance on several well-known deep neural networks.

Keywords: Pathology image classification · Computer-aided diagnosis · Deep learning · Transfer learning

1 Introduction

Cancer is acknowledged as one of the most serious threats to human health. Amongst cancer diagnostic techniques, advanced image diagnosis technologies such as CT, MRI and PET, along with increasingly credible biomarkers, are evolving rapidly and becoming

A. Roque et al. (Eds.): BIOSTEC 2019, CCIS 1211, pp. 105–119, 2020.
https://doi.org/10.1007/978-3-030-46970-2_6

widely used. Nevertheless, pathology diagnosis is still recognized as the gold standard for the final assessment of cancer presence, type, and degree of malignance. However, there is a major shortage of pathologists with the expertise to perform pathological diagnostic examinations [1]. Although digital pathology has been widely popularized over the past decade or so [2], a pathology diagnosis depends entirely on the pathologist's observation and judgment. As a result, diagnostic accuracy and pathologist workload alleviation remain significant challenges [3–5].

In order to provide a substantial solution to these issues, an increasing number of researchers are focusing on improving digital assistance. Amongst the research, computer-aided diagnosis (CAD) such as pre-diagnosis "screening" and post-diagnosis "double check" based on image classification technologies are expected to play a key role in facilitating smarter pathology diagnoses. In previous research, several approaches using specified pathological features or generalized texture handcrafted features combined with statistical classifiers have presented some degree of applicability, but such features generally limit the variability of pathological images. Recently, with the development of deep learning techniques, high expectations have been placed on deep learning-based approaches to CAD for pathology imaging. While deep convolutional neural networks (DCNNs) can solve highly challenging problems, they require large amounts of data for training; however, because of the extremely high cost of pathologists' professional work, it is difficult to obtain sufficient pathology image data labeled with diagnostic results.

Transfer learning is a good solution to improving pathology image classification with limited labeled data by passing knowledge from the source domain to the target domain. However, the relevance between these domains is generally weak and leads to less effective transfers. Inspired by the gradual human learning and inference process using information with little relevance, we propose a stepwise transfer learning approach for DCNNs. To connect the two weakly related domains, the proposed stepwise transfer learning establishes a systematic procedure by introducing intermediate domains to form a bridge between the source and target domains. Initially, DCNNs acquire knowledge of the general object classification domain from open datasets such as ImageNet and CIFAR, which are very large and easy to access. Next, trained by intermediate datasets which are classified based on various pathology features, the DCNNs are expected to acquire pathology-related knowledge. As a result, the learned DCNNs will more accurately solve the final task using rich fundamental and specific knowledge. Intermediate datasets consist of unlabeled data, making the data demanded in the proposed approach relatively inexpensive and abundant. To realize the proposed conception, we also introduced several methods to generate target domain-related intermediate datasets.

In the following, some related works will be introduced in Sect. 2, and the details the stepwise transfer learning scheme and the generation methods of intermediate datasets will be provided in Sect. 3. Following this, experiments will be organized to evidence our proposed scheme in Sect. 4.

2 Related Works

2.1 Pathology Image Classification

Many early pathology image classification methods employed specified pathological features, such as epithelium ratio and nuclei-cytoplasmic ratio, that were precisely calculated from their image processing and analysis system [6]. Benign or malignant classification was conducted by comparing these features with predefined criteria. However, cancer cells are often differently abnormally shaped, and defining all the morphological anomaly patterns is difficult. Moreover, image processing failures such as cell segmentation may also directly lead to classification failures.

In the 2000s, approaches using handcrafted image features and classifiers based on statistical models became an established trend. Compared to methods using pathological features, handcrafted image features seemed able to provide more robustness and adaptability to various morphological appearances. For example, Esgiar et al. [7] employed the grey-level co-occurrence matrix (GLCM) to obtain texture features corresponding to contrast, entropy, angular second moment, dissimilarity and correlation from a colon biopsy, and employed linear discriminate analysis (LDA) and the k-nearest neighbor algorithm (KNN) to realize the categorization of normal and cancer colon mucosa. Likewise, James Diamond et al. [8] employed Haralick features (a classification of texture features developed using the GLCM) to identify tissue abnormalities in prostate pathology images. Local binary patterns (LBP) is another strong contender; Masood et al. [9] proposed a scheme consisting of LBP and support vector machines (SVM), which were demonstrated to be effective for colon pathology images. In another study, Sertel et al. [10] similarly developed a classification method for neuroblastoma H&E stained whole-slide images using co-occurrence statistics and LBP. A recent report by Kather et al. [11] gave a relatively comprehensive investigation of texture analysis for colorectal cancer pathology imaging; besides LBP and GLCM, lower- and higher-order histogram features, Gabor filters and perception-like features were also utilized. In our earlier studies [12], higher-order local auto correlation (HLAC) texture features bonded with linear statistical models such as the principal component analysis (PCA) based subspace method were also shown to be capable of indicating the anomaly degree of gastric pathology images.

While all of these handcrafted feature-based approaches show promising feasibility, intractable issues still exist between the research and practical applications. One particular instance is that the confirmation of the suitability of handcrafted features for certain tasks is rather difficult [13]. Additionally, the uneven H&E staining among the pathology images may have a negative impact on image processing and feature extraction, making the tasks more challenging [14–16].

2.2 Deep Learning in Image Classification

Since 2012, deep learning-based approaches have consistently shown best-in-class performance in major computer vision competitions. In the 2012 ImageNet Large Scale Visual Classification Challenge (ILSVRC), the 8-layer convolutional neural networks (CNN) proposed by Hinton won over all the other approaches using non-deep-learning

[17]. Following this, the trend in image classification research has rapidly changed from the conventional image feature-based approaches to deep learning-based approaches. Furthermore, since 2015, newer deep learning approaches even achieved a higher classification accuracy than the human average.

Specifically within the pathology image domain, many researchers have been inspired to develop deep learning-based classification and segmentation approaches [15, 18–22]. In the CAMALYON 2016 Grand Challenge, to evaluate the accuracy of detecting metastases from whole-slide images of lymph node sections, around 70% of the participating methods took advantage of deep learning-based approaches, leaving a small number of those using classical machine learning approaches [23]. One representative approach [24], presented a typical processing flow of pathology image classification using deep learning. Apart from classification and segmentation approaches, deep learning methods are also utilized in new, expanded applications of pathology diagnosis, including staining normalization [25], assessment of tumor proliferation [26], and comprehensive multimodal mapping between medical images and diagnostic reports [27].

2.3 Issues and Challenges

With the development of deep learning techniques, high expectations have been placed on deep learning-based CAD for pathology imaging. While DCNNs efficiently solve the most challenging problems, they require a large amount of labeled data for training [28]. However, unlike natural image datasets such as ImageNet and CIFAR which can be acquired using the Internet and automated categorizing techniques, building up high-quality pathology image datasets requires professional observation and annotation by pathologists. Because of the shortage and tremendous workload of pathologists, pathology image data labeled with diagnosis result is very difficult and expensive to obtain. Thus, maximizing the classification performance with limited labeled data to avoid much more expensive data labeling efforts has become an urgent and challenging task.

3 Proposed Method

3.1 Stepwise Transfer of Domain Knowledge for Computer-Aided Diagnosis in Pathology

When there is a shortage of training data, transfer learning, a method that borrows knowledge from the source domain and applies it to the target domain, is an efficient solution [29]. Practically, in transfer learning, the CNN model pre-trained in the source domain is employed as an initial model for the target domain. Compared with the random initialized state of a deep learning network when learning from scratch, a task in the target domain shares the millions of parameters of a pre-trained model that have been trained to a stable state. As a result, the borrowed knowledge facilitates classification tasks in the target domain with shorter training time and significantly less labeling effort.

Transfer learning works efficiently when the source and target domains are related in terms of relevance in models or features. When the source and target domains are weakly related or unrelated, transfer learning produces little effect on improving the final task. In the source domain, large object classification datasets such as ImageNet are often adopted, and as to our task in target domain refers to benign/malignant classification in pathology image. Humans have the ability to connect two unrelated concepts through experience gained from other intermediate concepts. For instance, after learning to ride a bicycle, it may be easier to master operating a helicopter if the person intermediately learned how to drive a car. Similarly, before new medical learning to diagnose a pathology image, learning related knowledge such as the definition of a cell can improve results.

In this paper, we have proposed a stepwise transfer of domain knowledge for CAD in pathology based on this gradual inference method [38]. It is believed to be necessary and possible to make deep neural networks learn to understand pathology images in a rational manner. DCNNs are expected to gradually get optimized with knowledge related to the target task and finally become highly adaptive to the task. At first, DCNNs should understand the difference between general visual characteristics, such as color and texture. Such information is deemed acquirable from the natural image domain. Then, DCNNs may concentrate more on structural and morphological characteristics, such as the size of cell, the degree of nucleus distortion, and nuclear-cytoplasmic ratio considered to be involved. At this stage, professional pathology-related knowledge is supplied, and owing to the progressive transfer process, DCNNs finally gain the competence to classify benign and malignant images.

For an intuitive understanding, a practical model of the stepwise transfer of domain knowledge is shown in Fig. 1 [38]. The framework consists of three parts: source domain, intermediate domain and target domain. In the source domain, ImageNet is employed and defined as "low-level" data, meaning that its target-task correlation is relatively low. Meanwhile, the ultimate task, classification of benign/malignant pathology images called "high-level" data, is placed at the end. Between these two domains, intermediate domains classify unlabeled pathology image data according to some pathological features to create "mid-level" data. The knowledge transfer is conducted from the source to the intermediate and finally to the target domain.

Under this framework, the core is the type of pathology-related knowledge to be employed in the intermediate domain, and how the classification task design is managed for certain pathology-related knowledge. For the first problem, breakthrough diagnostic criteria can be found; as stated earlier, structural and morphological characteristics, such as the tissue distribution, cell size, degree of nucleus distortion, and nuclear-cytoplasmic ratio are regarded as promising clues in diagnosis. At the same time, the principle of the second problem is that the classification design must avoid pathologists' expensive work as far as possible.

Hence, we propose the following ideas. The first is to make use of the tissue structure, which is one of the existing natural characteristics based on human observation in pathological images. Labeling for classification tasks could be done by a nonprofessional annotator. The second is to take advantage of cell morphological characteristics, which also provide crucial clues for diagnosis. In order to generate morphology classifications, which are difficult to cluster directly, we raise an automatic measurement of cell morphology. The third is to extend pathology-related knowledge by combining the above intermediate domains in order.

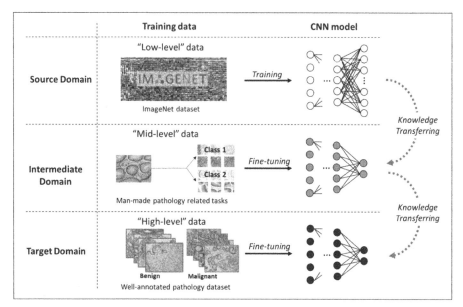

Fig. 1. Practical procedure of the proposed stepwise transfer of domain knowledge for computer-aided diagnosis in pathology [38].

3.2 Transfer of Pathological Knowledge Based on Human Observation

This section discusses the specific implementation of the first above-stated idea: to make use of the tissue structure as one of the existing natural characteristics in pathological images based on human observation. Based on investigation, this study presents a feasible stroma-epithelium dataset that can be made by non-professional annotator with minimal pathologist's direction. As naturally existing tissue structures, epithelium and stroma can be found in every organ [30, 31]. Epithelium is a type of tissue in which cells are packed into sheets to line the surfaces of structures throughout the body or organ, and stroma consists of all the parts of the tissue without specific organ functions. As shown in Fig. 2, the upper area encircled by dashed contours indicates epithelium issue, while the remaining lower area denotes stroma tissue. Although it is quite difficult to understand the two types of tissue for non-professional workers, it is found that stating the visual difference between them is fairly simple; such a distinct difference allows us to realize non-professional annotation. Without expensive pathologist's annotations, it would be advantageous if these tissue-wise (epithelium and stroma) data can impart pathology-related knowledge to DCNNs. We have experimentally collected a large number of images containing epithelium and stroma, after which they have been manually labeled according to the major presence of three classes (epithelium, stroma and background) in each image patch. An experiment for the idea transfer of pathological knowledge based on human observation of stroma-epithelium characteristics is shown in Sect. 4.

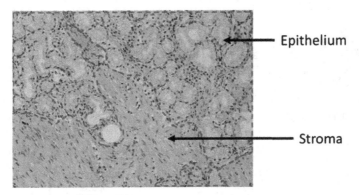

Fig. 2. Stroma and epithelium in a gastric pathology image.

3.3   Transfer of Pathological Knowledge Based on Automatic Measurement

Discussed here is another idea mentioned in Sect. 3.1: the extraction of cell morphological characteristics by automatic measurement. Cell-wise morphological characteristics, which may include the shape and size of the cell and the nuclei-cytoplasmic ratio, usually appear more miscellaneous than tissue-wise information. It is difficult to discern which parts of the images should be classified only by human observation, without any quantitative criteria. Therefore, to make use of this information, the proposed scheme introduces a specialized feature to measure morphological characteristics, and it performs classifications according to cell-wise morphological characteristics via unsupervised learning from a large quantity of data. This method achieves automatic classification; as a result, pathologists' work and even human annotation are avoided, and it becomes possible to generate "mid-level" data at almost zero cost from abundant unlabeled pathology data.

In order to build the automatic measurement, we attempt to evaluate cell-wise morphology through certain handcrafted features. According to our previous study [32], color index local auto-correlation (CILAC, [33]) has been evidenced as an independently competent handcrafted feature in pathology image classification. CILAC calculates the co-occurrence of certain color indexed regions, which are the background, nuclei and cytoplasm of the pathology image used. By quantifying the distribution among these regions, which are deemed to contain most of the crucial information for cell-wise morphological analysis, cell-wise morphology is also expected to be measured. Therefore, as shown in Fig. 3, CILAC based feature extraction is utilized for color-indexed images and cell-wise "mid-level" data are expected to be collected for fine-tuning.

Practically, we implement a string of automatic image pre-processing techniques including three-level quantization to obtain the color indexed background-nuclei-cytoplasm images. Afterwards, CILAC features are extracted from these three-level images, and PCA is used to reduce the dimensionality of the feature vector space. Next, unsupervised K-means clustering is employed to separate images into multiple clusters within the feature vector space. In order to feed DCNNs more explicit knowledge by using less obscure data, we set the number of clusters k = 3, and select the farthest two clusters within the coordinate space of principal components. Finally, the two clusters can be generated automatically.

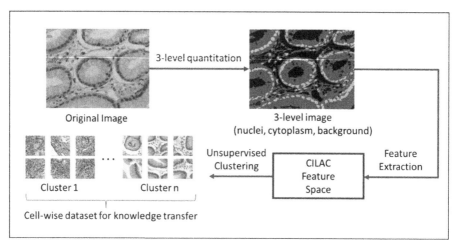

Fig. 3. Procedure of generating "mid-level" dataset with color index local auto-correlation (CILAC).

Specifically, the CILAC feature was developed on the basis of HLAC [34]. As shown in Fig. 4, CILAC consists of a set of local patterns that can calculate both the local auto-correlations of different color levels and their statistical distribution [38]. CILAC in order N ($N = 0, 1, 2$) is defined as

$$S_0(i) = \sum_r f_i(r) \tag{1}$$

$$S_1(i, j, a) = \sum_r f_i(r) f_j(r + a) \tag{2}$$

$$S_1(i, j, k, a, b) = \sum_r f_i(r) f_j(r + a) f_k(r + b) \tag{3}$$

where S_N denotes the Nth-order correlation. $f = \{e_1, e_2, e_3 \ldots, e_D\}$ is a D-dimensional vector standing for D color indexes of a color indexed image; r indicates the reference (central) pixel; a, b are different displacements of the surrounding inspected pixels, respectively, and f_i, f_j and f_k denote the pixels considered corresponding to all displacements. In this study, D is set to 3 according to three color indices of the three-level image. The zeroth order CILAC ($N = 0$) corresponds to an ordinary color histogram, and the first and second order CILAC ($N = 1$ and $N = 2$) represent the local co-occurrences of different color indices.

3.4 Stepwise Transfer of Multiple Domain Knowledge

Transfer of pathological knowledge based on direct human observation or automatic measurement has been proposed herein. Both proposed methods are conducted on a two-step transfer. However, stepwise transfer is not limited to the two-step way or a single intermediate domain. Just like the human learning process mentioned before, transfer knowledge of multiple intermediate domains step-by-step may lead to the CNN

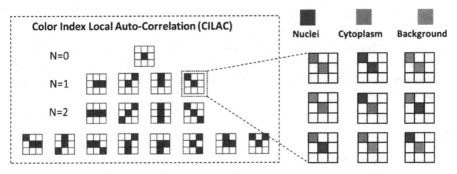

Fig. 4. CILAC mask patterns. (Color figure online)

models learning more and helping solve the final task. Therefore, to further strengthen the specialization of DCNNs, we verify the step-wise transfer of multiple domain knowledge (see Fig. 5).

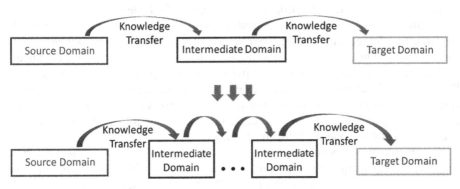

Fig. 5. Procedures of transfer of multiple domain knowledge.

Thus, after separately employing the two types of intermediate domain knowledge—tissue-wise and cell-wise knowledge—we will verify the feasibility of simultaneously using the two types of different knowledge to be transferred in one scheme. Although there are several combination ways of the two intermediate domains, to intuitively compare it with the two-step scheme, we execute a transfer in the order from tissue-wise knowledge to cell-wise knowledge as a representative. In practice, the CNN model pretrained by ImageNet is fine-tuned on the tissue-wise "mid-level" data in the first step. After that, cell-wise "mid-level" data are used to fine-tune the second step on the CNN model. Finally, the final classification task is conducted based on fine-tuning the third step of the CNN model trained with ImageNet, tissue-wise and cell-wise data.

4 Experiments and Discussions

To evaluate the effectiveness of our proposed scheme, with the tissue-wise and cell-wise "mid-level" data, stepwise knowledge transfer will be implemented on several representative CNN architectures, including VGG-16 [35], AlexNet [17], and GoogLeNet [36].

The performances of two-step domain transfer based on tissue-wise and cell-wise data will be compared to the commonly used one-step fine-tuning scheme in which knowledge transfer is directly conducted from a "low-level" domain to a "high-level" domain. Furthermore, a comparison will be drawn between the performance of our proposed multiple domain knowledge transfer, employing both tissue-wise and cell-wise data and the two-step method.

4.1 Data

This paper employs three types of data—"low-level", "mid-level" and "high-level" data— used for the initialization (pretraining), middle fine-tuning, and the final fine-tuning, respectively. In practice, ImageNet data containing approximately 1.2 million images in 1,000 separate categories are customarily utilized to initialize the CNN models. As for pathology data, we use data on gastric pathologies collected by two experienced pathologists, and some of the pathologies are annotated as either benign or malignant. All pathology images are cut off from entire pathology images into patches, each having a size of 256 × 256 pixels. All pathology data are listed in Table 1.

To investigate the performance of benign/malignant classification in the proposed step-wise transfer learning scheme, we make use of 5,400 benign and 5,400 malignant patches from the labeled data as "high-level" dataset in the target domain. Datasets in the intermediate domain are constructed from the remaining unlabeled pathology data. We manage to label the data manually as epithelium, stroma and background, and we considered 16,000 patches of each category as tissue-wise data. For cell-wise data, by adopting unsupervised clustering, we succeeded at obtaining 5,574 patches belonging to cluster 1 and 4,388 patches belonging to cluster 2.

Except from the former datasets, we additionally use a separated test dataset of 2,700 benign and 2,700 malignant patches to make a fair evaluation of the performance in each optional case. There is no overlap between the "mid-level" datasets and the "high-level" datasets; meanwhile, there is no overlap among the training, validation, and test datasets.

Table 1. Datasets used in the experiment.

	Category	Training	Validation	Test
Intermediate domain: Tissue-wise	Background	15,000	1,000	–
	Epithelium	15,000	1,000	–
	Stroma	15,000	1,000	–
Intermediate domain: Cell-wise	Cluster 1	5,016	558	–
	Cluster 2	3,949	439	–
Target domain	Benign	5,400	1,620	2,700
	Malignant	5,400	1,620	2,700

4.2   Results and Discussions

The performances of the benign/malignant classification task for different deep neural network architectures are demonstrated. This experiment concurrently adopts commonly used metrics in classification, area under the curve (AUC) of receiver operating characteristic (ROC) and F-score, as the evaluation criteria [37]. AUC of ROC provides an aggregate measure of performance across all possible classification thresholds. The F1 score is a measure of a test's accuracy at a certain classification threshold.

As shown in Table 2, AUC = 0.922 is achieved by learning-from-scratch approach adopting VGG-16 using the same "High-level" data. Both schemes using one-step and two-step knowledge transfer have achieved better performance almost at the same degree. It is confirmed that rather than learning from scratch, using large-scale data to initialize deep neural networks often leads to better accuracy. Furthermore, on comparing with the one-step transfer learning on ImageNet, the proposed two-step knowledge transfer using tissue-wise data and the one using cell-wise data both yielded notable promotion for all tree CNN architectures. Specifically, AUC value is raised from 0.936 to 0.963 and 0.957, respectively, in both two proposed methods, when CNN architectures VGG-16 is adopted. Besides, the F-score (for which we set the classification threshold to 0.5) also has a significant improvement. More intuitive comparisons are shown in Fig. 6 in terms of the ROC curves of VGG16. These results have illustrated that our proposed schemes are capable and are rarely dependent on the deep neural network's architecture.

Table 2. Performance of the one-step method vs. tissue-wise two-step method vs. cell-wise two-step method.

Scheme	CNN Architecture					
	VGG-16		AlexNet		GoogLeNet	
	AUC	F1	AUC	F1	AUC	F1
Learning-from-scratch	0.922	–	–	–	–	–
One-step on ImageNet	0.936	0.81	0.867	0.795	0.881	0.785
Two-step: Tissue-wise	0.963	0.885	0.92	0.84	0.934	0.86
Two-step: Cell-wise	0.957	0.87	0.923	0.845	0.939	0.865

In addition, a set of filter responses for a gray image exported by the final model of each approach is displayed in Fig. 7. We investigate on VGG-16 and obtain some outcomes of the first convolution layers (cov1) as a representative. These intuitive results would help us obtain a better understanding of how the proposed approaches work. Usually, the lower convolution layers are responsible for capturing the interpretable low-level features such as edges, texture, and gradient orientation. From Fig. 7, we can see that the interior of deep neural network changes depending on which of the four approaches is used. Compared to learning-from-scratch and one-step transfer learning on ImageNet, the CNN models in proposed two-step knowledge transfer (c) (d) extracts more morphological features. In Fig. 7(c), some assemble of cells appear in the left

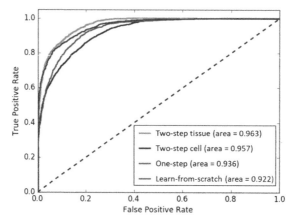

Fig. 6. ROC curves of the four schemes in VGG16.

middle and left bottom filter responses. We speculate that the CNN model focuses on more structural features by introducing structural information in two-step transfer based on tissue-wise data. In Fig. 7(d), some cell-like shapes can be observed in the right filter response images. It is considered that more cell morphological features are extracted by the CNN model after introducing the two-step transfer based on cell-wise data. Therefore, the feasibility of our proposed method using both tissue-wise and cell-wise-based data were proved to a certain extent.

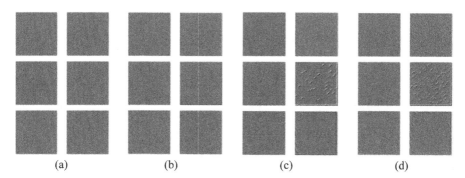

Fig. 7. Set of filter response (cov1) outputted by the VGG-16 model: (a) learning-from-scratch; (b) one-step; (c) two-step based on tissue-wise data; (d) two-step based on cell-wise data.

In this experiment, we execute a three-step transfer and employ two intermediate domains in the order from tissue-wise to cell-wise domain. The experiment is conducted on the VGG-16 model and evaluated by AUC. For a fair comparison of the two-step method and three-step method based on their combination, the total amount of training data employed in each method is set to 8,000 patches. As shown in Table 3, we can easily conclude that the three-step method transferring the tissue-wise to cell-wise domain in order brings about an improvement in performance improvement compared to the two-step method without adding new data into the intermediate domain. As the result, transferring multiple domain knowledge step by step is demonstrated to be feasible.

Table 3. Results of multiple domain knowledge transfer (three-step) vs. two-step method.

Category	Two-step: Tissue-wise	Two-step: Cell-wise	Three-step: Tissue-wise + Cell-wise
Size of dataset	8,000	8,000	4,000 + 4,000
AUC	0.961	0.965	0.969

5   Conclusions

In this paper, we study the problem of lack of pathology image data labeled by pathologists as well as the high cost to label new data when building CAD for pathology image based on DCNN approaches. When transfer learning is adopted to overcome labeled data shortage, weak relevance between the source domain and the target domain often makes the transfer less effective. To solve these problems, we proposed a stepwise domain knowledge transfer scheme. Following the natural step-by-step process humans undertake to learn and make inferences, this scheme introduces intermediate domains to bridge the source and target domain knowledge. The intermediate domains take advantages of unlabeled pathology image data, and two types of knowledge to be transferred have been presented. One type of knowledge can be directly generated based on human observation, while another type is generated based on automatic measurement. Specifically, the knowledge generated based on human observation is inspired by the distinct appearance of natural morphology in pathology images. The classification of stroma and epithelium through simple annotation operations by a non-professional annotator with only the pathologist's initial direction is employed. In knowledge transfer based on automatic measurement, cell-pathology information is extracted with handcrafted feature CILAC. Comparative experiments have been performed among different deep neural networks, and the proposed two-step knowledge transfer scheme, based on tissue or cell-wise data, is observed to be effective at contributing to boosting the classification accuracy in line with the results.

Furthermore, this research has explored step-wise transfer of multiple domain knowledge by introducing both tissue-wise data and cell-wise data into the knowledge transfer process in order. As a result, sequential knowledge transfer has brought about further enhancement. With the proposed methods, the AUC has raised significantly from 0.922 in learning-from-scratch to 0.969 under the VGG16 model.

In this paper, we regarded the final classification accuracy as the only evaluation standard. However, the training performance of the intermediate domain data is expected to be considered in a future study. In addition, introducing a parallel transfer of multiple intermediate domains such as multi-task learning may be an interesting way to realize a more powerful step-wise knowledge transfer.

References

1. Ferlay, J., et al.: Cancer incidence and mortality worldwide: sources, methods and major patterns in GLOBOCAN 2012. Int. J. Cancer **136**(5), E359–E386 (2005)
2. Morrison, A.O., Gardner, J.M.: Microscopic image photography techniques of the past, present, and future. Arch. Pathol. Lab. Med. **139**(12), 1558–1564 (2015)
3. The Japanese society of pathology: the Japanese society of pathology guideline 2015, In: The Japanese Society of Pathology, p. 6 (2015)
4. Robboy, S.J., et al.: Pathologist workforce in the United States: I. Development of a predictive model to examine factors influencing supply. Arch. Pathol. Lab. Med. **137**(12), 1723–1732 (2013)
5. How telemedicine answers global pathology demands. https://proscia.com/blog/2015/07/14/global-crisis-digital-solution. Accessed 19 Mar 2018
6. Jondet, M., Agoli-Agbo, R., Dehennin, L.: Automatic measurement of epithelium differentiation and classification of cervical intraneoplasia by computerized image analysis. Diagn. Pathol. **5**(1), 7 (2010). https://doi.org/10.1186/1746-1596-5-7
7. Esgiar, A.N., Naguib, R.N., Sharif, B.S., Bennett, M.K., Murray, A.: Microscopic image analysis for quantitative measurement and feature identification of normal and cancerous colonic mucosa. IEEE Trans. Inf. Technol. Biomed. **2**(3), 197–203 (1998)
8. Diamond, J., Anderson, N.H., Bartels, P.H., Montironi, R., Hamilton, P.W.: The use of morphological characteristics and texture analysis in the identification of tissue composition in prostatic neoplasia. Hum. Pathol. **35**(9), 1121–1131 (2004)
9. Masood, K., Rajpoot, N.: Texture based classification of hyperspectral colon biopsy samples using CLBP. In: 2009 IEEE International Symposium on Biomedical Imaging: From Nano to Macro, pp. 1011–1014 (2009)
10. Sertel, O., Kong, J., Shimada, H., Catalyurek, U.V., Saltz, J.H., Gurcan, M.N.: Computer-aided prognosis of neuroblastoma on whole-slide images: classification of stromal development. Pattern Recogn. **42**(6), 1093–1103 (2009)
11. Kather, J.N., et al.: Multi-class texture analysis in colorectal cancer histology. Sci. Rep. **6**, 27988 (2016)
12. Qu, J., Nosato, H., Sakanashi, H., Terai, K., Hiruta, N.: Cancer detection from pathological images using higher-order local autocorrelation feature. In: 2012 IEEE 11th International Conference on Signal Processing, vol. 2, pp. 1198–1201 (2012)
13. Shen, D., Wu, G., Suk, H.I.: Deep learning in medical image analysis. Annu. Rev. Biomed. Eng. **19**, 221–248 (2017)
14. Raphaël, M.: The need for careful data collection for pattern recognition in digital pathology. J. Pathol. Inf. **8**(19) (2017)
15. Chen, H., Qi, X., Yu, L., Heng, P.A.: DCAN: deep contour-aware networks for accurate gland segmentation. In: Proceedings of the IEEE Conference on Computer Vision and Pattern Recognition, pp. 2487–2496 (2016)
16. Bejnordi, B.E., et al.: Stain specific standardization of whole-slide histopathological images. IEEE Trans. Med. Imaging **35**(2), 404–415 (2015)
17. Krizhevsky, A., Sutskever, I., Hinton, G.E.: Imagenet classification with deep convolutional neural networks. In: Advances in Neural Information Processing Systems, pp. 1097–1105 (2012)
18. Xu, Y., et al.: Large scale tissue histopathology image classification, segmentation, and visualization via deep convolutional activation features. BMC Bioinform. **18**(1), 281 (2017)
19. Hou, L., Samaras, D., Kurc, T.M., Gao, Y., Davis, J.E., Saltz, J.H.: Patch-based convolutional neural network for whole slide tissue image classification. In: Proceedings of the IEEE Conference on Computer Vision and Pattern Recognition, pp. 2424–2433 (2016)

20. Xu, J., Luo, X., Wang, G., Gilmore, H., Madabhushi, A.: A deep convolutional neural network for segmenting and classifying epithelial and stromal regions in histopathological images. Neurocomputing **191**, 214–223 (2016)
21. Sirinukunwattana, K., et al.: Gland segmentation in colon histology images: the glas challenge contest. Med. Image Anal. **35**, 489–502 (2017)
22. Ciompi, F., et al.: The importance of stain normalization in colorectal tissue classification with convolutional networks. In: 2017 IEEE 14th International Symposium on Biomedical Imaging (ISBI 2017), pp. 160–163 (2017)
23. Shah, M., Wang, D., Rubadue, C., Suster, D., Beck, A.: Deep learning assessment of tumor proliferation in breast cancer histological images. In: 2017 IEEE International Conference on Bioinformatics and Biomedicine (BIBM), pp. 600–603 (2017)
24. Zhang, Z., Xie, Y., Xing, F., McGough, M., Yang, L.: MDNet: a semantically and visually interpretable medical image diagnosis network. In: Proceedings of the IEEE Conference on Computer Vision and Pattern Recognition, pp. 6428–6436 (2017)
25. Han, Z., Wei, B., Zheng, Y., Yin, Y., Li, K., Li, S.: Breast cancer multi-classification from histopathological images with structured deep learning model. Sci. Rep. **7**(1), 4172 (2017)
26. CAMELYON16. https://camelyon16.grand-challenge.org/
27. Wang, D., Khosla, A., Gargeya, R., Irshad, H., Beck, A.H.: Deep learning for identifying metastatic breast cancer. arXiv preprint arXiv:1606.05718 (2016)
28. Mao, J., Xu, W., Yang, Y., Wang, J., Huang, Z., Yuille, A.: Deep captioning with multimodal recurrent neural networks (m-RNN). arXiv preprint arXiv:1412.6632 (2014)
29. Pan, S.J., Yang, Q.: A survey on transfer learning. IEEE Trans. Knowl. Data Eng. **22**(10), 1345–1359 (2009)
30. Guarino, M., Micheli, P., Pallotti, F.: Pathological relevance of epithelial and mesenchymal phenotype plasticity. Pathol. – Res. Pract. **195**(6), 379–389 (1999)
31. Wiseman, B.S., Werb, Z.: Stromal effects on mammary gland development and breast cancer. Science **296**(5570), 1046–1049 (2002)
32. Qu, J., Nosato, H., Sakanashi, H., Takahashi, E., Terai, K., Hiruta, N.: Computational cancer detection of pathological images based on an optimization method for color-index local autocorrelation feature extraction. In: 2014 IEEE 11th International Symposium on Biomedical Imaging (ISBI), pp. 822–825 (2014)
33. Kobayashi, T., Otsu, N.: Color image feature extraction using color index local autocorrelations. In: 2009 IEEE International Conference on Acoustics, Speech and Signal Processing, pp. 1057–1060 (2009)
34. Otsu, N., Kurita, T.: A new scheme for practical flexible and intelligent vision systems. In: MVA, pp. 431–435 (1988)
35. Simonyan, K., Zisserman, A.: Very deep convolutional networks for large-scale image recognition. arXiv preprint arXiv:1409.1556 (2014)
36. He, K., Zhang, X., Ren, S., Sun, J.: Delving deep into rectifiers: Surpassing human-level performance on imagenet classification. In: Proceedings of the IEEE International Conference on Computer Vision, pp. 1026–1034 (2015)
37. Sokolova, M., Lapalme, G.: A systematic analysis of performance measures for classification tasks. Inf. Process. Manag. **45**(4), 427–437 (2009)
38. Jia, Q., Nobuyuki, H., Kensuke, T., Hirokazu, N., Masahiro, M., Hidenori, S.: Enhanced deep learning for pathology image classification: a knowledge transfer based stepwise fine-tuning scheme. In: 6th International Conference on BIOIMAGING, pp. 92–99 (2019)

Simultaneous Segmentation of Retinal OCT Images Using Level Set

Bashir Isa Dodo[1]([✉]), Yongmin Li[1], Muhammad Isa Dodo[2], and Xiaohui Liu[1]

[1] Brunel University London, London UB8 3PH, UK
{Bashir.Dodo,Yongmin.Li,XiaoHui.Liu}@brunel.ac.uk
[2] Katsina State Institute of Technology and Management, Katsina, Nigeria
muhammaddodo40@gmail.com

Abstract. Medical images play a vital role in clinical diagnosis and treatments of various diseases. In the field of ophthalmology, Optical coherence tomography (OCT) has become an integral part of the non-invasive advanced eye examination by providing images of the retina in high resolution. Reliable identification of the retinal layers is necessary for the extraction of clinically useful information used for tracking the progress of medication and diagnosing various ocular diseases because changes to retinal layers highly correlate with the manifestation of eye diseases. Owing to the complexity of retinal structures and the cumbersomeness of manual segmentation, many computer-based methods are proposed to aid in extracting useful layer information. Additionally, image artefacts and inhomogeneity of pathological structures of the retina pose challenges by significantly degrading the performance of these computational methods. To handle some of these challenges, this paper presents a fully automated method for segmenting retinal layers in OCT images using a level set method. The method starts by establishing a specific Region of interest (ROI), which aids in handling over- and under-segmentation of the target layers by allowing only the layer and image features to influence the curve evolution. An appropriate level set initiation is devised by refining the edges from the image gradient. Then the prior understanding of the OCT image is utilised in constraining the evolution process to segment seven layers of the retina simultaneously. Promising experimental results have been achieved on 225 OCT images, which show the method converges close to the actual layer boundaries compared to the ground truth images.

Keywords: Image segmentation · Level set · Evolution constrained optimisation · Optical Coherence Tomography · Medical image analysis

1 Introduction

Medical images have an irrefutable role in health care by improving the process of diagnosing and treating a vast number of ailments [2]. Notably, the field of ophthalmology has witnessed a significant improvement since the introduction

© Springer Nature Switzerland AG 2020
A. Roque et al. (Eds.): BIOSTEC 2019, CCIS 1211, pp. 120–136, 2020.
https://doi.org/10.1007/978-3-030-46970-2_7

of Optical Coherence Tomography (OCT) [13], which is a non-invasive imaging technique used for retinal imaging with high acquisition speed, and a resolution of approximately 5–7 μm [1,14,20]. In current ophthalmology, identifying various layers of the retina on OCT has become a vital tool for diagnosing and tracking the progress of medication of various visual impairments [1]. There is a continuous intrigue in OCT image analysis because individual layer thicknesses provide useful diagnostic information that have been shown to correlate well with the measures of severity in major eye diseases, such as glaucoma, diabetic retinopathy, and age-related macular degeneration. However, since manual segmentation is not only tedious but also subjected to intra- and inter-grader variance [28], many automatic methods are proposed to assist with the segmentation process [22], which are critical for full utilisation of the available technology [16]. For this reason, much research is carried out on retinal layer segmentation to help eye specialists in diagnosing and preventing the most common causes of vision loss in the developed world. Research in computer-based retinal OCT segmentation aims to improve various aspects including computational time, computational complexity the number of layers segmented, and the use of prior knowledge. Generally, segmentation is partitioning based on some image characteristics. How these characteristics are defined determines the computation burden of the algorithm. In some cases, this computational burden is reduced through dynamic programming [4] or topology modification [17]. The number of questions (conditions) an algorithm has to check or satisfy is usually the most crucial factor.

Moreover, Markov Boundary Model [15], later extended by [3], geodesic distance [11], level sets [7,19,26], graph-based methods [4,6,8,12], and machine learning [16] have been used in the segmentation of retinal OCT images. Although the level sets method has automatic topological handling, the steps can be computationally expensive [21], while adding complex constraints in the segmentation method usually increases the complexity of an algorithm.

Furthermore, under and over-segmentation are both phenomenon to be avoided when dealing with medical images, as falling on either side may affect the outcome of the diagnosis. These phenomena are among the major challenges of target-based segmentation. Whereby more regions or objects are delineated by segmentation methods, which then complicates the proper identification of which region was segmented. In OCT image noise and artifacts can easily lure algorithms into segmenting the wrong features [8], because the intensity values are inhomogeneous and other features such as the vitreous cortex resemble the actual retinal layers.

This paper extends our previous work [10], which incorporates simple yet efficient topological constraints to the evolution process of the level set method, to improve accuracy and reduce the computational complexity for OCT image segmentation. The method is based on the following considerations: 1. The image gradients are used to initialise curves, which ensures appropriate image-specific initial contours for each image under investigation to handle under-segmentation and over-segmentation of the image; 2. The evolution of each initial curve is based on layer arrangements explicitly and the OCT topology implicitly. The method partitions an OCT image into 7 segments, relating to : Nerve Fibre Layer (NFL); Ganglion Cell Layer + Inner Plexiform Layer + Inner Nuclear Layer (GCL + IPL + INL); Outer Plexiform Layer (OPL); Outer Nuclear Layer to Inner Segment (ONL+IS), Outer Segment (OS) and Retinal Pigment Epithelium (RPE). Locations of these layers on an OCT image are shown in Fig. 1. The organisation of the rest of the paper is as follows. Section 2 discusses the details of the proposed method. Experimental results and discussions are treated in Sect. 3. Finally, conclusions are drawn in Sect. 4.

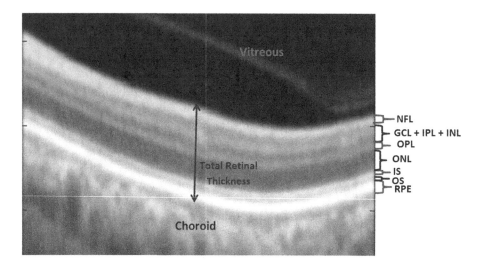

Fig. 1. Location of Nerve Fibre Layer (NFL); Ganglion Cell Layer + Inner Plexiform Layer + Inner Nuclear Layer (GCL + IPL + INL); Outer Plexiform Layer (OPL); Outer Nuclear Layer to Inner Segment (ONL + IS), Outer Segment (OS), Retinal Pigment Epithelium (RPE) and the total retinal thickness, on an OCT image [10].

2   Segmentation of OCT Images

A schematic depiction of the proposed method for segmenting retinal OCT images is illustrated in Fig. 2, and details of each step are elaborated in the succeeding subsections.

2.1   Pre-processing

The method establishes a distinct region of interest (ROI) to aid in the segmentation process. The preprocessing steps are employed to aid in plausible segmentation of the retinal layers, and a visual illustration of these steps is provided in Fig. 3. Initially, each OCT B-scan image I is enhanced with a Gaussian filter ($\sigma = 3$) to reduce the image noise. Referring to Fig. 1, the layers segmented in this study and most other segmentation methods, e.g. [4,9,18] lie within the total retinal thickness (TRT). The TRT starts from the boundary separating the retinal nerve fibre layer and the vitreous (ILM) at the top and ends with the boundary separating the RPE and the choroid (RPE) at the bottom of Fig. 1. As such, it is befitting to obtain a desired ROI with beneficial layer information solely. In retinal layer segmentation, it is commonly agreed that the NFL, IS-OS and RPE exhibit high reflectivity in an OCT image [4,18,23]. Also, based on experiments, the ILM and RPE exhibits the highest transitions from dark-bright and bright-dark, respectively [8]. Hence, the ILM and RPE are identified using the shortest path [5], by searching for the highest transitions on two separate adjacency matrices [4].

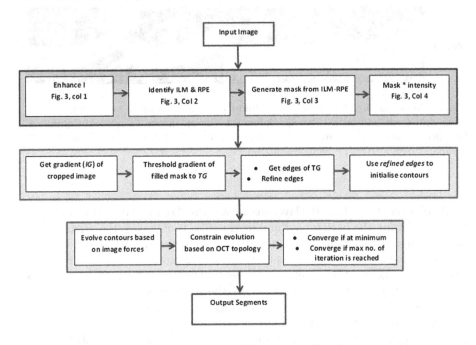

Fig. 2. Schematic representation of the proposed level set approach.

Further, the image is cropped to $I_{cropped}$ using the identified ILM and RPE points. This process is to assists in dealing with layer-like structures outside the ROI, and to reduce the computational cost associated with handling image background during segmentation. The preprocessing is vital in our segmentation process because only the actual layer properties impact the evolution of the curve. The next procedure is to generate a mask I_{mask} of the cropped image $I_{cropped}$. The I_{mask} is multiplied by the original image I to fill the (area in whit in Fig. 3, column 3) mask with actual intensity values of the original image I. The result of the multiplication is shown in Fig. 3, column 4, and expressed by the equation below:

$$I_{processed} = I_{mask} * I \tag{1}$$

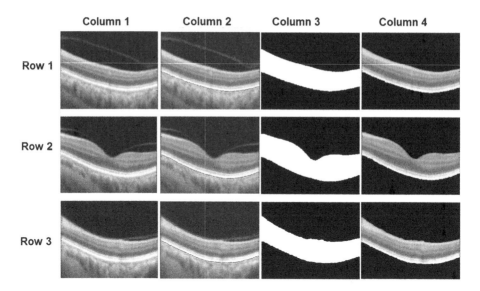

Fig. 3. Preprocessing steps showing: Column 1 - Enhanced images; Column 2 - identified ILM (red) and RPE (Green); Column 3 - image masks I_{mask}; and Column 4 - Cropped images $I_{cropped}$. Row 1 - Nasal region; Row 2 - Foveal Region; and Row 3 - Temporal region [10]. (Color figure online)

By observing Fig. 4(a), the layer-like area highlighted in red will be initialised, thereby allowing the background and image noise to influence the segmentation processes negatively. To avoid this negative effect, we establish the ROI based on the part of the image that contains useful information only, as shown in Fig. 4(b). Accordingly, the establishment of a distinct ROI is essential, considering that only the layer structures are obtained when the gradient of the image is acquired. Also, the ROI complements the thresholding and refinement processes in the layer initialisation stage. Additionally, it is imperative to consider the output of previous steps and their impact on subsequent steps in image analysis to enable robust performance. The employed preprocessing step is streamlined to eliminate the need for handling background as depicted in Fig. 4 and further discussed in the next few Subsects. 2.2 and 2.3. The size of the cropped image is used in subsequent processes to reduce computational time further and to eliminate the need for storing idle points.

2.2   Boundary Initialisation

Inherent of the nature of $I_{processed}$, it's vertical gradient $\nabla I_{processed}$ is obtained and then thresholded by a constant T, where T is set to 0.0018. The constant T should ideally have a low value to avoid getting more components, especially in the GCL - IPL regions, which will negatively impact the segmentation results. Based on the understanding that retinal layers span the image horizontally [4,8],

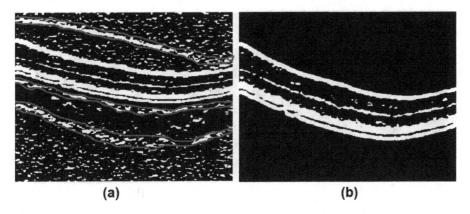

(a)   **(b)**

Fig. 4. Gradient of full image (Fig. 3 Column 1, Row 1) with background noise and layer-like structures in red (a), and thresholded gradient TG of preprocessed (Fig. 3 - Column 4, Row 1) with ROI only (b) [10]. (Color figure online)

the edges of the thresholded gradient TG image (Fig. 5(a)) are obtained and then refined in two simple steps. First, using area opening ([25], where any component (group of pixels) less than P pixels ($P = 30$ pixels) is removed from the TG image (most especially the GCL to IPL regions). Second, any fragmentary layer line is extrapolated to span the image horizontally by connecting broken lines to the most adjacent points. The consequence of the refinement is to ensure that each layer line starts from the first column and ends at the last column of the image (Fig. 5(b)). For this reason, only complete layer lines are initialised and evolved to ensure accurate segmentation further. In other words, neither merging nor splitting of boundaries is allowed, which limits under- or over-segmentation of the image. Generally, if the layers from the GCL to INL are to be segmented, then the refinement step can be overlooked. However, this will necessitate appropriate techniques for handling the splitting and merging of boundaries, and also alternative measures to rightly identify which layers are segmented. To proceed, the edges of the refined image serve as initial layer boundaries, such that in converging, the number of identified regions in the final output cannot exceed the number of the initialised curves. It is important to note that T is inversely proportional to P because the size of the small components remaining in Fig. 5(b) will increase with a smaller T. The level set function is initialised by representing each boundary curve C_b appropriately by a set of $C_b(x, y)$ on the image.

2.3   Boundary Evolution

The evolution of each initial boundary curve C_b is determined by a speed field F derived from the following differential equation [21]:

$$\frac{dC_b}{dt} = F\boldsymbol{N} \tag{2}$$

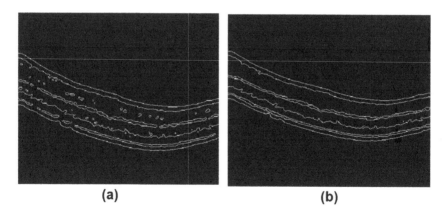

(a)   **(b)**

Fig. 5. Edges before refinement (a), and refined edges used for boundary initialisation (b) [10].

where N is the normal force of the curve pointing outward. The speed field F is comprised of an external speed from the image data and a characteristic speed based on C_b. Moreover, F could incorporate additional generated forces, such as the balloon force. We associate F and the ensuing evolution with a gradient descent solution based on the Mumford-Shah model [24]. Specifically, a curve C_b evolves until it gets to a local minimum C_{bmin} of the energy. In other words, a curve continues to evolve until it reaches static points of the dynamic equation (2). Adapting from [21], a layer boundary is uniquely represented by two lists of inside L_{in} and outside L_{out} points of C_b defined as follows:

$$L_{out} = \{x | \phi(x) > 0 \text{ and } \exists y \in N(x) : \phi(y) < 0\}$$
$$L_{in} = \{x | \phi(x) < 0 \text{ and } \exists y \in N(x) : \phi(y) > 0\}$$

where $N(x)$ is a distinct neighbourhood of x in the level set function ϕ at pixel x. Based on this definition, a positive force moves a point from L_{in} to L_{out} and a negative force moves a point from L_{out} to L_{in}. Each point (x, y) in level set function is defined in relation to the curve C_b as follows: [21]:

$$\phi = \begin{cases} 3, & \text{if } x, y \text{ is outside } C_b \text{ and } x, y \notin L_{out}; \\ 1, & \text{if } x, y \in L_{out}; \\ -3, & \text{if } x, y \text{ is inside } C_b \text{ and } x, y \notin L_{in}; \\ -1, & \text{if } x, y \in L_{in}. \end{cases} \quad (3)$$

Based on the representation of ϕ in equation (3), it is undemanding to recognise the position of a point (x, y) on the image in connection to C_b. We use a 2D list to represent initial boundary points and to save the positions of final boundary points, which facilitates mapping of the final image output. Alternatively, a 1-D list can be used to save the boundary points at position ϕ, as may be inferred from Liu et al. [17] who represented 3D with a 2D list. A boundary position (x, y)

of ϕ expands or shrinks based on the sign (+ or -) at the boundary position:

$$\begin{cases} \text{Expand}(x,y): & C_b(x,y) := C_b(x,y) + 1 \\[2ex] \text{Shrink}(x,y): & C_b(x,y) := C_b(x,y) - 1 \end{cases} \quad (4)$$

The evolution of each point is determined by the image forces computed by a fast gradient vector field [27] and controlled by topology constraints to be described in the subsequent Subsect. 2.4.

2.4   Boundary Topology Constrains

The ordering of the retinal layers is essential in the clinical application of OCT segmentation, and therefore must be preserved, as highlighted earlier in Subsect. 2.1. Taking into account the architectural appearance of the layers both naturally and on an OCT image, a boundary C_{b2} is always below C_{b1} for any given boundaries C_{b1} and C_{b2}. As such, a point (x,y) on the curve will neither Shrink nor Expand if it makes $C_{b1}(x,y) \leq C_{b2}(x,y)$. Hence, with the appropriate boundary initialisation, the layering topology requirement is enforced by carrying out this manageable topology validation before either shrinking or expanding any boundary point.

Furthermore, an intuitive approach is employed to better ensure the preservation of the layering topology, by additionally refining the above constraint in the vertical direction exclusively:

1. Because each layer boundary spans the image horizontally (one boundary point per column) we add a condition for evolving a boundary point $C_b(x,y)$ to a new boundary point $C_{bmin}(x,y)$. We restrict $Expand(x,y)$ if its neighbour points are u consecutive points above it; do not $Shrink(x,y)$ if its neighbour points are u consecutive points below it;
2. Looking at the sample of initial layer boundaries in Fig. 5, a boundary point $C_b(x,y)$ is limited to a maximum of v operations (either $Expand$ or $Shrink$) consecutively in the vertical direction. This condition restricts the region in which the method searches for a boundary.

The parameters u and v are two priors, which are set to 3 and 20, respectively. The parameter u aids with boundary smoothness and avoiding peaks for $Expand(x,y)$ or valleys for $Shrink(x,y)$ on the boundaries, while v further ensures the layered architecture is preserved. These constraints further indicate how a previous step complements the ensuing processes. Because with the befitting layer initialisation, the starting points for each layer are based on the individual image. Essentially, the topology constraints facilitate the evolution because the validation is performed before expanding or shrinking a boundary. Perhaps, this might not be ideal for abnormal structures, due to broken layers. However, considering the ordering of the layers where C_{b2} will always be below C_{b1} the layers will move together even in the case of abnormal retinal structure. The details of our algorithm from initialisation to convergence is illustrated in Algorithm 1. The segmentation pipeline ensures all targeted layers are segmented. Refined edges of TG are used in initialising the contours, which enables the differentiation of the segmented layers easily. The unique boundaries are constrained based on layer arrangements. Also, due to the understanding and unchanging nature of the OCT, a layer will always be above the one below it, even in unhealthy images, we can identify which layers were segmented in the output.

3   Results and Discussions

The images utilised in this study were captured using the Heidelberg SD-OCT Spectralis HRA imaging system (Heidelberg Engineering, Heidelberg, Germany) in Tongren Hospital, China. Non-invasive OCT imaging centred at the macular region was acquired from 13 subjects between the age of 20 to 85 years. Evaluation is carried out using 225 images, comprising of 75 images each from the temporal, nasal and foveal regions. The original size of each image is 512 by 992 pixels, with a resolution of 16 bits per pixel. We crop 15% of the image from the top to remove part of the image with no features of interest. In our experiments $N(x) = 8$ neighbourhood, mainly, because only the layers are remaining in the cropped image and the effect of inhomogeneity is reduced. Experimental results show that our method successfully segments seven layers of the retina. Visual outputs of the method from the three regions are shown in Fig. 6. Three criteria, namely the Dice (score or coefficient), accuracy, sensitivity (true positive rate (TPR)) were chosen to evaluate the method's performance, which are computed using equation (5), below:

$$
\begin{aligned}
Accuracy &= \frac{TP + TN}{(TP + FP + FN + TN)} \\
Sensitivity(TPR) &= \frac{TP}{(TP + FN)} \\
Dice &= \frac{2TP}{2TP + FP + FN}
\end{aligned}
\tag{5}
$$

where TP, TN, FP and FN refers to true positive, true negative, false positive and false negative respectively. TP represents the number of pixels which are part of the region that are labeled correctly by both the method and the ground truth. TN represents the number of pixels which are part of the background region and labeled correctly by both the method and the ground truth. FP represents the number of pixels labeled as a part of the region by the method but labeled as a part of the background by the ground truth. The average of these evaluation criteria (from equation (5)) with their respective standard deviations compared to the ground truth labelling is shown in Table 1. As can be inferred from the evaluation matrix in Table 1, promising results have been achieved by the method in converging at curves C_{bmin} very close to the actual layer boundaries.

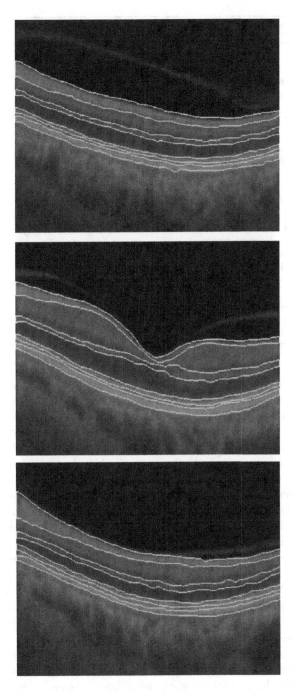

Fig. 6. From top to Bottom: Sample results from Nasal, Foveal and Temporal regions respectively [10].

Algorithm 1. Boundary Evolution.

1: Initialise Boundaries
2: **procedure** LOOP
3:     **if** evolution will not make $C_{b1}(x, y) \leq C_{b2}(x, y)$ **then**
4:         %% Shrink Boundary
5:         **if** neighbours of $C_b(x, y) \neq$ consecutive u points below it **then**
6:             **if** $C_b(x, y)$ has not moved v consecutive points in the vertical direction **then**
7:                 **if** force at point is negative **then**
8:                     $Shrink(x, y)$
9:                 **end if**
10:             **end if**
11:         **end if**
12:         %% Expand Boundaries.
13:         **if** neighbours of $C_b(x, y) \neq$ consecutive u points above it **then**
14:             **if** $C_b(x, y)$ has not moved v consecutive points in the vertical direction **then**
15:                 **if** force at point is positive **then**
16:                     $Expand(x, y)$
17:                 **end if**
18:             **end if**
19:         **end if**
20:     **end if**
21:     %% $C_b(x, y)$ are at relative local minima.
22:     %% break if no changes are made to boundaries.
23: **end procedure**

In contrast, the method segments seven layers efficiently, but slightly different from those segmented in [4,8]. This difference in segmented layers is mainly because the imposed topology constraints in the proposed method differ from the region limitation in the methods [4,8]. Mainly, due to fragile boundaries within the GCL+IPl and INL region, the method converges better at the INL region, unlike the other methods that are capable of identifying the IPL and INL, separately. On the other hand, the proposed method can handle the OS region better because the two other layers, i.e. the IS and RPE are the brightest. Consequently, the level set topology constraint can handle that challenge, as it evolves from the brighter part (boundaries initialised from gradient edges) of the layers to where the layer boundaries transitions.

Moreover, it can be deduced that the proposed method is consistent in identifying the layer boundaries from the distribution of the values in Fig. 7. Considering the second quarterlies of the NFL, IS and RPE begin at $\geq .900$ further attests to the reassuring performance of the method, except for few instances in the GCL+IPL+INL and OPL layers, where the Dice is below 0.800. Also, in a few instances, the method could not correctly identify the GCL-INL and the OPL due to some of the small components not been removed. The method avoids over and under segmentation, due to our layer initialisation and topological constraint, which prevents merging or splitting of boundaries, as can be seen in Fig. 6.

Furthermore, the proposed method is compared to another level set method [7], and the performance matrix of this comparison is shown in Table 2. We are

Table 1. Performance evaluation using Dice, Accuracy and Sensitivity with respective standard deviation (SD) in segmenting seven retinal layers on 225 images.

Retinal layer	Dice (SD)	Accuracy (SD)	Sensitivity (SD)
NFL	0.942 (0.025)	0.917 (0.038)	0.922 (0.029)
GCL + IPL + INL	0.875 (0.032)	0.889 (0.045)	0.892 (0.034)
OPL	0.894 (0.032)	0.883 (0.036)	0.906 (0.040)
ONL	0.905 (0.030)	0.899 (0.032)	0.908 (0.031)
IS	0.929 (0.021)	0.911 (0.028)	0.928 (0.020)
OS	0.921 (0.029)	0.909 (0.038)	0.913 (0.032)
RPE	0.933 (0.020)	0.928 (0.022)	0.930 (0.024)

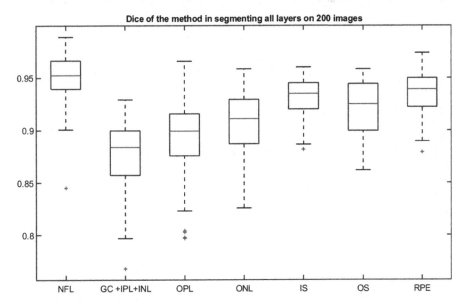

Fig. 7. Box plot of the Dice distribution for the 7 layers on 200 images. [10]

able to compare the methods based on six layers appropriately, i.e. layers that are segmented individually by the methods segment. In other words, the layers from GCL to INL are not included in the comparison, because they are not segmented individually by the proposed method, and could therefore not provide a fairground for evaluating the performance. The proposed method outperforms the other method in segmenting all the targeted layers. In particular, within the OS and RPE region, the method [7] has higher false positives due to the proximity within the layers. The proposed method is able to handle this challenge, as it evolves from the bright side of the layers, to where the layers actually transitions. Also, due to the topology constraints, the layers merging of the layers is prevented.

Table 2. Performance evaluation: Dice (Standard Deviation (SD)) in segmenting **6 layers (excluding GCL to INL)** on 200 B-Scan images.

Retinal layer	Region competition [7]	Proposed method
NFL	0.929 (±0.034)	0.951 (±0.022)
OPL	0.884 (±0.031)	0.892 (±0.032)
ONL	0.899 (±0.041)	0.907 (±0.030)
IS	0.908 (±0.030)	0.932 (±0.017)
OS	0.919 (±0.028)	0.920 (±0.028)
RPE	0.934 (±0.021)	0.964 (±0.014)

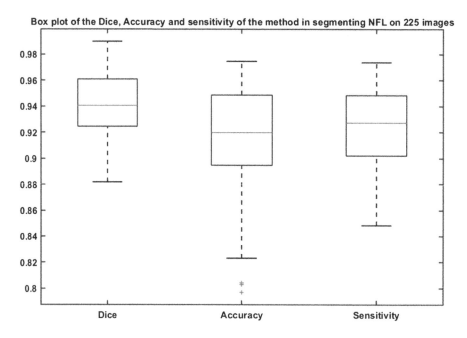

Fig. 8. Distribution of the Dice, Accuracy and sensitivity distribution for NFL on 225 images from Table 1.

Noteworthy is the importance of the RNL thickness in diagnosing major eye diseases such as glaucoma, and we evaluate the method further on this layer. The mean Dice, Accuracy and sensitivity of approximately 0.94, 0.92 and 0.92 from Table 1, respectively for this layer is reassuring. By observing Fig. 8, the first quartile for all images and evaluation criteria starts from about 0.80. There are few outliers, which are results of images from the foveal region, as can be seen in Fig. 9. This has to do with the boundary being smooth, making it more challenging to segment the boundary separating the Nerve Fibre Layer and the Ganglion Cell Layer.

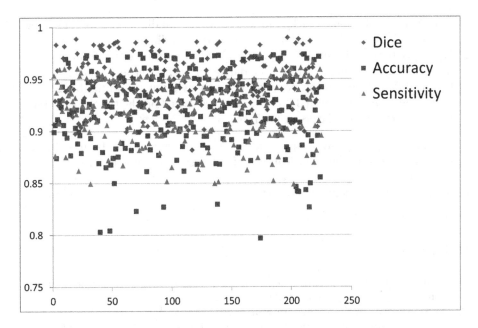

Fig. 9. Distribution of the Dice, Accuracy and sensitivity for the NFL on 225 images from Table 1.

The scheme of the method suggests it may perform well on unhealthy images, although we are unable to perform such tests on an unhealthy dataset due to limited access to data. The main reason for this assertion is that the layering topology restricts the search region. The level set method also is capable of handling such inconsistencies within a limited region.

In summary, the method segments seven layers of the retina simultaneously. The method starts by establishing a specific region of interest, which ensures the evolution of the initial layer boundaries is influenced by the actual layer properties solely. The method utilises edges from the OCT image gradients to represent initial layer boundary contours. Then constraints based on the OCT layer topology are deployed to manage the evolution of the initial contours to the actual layer boundaries. The method can handle edge leaks, which is a common challenge for standard level set methods. The method also converges quickly, as it carries out the topology checks before a boundary point expands or shrinks.

4   Conclusions

We have presented a fully automated and simultaneous method for plausible segmentation of seven non-overlapping retinal layers from optical coherence tomography images. Our approach has explored image segmentation using level set from the point of appropriate initialisation, and parameterisation for constraining the boundary evolution based on retinal layer architecture explicitly. Specifically, the main contributions of this paper can be summarised as follows:

1. Removal of all image background to aid in handling under- and over-segmentation, based on the OCT image understanding.
2. Appropriate level set initialisation technique by refining edges from gradient images to ensure unique initial boundaries for each layer and image.
3. Constraining the evolution process to effectively guide the initial boundaries (from 2 above) to the actual layer boundaries, based on the topological architecture of the retinal layers in OCT scans.

The combination of these components ensures the boundaries obtained by the method are close to the true features of interest. Experimental results show that the proposed approach successfully segmented the target layers from OCT images. Also, the segmentation results are close to the manually labelled ground-truth.

References

1. Adhi, M., Duker, J.S.: Optical coherence tomography-current and future applications. Curr. Opin. Ophthalmol. **24**(3), 213 (2013)
2. Al-Ayyoub, M., AlZu'bi, S., Jararweh, Y., Shehab, M.A., Gupta, B.B.: Accelerating 3D medical volume segmentation using GPUs. Multimedia Tools Appl. **77**(4), 4939–4958 (2018)
3. Boyer, K.L., Herzog, A., Roberts, C.: Automatic recovery of the optic nervehead geometry in optical coherence tomography. IEEE Trans. Med. Imaging **25**(5), 553–570 (2006). https://doi.org/10.1109/TMI.2006.871417
4. Chiu, S.J., Li, X.T., Nicholas, P., Toth, C.A., Izatt, J.A., Farsiu, S.: Automatic segmentation of seven retinal layers in SDOCT images congruent with expert manual segmentation. Opt. Express **18**(18), 19413–19428 (2010). https://doi.org/10.1364/OE.18.019413
5. Dijkstra, E.W.: A note on two problems in connexion with graphs. Numerische mathematik **1**(1), 269–271 (1959)
6. Dodo, B.I., Li, Y., Liu, X.: Retinal oct image segmentation using fuzzy histogram hyperbolization and continuous max-flow. In: 2017 IEEE 30th International Symposium on Computer-Based Medical Systems (CBMS), pp. 745–750. IEEE (2017)
7. Dodo, B.I., Li, Y., Tucker, A., Kaba, D., Liu, X.: Retinal oct segmentation using fuzzy region competition and level set methods. In: 2019 IEEE 32nd International Symposium on Computer-Based Medical Systems (CBMS), pp. 93–98. IEEE (2019)
8. Dodo, B.I., Li, Y., Eltayef, K., Liu, X.: Graph-cut segmentation of retinal layers from oct images. In: Proceedings of the 11th International Joint Conference on Biomedical Engineering Systems and Technologies - BIOIMAGING, vol. 2, pp. 35–42. INSTICC, SciTePress (2018). https://doi.org/10.5220/0006580600350042
9. Dodo, B.I., Li, Y., Eltayef, K., Liu, X.: Min-Cut segmentation of retinal OCT images. In: Cliquet Jr., A., et al. (eds.) BIOSTEC 2018. CCIS, vol. 1024, pp. 86–99. Springer, Cham (2019). https://doi.org/10.1007/978-3-030-29196-9_5
10. Dodo., B.I., Li., Y., Liu., X., Dodo., M.I.: Level set segmentation of retinal oct images. In: Proceedings of the 12th International Joint Conference on Biomedical Engineering Systems and Technologies - BIOIMAGING, vol. 2, pp. 49–56. INSTICC, SciTePress (2019). https://doi.org/10.5220/0007577600490056

11. Duan, J., Tench, C., Gottlob, I., Proudlock, F., Bai, L.: Automated segmentation of retinal layers from optical coherence tomography images using geodesic distance. Pattern Recogn. **72**, 158–175 (2017). https://doi.org/10.1016/j.patcog.2017.07.004. http://www.sciencedirect.com/science/article/pii/S0031320317302650

12. Garvin, M.K.: Automated 3-D segmentation and analysis of retinal optical coherence tomography images. PhD thesis - The University of Iowa (2008)

13. Huang, D., et al.: Optical coherence tomography. Science **254**(5035), 1178–1181 (1991). https://doi.org/10.1002/jcp.24872. (New York, N.Y)

14. Jaffe, G.J.: OCT of the Macula: an expert provides a primer on useful scans, identifying artifacts and time domain vs. spectral domain technology. In: Reinal Physician, pp. 10–12 (2012)

15. Koozekanani, D., Boyer, K., Roberts, C.: Retinal thickness measurements from optical coherence tomography using a Markov boundary model. IEEE Trans. Med. Imaging **20**(9), 900–916 (2001). https://doi.org/10.1109/42.952728

16. Lang, A., et al.: Retinal layer segmentation of macular OCT images using boundary classification. Biomed. Opt. Express **4**(7), 1133–1152 (2013). https://doi.org/10.1364/BOE.4.001133

17. Liu, Y., Carass, A., Solomon, S.D., Saidha, S., Calabresi, P.A., Prince, J.L.: Multilayer fast level set segmentation for macular oct. In: 2018 IEEE 15th International Symposium on Biomedical Imaging (ISBI 2018), pp. 1445–1448, April 2018

18. Lu, S., Yim-liu, C., Lim, J.H., Leung, C.K.S., Wong, T.Y.: Automated layer segmentation of optical coherence tomography images. In: Proceedings - 2011 4th International Conference on Biomedical Engineering and Informatics, BMEI 2011, vol. 1, no. 10, pp. 142–146 (2011). https://doi.org/10.1109/BMEI.2011.6098329

19. Novosel, J., Vermeer, K.A., Thepass, G., Lemij, H.G., Vliet, L.J.V.: Loosely coupled level sets for retinal layer segmentation in optical coherence tomography. In: IEEE 10th International Symposium on Biomedical Imaging, pp. 998–1001 (2013)

20. Raftopoulos, R., Trip, A.: The application of optical coherence tomography (OCT) in neurological disease. Adv. Clin. Neurosci. Rehabil. **12**(2), 30–33 (2012)

21. Shi, Y., Karl, W.C.: A fast level set method without solving pdes [image segmentation applications]. In: Proceedings (ICASSP 2005) IEEE International Conference on Acoustics, Speech, and Signal Processing, 2005, vol. 2, pp. ii/97-ii100, March 2005. https://doi.org/10.1109/ICASSP.2005.1415350

22. Sun, Y., Zhang, T., Zhao, Y., He, Y.: 3D automatic segmentation method for retinal optical coherence tomography volume data using boundary surface enhancement. J. Innov. Opt. Heal. Sci. **9**(02), 1650008 (2016)

23. Tian, J., Varga, B., Somfai, G.M., Lee, W.H., Smiddy, W.E., DeBuc, D.C.: Real-time automatic segmentation of optical coherence tomography volume data of the macular region. PLoS ONE **10**(8), 1–20 (2015). https://doi.org/10.1371/journal.pone.0133908

24. Tsai, A., Yezzi, A., Willsky, A.S.: Curve evolution implementation of the mumford-shah functional for image segmentation, denoising, interpolation, and magnification. IEEE Trans. Image Process. **10**(8), 1169–1186 (2001). https://doi.org/10.1109/83.935033

25. Vincent, L.: Morphological area openings and closings for grey-scale images. In: O, Y.L., Toet, A., Foster, D., Heijmans, H.J.A.M., Meer, P. (eds.) Shape in Picture. NATO ASI Series (Series F: Computer and Systems Sciences), vol. 126, pp. 197–208. Springer, Heidelberg (1994). https://doi.org/10.1007/978-3-662-03039-4_13

26. Wang, C., Wang, Y., Kaba, D., Wang, Z., Liu, X., Li, Y.: Automated layer segmentation of 3D macular images using hybrid methods. In: Zhang, Y.-J. (ed.) ICIG 2015. LNCS, vol. 9217, pp. 614–628. Springer, Cham (2015). https://doi.org/10.1007/978-3-319-21978-3_54

27. Wang, Q., Boyer, K.L.: The active geometric shape model: a new robust deformable shape model and its applications. Comput. Vis. Image Underst. **116**(12), 1178–1194 (2012)

28. Yazdanpanah, A., Hamarneh, G., Smith, B.R., Sarunic, M.V.: Segmentation of intra-retinal layers from optical coherence tomography images using an active contour approach. IEEE Trans. Med. Imaging **30**, 484–496 (2011). https://doi.org/10.1109/TMI.2010.2087390

Bioinformatics Models, Methods and Algorithms

Machine Learning and Combinatorial Optimization to Detect Gene-gene Interactions in Genome-wide Real Data: Looking Through the Prism of Four Methods and Two Protocols

Hugo Boisaubert and Christine Sinoquet[✉]

Nantes University, LS2N, UMR CNRS 6004, 2 rue de la Houssinière, Nantes, France
hugo.boisaubert@etu.univ-nantes.fr, christine.sinoquet@univ-nantes.fr

Abstract. For most genetic diseases, a wide gap exists between the heritability estimated from familial data and the heritability explained through standard genome-wide association studies. One of the incentive lines of research is epistasis - or gene-gene interaction -. However, epistasis detection poses computational challenges. This paper presents three contributions. Our first contribution aims at filling the lack of feedback on the behaviors of published methods dedicated to epistasis, when applied on real-world genetic data. We designed experiments to compare four published approaches encompassing random forests, Bayesian inference, optimization techniques and Markov blanket learning. We included in the comparison the recently developed approach SMMB-ACO (Stochastic Multiple Markov Blankets with Ant Colony Optimization). We used a published dataset related to Crohn's disease. We compared the methods in all aspects: running times and memory requirements, numbers of interactions of interest (statistically significant 2-way interactions), p-value distributions, numbers of interaction networks and structure of these networks. Our second contribution assesses whether there is an impact of feature selection, performed upstream epistasis detection, on the previous statistics and distributions. Our third contribution consists in the characterization of SMMB-ACO's behavior on large-scale real data. We report a great heterogeneity across methods, in all aspects, and highlight weaknesses and strengths for these approaches. Moreover, we conclude that in the case of the Crohn's disease dataset, feature selection implemented through a random forest-based technique does not allow to increase the proportion of interactions of interest in the outputs.

Keywords: Epistasis detection · Machine learning · Markov blanket · Markov chain Monte Carlo · Random forest · Ant colony optimization · Feature selection · Data-dimension reduction · Extensive comparative analysis

---

HB and CS are the two joint first co-authors.

A. Roque et al. (Eds.): BIOSTEC 2019, CCIS 1211, pp. 139–169, 2020.
https://doi.org/10.1007/978-3-030-46970-2_8

1   Introduction

Within two decades, genome-wide association studies (GWASs) have introduced a new paradigm in the field of complex disease genetics. GWASs' purpose is to detect statistical dependences, also called associations, that exist between genetic variants and some phenotype of interest, in a population under study. For example, in case-control studies, the phenotype of interest is the affected/unaffected status. Typically, a GWAS considers between a few thousand to ten thousand individuals in a population, for which high-throughput technologies allow to measure DNA variation at characterized *loci* distributed over the whole genome. Single nucleotide polymorphism (SNP) is a type of DNA variation widely-used in GWASs. Hereafter, we will only consider SNP-based association studies. Depending on the genotyping microarray used, GWASs analyze between a few hundred thousand to a few million SNPs. Standard GWASs test each of the SNPs one at a time, to identify a difference between case and control cohorts.

GWASs have allowed a greater understanding of the genetic architecture underlying complex phenotypes [38]. By fostering prevention and design of more efficient drug therapies depending on the genetic profiles of patients, GWASs have contributed to pave the way to personalized medicine. However, despite GWASs' successes, a wide gap exists between the heritability estimated from familial data and the heritability explained by genetic variants *via* standard GWASs, for most phenotypes investigated so far. To close this so-called 'missing heritability' gap [37], complementary venues of research actively investigate alternative heritable components of complex phenotypes. These alternatives encompass additivity of small effects from myriads of common variants, rare variants, structural variants, epigenetics, gene-environment interactions and genetic interactions [44].

This paper focuses on computational approaches designed to detect genetic interactions, also named *epistasis*. Nowadays, the term "epistasis" is widely used to refer to the situation in which genes interact together to determine some phenotype, whereas each of them alone is not influential on this phenotype: the contribution of one gene to a phenotype depends on the genetic profile of the organism under study. To note, the latter phenotype is not directly observed in case-control studies, in which a physiological quantitative phenotype underlies the unaffected/affected phenotypic status expressed. Epistasis can be seen as the result of physical interactions among biomolecules involved in biochemical pathways and gene regulatory networks, in an organism [29].

To illuminate where part of the missing heritability lies, the role of gene interactions is substantiated by a persuasive body of evidence: biomolecular interactions are omnipresent in gene regulation, signal transduction, biochemical networks and physiological pathways [9,12]. These interactions play a key role in transcriptional and post-translational regulations, interplay between proteins as well as intercellular signaling. Biological evidence for epistasis has been documented in the literature (*e.g.*, [10,11,18,27]). In regard of the ubiquitous character of gene-gene interactions, the relatively limited number of findings published is arguably explained by the computational issue raised by epistasis detection.

In the remainder of this article, a combination of SNPs that interact to determine a phenotype is called an interaction. A k-way interaction is a combination of k interacting SNPs. A 2-way interaction will also be called a gene-gene interaction (with SNPs either in exons or introns).

A key motivation for the large-scale comparative study reported in this paper lies in the following observation: we miss feedback about the respective behaviors of methods designed to implement GWASs on *real-world data*. This observation extends to Genetic Association Interaction Studies (GAISs), and *a fortiori* to genome-wide AISs (GWAISs). This paper contributes to fill this lack. Besides, we recently extended our work to assess the impact of feature selection, when applied upstream epistasis detection. Another strong motivation for our work was to analyze how SMMB-ACO [32], a method proposed most recently, compares with other approaches, on *real* GWAIS data. The remainder of the paper is organized as follows. Section 2 presents a succinct overview of the recent state-of-the-art of the domain. Section 3 provides the motivations for our study and sketches our main contributions. Section 4 depicts the five methods involved in our study, in a broad-brush way for the four reference methods chosen, and in more details for the recently developed SMMB-ACO. Section 5 focuses on the two experimental protocols involved, the real-world datasets analyzed, the implementation and parameter adjustment of the five methods. The experimental results, discussion and feedback gained are presented in the last section.

2   A Brief State-of-the-Art in the Computational Landscape of Gene-gene Interactions

This section provides an overview of the various categories of methods designed to address epistasis detection issues.

2.1   Exhaustive Approaches

The detection of gene-gene interactions is no easy task, especially for large datasets. High level interactions, which involve more than two *loci*, pose a formidable computational challenge. For instance, the number of potential pairwise interactions in a dataset of 500,000 SNPs amounts to 12.5×10^{11}; in the same dataset, the number of potential 3-way interactions rises to 2.08×10^{16}, Hereafter, we will describe the main classes of methods and provide an illustration for each, with a highlight on the scalabilities of the methods cited as illustrations.

In the class of **statistical approaches, linear generalized regression** (LGR) offers a framework to model the relationship between an outcome variable y and multiple interacting predictors $x_1, x_2, ..., x_q$ (continuous or categorical), such as in $f(y) \sim \beta_0 + \beta_1\, x_1 + \beta_2\, x_2 + \beta_{12}\, x_1 x_2$, with $q = 2$. In this framework, two ingredients allow to escape from the pure linear scheme ($y \sim \beta_0 + \beta_1\, x_1 + \beta_2\, x_2$), in the case of two predictors). On the one hand, interaction terms β_{ij} capture potential interplay between predictors. On the other hand, the *link* function f is used to transform the outcome y, to match the real distribution of y. Obviously, LGR cannot be used straightforwardly to analyze data on the genome scale: the exhaustive enumeration and test of potential q-way interactions is prohibitive, and this task should be performed for q comprised between 2 and r, where r is an upper bound arbitrarily set by the user. Furthermore, identifying an appropriate link function f may not be trivial. Nevertheless, **logistic regression** (LR) is a widely-used specific case of LGR in which the link function is known, to model a binary outcome: in case control studies, with p representing the probability to be affected by the pathology of interest, the LR model with two interacting predictors writes: $logit(p) = ln(\frac{p}{1-p}) = \beta_0 + \beta_1 \ x_1 + \beta_2 \ x_2 + \beta_{12} \ x_1 x_2$. We will further specify to which aim and how LR is used in the comparative study reported here.

Penalized regression (PR) implemented through Lasso, Ridge or Elastic Net regression can be used for the purpose of epistasis detection [2]. The computational burden of these methods is particularly heavy. The approach described in [5] attempts to palliate this issue through a two-stage procedure. First, pairwise interactions are searched for within each gene, using Randomized Lasso and penalized Logistic Regression (RLLR). Second, pairwise interactions across genes are assessed considering the SNPs obtained in the first stage. RLLR is again used in this second stage. In [33], interactions are searched for each pair of genes. A Group Lasso approach is employed, in which groups comprise either the SNPs of a given gene, or interaction terms relative to a given pair of genes. Though such approaches seem appealing to capture cross-gene epistasis, they each feature a major drawback. In [5], the biological motivation for the data dimension reduction performed *via* the first stage is questionable since 2-way interactions within genes are not necessarily connected to cross-gene interactions. On the other hand, the approach in [33] could only be run on a pre-selected set of a few dozen genes, for each of three real GWAS datasets. These genes were pre-selected based on an univariate analysis, which introduces a bias.

A step further, model-free data mining methods in the line of **multifactor-dimensionality reduction** (MDR) categorize the observed genotypes into high-risk and low-risk groups, for each q-way potential interaction [13]. Since enumerating all potential q-way interactions is required, MDR-based approaches fail to handle large-scale data. An exception is the case when GPU calculation is used [43].

2.2   Dimension Reduction Upstream of Epistasis Detection

A direct way to reduce the search space is to decrease the dataset size. **Filtering based on extrinsic biological knowledge** is expected to yield meaningful and biologically relevant results. However, exploiting additional knowledge such as protein-protein interaction networks or pathways is questionable. Online databases are incomplete and our understanding of biological pathways is limited. Therefore, relying on such knowledge for data dimension purpose would result in a biased analysis in the majority of cases.

In the category of machine learning and data mining approaches, feature selection techniques rely on properties intrinsic to the data, to select SNPs potentially relevant for epistasis detection.

A number of variants were proposed around Relief [36]. The first step in **Relief-based approaches** (RBAs) is to compute pairwise (genetical) similarities between subjects. A nearest neighbor technique is further applied, to assess importances for SNPs with respect to the phenotype of interest. Basically, the method identifies SNPs not sharing the same values between a subject and its nearest neighbors. If this situation arises when the subject and its nearest neighbors neither share the same phenotype, the SNPs' importances are increased; otherwise, the importances are decreased. This step is only repeated over a user-defined number of subjects, which nonetheless requires the costly computation of pairwise similarities. Moreover, Relief-based approaches are prone to pre-select SNPs marginally associated with the phenotype.

Random forest (RF) approaches implement high-dimensional non-parametric predictive models relying on ensemble features. In RFs, bootstrap aggregating [4] allows to convert a collection of weak learners (decision trees in this case) into a strong learner. The decision trees (classification trees for a categorical outcome, regression trees for a continuous outcome) are grown recursively from bootstrap samples of observations. At each node in each tree, the observations (*e.g.*, individuals) that have percolated down this node are splitted relying on an optimal cut-point. A cut-point is a pair involving one of the available variables (*e.g.*, SNPs) and a value in the variable's domain. Over all available variables, the optimal cut-point best discriminates the observations with respect to the outcome of interest (*e.g.*, phenotype). In RFs, the optimal cut-point is determined using a random subset of the initial variables. RFs produce a ranking of the variables, by decreasing importance measure. This measure quantifies the impact of a variable in predicting the outcome and thus potentially reflects a causal effect. RF-based approaches were shown efficient in ranking simulated disease-associated SNPs, to detect gene-gene interactions [24,25]. Computational cost and memory inefficiency were severe impediments to RF learning in high-dimensional settings. In this respect, the advances reported in [30] and [40] render RF-based feature selection practicable for epistasis detection at large scale.

In association studies, feature selection yields a ranking for the SNPs in the initial available dataset. A procedure is required downstream such methods as Relief-based approaches and Random Forests, to generate gene-gene interactions from the top ranking SNPs. Such procedure may boil down to assessing potential interactions through statistical tests. In contrast, a specific approach designed to detect epistasis may be used. We explored both modalities in the work reported here.

2.3 Sampling from Probability Distributions

The popular BEAM algorithm (Bayesian Epistasis Association Mapping) [42] relies on a **Markov Chain Monte Carlo** (MCMC) process to test iteratively each SNP, conditional on the current status of other SNPs. For each SNP, the algorithm outputs its posterior probability of association with disease. BEAM then partitions the SNPs into three categories. One category contains SNPs with no impact on the disease. A second category contains SNPs that contribute independently to the disease. The third category highlights SNPs assumed to jointly influence the disease given particular variant combinations of some other SNPs. BEAM was reported to handle datasets with half a million of SNPs, at the cost of high running times (up to a week and even more).

2.4 Machine Learning Techniques

To detect epistasis, machine learning approaches represent appealing alternatives to parametric statistical methods. Such approaches build non-parametric models to compile information further used for gene-gene interaction detection.

Standard supervised machine learning and data mining techniques can be employed directly for the purpose of epistasis detection. **Support vector machines** (SVMs) separate interacting and non-interacting groups of SNPs using a hyperplane in multi-dimensional space. The work in [31] reports an SVM-based study of 2-way interactions conducted at the genome scale. On the other hand, **artificial neural networks** (ANNs) allow to model non-linear feature interactions. To this aim, non-linear activation functions are used, in conjunction with a sufficient number of hidden layers. Advanced stochastic gradient descent techniques brought a remarkable breakthrough in training feedforward networks with many hidden layers, thereby paving the way to deep neural networks (DNNs). However, so far, DNNs were confined to process small datasets. In [35], a DNN was learned from small datasets (no more than 1,600 subjects, a few dozen SNPs). The DNN used in [8] was learned from around 1,500 subjects and 5,000 SNPs, downstream a filtering stage consisting in logistic regression.

Bayesian Networks (BNs) allow to model patterns of probabilistic dependences between variables represented as nodes in a directed acyclic graph. In the context of epistasis detection, BNs offer an incentive framework to discover the best scoring graph structure connecting SNPs to the disease variable. In [15], a branch and bound heuristic allowed to handle a relatively limited dataset, a published AMD (Age Macular Degenerated) dataset (150 individuals, around 110,000 SNPs). In [19], a greedy search implements a forward phase consisting in edge addition followed by a backward phase orchestrating edge removal. The tractability issue is addressed by starting the greedy search with one pair of interacting SNPs which are each influential on the disease status. This approach is therefore limited to the detection of a specific case of epistasis, named *embedded* epistasis.

In Bayesian networks, the concept of Markov blanket [28] offers an appealing line of investigation for epistasis detection. Given a BN built over the variables of a dataset V, the Markov Blanket (MB) of a target variable T, $MB(T)$, is defined as a minimal set of variables that renders any variable outside $MB(T)$ probabilistically independent of T, conditional on $MB(T)$. Otherwise stated, $MB(T)$ is theoretically the optimal set of variables to predict the value of T [22]. In the GAIS context, the purpose is to build a MB for the variable representing the affected/unaffected status. Feature subset selection stated as **Markov blanket** learning was thus explored and produced FEPI-MB (Fast epistatic interactions detection using Markov blanket) [16] and DASSO-MB (Detection of ASSOciations using Markov Blanket) [17]. Both approaches were able to process the above mentioned AMD dataset.

2.5   Combinatorial Optimization Approaches

In the **optimization** field, techniques dedicated to AISs browse through the search space of solutions (combinations of potentially interacting SNPs). Various heuristics were proposed, to identify the more relevant combinations of SNPs. In the line of genetic algorithms, the approach described in [1] relies on an **evolutionary-based** heuristic. This method allowed to process around 1,400 subjects and 300,000 SNPs. **Ant colony optimization** (ACO) was exploited by several proposals such as AntEpiSeeker [39], MACOED [20] and EpiACO [34]. The widely cited reference AntEpiSeeker consists in the straightforward adaptation of classical ACO to epistasis detection and is tractable on the genome scale. MACOED, a multi-objective approach employing the Akaike information criterion (AIC) score and a BN-based score, was able to process 1,411 individuals described by 312,316 SNPs (late-onset Alzheimer's disease (LOAD) dataset). Since MACOED needs unaffordable running times to obtain results, the analysis focused on separate chromosome datasets. The unique objective function used in EpiACO combines a mutual information measure with a BN-based score. EpiACO was able to handle the above cited AMD dataset.

3   Motivations and Contributions of Our Study

The critical analysis of the specialized literature led us to draw several remarks about the evaluation and comparison of computational approaches dedicated to epistasis detection.

First, evaluating the effectiveness of a method requires the generation of multiple synthetic datasets, for instance 100, under some controlled assumption. The points to control are the number of interacting SNPs and the strength of the joint effect of simulated influential SNPs on the disease status. When evaluating a non-deterministic method, we have to compute a performance for each synthetic dataset, which is a function of the numbers of true positives, false positives and false negatives recorded through multiple runs of the same method on the same dataset (*e.g.,* power, F-measure). Unfortunately, tractability reasons compell methods' authors to generate simulated datasets whose size remains compatible with the computing and storage resources available to these authors.

Thus, an overwhelming majority of publications rely on synthetic datasets that describe 100 SNPs, a few thousand SNPs at best, for a few thousand subjects. A notable exception is the study reported in [6]. This practical limitation renders questionable the significance of the evaluation and comparison of methods on such small simulated datasets: in no way do such experimentations reflect real-world GWAIS analyses.

Besides, as regards real-world GWAIS analyses, the overwhelming trend in publications is to submit a unique genome-wide dataset to the proposed method. No comparison is performed with other methods. Again, the reason lies in tractability. Comparing several methods at this scale requires authors to adjust a list of parameters for each method. Ideally, adjusting parameters for any approach resorting to supervised machine learning would need running ten times a GWAIS (in a 10-fold cross-validation procedure) in each of the parameter instantiations of a parameter grid. Optimizing the parameters for any heuristics in the field of combinatorial optimization also requires unaffordable running times in general.

A third remark is that running times are but exceptionally reported in publications describing a novel method. If so, they are only reported for small simulated datasets. Instead, assessing orders of magnitude for running times across methods would be far more informative (*e.g.*, for practitioners), if the methods were applied on datasets of realistic scale.

A fourth remark arises from the observed lack of comparative studies focused on epistasis detection methods applied at the genome scale: it is questionable whether the lists of gene-gene interactions output by these methods overlap, and if so, by which overlapping rate.

The works presented in this paper were designed with the four previous points in mind and with the five following related objectives: (i) perform an unprecedented comparative analysis on real-world GWAS data, for a selection of methods dedicated to GWAIS, (ii) assess the respective requirements of these methods, in terms of running times and memory resources, (iii) characterize the solutions respectively output by these methods, (iv) examine the pairwise intersections of solutions output by these methods and possible intersections between more than two methods. A first presentation of these works was published in [3], of which the present paper is an extended version. In addition to the extensive comparative study reported in [3], we have started afresh a novel comparative study. This time, we have run each method compared, after a common feature selection procedure was applied on each of the chromosome-wide datasets considered. The additional three contributions highlighted in this extended version are the following: (v) include additional criteria to characterize the solutions output by the methods compared, namely around the connectivity between SNPs involved in multiple interactions, (vi) characterize the solutions respectively output by the methods in previous and novel experimental conditions, that is without and with the filtering stage, (vii) provide an illustration focused on a network of interactions, and give corresponding biological insights.

4   The Approaches Selected for the Extensive Comparison

To analyze the epistasis detection task in real-world conditions, we selected five approaches illustrating various techniques.

Data dimension reduction upstream of epistasis detection is illustrated through ranger [40] coupled with logistic regression. The reference ranger software is a fast implementation for random forest-based feature selection; it was specifically designed to cope with high-dimensional data. A further argument for including ranger in our comparative study is that, so far, any novel method proposed was generally compared to Random Jungle [30], the precursor of ranger.

BEAM3 [41], the successor of the reference software BEAM [42], implements Bayesian inference *via* the sampling of probability distributions. An MCMC simulation allows to assign a statistical significance to each SNP, thus avoiding expensive permutation-based tests.

In the field of machine learning, feature subset selection stated as **Markov blanket** learning is implemented through DASSO-MB [17]. For didactical reasons, the sketch of DASSO-MB will be provided together with that of the fifth approach selected.

The reference method AntEpiSeeker [39] was incorporated in our study to represent combinatorial optimization heuristics. The ant colony optimization (ACO) technique behind AntEpiSeeker is as follows: in each iteration, the ants each sample a SNP set of user-defined size from the initial dataset, based on a probability distribution $\mathbb{P}$; each ant then assesses the dependence of the SNP set S sampled with the affected/unaffected status through a statistical test (χ^2). The SNP sets showing the highest dependence scores are kept. The pheromone level of each SNP s thus highlighted is computed based on the dependence of the set S that contains s. A standard ACO scheme uses the pheromone levels to update the probability distribution $\mathbb{P}$ of each SNP. At the end of a user-defined number of ACO iterations, a pre-specified number of best SNP sets is available, together with a list $\mathcal{L}$ of SNPs characterized by the highest pheromone levels. The final step of AntEpiSeeker then examines each best SNP set S as follows: given q, the size of the epistatic interactions to be uncovered, each subset of S of size q is kept as an epistatic interaction, provided all its SNPs belong to $\mathcal{L}$. It may happen that two interactions overlap, in which case the one with the smallest p-value is kept.

The selection of DASSO-MB and AntEpiSeeker was no innocent choice. Indeed, the fifth approach included in our comparative study, SMMB-ACO (Stochastic Multiple Markov Blankets with Ant Colony Optimization) [32], is a recent method that borrows from Markov blanket learning and ant colony optimization techniques. In the previous paragraph, we have explained the ACO mechanism behind AntEpiSeeker.

We now highlight the differences between the deterministic DASSO-MB approach and the stochastic and ensemble feature-based SMMB-ACO approach. DASSO-MB chains a forward phase and a backward phase. Starting from an empty Markov blanket (MB), the forward phase adds a SNP to the growing MB based on two conditions: (i) the dependence between this SNP and the target variable (affected/unaffected status in our case) is the highest, conditional on the MB, when compared to all other SNPs; (ii) this dependence is statistically significant. The backward phase successively examines the SNPs belonging to the current MB; a SNP is removed from the MB based on (statistically significant) conditional independence. To discard false positives as soon as possible, DASSO-MB triggers a full backward phase after a SNP has been added during the forward phase. In each iteration of SMMB-ACO, the ants each learn a suboptimal Markov blanket from a subset of SNPs sampled from the initial set. The MB learning scheme in SMMB-ACO relies on a forward phase intertwined with backward phases. In this respect, MB learning in SMMB-ACO is quite similar to that in DASSO-MB. However, SMMB-ACO and DASSO-MB's forward steps fundamentally differ: DASSO-MB attempts to add the SNP showing the strongest dependence with the target variable; in contrast, SMMB-ACO seeks to stochastically add a group of SNPs highly dependent with the target variable. The stochastic feature of SMMB-ACO is implemented through the sampling of groups of SNPs, and relies on a probability distribution $\mathbb{P}$ updated based on pheromone levels. To note, a specific operating mode may be specified for SMMB-ACO, to handle high-dimensional data: a two-pass procedure is then triggered. DASSO-MB and SMMB-ACO are sketched and commented in Fig. 1.

5   Extensive Experimentation Framework

This section starts with the presentation of the experimental road map designed. Second, the real-world datasets used are briefly depicted. Finally, the section focuses on implementation aspects, including parameter adjustment of the approaches compared.

5.1   Experimental Road Map

In the so-called additive model, the SNPs are coded with 0, 1 and 2, which respectively denote major homozygous, heterozygous and minor homozygous. The allele with minor frequency is the disease susceptibility allele. The notion of **interaction of interest** (IoI) is central to our study. An IoI is a 2-way interaction for which logistic regression ($y \sim \beta_0 + \beta_1 \ x_1 + \beta_2 \ x_2 + \beta_{12} \ x_1 x_2$) provides a significant p-value for the interaction coefficient β_{12}, given some specific significance threshold, whereas no significant p-value is obtained for the regression of the target variable on each individual SNP. Our experimental protocol was two-fold.

To use the random forest-based approach ranger for epistatic detection purpose, we generated 2-way interactions from the top most important SNPs returned by ranger. For tractability reasons, the 2-way interaction candidates were generated from the 20 most important SNPs selected. Thus, C_{20}^2 2-way interactions were submitted to logistic regression. To characterize IoIs, the significance threshold 5×10^{-4} was chosen. In our comparative study, we put all approaches on an equitable basis. Therefore, we filtered the interactions obtained from BEAM3, AntEpiSeeker, and DASSO-MB as well as the results obtained

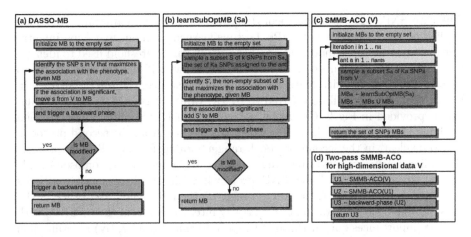

Fig. 1. Sketches of the DASSO-MB and SMMB-ACO algorithms. (Figure published in [3]). (a) DASSO-MB. (b) SMMB-ACO stochastic procedure to learn a suboptimal Markov blanket. (c) SMMB-ACO top-level algorithm. (d) Two-pass SMMB-ACO procedure adapted to high-dimensional data. MB: Markov blanket. V is the initial set of SNPs. (a) DASSO-MB adds SNPs one at a time, which hinders the epistasis detection task: since the dependence test achieved at first iteration is conditioned on the empty Markov blanket, this test is indeed a marginal test of dependence; therefore, a SNP marginally dependent with the target variable is added at the outset, which skews the whole MB learning. (b) SMMB-ACO addresses this issue by adding groups of SNPs. For this purpose, each forward step starts with the sampling of a set S of k SNPs, from the subset S_a of size K_a that was assigned to the ant in charge of the suboptimal MB learning. For each non-empty subset S' of S, a score is computed, which measures the association strength between S' and the target variable, conditional on the MB under construction. The subset S' with the highest association score is added to the MB if the association is statistically significant. (c) SMMB-ACO returns the set of SNPs obtained as the union of all suboptimal MBs generated throughout all iterations. (d) In the two-pass procedure adapted to high-dimensional data, SMMB-ACO is first applied on the initial set of SNPs V, which produces the set of SNPs U_1. In the second pass, SMMB-ACO is applied on U_1. This time, the resulting set U_2 is submitted to a backward phase, to yield U_3, a set of SNPs.

from the modified post-processing phase of SMMB-ACO (Details about this modification will be provided in Sect. 5.3). This filtering stage kept the IoIs with significance threshold 5×10^{-2}. The use of two significance thresholds will be substantially justified further (see Subsect. 5.3). For now, the reader needs only keep in mind that AntEpiSeeker, DASSO-MB and SMMB-AC0 *already intrinsically* rely on a significance threshold.

In addition to the experimental protocol just described, we designed afresh novel experimentations. This time, a feature selection procedure was first run on the datasets considered. The second experimental protocol started with feature selection carried out through ranger. For each of the 50 runs of ranger on a given chromosome dataset, the 5,000 SNPs with the highest importances were memorized. The set of 25,000 SNPs thus obtained was then processed to discard duplicate SNPs. The first protocol described in previous paragraph was then applied on the reduced set of SNPs. Lessons learned from our first experimentations [3] motivated the modification of the significance threshold used to identify IoIs with ranger (see Subsect. 5.3). From now on, we will use the symbol "*" to refer to the protocol with feature selection. For instance, the use of BEAM3 in the two frameworks will be referred to by BEAM3 and BEAM3*. A recapitulation is provided in Fig. 2. Given the poor results of DASSO-MB obtained when applying the first protocol, we discarded this method from the second protocol.

To be clear, in the second protocol, ranger* stands for the following process: (i) off-line feature selection by ranger applied 50 times on a chromosome-wide dataset, to provide $50 \times 5,000$ SNPs from which the resulting set of n_{fs} SNPs with no duplicates is kept, (ii) run of ranger on the reduced dataset of n_{fs} SNPs thus obtained, (iii) generation of $C_{n_r}^2$ 2-way interactions from the n_r SNPs with highest importances output through the second run of ranger, (iv) identification of the IoIs in the $C_{n_r}^2$ 2-way interactions using logistic regression. We highlight here that we set n_r to 20, for consistency with the first protocol.

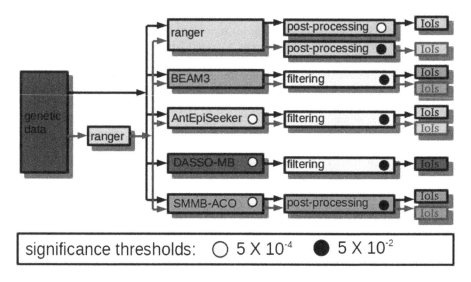

Fig. 2. Flow diagram for the two extensive comparative analyses performed. The data flows relative to first and second experimental protocols respectively appear in black and blue arrows. (Color figure online)

Table 1. Implementations for the five software programs used in the two comparative studies. (Table published in [3]).

Ranger	http://dx.doi.org/10.18637/jss.v077.i01
BEAM3	http://www.mybiosoftware.com/beam-3-disease-association-mapping.html
AntEpiSeeker	http://nce.ads.uga.edu/~romdhane/AntEpiSeeker/index.html
DASSO-MB	Not distributed by its authors, reimplemented
SMMB-ACO	https://ls2n.fr/listelogicielsequipe/DUKe/130/SMMB-ACO

5.2 Real-World Datasets

We applied the two experimental protocols above described to a Crohn's disease (CD) dataset. This data was made available by the Wellcome Trust Case Control Consortium (WTCCC, https://www.wtccc.org.uk/). The choice of this dataset was motivated by the insights generated by advancements in human genetics into the mechanisms driving inflammatory conditions of the colon and small intestine. Notably, major pathways involved in Crohn's disease and ulcerative colitis have emerged from standard single-SNP GWASs [14]. We relied on the cohort of cases affected by CD and two cohorts of unaffected (controls) provided by the WTCCC, to generate 23 datasets related to the 23 human chromosomes. We followed the quality control protocol specified by the WTCCC. In particular, we excluded subjects having more than 5% of missing data together with SNPs having more than 1% of missing data and excessive Hardy-Weinberg disequilibrium (5.7×10^{-7} threshold). After quality control, we obtained a population of $4,686$ subjects composed of $1,748$ affected and $2,938$ unaffected. We imputed data using a k-nearest neighbor procedure, in which the missing variant of subject s is assigned the variant most frequent in the nearest neighbors of s. The average number of SNPs per chromosome is $20,236$; the minimum and maximum numbers are $5,707$ and $38,730$, respectively.

5.3 Implementation of the Two Comparative Analyses

This subsection first focuses on the intensive computing aspects. Then it describes parameter adjustment for the five methods involved in the experimentations.

Intensive Computing. Except for DASSO-MB, all software programs are available on the Internet (Table 1); they are coded in C++. We recoded DASSO-MB in C++. As mentioned in Sect. 5.1, to include SMMB-ACO in our experimental protocol, we modified the post-processing phase of the native SMMB-ACO algorithm [32]. The native algorithm outputs as an interaction any suboptimal Markov blanket generated (*via* procedure learnSubOPtMB, see Fig. 1 (b)) if all its SNPs belong to the set U_3 (see Fig. 1 (d)) obtained as the final result of the two-pass modality. The adapted post-processing phase of SMMB-ACO consists in the generation of interactions of interest (IoIs), as defined in Subsect. 5.1, from the set U_3.

DASSO-MB is the only deterministic approach of our selection of methods. Each other (stochastic) method was run several times on each dataset. In the first experimental protocol, this number was set to 10 for tractability reasons. For a fair comparison, this number was kept to 10 in the second protocol involving data dimension reduction.

The extensiveness of our two comparative studies required intensive computing resources from a Tier 2 data centre (Intel 2630v4, 2×10 cores 2,2 Ghz, 20×6 GB). On the one hand, we benefitted from the OpenMP intrinsical parallelization of the C++ implementations of ranger, BEAM3 and SMMB-ACO. In addition, we exploited data-driven parallelization to run each stochastic method 10 times on each dataset. To cope with running time heterogeneity across the methods, together with the occurrence of memory shortages, we had to balance the workload distribution between two strategies. One strategy was to sequentially process the 23 chromosome datasets for one method on one node, and to repeat this task 9 times on other nodes. The alternative strategy was to process a single chromosome dataset 10 times for one method on one node, and to repeat this task for the remaining chromosomes (on other nodes). We managed the workload using the three following modalities: short, medium and long, for expected calculation durations respectively below 1, 5 and 30 days. When a time-out or shortage event occurred in a node, depending on the degree of completion of the task, we either switched to the first strategy with higher time limit or to a chromosome by chromosome management.

The first batch of experimentations involved 943 chromosome-wide association studies. The second batch involved as many analyses, together with the prior feature selection performed chromosome by chromosome. This pre-processing step involved 50 runs of ranger for each of the 23 chromosome datasets. In total, we run 3,036 chromosome-wide analyses.

Finally, it is important to note that generating all 2-way interactions from a set of t SNPs (as is done when ranger is used for epistasis detection) may be computationally expensive. For example, the exhaustive generation and assessment of dependence with the disease status through logistic regression takes around 30 h for $t = 20$ SNPs.

Parameter Adjustment. In the machine learning and combinatorial optimization fields, adjusting methods' parameters is a recurring issue. Table 7 in Appendix recapitulates the main parameters of the software programs used in the two batches of experimentations.

The software program ranger is a fast implementation of the random forest technique, to cope with high-dimensional data. We therefore left unchanged the default value of 500 for the number of trees in the forest. In a preliminary study (results not shown), we tried various values of mtry between $\sqrt{n}$ and n, the total number of SNPs. On the datasets considered, the optimal value was shown to be $\frac{5}{8}n$. This setting was adopted for ranger used in the first protocol, ranger employed for feature selection in the second protocol as well as for ranger run downstream feature selection in the second protocol. Importantly, a greater computational effort was devoted to the feature selection task carried out by ranger in the second protocol: the number of trees was set to $1,000$ instead of 500.

To attempt to diminish the large number of interactions output by AntEpiSeeker, we conducted a preliminary study. The product "number of ACO iterations $\times$ number of ants" impacts this number of interactions. In the preliminary study, the number of ACO iterations was kept to AntEpiSeeker's default value (450); the number of ants was varied between 500 and 5,000 (step 500).

Using 1,000 ants still allows to control the number of interactions output below 15,000, while still guaranteeing a coverage of 10 for each SNP in the largest chromosome-wide dataset. For a fair comparison, this parameter setting was kept in the second experimental protocol.

To set the numbers of iterations of the burn-in and stationary phases of BEAM3, we followed the recommendation of its author. This setting was made in adequacy with the dimension of the data handled in the first protocol. For an unbiased comparison, this setting was also applied to the second protocol.

The first reflex would be to set the product $n_{it} \times n_{ants}$ (number of ACO iterations $\times$ number of ants) in SMMB-ACO to the value chosen for AntEpiSeeker. However, two points must be emphasized. On the one hand, AntEpiSeeker software program is not parallelized, whereas SMMB-ACO is: during each of the n_{it} SMMB-ACO iterations, n_{ants} Markov blankets are learned in parallel. On the other hand, an iteration in AntEpiSeeker is far less complex than an iteration in SMMB-ACO: in AntEpiSeeker, each ant samples a set of SNPs and computes the corresponding χ^2 statistic; in SMMB-ACO, each ant grows a Markov blanket via a forward phase intertwined with full backward phases. We adjusted SMMB-ACO parameters n_{it}, n_{ants} and K_a (number of SNPs drawn by each ant), to expect that each SNP of the initial dataset would be drawn a sufficient number of times during a single run of SMMB-ACO. The parameter setting adopted $(n_{it}, n_{ants}, K_a) = (360, 20, 160)$ guarantees in theory a coverage of 30 for the largest datasets, in a single run. We recall that 10 runs are performed for each stochastic method.

A type I error threshold is required for the statistical independence tests triggered by AntEpiSeeker and the statistical conditional independence tests run in DASSO-MB and SMMB-ACO. We set a common threshold value of 5×10^{-4} for these three methods. Consistently, in the first protocol implemented in [3], we fixed the same threshold for the logistic regression used downstream ranger execution. On the other hand, we recall that logistic regression is used to identify IoIs from the results output by BEAM3, DASSO-MB, AntEpiSeeker and SMMB-ACO. A less stringent threshold of 5×10^{-2} was chosen for this purpose. Importantly, one of the conclusions of the work reported in [3] highlighted the necessity to relax the threshold of 5×10^{-4} used downstream a run of ranger, to identify more IoIs. Therefore, in the second protocol, the second pass of ranger is followed by IoI identification at 5×10^{-2} significance threshold. This information about the various thresholds used in the two protocols is provided in Fig. 2.

6   Results and Discussion

We first compare the five approaches with respect to running times and memory occupancies. Second, we compare the numbers of interactions of interest (IoIs) identified by these approaches, and we thoroughly analyze the distributions of p-values obtained. Third, we provide insights regarding whether some IoIs were jointly detected by several approaches. A fourth subsection is devoted to the analysis of the networks of IoIs that could be identified by the methods. A fifth subsection provides an illustration focused on a network of 19 IoIs detected *via* SMMB-ACO, and gives corresponding biological insights. This section ends with a discussion.

6.1   Computational Running Times and Memory Occupancies

Table 2 highlights a great heterogeneity between the methods compared.

We first comment the complexities observed when chromosome-wide datasets are input to the methods (first protocol). DASSO-MB is both much faster and far less greedy in memory than its competitors. A salient feature of AntEpiSeeker is that it shows low running times across all chromosomes. The software program ranger is fast (around 14 mn for the 10 runs on a chromosome). However, this quickness is hindered by the exhaustive generation of C_{20}^2 2-way interactions further submitted to logistic regression (between 40 and 80 mn cumulated over the 10 runs on a chromosome). The trends observed for BEAM3 and SMMB-ACO are respectively extremely disparate across the datasets. When processing the largest chromosomes with BEAM3, we first experienced timeouts. We therefore specified the highest timeouts possible (30 days), with the consequence of longer waiting times in job queues. Indeed, in BEAM3, the cumulative running time may exceed 8 days for the largest chromosomes, which is over the "medium" timeout of 5 days. Besides prohibitive running times, BEAM3 si also the approach most greedy in memory on average for the datasets considered. Nonetheless, BEAM3 never ran out of memory.

As regards SMMB-ACO, a great heterogeneity in running times was also observed across the chromosome-wide datasets. SMMB-ACO is faster than BEAM3. However, the stochastic feature of SMMB-ACO translates into an extreme heterogeneity of memory occupancies across the chromosomes, even across the 10 executions on a given chromosome. In particular, we observed memory shortages, even for short chromosomes (for a limitation of 120 GB per node). Because of these shortages, for around the third of the datasets, we had to launch additional runs (up to 5), to obtain the 10 runs required by our protocol. Nevertheless, the processing of all chromosomes by SMMB-ACO remains feasible within 5 days, on 10 nodes.

We recall that a crucial step in the second protocol is the dimensionality reduction task: an off-line feature selection driven by ranger is applied 50 times on each chromosome-wide dataset, to provide $50 \times 5,000$ SNPs from which the resulting set of n_{fs} SNPs with no duplicates is kept. We emphasize that for each chromosome, the 5,000 top ranked SNPs were remarkably well conserved throughout the 50 executions of ranger. Namely, n_{fs} varied between 5,000 and 5,150.

Table 2. Trends observed for the running times and memory occupancies for the methods compared, in the two protocols. Otherwise stated, the average running time indicated is computed over the 23 chromosome-wide datasets (it measures the average for the running time cumulated over 10 executions, for a chromosome-wide dataset). FS: off-line feature selection driven by ranger.

Method	First protocol		Second protocol	
	Average running time	Memory occupancy	Average running time	Memory occupancy
ranger			FS: 11 h ± 5.5	4 GB
	1.3 h ± 27 mn	2 GB ± 0.6	19.6 mn ± 7	120 MB ± 20
BEAM3	Chr7 to Chr23: 54 s ± 66	79 GB ± 46	Chr7 to Chr23: 24.1 h ± 0.1	800 MB ± 200
	Chr6: 22.4 h		Chr6: 38.9 h	
	Chr1 to Chr5: above 8 days		Chr1 to Chr5: below 5 days	
AntEpiSeeker	16 mn ± 3	0.5 GB ± 0.2	15 mn ± 4	70 MB ± 5
DASSO-MB	82 s ± 22	1.5 GB ± 0.7	—	—
SMMB-ACO	Chr7 to Chr23: 30 mn ± 17	43 GB ± 17	17.3 h ± 3.3	700 MB ± 150
	Chr1 to Chr6: up to 3 days	Many execution abortions		

The running times obtained in the second protocol, in which reduced sets of n_{fs} SNPs are processed, give rise to several comments.

As expected, the cumulative running time for ranger diminishes with the size of the dataset (at most one hour an a half for a chromosome-wide dataset *versus* half an hour at most for a reduced dataset). The renown scalability of ranger is confirmed by our study [40].

In the MCMC-based software BEAM3, the cumulative running time shows an unexpected trend, on average, for chromosomes 7 to 23: the average was around one minute on a chromosome-wide dataset; it is around one day after dimension reduction. For chromosome 6, for instance, we still observe a higher running time for the reduced dataset than for the chromosome-wide dataset (38.9 h *versus* 22.4 h), but this time, the orders of magnitude are quite similar. In contrast, the expected ratio is observed for chromosomes 1 to 5 (above 8 days *versus* 5 days). For instance, the cumulative running time over 10 BEAM3 runs took 2 days and 18 h for chromosome 4, in the second protocol, whereas this cumulative time was above a week in the first protocol. To explain the unexpected high running times likely to be observed on the reduced datasets, we contacted BEAM3's author. The slowdown observed can be explained by BEAM3 having to deal with a lot of dependences, in order to find independent signals. This becomes particularly acute when SNP selection is applied. In contrast, if the SNP pool is *relatively* large, the program may converge faster because many more SNPs are independent.

For the same parameterization of AntEpiSeeker, the respective running times relative to two datasets of different sizes are not expected to differ. This fact is confirmed in Table 2.

In the first protocol applied to SMMB-ACO, we highlighted a great heterogeneity across chromosomes, with cumulative running times frequently reaching 3 days. In contrast, on the reduced datasets, a series of 10 SMMB-ACO runs can be processed at ease within a day.

Finally, BEAM3 remained the most greedy algorithm in the second protocol, closely followed by SMMB-ACO.

6.2   Interactions of Interest

Number of Interactions of Interest and Spatial Distribution over the Chromosomes. Table 3 highlights contrasts between the approaches. First, with only 18 interactions obtained *via* the first protocol, DASSO-MB was not expected to output IoIs, which is confirmed. We therefore excluded DASSO-MB from the second protocol. In the remainder of this article, we will not mention this method anymore. Second, a salient feature is the great heterogeneity in the numbers of IoIs detected by the four other methods. In the first protocol, these numbers scale in a ten thousands, a thousand, a hundred and a few tens for AntEpiSeeker, SMMB-ACO, BEAM3 and ranger respectively.

Table 3. Comparison of the numbers of interactions detected by ranger, BEAM3, AntEpiSeeker and SMMB-ACO, in the two protocols. N_t: total number of interactions identified by a method; N_{IoIs}: number of interactions of interest identified from the N_t previous interactions.

	First protocol		Second protocol	
	N_t	N_{IoIs}	N_t	N_{IoIs}
ranger	34	(**34**) (100%)	180	**180** (100%)
BEAM3	1,082	**131** (12.1%)	130	**11** (8.5%)
AntEpiSeeker	14,670	**13,062** (89.0%)	8,647	**7,633** (88.7%)
DASSO-MB	18	0	—	—
SMMB-ACO	6,346	**1,142** (18.0%)	498	**88** (17.7%)

Table 3 shows an impact of dimension reduction in the decrease of the total number of interactions output, N_t: the ratio of N_t measured for the first protocol to N_t observed for the second protocol is around 8 for BEAM3, close to 1.5 for AntEpiSeeker, and nearly 13 for SMMB-ACO. In the second protocol, AntEpiSeeker still outputs over 7,000 IoIs, whereas BEAM3 and SMMB-ACO respectively generate a dozen and less than a hundred IoIs. The situation of ranger

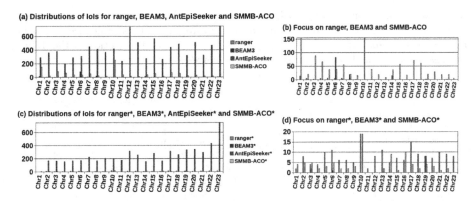

Fig. 3. Distributions of *interactions of interest* detected by ranger, BEAM3, AntEpiSeeker and SMMB-ACO, in the two protocols. "method*" denotes an approach with feature selection. AntEpiSeeker detected 13,062 IoIs which are spread over the 23 chromosomes (smallest number of IoIs for a chromosome: 202; median number: 380). Moreover, IoIs are overly abundant in chromosome X, whose presence is not known to bias Crohn's disease onset (4,427 IoIs representing 34.9% of AntEpiSeeker's IoIs; the corresponding bar is truncated in subfigure (a)). These observations comfort the hypothesis of a high rate of false positives. AntEpiSeeker* detected 7,633 IoIs distributed over all chromosomes but Chr1. An excess of IoIs in chromosome X is still observed for AntEpiSeeker* (35.2% of AntEpiSeeker's IoIs). SMMB-ACO identified 1,142 IoIs distributed across all chromosomes except chromosome X (smallest number of IoIs for a chromosome: 8; median number: 38; largest number: 251; the corresponding bar (Chr10) is truncated in subfigure (b)). SMMB-ACO* highlighted 88 IoIs spread over all chromosomes except Chr11, Chr12 and ChrX (smallest number of IoIs for a chromosome: 1; median number: 3; largest number: 19). The 131 IoIs detected by BEAM3 are located within 5 chromosomes only: Chr1, Chr6, Chr7, Chr8 and Chr14 respectively harbour 13, 83, 2, 18 and 15 IoIs. The 11 IoIs detected by BEAM3* are confined to Chr3 (2 IoIs), Chr6 (1 IoI) and Chr19 (8 IoIs). The 34 IoIs identified by ranger are distributed across 10 chromosomes: Chr2 to Chr7, Chr9, Chr19, Chr22 and Chr23 (minimum number of IoIs for these 10 chromosomes: 1; maximum number: 6). In contrast, the 180 IoIs highlighted by ranger* are spread over all chromosomes (smallest number of IoIs for a chromosome: 2; largest number: 19; median: 8).

is specific (five-fold increase): indeed, the relaxation of the significance threshold, from 5×10^{-4} (first protocol) to 5×10^{-2} (second protocol) was intended to put ranger on equal footing with the other methods' post-processings.

By construction of the protocols, the ratio of the number of IoIs to the total number of interactions is 100% for ranger. For the other methods, the feature selection does not allow to densify the number of IoIs in the outputs generated: the above ratio is constant through the two protocols, for each of the other methods: around 10% for BEAM3, close to 20% for SMMB-ACO and around 90% for AntEpiSeeker. This conclusion, which holds for three methods, is an important contribution of our study: it was not foreseeable that the much-vaunted credentials of feature selection for highlighting SNPs in epistasis detection would be undermined.

Table 4. Comparison of the distributions of p-values for the *interactions of interest* detected with the five approaches, in the two protocols. Four significance intervals are shown for $-log_{10}$(p-value). $-log_{10}(5 \times 10^{-2}) = 1.5$. The top section of the Table presents counts. The bottom section shows the corresponding percentages.

	First protocol					Second protocol			
	$\geq$20	[10, 20[	[5, 10[	[1.5, 5[		$\geq$20	[10, 20[	[5, 10[	[1.5, 5[
ranger	10	12	6	6	ranger*	3	3	1	173
BEAM3	0	0	0	131	BEAM3*	0	0	0	11
AntEpiSeeker	13	13	458	12,578	AntEpiSeeker*	10	8	315	7300
SMMB-ACO	0	0	6	1,136	SMMB-ACO*	0	0	2	86
ranger	29.40%	35.30%	17.65%	17.65%	ranger*	1.67%	1.67%	0.56%	96.10%
BEAM3	0%	0%	0%	100%	BEAM3*	0%	0%	0%	100%
AntEpiSeeker	0.10%	0.10%	3.51%	96.29%	AntEpiSeeker*	0.13%	0.11%	4.13%	95.63%
SMMB-ACO	0%	0%	0.53%	99.47%	SMMB-ACO*	0%	0%	2.27%	97.73%

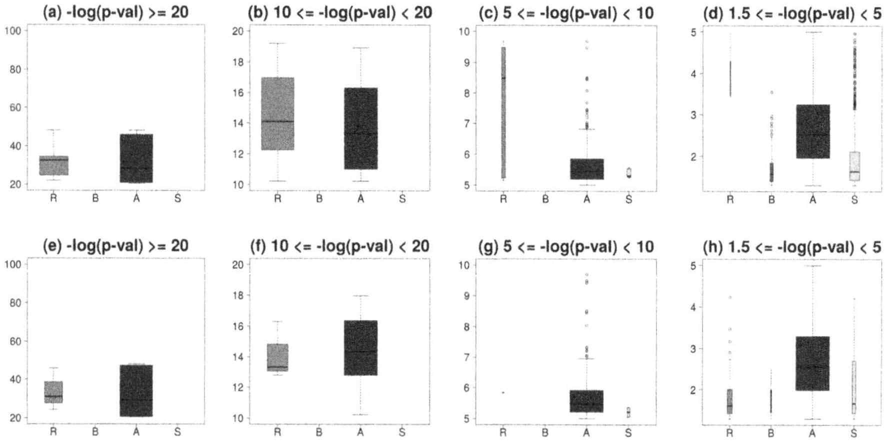

Fig. 4. Distributions of p-values for the *interactions of interest* detected by ranger, BEAM3, AntEpiSeeker and SMMB-ACO, in the two protocols. IoIs: interactions of interest. R: ranger. B: BEAM3. A: AntEpiSeeker. S: SMMB-ACO. $-log_{10}(5 \times 10^{-2}) = 1.5$.

Figure 3 focuses on the distribution of IoIs across the chromosomes. In the first protocol, a sharp contrast exists between AntEpiSeeker and SMMB-ACO, whose IoIs are abundantly present in nearly all chromosomes, and BEAM3 and ranger, whose IoIs are confined to ten and five chromosomes respectively. Besides, the number of IoIs in BEAM3, around four times higher than in ranger, is circumscribed to a number of chromosomes that is two times less than for ranger. In the second protocol, the IoIs respectively detected by SMMB-ACO, AntEpiSeeker and ranger are present in nearly all chromosomes. The relaxation of the significance threshold explains the increase of IoIs in ranger. Again, the IoIs detected by BEAM3 are located in a few chromosomes (three chromosomes in the second protocol *versus* ten chromosomes in the first protocol).

Distributions of P-Values. Figure 4 and Table 4 allow to compare the distributions of IoI p-values obtained across ranger, BEAM3, AntEpiSeeker and SMMB-ACO, in the two protocols. We consider four intervals for the p-values.

We observe great discrepancies between the methods. A first remark is that AntEpiSeeker and ranger are the only two methods for which the p-values spread over the four intervals, for the two protocols: in contrast to the two other methods, AntEpiSeeker and ranger show p-values within the two first intervals (*i.e.*, below 10^{-10}) (subfigures (a), (b), (e) and (f)). A second observation is that BEAM3 is the only method whose 131 p-values (first protocol) and 11 p-values (second protocol) are all contained in the fourth interval (and are even confined to $[10^{-3.5}, 5 \times 10^{-2}]$ (subfigure (d)) and $[10^{-2.5}, 5 \times 10^{-2}]$ (subfigure (h)) for first and second protocols respectively. The overwhelming majority of IoIs detected by SMMB-ACO are also confined in the fourth interval. However, SMMB-ACO is able to highlight more significant IoIs than BEAM3: the SMMB-ACO p-values fall within ranges $[10^{-5}, 5 \times 10^{-2}]$ and $[10^{-4.4}, 5 \times 10^{-2}]$, respectively for the first and second protocols.

Besides, we already observed in Subsect. 6.2 that for each method except ranger, the percentages of IoIs (in the total set of interactions generated by the method) are identical for the two protocols. Again, the two protocols applied on the same method output close p-value distributions. The second conclusion to draw here is as follows: not only does feature selection not increase the rate of IoIs in the interactions generated by a method, feature selection does not enrich the IoIs generated with still more statistically significant IoIs.

6.3   Interactions of Interest Jointly Identified by Several Approaches

None of the 131 IoIs identified by BEAM3 is detected by another method. On the contrary, 32 of the 34 IoIs detected by ranger were also detected by AntEpiSeeker. AntEpiSeeker and SMMB-ACO detected 16 common IoIs. SMMB-ACO and ranger have only 3 IoIs in common. One IoI was jointly identified by AntEpiSeeker, ranger and SMMB-ACO. Under the second protocol, 4 IoIs were jointly identified by ranger* and AntEpiSeeker*.

Given the number of interactions output by AntEpiSeeker, an overlap was expected between AntEpiSeeker and some other method. However, an overlap was only observed between ranger and AntEpiSeeker. On the other hand, our study indicates that the mechanisms behind BEAM3, AntEpiSeeker and SMMB-ACO explore different sets of solutions. Finally, we observe that the selection discarded most of the SNPs that belonged to IoIs jointly identified by ranger and AntEpiSeeker. We emphasize here this impact of the feature selection: in the second protocol, ranger was run with a relaxed threshold (5×10^{-2} instead of 5×10^{-4}); we would therefore expect a larger overlap between AntEpiSeeker and ranger (which we did not check), but we verified that ranger* and AntEpiseeker* do not overlap much when the input dataset is reduced by feature selection.

Table 5. Statistics on the networks of *interactions of interest*, across all chromosomes, for ranger, BEAM3, AntEpiSeeker and SMMB-ACO, in the two protocols. "method*" denotes an approach with feature selection. IoI: interaction of interest. n_{IoIs}: total number of IoIs detected by a method; nb_{chr}: number of chromosomes in which IoI networks were found; nb_{net}: number of such IoI networks; N_i, N_g and N_s: respectively, number of IoIs, genes and SNPs in a network. Q1, Q2 and Q3 respectively denote the first quartile, the median and the third quartile.

Method	n_{IoIs}	nb_{chr}	nb_{net}	N_i			N_g			N_s		
				Q1	Q2	Q3	Q1	Q2	Q3	Q1	Q2	Q3
ranger	34	7	8	2	3.5	4	0	0.5	1	3	4.5	5
ranger*	180	23	25	4	6	8	2	3	6	5	7	9
BEAM3	131	4	4	14.3	16.5	33.8	10	10.5	13.8	12	13	22
BEAM3*	11	1	1	8	8	8	6	6	6	8	8	8
AntEpiSeeker	13,062	23	929	2	3	4	2	3	4	3	4	5
AntEpiSeeker*	7,633	23	611	2	3	4	1	2	4	3	4	5
SMMB-ACO	1,142	22	87	2	4	8.5	2	4	8	3	5	9.5
SMMB-ACO*	88	20	15	2	2	3	1.8	3	4	3	3	4

6.4 Networks of Interactions of Interest

This subsection is devoted to the detection of networks of interactions of interest (IoIs). Some statistics on the number of networks identified per method are first provided. Then we focus on the distributions of the networks' sizes. We end this subsection by comparing across all methods the spatial distributions of the networks of IoIs across chromosomes.

Number of Networks Detected and Distribution of Their Sizes. For each method and for each chromosome, we have identified all pairs of IoIs whose members share a SNP. This led us to build networks of IoIs. Table 5 allows to compare the four methods, in the two protocols, with respect to the numbers of IoIs, genes and SNPs involved in each of the networks identified across all chromosomes. We used the R package biomaRt to identify the genes associated with SNPs [7]. We could only identify genes for SNPs whose RefSNP label (*e.g.*, rs1996546) is known for the corresponding SNP provided by the WTCCC Consortium. For example, a network involving 6 IoIs and 7 SNPs was identified in chromosome 5 through ranger; however, none of the corresponding genes could be retrieved in this case.

We first observe that the number of IoI networks is more or less related to the total number of IoIs detected by the method considered. This observation was expected for statistical reasons. The second remark to draw from Table 5 is the existence of a contrast between the networks in ranger*, BEAM3* and BEAM3, and the networks in the other methods. For the three former methods, the medians for the number of IoIs in a network are respectively 6, 8 and 16.5. All the other methods show a median in interval [2, 4]. The maxima observed for the 25, 1 and 4 networks respectively identified in ranger*, BEAM3* and BEAM3 are respectively 18, 8 and 81 IoIs in a network.

The explanation for these high medians lies in the small number of networks identified, which gives weight to the few networks of large sizes. Indeed, ranger and SMMB-ACO* only detected 8 and 15 IoI networks respectively, but no outlier exists for ranger (maximum number of IoIs in a network: 6), or only one exists for SMMB-ACO* (maximum number of IoIs in a network: 9). On the other hand, it is remarkable that the *median* number of IoIs in a network is not inflated for SMMB-ACO, AntEpiSeeker* and AntEpiSeeker, which yielded over a thousand IoIs. Therefore, we conclude that the number of IoIs detected by a method impacts the number of IoI networks identified, but not the size of the networks identified.

Besides, as highlighted in Sect. 6.2 (caption of Fig. 3), a specific behavior was shown for AntEpiSeeker and AntEpiSeeker*: they detected a third of their IoIs in chromosome X. Again, a specific characteristic is shown: the first method identified a *single* network containing 4,330 IoIs, whereas the second method detected a *unique* network of size 2,575 IoIs. All the remarks provided in this paragraph hold when we consider N_s, the number of SNPs, to measure the size of an IoI network. The conclusions are similar if we consider N_g, the number of genes, except that we could not list genes related to SNPs with unknown RefSNP labels, on the one hand, and that some SNPs are connected to several genes, on the other hand.

Spatial Distribution of the Interactions of Interest Detected Across Chromosomes. Figure 5 allows the visual comparison of the spatial distributions of IoIs across chromosomes, for ranger, BEAM3, AntEpiSeeker and SMMB-ACO, in the two protocols. As an illustration, Fig. 6 focuses on SMMB-ACO, for which a SNP may belong to 10 IoIs and even up to 19 (chromosome 10). These two latter figures were drawn using the R software package circos dedicated to data visualization through circular layouts [23].

Illustration with a Network Detected by SMMB-ACO, and Biological Insights. As an illustration, we show in Table 6 the 19 IoIs constituting one of the networks identified in chromosome 10 by SMMB-ACO run downstream feature selection. This network involves 13 SNPs and is related to 6 known genes. It is beyond the scope of this study focused on methodological and computational aspects, to bring deeper biological insights on the potential mechanisms involved in the networks and IoIs.

Besides a number of standard single-SNP GWASs, the few AISs devoted to Crohn's disease (CD) focus on genes or pathways already known to contribute to the disease onset, such as NOD on Chr16, CCNY and NKX2-3 on Chr10, LGALS9 and STAT3 on Chr17, and SBNO2 on Chr19 [21,26]. It is not a surprise that among the six genes highlighted in the network of Fig. 7, two genes are already known to impact CD onset: CCNY and NKX2-3. It was also expected that our protocol designed for AIS investigation without prior biological knowledge would detect novel interaction candidates, which it does.

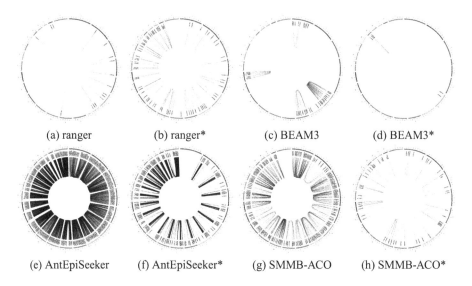

| (a) ranger | (b) ranger* | (c) BEAM3 | (d) BEAM3* |

| (e) AntEpiSeeker | (f) AntEpiSeeker* | (g) SMMB-ACO | (h) SMMB-ACO* |

Fig. 5. Spatial distributions of the *interactions of interest* detected across the chromosomes, for ranger, BEAM3, AntEpiSeeker and SMMB-ACO under the two protocols. "method*" denotes an approach with feature selection.

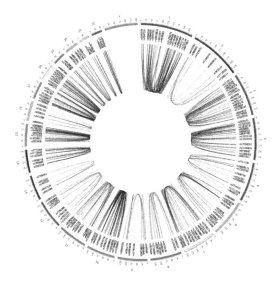

Fig. 6. Spatial distribution of the interactions of interest detected across the chromosomes, for SMMB-ACO.

6.5   Discussion

We gained considerable and unforeseeable insights from our study. First, on the CD dataset, DASSO-MB is of no help. The verbose AntEpiSeeker provides a

Table 6. Network of 19 interactions of interest, 13 SNPs and 6 known genes, identified by SMMB-ACO* in chromosome 10. "SMMB-ACO*" denotes the approach with feature selection. A letter in first column and a letter in second column denote an interaction (for instance, G-F in first line). iv: intron variant; gutv: genic upstream transcript variant; utv: upstream transcript variant; gdtv: genic downstream transcript variant; nctv: non coding transcript variant; 3puv: 3 prime UTR variant. CREM encodes a transcription factor that binds to the cAMP responsive element found in many cellular promoters. Alternative promoter and translation initiation site usage enables CREM to exert spatial and temporal specificity in cAMP-mediated signal transduction. This gene is broadly expressed (36 tissues including colon, small intestine and appendix). CUL2 is a major component of multiple cullin-RING-based ECS (ElonginB/C-CUL2/5-SOCS-box protein) E3 ubiquitin-protein ligase complexes; these complexes mediate the ubiquitination of target proteins. CUL2 is ubiquitous (27 tissues, including colon, small intestine and appendix). NKX2-3 is a member of the NKX family of homeodomain-containing transcription factors; the latter are involved in many aspects of cell type specification and maintenance of differentiated tissue functions. LINC01475 (long intergenic non-protein coding RNA 1475) is expressed in 7 tissues including colon, small intestine, duodenum and appendix. CPXM2, a protein of the carboxypeptidase X, M14 family member 2, is broadly expressed in 21 tissues. CCNY belongs to the cyclins, which control cell division cycles and regulate cyclin-dependent kinases (27 tissues including colon, small intestine, duodenum and appendix).

SNP	RefSNP label	Location	Gene	SNP	RefSNP label	Location	Gene
G	rs7095491	99514301	—	F	rs2505639	35185493	CREM (gutv, gdtv, iv)
				H	rs11010067	35006503	—
				I	rs4934709	35050396	CUL2 (iv)
				K	rs17582416	34998722	—
				D	rs10761659	62685804	—
D	rs10761659	62685804	—	E	rs7078219	99514608	—
				J	rs10883371	99532698	NKX2-3, LINC01475 (utv)
				L	rs1548964	99529896	LINC01475 (iv)
				B	rs7067790	123917521	CPXM2 (gutv, iv)
				M	rs3936503	35260329	CCNY (gutv, iv)
L	rs1548964	99529896	LINC01475 (iv)	F	rs2505639	35185493	CREM (gutv, gdtv, iv)
				I	rs4934709	35050396	CUL2 (iv)
				A	rs10995271	62678726	—
B	rs7067790	123917521	CPXM2 (gutv, iv)	A	rs10995271	62678726	—
				C	rs6601764	3820350	—
J	rs10883371	99532698	NKX2-3, LINC01475 (utv)	F	rs2505639	35185493	CREM (gutv, gdtv, iv)
				I	rs4934709	35050396	CUL2 (iv)
I	rs4934709	35050396	CUL2 (iv)	A	rs10995271	62678726	—
M	rs3936503	35260329	CCNY (gutv, iv)	E	rs7078219	99514608	—

wealth of results, in which we suspect a high rate of false positives. Moreover, under each protocol, 30% of the IoIs generated by AntEpiSeeker are discovered in chromosome X, a chromosome not related to Crohn's disease. Besides, it appears

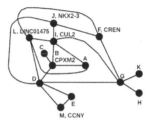

Fig. 7. Network of 19 interactions of interest, 13 SNPs and 6 known genes, identified by SMMB-ACO* in chromosome 10. See Table 6 for complementary information.

that the only way to reduce this verbosity is decreasing the p-value threshold. The widely cited software BEAM3 cannot pinpoint IoIs with p-values lower than $10^{-3.5}$. In this respect, SMMB-ACO seems more promising than the renowned BEAM3, on the CD dataset. The reason lies in BEAM3's low number of 2-way interactions. In contrast, SMMB-ACO notably detects IoIs in chromosome 10, a chromosome which harbours genes connected to CD. Besides, in spite of dimension reduction, this result holds when feature selection is applied upstream SMMB-ACO. To note, ranger is the only method in the first protocol to output a high proportion (around 65%) of IoIs with low p-values (below 10^{-10}). However, with a relaxed threshold and upstream feature selection, this phenomenon is marginal.

The case of ranger set apart, feature selection does not help increase the rate of IoIs (significant 2-way interactions) in the interactions generated by any method. In BEAM3, AntEpiSeeker and SMMB-ACO, the ratio of the number of IoIs to the total number of interactions detected remains constant through the two protocols: around 10% for BEAM3, around 90% for AntEpiSeeker, and close to 20% for SMMB-ACO. This conclusion is an important contribution of our study since feature selection is often put forth as a means to not only reduce the search space, but reduce it to a subspace of interest. In the case of the CD dataset, feature selection just implemented data dimension reduction. Besides, the three methods differ in the ratios of IoIs identified, which shows that these methods do not explore the same solution space. Moreover, feature selection does not enrich the IoIs generated with still more statistically significant IoIs.

Finally, the number of IoIs detected by a method impacts the number of IoI networks identified, but not the size of the networks identified.

The two experimental protocols implemented in this extensive analysis allow us to highlight a great heterogeneity between the methods compared, in all domains: running times, numbers of IoIs detected, distributions of p-values for the IoIs identified, numbers of IoI networks and distributions of the sizes of the latter. Some methods, which fall into the category of widely cited approaches in the literature, however showed weaknesses. BEAM3 is extremely time consuming for large chromosome datasets. At the opposite, a flaw was also evidenced since BEAM3 produced surprisingly high running times for small datasets obtained *via* feature selection. The verbosity of AntEpiSeeker, even on reduced datasets of around 5,000 SNPs, renders its use questionable for practitioners: it is not affordable to biologically validate IoIs whose number scales in thousands. Thus, the quickness of AntEpiSeeker is impeded by this verbosity. The more recent approach SMMB-ACO, a complex method, is nonetheless faster than the reference software BEAM3. However, SMMB-ACO still requires memory management improvements since it was shown to consume fluctuating memory across several runs on the same large dataset.

7   Conclusion and Further Work

For computational reasons, in the GWAS field, simulations are performed using data whose dimension is not comparable with real genome-wide datasets'. Consequently, these simulations reveal nothing about the effectiveness and efficiency of methods in true conditions. Moreover, the ratio between the number of SNPs and the number of subjects observed is not comparable between simulated and real datasets.

This work departs from the standard framework in genetic association studies as it reports an unprecedented extensive comparative analysis of five approaches on large-scale real data, following two experimental protocols. In the first protocol, the native methods are used straightforwardly. In the second protocol, feature selection is performed upstream of these methods. Our analysis rapidly discarded DASSO-MB, to focus on the two remaining state-of-the-art approaches designed to detect epistasis from scratch, AntEpiSeeker and BEAM3. An unavoidable reference in GWAS, ranger was used in combination with logistic regression, to detect epistasis. A more recent approach, SMMB-ACO, was included in the comparison. We designed the two experimental protocols, taking care to output comparable sets of (2-way) interactions across the approaches. In the second protocol, ranger was used upstream any of the former methods (including ranger itself), to implement feature selection. Using 23 chromosome-wide case control datasets related to Crohn's disease, we achieved 1,150 feature selection phases together with 1,886 genetic analyses. We observed a great heterogeneity across methods in all aspects: running times and memory requirements, numbers of interactions of interest (IoIs) output, p-value ranges, numbers of IoI networks and distributions of the sizes of the latter.

The insights gained in the present work will lead us to discart feature selection in our future work. We plan to extend the comparative analysis to six additional genome-wide real datasets. At this scale (10,441 chromosome-wide analyses on 161 datasets), we will be able to confirm or infirm the trends observed for the CD dataset. We also plan to consider various genetic models.

Acknowledgment. This work was supported by the GRIOTE Research project funded by the Pays de la Loire Region. In this study, we have processed real-world data generated by the Wellcome Trust Case Control Consortium. The experiments reported in this paper were performed at the CCIPL (Centre de Calcul Intensif des Pays de la Loire).

Appendix

Table 7. Parameter adjustment for the five methods. (Table published in [3]).

Software	Parameter description	Value
Ranger	**num.trees** Number of trees	500
	mtry Number of variables to possibly split at in each node, with n, the total number of variables	$5/8\,n$
	impmeasure Type of importance measure	Gini Index
BEAM3	**itburn** Number of iterations in burn-in phase	50
	itstat Number of iterations in stationary phase	50
AntEpiSeeker	**iAntCount** Number of ants	1000
	iItCountLarge Number of iterations for the large haplotypes	150
	iItCountSmall Number of iterations for the small haplotypes	300
	iEpiModel Number of SNPs in an epistatic interaction	2
	pvalue p-value threshold (after Bonferroni correction)	5×10^{-4}
	alpha Weight given to pheromone deposited by ants	1
	phe Initial pheromone rate for each variable	100
	rou Evaporation rate in ant colony optimization	0.05
DASSO-MB	**alpha** Global type I error threshold	5×10^{-4}
SMMB-ACO	$\mathbf{n_{it}}$ Number of ACO iterations	360
	$\mathbf{n_{ants}}$ Number of ants	20
	$\mathbf{K_a}$ Size of the subset of variables sampled by each ant	160
	k Size of a combination of variables sampled amongst the K_a above variables ($k < K_a$)	3
	α' Global type I error threshold	5×10^{-4}
	τ_0 Constant to initiate pheromone rates	100
	ρ and λ Two constants used to update pheromone rates	0.05 0.1
	η Vector of weights, to account for prior knowledge on the variables	1
	α and β Two constants used to adjust the relative importance between pheromone rate and Prior knowledge on the variables	1 1

References

1. Aflakparast, M., Salimi, H., Gerami, A., Dubé, M.-P., Visweswaran, S., et al.: Cuckoo search epistasis: a new method for exploring significant genetic interactions. Heredity **112**, 666–764 (2014)
2. Ayers, K., Cordell, H.: SNP selection in genome-wide and candidate gene studies via penalized logistic regression. Genet. Epidemiol. **34**(8), 879–891 (2010)
3. Boisaubert, H., Sinoquet, C.: Detection of gene-gene interactions: methodological comparison on real-world data and insights on synergy between methods. In: Proceedings of the 12th International Joint Conference on Biomedical Engineering Systems and Technologies (BIOSTEC 2019), vol. 3, pp. 30–42. BIOINFORMATICS (2019)
4. Breiman, L.: Bagging predictors. Mach. Learn. **24**(2), 123–140 (1996). https://doi.org/10.1023/A:1018054314350
5. Chang, Y.-C., Wu, J.-T., Hong, M.-Y., Tung, Y.-A., Hsieh, P.-H., et al.: GenEpi: gene-based epistasis discovery using machine learning (2018). bioRXiv, https://doi.org/10.1101/421719
6. Chatelain, C., Durand, G., Thuillier, V., Augé, F.: Performance of epistasis detection methods in semi-simulated GWAS. BMC Bioinform. **19**(1), 231 (2018)
7. Durinck, S., Moreau, Y., Kasprzyk, A., Davis, S., Moor, B.D., et al.: Biomart and Bioconductor: a powerful link between biological databases and microarray data analysis. Bioinformatics **21**, 3439–3440 (2005)
8. Fergus, P., Montanez, C., Abdulaimma, B., Lisboa, P., Chalmers, C.: Utilising deep learning and genome wide association studies for epistatic-driven preterm birth classification in African-American women (2018). arXiv preprint, arXiv:1801.02977
9. Furlong, L.: Human diseases through the lens of network biology. Trends Genet. **29**, 150–159 (2013)
10. Gao, H., Granka, J., Feldman, M.: On the classification of epistatic interactions. Genetics **184**(3), 827–837 (2010)
11. Gibert, J.-M., Blanco, J., Dolezal, M., Nolte, V., Peronnet, F., Schlötterer, C.: Strong epistatic and additive effects of linked candidate SNPs for Drosophila pigmentation have implications for analysis of genome-wide association studies results. Genome Biol. **18**, 126 (2017)
12. Gilbert-Diamond, D., Moore, J.: Analysis of gene-gene interactions. Current Protocols in Human Genetics, 0 1: Unit1.14 (2011)
13. Gola, D., Mahachie John, J., van Steen, K., König, I.: A roadmap to multifactor dimensionality reduction methods. Briefings Bioinform. **17**(2), 293–308 (2016)
14. Graham, D., Xavier, R.: From genetics of inflammatory bowel disease towards mechanistic insights. Trends Immunol. **34**, 371–378 (2013)
15. Han, B., Chen, X.-W.: bNEAT: a Bayesian network method for detecting epistatic interactions in genome-wide association studies. BMC Genomics **12**(Suppl. 2), S9 (2011)
16. Han, B., Chen, X.-W., Talebizadeh, Z.: FEPI-MB: identifying SNPs-disease association using a Markov blanket-based approach. BMC Bioinform. **12**(Suppl. 12), S3 (2011)
17. Han, B., Park, M., Chen, X.-W.: A Markov blanket-based method for detecting causal SNPs in GWAS. BMC Bioinform. **11**(Suppl. 3), S5 (2010)
18. Hohman, T., Bush, W., Jiang, L., Brown-Gentry, K., Torstenson, E., et al.: Discovery of gene-gene interactions across multiple independent datasets of Late Onset Alzheimer Disease from the Alzheimer Disease Genetics Consortium. Neurobiol. Aging **38**, 141–150 (2016)

19. Jiang, X., Neapolitan, R., Barmada, M., Visweswaran, S., Cooper, G.: A fast algorithm for learning epistatic genomic relationships. In: Proceedings of the Annual American Medical Informatics Association Symposium (AMIA 2010), pp. 341–345 (2010)

20. Jing, P., Shen, H.: MACOED: a multi-objective ant colony optimization algorithm for SNP epistasis detection in genome-wide association studies. Bioinformatics **31**(5), 634–641 (2015)

21. Khor, B., Gardet, A., Ramnik, J.: Genetics and pathogenesis of inflammatory bowel disease. Nature **474**(7351), 307–317 (2011)

22. Koller, D., Sahami, M.: Toward optimal feature selection. In: Proceedings of the 13th Conference on Machine Learning (ICML 1996), pp. 284–292. Morgan Kaufmann, San Fransisco (1996)

23. Krzywinski, M., Schein, J., Birol, I., Connors, J., Gascoyne, R., et al.: Circos: an information aesthetic for comparative genomics. Genome Res. **19**(9), 1639–1645 (2009)

24. Li, J., Malley, J., Andrew, A., Karagas, M., Moore, J.: Detecting gene-gene interactions using a permutation-based random forest method. BioData Min. **9**, 14 (2016)

25. Lunetta, K., Hayward, L., Segal, J., Eerdewegh, P.V.: Screening large-scale association study data: exploiting interactions using random forests. BMC Genet. **5**, 32 (2004)

26. McGovern, D., Kugathasan, S., Cho, J.: Genetics of inflammatory bowel diseases. Gastroenterology **149**(5), 1163–1176 (2015)

27. Nicodemus, K., Law, A., Radulescu, E., Luna, A., Kolachana, B., et al.: Biological validation of increased schizophrenia risk with NRG1, ERBB4, and AKT1 epistasis via functional neuroimaging in healthy controls. Arch. Gen. Psychiatry **67**(10), 991–1001 (2013)

28. Pearl, J.: Probabilistic Reasoning in Intelligent Systems: Networks of Plausible Inference. Morgan Kaufmann Publishers Inc., San Francisco (1988)

29. Sackton, T., Hartl, D.: Genotypic context and epistasis in individuals and populations. Cell **166**(2), 279–287 (2016)

30. Schwarz, D., König, I., Ziegler, A.: On safari to random jungle: a fast implementation of random forests for high-dimensional data. Bioinformatics **26**(14), 1752–1758 (2010)

31. Shen, Y., Liu, Z., Ott, J.: Support vector machines with L1 penalty for detecting gene-gene interactions. Int. J. Data Min. Bioinform. **6**, 463–470 (2012)

32. Sinoquet, C., Niel, C.: Enhancement of a stochastic Markov blanket framework with ant colony optimization, to uncover epistasis in genetic association studies. In: Proceedings of the 26th European Symposium on Artificial Neural Networks, Computational Intelligence and Machine Learning (ESANN 2018), pp. 673–678 (2018)

33. Stanislas, V., Dalmasso, C., Ambroise, C.: Eigen-Epistasis for detecting gene-gene interactions. BMC Bioinform. **18**, 54 (2017). https://doi.org/10.1186/s12859-017-1488-0

34. Sun, Y., Shang, J., Liu, J.-X., Li, S., Zheng, C.-H.: epiACO - a method for identifying epistasis based on ant colony optimization algorithm. BioData Min. **10**, 23 (2017)

35. Uppu, S., Krishna, A., Gopalan, R.: Towards deep learning in genome-wide association interaction studies. In: Proceedings of the 20th Pacific Asia Conference on Information Systems (PACIS2016), p. 20 (2016)

36. Urbanowicz, R., Meeker, M., LaCava, W., Olson, R., Moore, J.: Relief-based feature selection: introduction and review. J. Biomed. Inform. **85**, 189–203 (2018)
37. Vineis, P., Pearce, N.: Missing heritability in genome-wide association study research. Nat. Rev. Genet. **11**, 589–589 (2010)
38. Visscher, P., Wray, N., Zhang, Q., Sklar, P., McCarthy, M., et al.: 10 years of GWAS discovery: biology, function, and translation. Am. J. Hum. Genet. **101**(1), 5–22 (2017)
39. Wang, Y., Liu, X., Robbins, K., Rekaya, R.: AntEpiSeeker: detecting epistatic interactions for case-control studies using a two-stage ant colony optimization algorithm. BMC Res. Notes **3**, 117 (2010)
40. Wright, M., Ziegler, A.: ranger: a fast implementation of random forests for high dimensional data in C++ and R. J. Stat. Softw. **77**(1), 1–17 (2017)
41. Zhang, Y.: A novel Bayesian graphical model for genome-wide multi-SNP association mapping. Genet. Epidemiol. **36**(1), 36–47 (2012)
42. Zhang, Y., Liu, J.: Bayesian inference of epistatic interactions in case-control studies. Nat. Genet. **39**, 1167–1173 (2007)
43. Zhu, Z., Tong, X., Zhu, Z., Liang, M., Cui, W., et al.: Development of MDR-GPU for gene-gene interaction analysis and its application to WTCCC GWAS data for type 2 diabetes. PLOS ONE **8**(4), e61943 (2013)
44. Zuk, O., Hechter, E., Sunyaev, S., Lander, E.: The mystery of missing heritability: genetic interactions create phantom heritability. Proc. Nat. Acad. Sci. **109**, 1193–1198 (2012)

The Properties of the Standard Genetic Code and Its Selected Alternatives in Terms of the Optimal Graph Partition

Daniyah A. Aloqalaa[1], Dariusz R. Kowalski[2,4], Paweł Błażej[3], Małgorzata Wnętrzak[3], Dorota Mackiewicz[3], and Paweł Mackiewicz[3(✉)]

[1] Department of Computer Science, University of Liverpool, Liverpool, UK
d.aloqalaa@gmail.com
[2] SWPS University of Social Sciences and Humanities, Warsaw, Poland
dariusz.kowalski@swps.edu.pl
[3] Faculty of Biotechnology, University of Wrocław, Wrocław, Poland
pawel.blazej@uwr.edu.pl, earine2909@gmail.com,
{dorota,pamac}@smorfland.uni.wroc.pl
[4] School of Computer and Cyber Sciences, Augusta University, Augusta, USA

Abstract. The standard genetic code (SGC) is a system of rules, which assigns 20 amino acids and stop translation signal to 64 codons, i.e triplets of nucleotides. The structure of the SGC shows some properties suggesting that this code evolved to minimize deleterious effects of mutations and translational errors. To analyse this issue, we presented the structure of the SGC and its natural alternative versions as a graph, in which vertices corresponded to codons and edges to point mutations between these codons. The mutations were weighted according to the mutation type, i.e. transitions and transversions. Under this representation, each genetic code is a partition of the set of vertices into 21 disjoint subsets, while its resistance to the mutation consequences can be reformulated into the optimal graph clustering task. In order to investigate this problem, we developed an appropriate clustering algorithm, which searched for the codes showing the minimum average calculated for the set conductance of codon groups. The algorithm found three best codes for various ranges of the weights for the mutations. The average weighted-conductance of the studied genetic codes was the most similar to that of the best codes in the range of weights corresponding to the observed transversion/transition ratio in natural mutational pressures. However, it should be noted that the optimization of the codes was not as perfect as the best codes and many alternative genetic codes performed better than the SGC. These results may suggest that the evolution of the SGC was driven not only by the selection for the robustness to mutations or mistranslations.

Keywords: Code degeneracy · Graph theory · Mutation · Set conductance · Standard genetic code · Transition · Transversion

Supported by the National Science Centre, Poland (Narodowe Centrum Nauki, Polska) under Grants number UMO-2017/27/N/NZ2/00403 and UMO-2017/25/B/ST6/02553.

© Springer Nature Switzerland AG 2020
A. Roque et al. (Eds.): BIOSTEC 2019, CCIS 1211, pp. 170–191, 2020.
https://doi.org/10.1007/978-3-030-46970-2_9

1   Introduction

The origin and the structure of the standard genetic code (SGC) have puzzled biologists since the first assignments of codons to amino acids were discovered [46,63]. The code is a universal set of rules responsible for transmitting genetic information encoded in DNA molecules into the protein world. Specifically, the code uses all possible 64 nucleotide triplets, i.e. codons, to encode 20 canonical amino acids and also the signal for stopping the protein synthesis, i.e. translation.

Since the total number of codons is greater than the number of encoded items, the code have to be degenerated. It means that there are amino acids that are encoded by more than one codon. These redundant codons, called synonymous, are organized in characteristic groups. In most cases, the groups include codons that differ in the third position, which is called a degenerate position. These positions can show various level of redundancy described as n-fold degeneracy, where n is the number of nucleotides out of four possible (A, C, G, T) that specify the same amino acid at this position. The high degeneracy level of the third codon position suggested to Francis Crick that only the first two codon positions were important in a primordial code [21].

The redundancy of the genetic code entails important consequences related to the process of single nucleotide mutations. If these changes occur in the degenerate codon position, the originally encoded amino acid will not be changed. These mutations are called synonymous or silent, whereas those that change the encoded amino acid or stop translation signal are named nonsynonymous. In the case of four-fold degenerated positions, all possible single nucleotide changes are synonymous and do not affect the coded amino acid. In almost all two-fold degenerated positions, the synonymous character is shown by transitions, i.e. when a purine nucleotide, i.e. adenine or guanine, mutates to another purine (A↔G), or a pyrimidine nucleotide, i.e. cytosine or thymine, changes into another pyrimidine (C↔T). Another types of point mutations are transversions, when a purine mutates to a pyrimidine or *vice versa* (A↔C, A↔T, G↔C, G↔T).

There are four possible transitions and eight possible transversions, but transitions are more often observed in sequences than transversions in biological sequences [31,39,49,55,56,67,68,77]. It may result from a higher mutation rate of transitions than transversions in nucleic acids due to the greater physico-chemical similarity between nucleotides of the same type, less distinguished by enzymes processing DNA and RNA. Moreover, transitions are accepted with a greater probability because they rarely lead to amino acid substitutions in encoded proteins due to the specific degeneracy of codons, especially two-fold degenerated. The transitions occur also more frequently during protein synthesis [34].

It must be emphasized, however, that the synonymous substitutions do not have to be completely neutral mutations, even though they do not change a coded amino acid. The specific codon usage can be associated with co-translational modifications of amino acids, efficiency and accuracy of translation as well as co-translational folding of synthesized proteins [18,44,85]. The synonymous codon usage can be also under the influence of selection at the amino acid level [7,61].

The SGC structure shows a tendency to minimize the number of nonsynony-mous substitutions, which suggested that this code could have evolved to mini-mize harmful consequences of mutations and translational errors [3,4,28,30,33–38,40–42,79]. Since ancestral forms of the current genetic code did not survive to modern times, it is not easy to reconstruct the primordial stages of the SGC evolution. Therefore, it is especially interesting to investigate the properties of the SGC in comparison with its alternative variants called alternative genetic codes (AGCs), because such study can reveal general tendencies in the genetic code evolution. AGCs operate mainly in bacterial [17,54,59] and organellar genomes [1,20,22,23,45,47,51,65,75], but were also found in nuclear genomes of eukaryotes [43,62,66,70,73,74,84]. AGCs are particularly characteristic of small genomes containing a limited number of protein-coding sequences, which facili-tates the evolution of alternative codes, because potential codon reassignments may not as deleterious as in huge genomes encoding many proteins. Some com-parisons of the SGC and the AGCs showed that the latter were not selected for robustness against mutations [36,50,69], but others revealed that they became better optimized in this respect [5,13,60].

Since the genetic code is a set of codons, which are related, e.g. by nucleotide mutations, the general structure of this code can be well described by the methodology taken from graph theory [6,52]. Similarly to [10,76], we assume that the code encodes 21 items, i.e. 20 amino acids and stop translation signal, and all 64 codons create the set of vertices of the graph, in which the set of edges corresponds to all possible single nucleotide mutations occurring between the codons. This graph is undirected, unweighted and regular. Moreover, accord-ing to this representation, each genetic code is a partition of the set of vertices into 21 disjoint subsets. Therefore, the question about the potential genetic code optimality in regard to the mutations can be reformulated into the optimal graph clustering problem.

The present study is a continuation of our previous work [2] and investigates the properties of the SGC in comparison with selected AGCs, which are gathered at the NCBI database (http://www.ncbi.nlm.nih.gov/Taxonomy/Utils/wprint. cgi). In total, we tested 15 AGCs that differ from the SGC in at least one codon reassignment. In the Table 1, we presented the tested alternative codes and the number of codon reassignments compared with the SGC.

The applied graph representation of the genetic code is a general model, because includes transition to transversion ratio, which was not considered pre-viously by [10,76]. From the mathematical point of view, the analyzed repre-sentation of the genetic code is the weighted graph, in which all weights were dependent on the nucleotide substitution type. To quantify robustness of the codes to mutations, we adjusted the set conductance measure. It is widely used in the graph theory [52] and has many practical interpretations, for example in the theory of random walks [53] and social networks [16]. In the task considered here, the conductance of a codon group is the ratio of the weights of nonsyn-onymous mutations to the weights of all possible single nucleotide mutations, which affect codons in this group. Thus, this parameter can measure robustness

Table 1. Alternative genetic codes.

Full name	Abbreviation	Num. of reassign
Alternative Flatworm Mitochondrial Code	AFMC	4
Alternative Yeast Nuclear Code	AYNC	1
Ascidian Mitochondrial Code	AMC	4
Chlorophycean Mitochondrial Code	CMC	1
Euploid Nuclear Code	ENC	1
Echinoderm and Flatworm Mitochondrial Code	FMC	4
Candidate Division SR1 and Gracilibacteria Code	GC	1
Ciliate, Dasycladacean and Hexamita Nuclear Code	HNC	2
Invertebrate Mitochondrial Code	IMC	4
Mold, Protozoan, and Coelenterate Mitochondrial Code and the Mycoplasma/Spiroplasma Code	PrMC	1
Pterobranchia Mitochondrial Code	PtMC	3
Scenedesmus obliquus Mitochondrial Code	SMC	2
Pachysolen tannophilus Nuclear Code	TNC	1
Trematode Mitochondrial Code	TMC	5
Vertebrate Mitochondrial Code	VMC	4

of the genetic codes against the potential changes in protein-coding sequences. Basing on the methodology described in detail by [10], we found the genetic code structures that are solutions of the optimal graph clustering problem.

2 Preliminaries

2.1 Model Description

We developed a graph representation of the genetic code to study properties of its general structure. Let $G(V, E)$ be a graph in which V is the set of vertices representing all possible 64 codons, while E is the set of edges connecting these vertices. All connections fulfil the property that the vertices, i.e. codons $u, v \in V$ are connected by the edge $e(u, v) \in E$ ($u \sim v$), if and only if the codon u differs from the codon v in exactly one position. From a biological perspective, the set of edges represents all possible single nucleotide substitutions, which occur between codons in a DNA sequence. What is more, this model includes two important types of mutations, transitions and transversions. We assume that all transitions are given a weight, which equals always to one, while the transversions have a weight W, where $W \in [0, \infty)$. The larger weight indicates that the transversions are more important than transitions in the model. The weight can be interpreted as transversion to transition ratio. Hence, the graph G is undirected, weighted and regular with the vertices degree equal to 9.

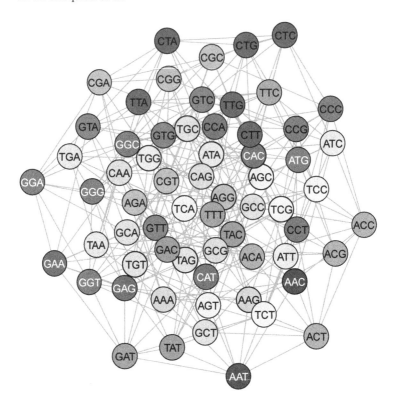

Fig. 1. The standard genetic code as an example of the partition of the graph $G(V, E)$. Every group of vertices with the same colour corresponds to the respective set of codons, which code for the same amino acid or stop translation signal. The edges represent all possible single nucleotide substitutions. According to [2]. (Color figure online)

Following the methodology presented in [10], each potential genetic code C, which encodes 20 amino acids and stop translation signal is a partition of the set V into 21 disjoint subsets, i.e. groups of codons, S. Thus, we obtain the following representation of the genetic code C:

$$C = \{S_1, S_2, \cdots, S_{20}, S_{21} : S_i \cap S_j = \emptyset, S_1 \cup S_2 \cup \cdots \cup S_{21} = V\}.$$

Figure 1 shows an example of the partition of the graph G, which corresponds to the standard genetic code. From a biological point of view, it is interesting to study the code structure according to the types and the number of connections between and within the codon groups, because these connections correspond to nonsynonymous and synonymous substitutions, respectively. The former have a more harmful effect on coded proteins than the latter. It should be noted that each potential genetic code that minimizes the number of the nonsynonymous substitutions is regarded the best in terms of decreasing the biological consequences of mutations. Therefore, the conditions under which the partitions of the graph vertices describe the best genetic code, are worth finding.

There are many methods of the optimal graph partitioning, which are based on different approaches. Here, we decided to use the set conductance measure, which is important in the spectral graph clustering method. This measure enabled us to investigate the theoretical features of genetic codes in terms of the connections between the codon groups. The definition of the set W-conductance measure including weights for edges is as follows [2]:

Definition 1. *For a given weighted graph G let W be a weight of transversion connections in G and S be a subset of V. The W-conductance of S is defined as:*

$$\phi_S(W) = \frac{E_{tr}(S, \overline{S}) + E_{trv}(S, \overline{S}) \cdot W}{|S| \cdot (3 + 6W)} \, ,$$

where $E_{tr}(S, \overline{S})$ is the total number of transition edges going from S to its complement $\overline{S}$, whereas $E_{trv}(S, \overline{S})$ is the total number of transversion edges going from S to its complement $\overline{S}$, and $|S|$ is the number of vertices belonging to S.

The definition of the set W-conductance is a good staring point to describe a quality measure of a given codon group. Large values of this measure mean that a substantial fraction of substitutions, in which these codons are involved, are nonsynonymous, i.e. they change one amino acid to another. From the robustness point of view, small values are desirable because in this case many substitutions are neutral (synonymous) and do not change coded amino acids.

Following the definition of the set W-conductance, we can calculate the average W-conductance of a genetic code, which is useful to characterize the properties of the genetic codes as a whole.

Definition 2. *The average W-conductance of a given genetic code C and a given weight W is defined as:*

$$\Phi_C(W) = \frac{1}{21} \sum_{S \in C} \phi_S(W) \, .$$

Low Φ_C values indicates that the code consists of codon groups that show a tendency to minimize nonsynonymous mutations. Thus, such code can buffer consequences of point mutations in protein-coding sequences.

Using the definition presented above, we are able to describe the best code in terms of the average W-conductance, which is defined as follows:

$$\Phi_{min}(W) = \min_C \Phi_C(W) \, .$$

$\Phi_{min}(W)$ gives us the lower bound of the genetic code robustness measured in terms of the average code W-conductance.

Algorithm 1. The clustering algorithm [2].

1: **function** AVERAGECONDUCTANCE($A, B, W, iterations$)
2:     $D = A - B$ ▷ Create transversion matrix
3:     $M = B + (W \cdot D)$ ▷ Create matrix M
4:     min-ave-cond ← 2
5:     **for** each iteration **do**
6:         $g = [(\text{node, edges}) \text{ for each node in M}]$ ▷ List g stores each node i in M and its edges
7:             **while** ($len(g) > 21$ nodes) **do** ▷ Keep picking and merging nodes until we have 21 clusters
8:                 $u ←$ PICKFIRSTNODE(g)
9:                 $v ←$ PICKSECONDNODE(g)
10:                Merge nodes u and v
11:            conductance = compute conductance for each cluster in g ▷ List conductance stores conductance of 21 clusters using $\phi_S(W)$ formula in Definition 1
12:            **if** min-ave-cond>sum(conductance)/len(conductance) **then**
13:                min-ave-cond = sum(conductance)/len(conductance)
14:                clusterings-min-ave-cond = g ▷ Stores the structure of the genetic code
15:        **return** min-ave-cond, clusterings-min-ave-cond
16: **function** PICKFIRSTNODE(g)
17:     $cond ← [(i, \phi_i(W)) \text{ for each node } i \text{ in } g]$ ▷ List to store conductance for each node i in g
18:     **for** for each node i in $cond$ **do**
19:         $weight[i] ← (i, cond[i]^{20})$ ▷ List to store weight for each node i in $cond$ list
20:     **for** for each node i in $weight$ **do**
21:         $prob[i] ← (i, \frac{weight[i]}{sum(weight)})$ ▷ List to store probability of selecting each node i in $weight$ list
22:     $R ←$ Generate a random number between 0 and 1
23:     $j ← 0$
24:     $a ← prob[0]$
25:     **while** ($R > a$) **do**
26:         $j ← j + 1$
27:         $a ← a + prob[j]$
28:     **return** j
29:     $u ← cond[j]$ ▷ Select the jth node in the $cond$ list
30:     **return** u
31: **function** PICKSECONDNODE(g)
32:     $cond1 ← cond - u$ ▷ Copy $cond$ list without the selected node u
33:     **for** for each node i in $cond1$ **do**
34:         $edges[i] ← (i, \#\text{edges between } i \text{ and } u)$
35:     **for** for each node i in $cond1$ **do**
36:         $weight[i] ← (i, (edges[i] + 1)^{10} \cdot cond1[i]^{20})$ ▷ List to store weight for each node i in $cond1$ list
37:     **for** for each node i in $weight$ **do**
38:         $prob[i] ← (i, \frac{weight[i]}{sum(weight)})$ ▷ List to store probability of selecting each node i in $weight$ list

```
39:     R ← Generate a random number between 0 and 1
40:     j ← 0
41:     a ← prob[0]
42:     while (R > a) do
43:         j ← j + 1
44:         a ← a + prob[j]
45:     return j
46:     v ← cond1[j]                        ▷ Select the j^{th} node in the cond1 list
47:     return v
```

Table 2. Input parameters and output variables for Algorithm 1 [2].

Input parameters:
1 Adjacent matrix of 64 codons, called A, where $A[i, j]$ can take:
$$A[i,j] = \begin{cases} 1 & \text{if } i \neq j \text{ and } \iff i \text{ differs from } j \text{ in exactly one position} \\ 0 & \text{otherwise} \end{cases}$$
2 Adjacent transition matrix of codons, called B, where $B[i, j]$ can take 1 only with transition connections i.e. A↔G, C↔T, otherwise 0
3 $W \in [0, \infty)$
4 #iterations ← 20,000
Output variables:
1 The minimum average conductance
2 The structure of the best genetic code that gives the minimum average conductance

2.2   The Clustering Algorithm

In order to find the optimal genetic code with respect to the minimum average W-conductance, we applied a new randomized clustering algorithm [2]. Its more formal description (Algorithm 1) provides the structure of the clustering algorithm. The generic structure of the clustering algorithm contains inputs, outputs (cf. input parameters and output variables in Table 2), and three functions, namely: AVERAGECONDUCTANCE, PICKFIRSTNODE, and PICKSECONDNODE. The main function is the AVERAGECONDUCTANCE function, which aims to find the optimal genetic code with the minimum average W-conductance. The function includes nested loops of two levels. The main loop (lines 5–14) counts the average conductance for each iteration. The second level loop (lines 7–14) picks and merges nodes of the graph until 21 clusters (super nodes) are achieved. The AVERAGECONDUCTANCE terminates when the graph is clustered to 21 clusters for each iteration and returns the best genetic code with the minimum average conductance from all independent iterations. The PICKFIRSTNODE (lines 16–30) and the PICKSECONDNODE (lines 31–47) associate a probability with each node in the graph and each function picks a node randomly.

3 Results and Discussion

The main goal of the presented work is to find the optimal genetic codes in terms of the average W-conductance $\Phi_{min}(W)$ and compare their properties with the standard genetic code and selected natural variants. The results are interesting from the biological point of view, because they can reveal interesting structural properties and evolution of the SGC.

We run the clustering algorithm (Algorithm 1) 20,000 times independently to find the genetic code showing the minimum of the W-average conductance. We carried out the calculations for the transversion weight $W \in [0, 10]$. These weights can be interpreted as a relative ratio between transversions and transitions. Smaller weights mean that transitions are more frequent than transversions, while larger weights indicate that the transversions dominate over transitions.

The algorithm found three genetic codes named $C1$, $C2$ and $C3$ that were best for different ranges of $W \in [0, \infty]$. The genetic code $C1$ was best for every $W \in [0, \frac{37}{70}]$, the code $C2$ for every $W \in [\frac{37}{70}, 1]$, while the code $C3$ for every $W \in [1, \infty]$. The average W-conductance for these codes in the function of weight W is $\Phi_{C1}(W) = \frac{1}{21} \cdot \frac{126W+31}{6W+3}$, $\Phi_{C2}(W) = \frac{1}{21} \cdot \frac{308W+130}{9(2W+1)}$, and $\Phi_{C3}(W) = \frac{1}{21} \cdot \frac{94W+52}{6W+3}$ for every $W \in [0, \frac{37}{70}], [\frac{37}{70}, 1]$, and $[1, \infty]$, respectively. Since the algorithm was repeated the large number of times to reduce the probability of finding sub-optimal solutions, we can assume that the found codes are optimal in the corresponding ranges of weights describing the transversion/transition ratio. Nevertheless, the formal proof of its optimality is an open question.

Figure 2 shows the average W-conductance for the best codes and the SGC depending on the transversion weight. Generally, the average conductance for the codes $C1$ and $C2$ that occurred best for $W < 1$ increases rapidly with W and then stabilizes for large values. In the case of the best code $C3$, its conductance decreases for small weights and then also approaches a certain value, which is much smaller than for the codes $C1$ and $C2$. Taking the minimum of the best codes, we can state that the average conductance is the smallest for the code $C1$, when W values are smaller, and for code $C3$, when the values are larger. For the small value range $[\frac{37}{70}, 1]$, the average conductance is smallest for the code $C2$. The code $C1$ is characterized by the biggest difference between its average conductance values through the studied weight range. In other words, this code is very well optimized to minimize nonsynonymous mutations for the excess of transitions over transversions, but performs poorly, when transversions dominate over transitions. In contrast to that, the code $C3$ shows the smallest variation in the average conductance and is better optimized for the larger transversion weights.

The average W-conductance of the SGC shows the general course similar to that of the $C1$ and $C2$ codes. Its conductance increases with the transversion weight, which indicates that the SGC is better optimized for more frequent transitions than transversions.

In Fig. 2, we also compared the relationship between the average conductance and transversion weights for AGCs and $C1, C2, C3$. The conductance of

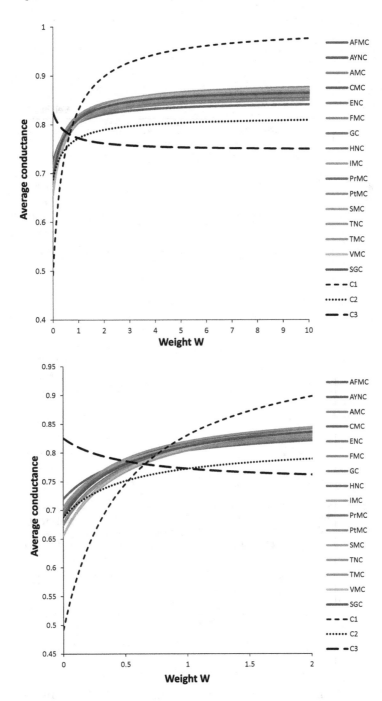

Fig. 2. The average conductance for the best codes $C1, C2, C3$, as well as the standard genetic code (SGC) and selected alternative genetic code for the weights of transversions $W \in [0, 10]$ and $W \in [0, 2]$.

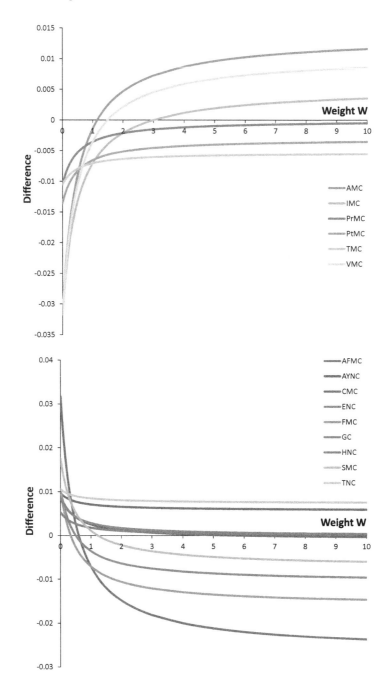

Fig. 3. The difference between the average conductance for the alternative genetic codes and the standard genetic code (SGC) for the weights of transversions $W \in [0, 10]$.

individual AGCs shows generally very similar course to the SGC and also better optimized for more frequent transitions than transversions. Hoverer, it is possible to find codes that have smaller as well as larger conductance values than the SGC depending on the transversion weight (Fig. 3). Three alternative codes (PrMC, PtMC and TMC) have the average conductance smaller than the SGC for the whole studied range of the transversion weight W, i.e. from 0 to 10. Additional three codes (AMC, VMC and IMC) have the smaller conductance than the SGC for W from 0 to 1.2, 1.5 and 3, respectively. Four codes (FMC, ENC, AFMC, SMC and CMC) show the smaller average conductance than the SGC for W from respectively 0.3, 0.5, 0.6, 1.2 and 6 to 10. Only AYNC, GC, HNC and TNC perform worse than the SGC for the studied weight range in terms of the conductance.

In order to compare the properties of the natural codes with the optimal ones, we computed functions $f1, f2, f3$, which are differences between the average W-conductance obtained for: (i) each natural code under study, $\Phi_{code}(W)$, and (ii) the best codes $(C1, C2, C3)$ found by the algorithm (Table 3).

Besides the general formulas, we gave values of these functions for the critical weights, 0, $\frac{37}{70}$, 1 and 10. We also calculated the derivatives $f1', f2', f3'$ for each functions. The real codes can obtain the same average W-conductance as each of the optimized codes but for different transversion weights. Nevertheless, the W is always smaller than 1 in these cases. The minimum distance between the SGC and the best genetic codes in terms of the average conductance is 0.03 for $W = \frac{37}{70} = 0.53$ (Table 3, Fig. 4). Majority of AGCs also show the minimum distance for this weight with the exception of AFMC, for which the minimum distance is for the range of W from $\frac{37}{70}$ to 1. This distance depends on the codes and is from 0.017 (for IMC) to 0.039 (for TNC). Seven alternative codes (AMC, FMC, IMC, PrMC, PtMC, TMC and VMC) have the distance smaller than the SGC, which suggests that can be more robust to mutations for 0.53 transversion rate.

Since there are twice as many possible transversions as transitions, the theoretical expected ratio should be 2, if all nucleotide substitutions happen with the same probability. Interestingly, the weights for which the average conductance Φ_{code} is close to Φ of the best codes is in the range of the transversion/transition ratio observed in genomic mutational pressures, i.e. from 1.44 to 0.10 [12,48]. However, for each transversion weight, it is possible to find a code better optimized than the SGC or AGC in terms of the average W-conductance, which means that the natural codes are not perfectly optimized. Comparing the SGC with AGCs, we can also state that more of the alternatives minimize the number of nonsynonymous substitutions in terms of the conductance better that the standard code for the transversion/transition ratio observed in genomes.

The structure of the best genetic codes is presented in Table 4. Although the code $C1$ and $C3$ are best for different and extreme W values, they have the same number of two- and four-codon groups, 10 and 11, respectively. The code $C2$ has in addition 3 groups consisting of three codons as well as 8 two-codon groups and 9 four-codon groups. The SGC is more diversified in this respect, because it

Table 3. Comparison between the best codes ($C1, C2, C3$) the standard genetic code (SGC) and the alternative genetic codes (AGCs).

code	Φ_{code}	$f1(W) = \Phi_{code} - \Phi_{C1}$	$f1'(W)$	$f1(0)$	$f1(\tfrac{37}{70})$	$f2(W) = \Phi_{code} - \Phi_{C2}$	$f2'(W)$	$f2(\tfrac{37}{70})$	$f2(1)$	$f3(W) = \Phi_{code} - \Phi_{C3}$	$f3'(W)$	$f3(1)$	$f3(10)$
		1				**2**				**3**			
SGC	$\dfrac{1}{21}\cdot\dfrac{10(33W+13)}{9(2W+1)}$	$\dfrac{37-48W}{21(18W+9)}$	$-\dfrac{122}{189(2W+1)^2}$	0.19	0.03	$\dfrac{22W}{21(18W+9)}$	$\dfrac{22}{189(2W+1)^2}$	0.03	0.04	$\dfrac{48W-26}{21(18W+9)}$	$\dfrac{100}{189(2W+1)^2}$	0.04	0.11
AFMC	$\dfrac{8(40W+17)}{189(2W+1)}$	$\dfrac{58W-43}{378W+189}$	$-\dfrac{16}{21(2W+1)^2}$	0.23	0.03	$\dfrac{2}{63}$	0	0.03	0.03	$\dfrac{38W-20}{378W+189}$	$\dfrac{26}{63(2W+1)^2}$	0.03	0.09
AYNC	$\dfrac{2(5813W+2307)}{6615(2W+1)}$	$\dfrac{1604W-1359}{13230W+6615}$	$\dfrac{4322}{6615(2W+1)^2}$	0.21	0.04	$\dfrac{846W+64}{13230W+6615}$	$\dfrac{718}{6615(2W+1)^2}$	0.04	0.05	$\dfrac{1756W-846}{13230W+6615}$	$\dfrac{3448}{6615(2W+1)^2}$	0.05	0.12
AMC	$\dfrac{4(419W+155)}{945(2W+1)}$	$\dfrac{214W-155}{1890W+945}$	$\dfrac{524}{945(2W+1)^2}$	0.16	0.02	$\dfrac{136W-30}{1890W+945}$	$\dfrac{28}{135(2W+1)^2}$	0.02	0.04	$\dfrac{266W-160}{1890W+945}$	$\dfrac{586}{945(2W+1)^2}$	0.04	0.13
CMC	$\dfrac{2(1154W+461)}{1323(2W+1)}$	$\dfrac{338W-271}{2646W+1323}$	$\dfrac{880}{1323(2W+1)^2}$	0.20	0.03	$\dfrac{152W+12}{2646W+1323}$	$\dfrac{128}{1323(2W+1)^2}$	0.03	0.04	$\dfrac{334W-170}{2646W+1323}$	$\dfrac{674}{1323(2W+1)^2}$	0.04	0.11
ENC	$\dfrac{2(163W+66)}{189(2W+1)}$	$\dfrac{52W-39}{378W+189}$	$-\dfrac{130}{189(2W+1)^2}$	0.21	0.03	$\dfrac{18W+2}{378W+189}$	$\dfrac{2}{27(2W+1)^2}$	0.03	0.04	$\dfrac{44W-24}{378W+189}$	$\dfrac{92}{189(2W+1)^2}$	0.04	0.10
FMC	$\dfrac{4(27W+11)}{63(2W+1)}$	$\dfrac{18W-13}{126W+63}$	$-\dfrac{44}{63(2W+1)^2}$	0.21	0.027	$\dfrac{16W+2}{378W+189}$	$\dfrac{4}{63(2W+1)^2}$	0.027	0.032	$\dfrac{14W-8}{126W+63}$	$\dfrac{10}{21(2W+1)^2}$	0.032	0.1
GC	$\dfrac{2(825W+329)}{945(2W+1)}$	$\dfrac{240W-193}{1890W+945}$	$-\dfrac{626}{945(2W+1)^2}$	0.2	0.03	$\dfrac{110W+8}{1890W+945}$	$\dfrac{94}{945(2W+1)^2}$	0.03	0.04	$\dfrac{240W-122}{1890W+945}$	$\dfrac{484}{945(2W+1)^2}$	0.04	0.11
HNC	$\dfrac{330W+131}{189(2W+1)}$	$\dfrac{48W-38}{378W+189}$	$-\dfrac{124}{189(2W+1)^2}$	0.2	0.03	$\dfrac{22W+1}{378W+189}$	$\dfrac{20}{189(2W+1)^2}$	0.03	0.04	$\dfrac{48W-25}{378W+189}$	$\dfrac{14}{27(2W+1)^2}$	0.04	0.11
IMC	$\dfrac{4(83W+31)}{189(2W+1)}$	$\dfrac{46W-31}{378W+189}$	$-\dfrac{4}{7(2W+1)^2}$	0.16	0.02	$\dfrac{8W-2}{126W+63}$	$\dfrac{4}{21(2W+1)^2}$	0.02	0.03	$\dfrac{50W-32}{378W+189}$	$\dfrac{38}{63(2W+1)^2}$	0.03	0.12
PrMC	$\dfrac{2(165W+64)}{189(2W+1)}$	$\dfrac{48W-35}{378W+189}$	$-\dfrac{118}{189(2W+1)^2}$	0.19	0.02	$\dfrac{22W-2}{378W+189}$	$\dfrac{26}{189(2W+1)^2}$	0.02	0.04	$\dfrac{48W-28}{378W+189}$	$\dfrac{104}{189(2W+1)^2}$	0.04	0.11
PtMC	$\dfrac{2(1151W+446)}{1323(2W+1)}$	$\dfrac{344W-241}{2646W+1323}$	$-\dfrac{118}{189(2W+1)^2}$	0.18	0.02	$\dfrac{146W-18}{2646W+1323}$	$\dfrac{26}{189(2W+1)^2}$	0.02	0.03	$\dfrac{328W-200}{2646W+1323}$	$\dfrac{104}{189(2W+1)^2}$	0.03	0.11
SMC	$\dfrac{2(5728W+2333)}{6615(2W+1)}$	$\dfrac{1774W-1411}{13230W+6615}$	$-\dfrac{1532}{2205(2W+1)^2}$	0.21	0.03	$\dfrac{676W+116}{13230W+6615}$	$\dfrac{148}{2205(2W+1)^2}$	0.03	0.04	$\dfrac{1586W-794}{13230W+6615}$	$\dfrac{1058}{2205(2W+1)^2}$	0.04	0.11
TNC	$\dfrac{4(416W+165)}{945(2W+1)}$	$\dfrac{226W-195}{1890W+945}$	$-\dfrac{88}{135(2W+1)^2}$	0.2	0.04	$\dfrac{124W+10}{1890W+945}$	$\dfrac{104}{945(2W+1)^2}$	0.04	0.05	$\dfrac{254W-120}{1890W+945}$	$\dfrac{494}{945(2W+1)^2}$	0.05	0.12
TMC	$\dfrac{8(41W+16)}{189(2W+1)}$	$\dfrac{50W-35}{378W+189}$	$-\dfrac{40}{63(2W+1)^2}$	0.19	0.02	$\dfrac{20W-2}{378W+189}$	$\dfrac{8}{63(2W+1)^2}$	0.02	0.03	$\dfrac{46W-28}{378W+189}$	$\dfrac{34}{63(2W+1)^2}$	0.03	0.11
VMC	$\dfrac{2(167W+62)}{189(2W+1)}$	$\dfrac{44W-31}{378W+189}$	$-\dfrac{106}{189(2W+1)^2}$	0.16	0.02	$\dfrac{26W-6}{378W+189}$	$\dfrac{38}{189(2W+1)^2}$	0.02	0.03	$\dfrac{52W-32}{378W+189}$	$\dfrac{116}{189(2W+1)^2}$	0.03	0.12

Table 4. The structure of the best genetic codes $C1, C2$, and $C3$ for $W \in [0, \frac{37}{70}]$, $W \in [\frac{37}{70}, 1]$, and $W \in [1, \infty]$, respectively. Each row describes the codon group for a cluster. According to [2].

	$C1$	$C2$	$C3$
1	$\{AAA, AAG, AGG, AGA\}$	$\{AAG, ACG, ATG\}$	$\{ATA, AAA, AGA, ACA\}$
2	$\{ATT, ATC\}$	$\{AGA, AGG\}$	$\{AGC, ACC\}$
3	$\{TAG, TAA\}$	$\{AGC, ATC, AAC, ACC\}$	$\{ACT, TCT\}$
4	$\{TAC, TAT, TGT, TGC\}$	$\{ACA, AAA, ATA\}$	$\{ACG, AAG, ATG, AGG\}$
5	$\{TTT, CTT\}$	$\{TAA, TAG\}$	$\{TTA, TAA\}$
6	$\{TGA, TGG\}$	$\{TAC, CAC\}$	$\{TTC, TAC, TCC, TGC\}$
7	$\{TCT, CCT\}$	$\{TTA, CTA, GTA\}$	$\{TGG, TAG, TCG, TTG\}$
8	$\{TCG, TTG, TTA, TCA\}$	$\{TTG, CTG\}$	$\{TCA, TGA\}$
9	$\{TCC, TTC, CTC, CCC\}$	$\{TGA, TGG, TGC, TGT\}$	$\{GAT, AAT, TAT, CAT\}$
10	$\{GTA, ATA, GTG, ATG\}$	$\{TCA, TCT, TCC, TCG\}$	$\{GTT, ATT, TTT, CTT\}$
11	$\{GTC, GTT\}$	$\{GAT, AAT, TAT, CAT\}$	$\{GGA, GCA, GAA, GTA\}$
12	$\{GGA, GAA, GAG, GGG\}$	$\{GAC, GGC, GCC, GTC\}$	$\{GGT, CGT, AGT, TGT\}$
13	$\{GGT, GAT, AGT, AAT\}$	$\{GTG, GAG, GGG, GCG\}$	$\{GCG, GAG, GGG, GTG\}$
14	$\{GGC, AGC, AAC, GAC\}$	$\{GGT, AGT\}$	$\{GCC, GTC, GAC, GGC\}$
15	$\{GCG, GCA, ACA, ACG\}$	$\{GCA, GGA, GAA\}$	$\{CAA, CTA\}$
16	$\{GCC, ACC, GCT, ACT\}$	$\{GCT, ACT\}$	$\{CAC, AAC\}$
17	$\{CAT, CGT, CGC, CAC\}$	$\{CAG, CAA\}$	$\{CTG, CGG, CAG, CCG\}$
18	$\{CTA, CTG\}$	$\{CTT, GTT, ATT, TTT\}$	$\{CTC, ATC\}$
19	$\{CGA, CAA\}$	$\{CTC, TTC\}$	$\{CGC, CCC\}$
20	$\{CGG, CAG\}$	$\{CGC, CGG, CGT, CGA\}$	$\{CCA, CGA\}$
21	$\{CCG, CCA\}$	$\{CCA, CCC, CCT, CCG\}$	$\{CCT, GCT\}$

has 2 one-codon groups, 9 two-codon groups, 2 three-codon groups, 5 four-codon groups and 3 six-codon groups. Thereby, it is more similar to the code $C2$.

The code $C1$ is best for smaller weights of transversions. Therefore, such mutations are preferably involved in changes between codon groups of this code in order to minimize these changes. Consequently, all synonymous substitutions in this code are transitions. In the case of the code $C3$, which is best for larger weights, transversions were eliminated from changes between codon groups as much as possible to increase the number of transitions. In consequence, all changes within two-codon groups of this code are transversions. Since there are only two purines and two pyrimidines, it is not possible to create four-codon groups that can change to each other by only transversions. Therefore, changes within such groups are both transitions and transversions. The code $C2$ is a mixture in this respect, because codons in its two-codon groups can change to each other only by transitions, while in other groups by both by transitions and transversions. Considering only one point mutations in the SGC, all changes within two-codon groups are also transitions and within other groups both transitions and transversions with exception to the stop codon group, which also

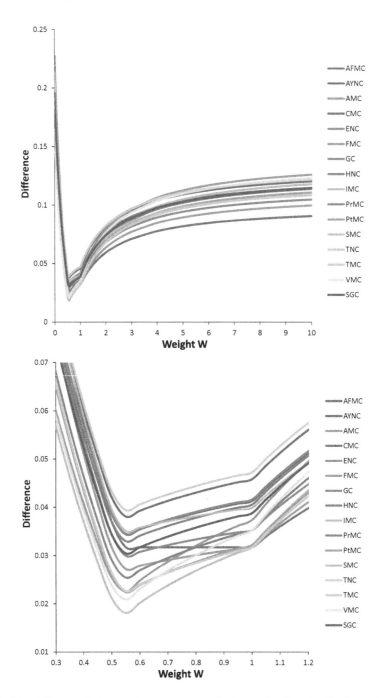

Fig. 4. The difference between the average conductance for the standard genetic code (SGC), alternative genetic codes (Φ_{SGC}) and the best codes (Φ_{min}) for the weights of transversions $W \in [0, 10]$ and $W \in [0.3, 1.2]$.

involves only transitions. Then the SGC is again more similar to the code $C2$ in this respect.

The changes between codons in one group of the code $C3$ can occur only in one fixed codon position, the first or the second one. The third codon position can also be mutated in the code $C2$. However, the code $C1$ contains also the groups in which any two codon positions can be changed. The SGC contains many codon groups with synonymous mutations in the third codon position, but there are also three codon groups involving single changes in two codon positions.

The comparison of structures of the genetic codes show that the assignments of amino acids to codons is not ideally optimized in the SGC. Some similarity of the SGC to the code $C2$ suggests that the standard genetic code could evolve under the transversion/transition for which the code $C2$ is best.

In AGCs we can find structural changes that improve their robustness to mutations compared with the SGC. The most commonly observed change refers to the creation of new codon block including two codons for tryptophan, namely TGA and TGG, at the expense of the loss of termination signal assignment to TGA. Such change is observed in many codes, which are better than the SGC for the wide ranges of transversion weights: PrMC, PtMC, TMC, AMC, VMC, IMC, FMC and AFMC. In addition, four codes, TMC, AMC, VMC and IMC, show the reassignment of ATA, originally coded isoleucine, to methionine. These two types of changes generate two-codon blocks, which substantially decrease the average conductance of these codes. Moreover, in TMC and IMC codes, there occurs the AGN-codon block for serine. Such four-codon group is characterized by the smallest set conductance. In contrast to that, the codes worse than the SGC have the split of four-codon block for leucine by reassignment of serine (AYNC code) or alanine (TNC code) to CTG.

4   Conclusions

Our results show that the general structure of the genetic code and its optimality can be successfully reformulated using a methodology adapted from graph theory in the context of optimal clustering of a specific graph. To evaluate the quality of the genetic code, we calculated the average code W-conductance including weights for mutation types distinguishing transitions and transversions. From the biological point of view, this measure describes the robustness of the genetic code against amino acid and stop translation signal replacements resulting from single nucleotide substitutions between codons.

We found three best codes with respect to the average code conductance for various ranges of the applied weight. The W-conductance of tested genetic code, the SGC and its natural alternatives, was the most similar to that of the best codes in the range of weights corresponding to the observed small transversion/transition ratio in the mutational pressure. This is in line with other studies which also showed that the genetic code performs better for the excess of transitions over transversions [34,35]. It indicates that the code is optimized

to some extent in terms of the minimization of amino acid and stop translation replacements. However, the optimization is not ideal and better theoretical
codes could be found for each weight. In agreement with that, other investigations also showed that the SGC is not perfectly robust against point mutations or mistranslations [9,14,15,58,64,71,72,78]. The alternative genetic codes
show the relationship between their average conductance and the transversion
weight similar to that of the SGC, but there are many AGCs more robust to
mutational errors than the SGC. These codes possess assignment that generate
codon blocks that improve the set conductance. Nevertheless, the structure of
the natural codes is different from that of the best theoretical codes. Therefore,
most likely, the robustness to single point mutations was not the main force that
drove the evolution of the genetic code and amino acids were assigned to codons
according to expansion of biosynthetic pathways synthesizing amino acids [24–
27,29,80–82]. In this case, the potential minimization of mutation errors could
have occurred by the direct optimization of the mutational pressure around the
established genetic code [8,11,12,32,57].

The results can have practical consequences in the context of designing modified or extended genetic codes [19,83]. The aim of this engineering is to produce
peptides or proteins containing unnatural amino acids and showing an improved
activity or completely new functions.

References

1. Abascal, F., Posada, D., Knight, R.D., Zardoya, R.: Parallel evolution of the genetic code in arthropod mitochondrial genomes. PLoS Biol. **4**(5), 711–718 (2006)
2. Aloqalaa, D.A., Kowalski, D.R., Błażej, P., Wnetrzak, M., Mackiewicz, D., Mackiewicz, P.: The impact of the transversion/transition ratio on the optimal genetic code graph partition. In: Proceedings of the 12th International Joint Conference on Biomedical Engineering Systems and Technologies - Volume 3: BIOINFORMATICS, pp. 55–65. INSTICC, SciTePress (2019). https://doi.org/10.5220/0007381000550065
3. Ardell, D.H.: On error minimization in a sequential origin of the standard genetic code. J. Mol. Evol. **47**(1), 1–13 (1998). https://doi.org/10.1007/PL00006356
4. Ardell, D.H., Sella, G.: On the evolution of redundancy in genetic codes. J. Mol. Evol. **53**(4–5), 269–281 (2001). https://doi.org/10.1007/s002390010217
5. Błażej, P., Wnetrzak, M., Mackiewicz, P.: The importance of changes observed in the alternative genetic codes. In: Proceedings of the 11th International Joint Conference on Biomedical Engineering Systems and Technologies - Volume 4: BIOINFORMATICS, pp. 154–159 (2018)
6. Beineke, L.W., Wilson, R.J.: Topics in Algebraic Graph Theory. Cambridge University Press, Cambridge (2005)
7. Błażej, P., Mackiewicz, D., Wnętrzak, M., Mackiewicz, P.: The impact of selection at the amino acid level on the usage of synonymous codons. G3-Genes Genom. Genet. **7**(3), 967–981 (2017)
8. Błażej, P., Mackiewicz, P., Cebrat, S., Wańczyk, M.: Using evolutionary algorithms in finding of optimized nucleotide substitution matrices. In: Genetic and Evolutionary Computation Conference, GECCO 2013, pp. 41–42. Companion ACM (2013)

9. Błażej, P., Wnętrzak, M., Mackiewicz, D., Mackiewicz, P.: Optimization of the standard genetic code according to three codon positions using an evolutionary algorithm. PLoS One **13**(8), e0201715 (2018)
10. Błażej, P., Kowalski, D., Mackiewicz, D., Wnętrzak, M., Aloqalaa, D., Mackiewicz, P.: The structure of the genetic code as an optimal graph clustering problem. bioRxiv (2018).https://doi.org/10.1101/332478. https://www.biorxiv.org/content/early/2018/05/28/332478
11. Błażej, P., Mackiewicz, D., Grabinska, M., Wnętrzak, M., Mackiewicz, P.: Optimization of amino acid replacement costs by mutational pressure in bacterial genomes. Sci. Rep. **7**, 1061 (2017). https://doi.org/10.1038/s41598-017-01130-7
12. Błażej, P., Miasojedow, B., Grabinska, M., Mackiewicz, P.: Optimization of mutation pressure in relation to properties of protein-coding sequences in bacterial genomes. PLoS One **10**, e0130411 (2015). https://doi.org/10.1371/journal.pone.0130411
13. Błażej, P., Wnętrzak, M., Mackiewicz, D., Gagat, P., Mackiewicz, P.: Many alternative and theoretical genetic codes are more robust to amino acid replacements than the standard genetic code. J. Theor. Biol. **464**, 21–32 (2019). https://doi.org/10.1016/j.jtbi.2018.12.030
14. Błażej, P., Wnętrzak, M., Mackiewicz, D., Mackiewicz, P.: The influence of different types of translational inaccuracies on the genetic code structure. BMC Bioinf. **20**(1), 114 (2019)
15. Błażej, P., Wnętrzak, M., Mackiewicz, P.: The role of crossover operator in evolutionary-based approach to the problem of genetic code optimization. Biosystems **150**, 61–72 (2016)
16. Bollobás, B.: Modern Graph Theory. graduate Texts in Mathematics, vol. 184. Springer, Heidelberg (1998). https://doi.org/10.1007/978-1-4612-0619-4
17. Bove, J.M.: Molecular features of mollicutes. Clin. Infect. Dis. **17**(Suppl 1), S10–31 (1993)
18. Bulmer, M.: The selection-mutation-drift theory of synonymous codon usage. Genetics **129**(3), 897–907 (1991)
19. Chin, J.W.: Expanding and reprogramming the genetic code of cells and animals. Annu. Rev. Biochem. **83**, 379–408 (2014)
20. Clark-Walker, G.D., Weiller, G.F.: The structure of the small mitochondrial dna of kluyveromyces thermotolerans is likely to reflect the ancestral gene order in fungi. J. Mol. Evol. **38**(6), 593–601 (1994). https://doi.org/10.1007/BF00175879
21. Crick, F.H.: The origin of the genetic code. J. Mol. Biol. **38**(3), 367–379 (1968)
22. Crozier, R.H., Crozier, Y.C.: The mitochondrial genome of the honeybee apis mellifera: complete sequence and genome organization. Genetics **133**(1), 97–117 (1993)
23. Del Cortona, A., et al.: The plastid genome in cladophorales green algae is encoded by hairpin chromosomes. Curr. Biol. **27**(24), 3771–3782 e6 (2017)
24. Di Giulio, M.: The coevolution theory of the origin of the genetic code. J. Mol. Evol. **48**(3), 253–5 (1999)
25. Di Giulio, M.: An extension of the coevolution theory of the origin of the genetic code. Biol. Direct **3**, 37 (2008)
26. Di Giulio, M.: The lack of foundation in the mechanism on which are based the physico-chemical theories for the origin of the genetic code is counterposed to the credible and natural mechanism suggested by the coevolution theory. J. Theor. Biol. **399**, 134–40 (2016)
27. Di Giulio, M.: Some pungent arguments against the physico-chemical theories of the origin of the genetic code and corroborating the coevolution theory. J. Theor. Biol. **414**, 1–4 (2017)

28. Di Giulio, M.: The extension reached by the minimization of the polarity distances during the evolution of the genetic code. J. Mol. Evol. **29**(4), 288–293 (1989)

29. Di Giulio, M.: A discriminative test among the different theories proposed to explain the origin of the genetic code: the coevolution theory finds additional support. Biosystems **169**, 1–4 (2018)

30. Di Giulio, M., Medugno, M.: Physicochemical optimization in the genetic code origin as the number of codified amino acids increases. J. Mol. Evol. **49**(1), 1–10 (1999). https://doi.org/10.1007/PL00006522

31. Duchêne, S., Ho, S.Y., Holmes, E.C.: Declining transition/transversion ratios through time reveal limitations to the accuracy of nucleotide substitution models. BMC Evol. Biol. **15**(1), 36 (2015). https://doi.org/10.1186/s12862-015-0312-6

32. Dudkiewicz, A., et al.: Correspondence between mutation and selection pressure and the genetic code degeneracy in the gene evolution. Future Gener. Comput. Syst. **21**(7), 1033–1039 (2005)

33. Epstein, C.J.: Role of the amino-acid "code" and of selection for conformation in the evolution of proteins. Nature **210**(5031), 25–28 (1966)

34. Freeland, S.J., Hurst, L.D.: The genetic code is one in a million. J. Mol. Evol. **47**(3), 238–248 (1998). https://doi.org/10.1007/PL00006381

35. Freeland, S.J., Hurst, L.D.: Load minimization of the genetic code: history does not explain the pattern. Proc. Roy. Soc. London B: Biol. Sci. **265**(1410), 2111–2119 (1998)

36. Freeland, S.J., Knight, R.D., Landweber, L.F., Hurst, L.D.: Early fixation of an optimal genetic code. Mol. Biol. Evol. **17**(4), 511–518 (2000)

37. Freeland, S.J., Wu, T., Keulmann, N.: The case for an error minimizing standard genetic code. Orig. Life Evol. Biosph. **33**(4–5), 457–477 (2003). https://doi.org/10.1023/A:1025771327614

38. Gilis, D., Massar, S., Cerf, N.J., Rooman, M.: Optimality of the genetic code with respect to protein stability and amino-acid frequencies. Genome Biol. **2**(11), research0049-1 (2001)

39. Gojobori, T., Li, W.H., Graur, D.: Patterns of nucleotide substitution in pseudogenes and functional genes. J. Mol. Evol. **18**(5), 360–369 (1982). https://doi.org/10.1007/BF01733904

40. Goldberg, A.L., Wittes, R.E.: Genetic code: aspects of organization. Science **153**(3734), 420–424 (1966)

41. Goodarzi, H., Najafabadi, H.S., Torabi, N.: Designing a neural network for the constraint optimization of the fitness functions devised based on the load minimization of the genetic code. Biosystems **81**(2), 91–100 (2005)

42. Haig, D., Hurst, L.D.: A quantitative measure of error minimization in the genetic code. J. Mol. Evol. **33**(5), 412–417 (1991). https://doi.org/10.1007/BF02103132

43. Heaphy, S.M., Mariotti, M., Gladyshev, V.N., Atkins, J.F., Baranov, P.V.: Novel ciliate genetic code variants including the reassignment of all three stop codons to sense codons in condylostoma magnum. Mol. Biol. Evol. **33**(11), 2885–2889 (2016)

44. Hershberg, R., Petrov, D.A.: Selection on codon bias. Ann. Rev. Genet. **42**, 287–299 (2008)

45. Janouskovec, J., et al.: Split photosystem protein, linear-mapping topology, and growth of structural complexity in the plastid genome of chromera velia. Mol. Biol. Evol. **30**(11), 2447–62 (2013)

46. Khorana, H.G., et al.: Polynucleotide synthesis and the genetic code. In: Cold Spring Harbor Symposia on Quantitative Biology, vol. 31, pp. 39–49. Cold Spring Harbor Laboratory Press (1966)

47. Knight, R.D., Landweber, L.F., Yarus, M.: How mitochondria redefine the code. J. Mol. Evol. **53**(4–5), 299–313 (2001). https://doi.org/10.1007/s002390010220
48. Kowalczuk, M., et al.: High correlation between the turnover of nucleotides under mutational pressure and the DNA composition. BMC Evol. Biol. **1**(1), 13 (2001)
49. Kumar, S.: Patterns of nucleotide substitution in mitochondrial protein coding genes of vertebrates. Genetics **143**(1), 537–548 (1996)
50. Kurnaz, M.L., Bilgin, T., Kurnaz, I.A.: Certain non-standard coding tables appear to be more robust to error than the standard genetic code. J. Mol. Evol. **70**(1), 13–28 (2010). https://doi.org/10.1007/s00239-009-9303-9
51. Lang-Unnasch, N., Aiello, D.P.: Sequence evidence for an altered genetic code in the neospora caninum plastid. Int. J. Parasitol. **29**(10), 1557–62 (1999)
52. Lee, J.R., Gharan, S.O., Trevisan, L.: Multiway spectral partitioning and higher-order cheeger inequalities. J. ACM (JACM) **61**(6), 37 (2014)
53. Levin, D.A., Peres, Y., Wilmer, E.L.: Markov Chains and Mixing Times. American Mathematical Society, Providence (2009)
54. Lim, P.O., Sears, B.B.: Evolutionary relationships of a plant-pathogenic mycoplas-malike organism and acholeplasma-laidlawii deduced from 2 ribosomal-protein gene-sequences. J. Bacteriol. **174**(8), 2606–2611 (1992)
55. Lynch, M.: Rate, molecular spectrum, and consequences of human mutation. Proc. Natl. Acad. Sci. U.S.A. **107**(3), 961–968 (2010)
56. Lyons, D.M., Lauring, A.S.: Evidence for the selective basis of transition-to-transversion substitution bias in two rna viruses. Mol. Biol. Evol. **34**(12), 3205–3215 (2017)
57. Mackiewicz, P., et al.: Optimisation of asymmetric mutational pressure and selection pressure around the universal genetic code. In: Bubak, M., van Albada, G.D., Dongarra, J., Sloot, P.M.A. (eds.) ICCS 2008. LNCS, vol. 5103, pp. 100–109. Springer, Heidelberg (2008). https://doi.org/10.1007/978-3-540-69389-5_13
58. Massey, S.E.: A neutral origin for error minimization in the genetic code. J. Mol. Evol. **67**(5), 510–516 (2008). https://doi.org/10.1007/s00239-008-9167-4
59. McCutcheon, J.P., McDonald, B.R., Moran, N.A.: Origin of an alternative genetic code in the extremely small and GC-rich genome of a bacterial symbiont. Plos Genet. **5**(7), (2009)
60. Morgens, D.W., Cavalcanti, A.R.: An alternative look at code evolution: using non-canonical codes to evaluate adaptive and historic models for the origin of the genetic code. J. Mol. Evol. **76**(1–2), 71–80 (2013). https://doi.org/10.1007/s00239-013-9542-7
61. Morton, B.R.: Selection at the amino acid level can influence synonymous codon usage: implications for the study of codon adaptation in plastid genes. Genetics **159**(1), 347–358 (2001)
62. Muhlhausen, S., Findeisen, P., Plessmann, U., Urlaub, H., Kollmar, M.: A novel nuclear genetic code alteration in yeasts and the evolution of codon reassignment in eukaryotes. Genome Res. **26**(7), 945–955 (2016)
63. Nirenberg, M., et al.: The RNA code and protein synthesis. In: Cold Spring Harbor symposia on quantitative biology, vol. 31, pp. 11–24. Cold Spring Harbor Laboratory Press (1966)
64. Novozhilov, A.S., Wolf, Y.I., Koonin, E.V.: Evolution of the genetic code: partial optimization of a random code for robustness to translation error in a rugged fitness landscape. Biol. Direct **2**, 24 (2007)

65. Osawa, S., Ohama, T., Jukes, T.H., Watanabe, K.: Evolution of the mitochondrial genetic code. I. Origin of AGR serine and stop codons in metazoan mitochondria. J. Mol. Evol. **29**(3), 202–207 (1989). https://doi.org/10.1007/BF02100203

66. Panek, T., et al.: Nuclear genetic codes with a different meaning of the UAG and the UAA codon. BMC Biol. **15**(1), 8 (2017)

67. Petrov, D.A., Hartl, D.L.: Patterns of nucleotide substitution in drosophila and mammalian genomes. Proc. Natl. Acad. Sci. U.S.A. **96**(4), 1475–1479 (1999)

68. Rosenberg, M.S., Subramanian, S., Kumar, S.: Patterns of transitional mutation biases within and among mammalian genomes. Mol. Biol. Evol. **20**(6), 988–993 (2003)

69. Sammet, S.G., Bastolla, U., Porto, M.: Comparison of translation loads for standard and alternative genetic codes. BMC Evol. Biol. **10**, 178 (2010). https://doi.org/10.1186/1471-2148-10-178

70. Sanchez-Silva, R., Villalobo, E., Morin, L., Torres, A.: A new noncanonical nuclear genetic code: translation of UAA into glutamate. Curr. Biol. **13**(5), 442–447 (2003)

71. Santos, J., Monteagudo, Á.: Simulated evolution applied to study the genetic code optimality using a model of codon reassignments. BMC Bioinf. **12**, 56 (2011). https://doi.org/10.1186/1471-2105-12-56

72. Santos, J., Monteagudo, Á.: Inclusion of the fitness sharing technique in an evolutionary algorithm to analyze the fitness landscape of the genetic code adaptability. BMC Bioinf. **18**(1), 195 (2017). https://doi.org/10.1186/s12859-017-1608-x

73. Santos, M.A.S., Keith, G., Tuite, M.F.: Nonstandard translational events in candida-albicans mediated by an unusual seryl-transfer RNA with a 5'-CAG-3' (leucine) anticodon. EMBO J. **12**(2), 607–616 (1993)

74. Schneider, S.U., Leible, M.B., Yang, X.P.: Strong homology between the small subunit of ribulose-1,5-bisphosphate carboxylase oxygenase of 2 species of acetabularia and the occurrence of unusual codon usage. Mol. Gener. Genet. **218**(3), 445–452 (1989). am870 Times Cited:55 Cited References Count:45

75. Sengupta, S., Yang, X., Higgs, P.G.: The mechanisms of codon reassignments in mitochondrial genetic codes. J. Mol. Evol. **64**(6), 662–88 (2007). https://doi.org/10.1007/s00239-006-0284-7

76. Tlusty, T.: A colorful origin for the genetic code: information theory, statistical mechanics and the emergence of molecular codes. Phys. Life Rev. **7**(3), 362–376 (2010)

77. Wakeley, J.: The excess of transitions among nucleotide substitutions: new methods of estimating transition bias underscore its significance. Trends Ecol. Evol. **11**(4), 158–162 (1996)

78. Wnętrzak, M., Błażej, P., Mackiewicz, D., Mackiewicz, P.: The optimality of the standard genetic code assessed by an eight-objective evolutionary algorithm. BMC Evol. Biol. **18**, 192 (2018)

79. Woese, C.R.: On the evolution of the genetic code. Proc. Natl. Acad. Sci. U.S.A. **54**(6), 1546–1552 (1965)

80. Wong, J.T.: A co-evolution theory of the genetic code. Proc. Natl. Acad. Sci. U.S.A. **72**(5), 1909–12 (1975)

81. Wong, J.T., Ng, S.K., Mat, W.K., Hu, T., Xue, H.: Coevolution theory of the genetic code at age forty: pathway to translation and synthetic life. Life (Basel) **6**(1), E12 (2016)

82. Wong, J.T.F.: Coevolution theory of the genetic code: a proven theory. Orig. Life Evol. Biosph. **37**(4–5), 403–408 (2007)

83. Xie, J.M., Schultz, P.G.: Innovation: a chemical toolkit for proteins - an expanded genetic code. Nat. Rev. Mol. Cell Biol. **7**(10), 775–782 (2006)
84. Zahonova, K., Kostygov, A.Y., Sevcikova, T., Yurchenko, V., Elias, M.: An unprecedented non-canonical nuclear genetic code with all three termination codons reassigned as sense codons. Curr. Biol. **26**(17), 2364–9 (2016)
85. Zhou, T., Weems, M., Wilke, C.O.: Translationally optimal codons associate with structurally sensitive sites in proteins. Mol. Biol. Evol. **26**(7), 1571–1580 (2009)

Characteristic Topological Features of Promoter Capture Hi-C Interaction Networks

Lelde Lace, Gatis Melkus, Peteris Rucevskis, Edgars Celms, Kārlis Čerāns,
Paulis Kikusts, Mārtiņš Opmanis, Darta Rituma, and Juris Viksna[✉]

Institute of Mathematics and Computer Science, University of Latvia,
Rainis Boulevard 29, Riga, Latvia
{lelde.lace,gatis.melkus,peteris.rucevskis,
edgars.celms,karlis.cerans,paulis.kikusts,
martins.opmanis,darta.rituma,juris.viksna}@lumii.lv

Abstract. Current Hi-C technologies for chromosome conformation capture allow to understand a broad spectrum of functional interactions between genome elements. Although significant progress has been made into analysis of Hi-C data to identify the biologically significant features, many questions still remain open. In this paper we describe analysis methods of Hi-C (specifically PCHi-C) interaction networks that are strictly focused on topological properties of these networks. The main questions we are trying to answer are: (1) can topological properties of interaction networks for different cell types alone be sufficient to distinguish between these types, and what the most important of such properties are; (2) what is a typical structure of interaction networks and can we assign a biological significance to network structural elements or features?

We have performed analysis on a dataset describing PCHi-C genome-wide interaction networks for 17 types of haematopoietic cells. From this analysis we propose a concrete set *Base6* of network topological features (called metrics) that provide good discriminatory power between cell types. The identified features are clearly defined and simple topological properties – the presence and size of connected components and bi-connected components, cliques and cycles of length 2.

We have explored in more detail the component structure of the networks and show that such components tend to be well conserved within particular cell type subgroups and can be well associated with known biological processes. We also have assessed biological significance of network cliques using promoter level expression data and the obtained results indicate that for closely related cell types genes from the same clique tend to be co-expressed.

Keywords: PCHi-C networks · Cell type specificity · Graph-based metrics · Graph topology

The research was supported by ERDF project 1.1.1.1/16/A/135.

A. Roque et al. (Eds.): BIOSTEC 2019, CCIS 1211, pp. 192–215, 2020.
https://doi.org/10.1007/978-3-030-46970-2_10

1   Introduction

The spatial organization of a genome inside of a living cell's nucleus has long been recognised as an important determinant of genomic function. One of the most important experimental techniques for gaining insights into this spatial organization has been chromosome conformation capture (3C). In this method closely associated genomic fragments are cross-linked via formaldehyde treatment and then purified, permitting their closer analysis [7]. Since its initial introduction more that 10 years ago, the original 3C protocol has been adapted and combined with other methods. These include chromatin immunoprecipitation and next-generation sequencing to assist in broadening the scope and depth of individual experiments. Particularly noteworthy among these methods is Hi-C, which utilises a biotin-streptavidin purification in combination with next-generation sequencing technology to potentially create a complete, unbiased genomic library of chromatin interactions [2,17].

However, in practice Hi-C produces highly complex datasets in which analysis of genomic contacts below a resolution of 1 Mb is difficult. In order to simplify such studies an additional refinement, capture Hi-C (CHi-C) method, has been invented. The method adds an additional sequence capture step that reduces the range of interactions to a smaller subset associated with defined genomic regions ('baits') [9,19]. This allows for easier capture of a particular kind of interaction and has been successfully applied to study promoter-enhancer interactions (PEIs) specifically in a variant of the method called promoter capture Hi-C, or PCHi-C [12,19]. The single largest PCHi-C study to date was conducted by Javierre and colleagues [12] on a variety of human cells belonging to the haematopoietic lineage. This study found that each particular lineage of cells had noticeable differences in the distribution of its PEIs and that many of these interactions appeared to match up with putative genetic variations linked to disease and altered gene expression. Due to its excellent coverage of a range of closely related non-cancerous cell lineages the study provides an attractive target for further analysis, particularly for using computational methods to find patterns in chromatin dynamics.

For basic analysis methods of Hi-C datasets there are a number of well-established and well-documented methods [15]. Several methods exist by which the resolution of a Hi-C dataset can be theoretically improved through more sophisticated interaction calling algorithms. These include several algorithms with broadly comparable performances for general Hi-C data [10] and also more specific tools such as the CHiCAGO analysis pipeline meant specifically for cHi-C datasets [3]. These algorithms involve techniques ranging from modelling technical biases [1] to employing a deep convolutional neural network [30]. Another set of approaches are based on clustering methods by which the available 3C and Hi-C data are analysed with the aim of discovering functionally related modules of genes and regulatory elements. These include the use of δ-teams models for Hi-C data to identify both known and putative gene clusters [24], hard- and soft-clustering algorithms that could theoretically assist in the interpretation of combined metagenomic sequencing and 3C data [8], and also spectral clustering-based methods such as the Arboretum-Hi-C framework that was found to be useful in identifying chromatin features in mammalian Hi-C datasets at several levels of organization and pointed to the potential utility of graph-based clustering in both analysing and comparing Hi-C datasets in general [25].

In principle the advantages of analysing Hi-C interaction data in graph-related terms are already well recognised. For example, approaches by [25] or [3] explicitly discuss graph-based formalisms and their methods have been successfully applied when analysing new data sets [12]. However, these approaches remain largely focused only on the properties of interaction matrices (which can be considered as weighted graphs) as well as on some additional data (e.g. interaction segment distances and associations with known gene regulations). At the same time potential of analysis of topological features of these interaction graphs and assessment of their biological significance remains largely unexplored. (Although there are studies that explicitly mention 'topological features', the considered features are more related to the topology of chromosomes rather than interaction graphs – e.g. in [28] these features are interpreted as the distributions of interaction endpoints on chromosomes).

In this paper we explicitly focus on the topological properties (and only on such type of properties) of Hi-C interaction networks using for analysis one of the richest datasets available – genome-wide PCHi-C data obtained by [12] for 17 types of haematopoietic cells (thus practically covering the whole haematopoietic cell lineage) using a unified protocol. There are two main research questions we are trying to answer: (1) are topological properties of Hi-C interaction networks alone able to distinguish between different cell types and assign biologically meaningful distances between them; (2) what is a typical structure of Hi-C interaction networks and can we assign some biological significance to structural elements or features of these networks?

Some initial results on these research questions have already been obtained by the authors in [14]. In particular, we have proposed a set *Base11* of 11 topological features of networks that provide good discriminatory power for distinguishing between different cell types. We also have stated the hypothesis on biological significance of certain connected components of the networks and have provided some limited biological validation for this hypothesis.

In this paper we are more focusing on potential biological significance on topological features that are the most useful for distinguishing between different cell types. We start with a somewhat different set of the initial features (metrics) that allows to derive a smaller (6 instead of 11) *Base6* set of the most characteristic topological features. *Base6* set also has an improved discriminatory power and does not include any pairs of too closely related metrics. In particular, this allows quite clear and unambiguous identification of network topological features of potential significance – these are medium-sized connected components of networks, bi-connected components, cliques and cycles of length 2. Apart from bi-connected components, potential biological role of which remains unknown, it is possible to assign some biological explanation for other three types of topological features, although we by no means suggest that there are unique and/or uniform biological explanations of these. Here we also provide a new assessment the potential biological significance of network cliques using data from FANTOM5 promoter level expression atlas [18], with the results indicating that for PCHi-C interaction networks for closely related cell types genes from the same clique tend to be co-expressed.

2   Datasets and Graph Representations of PCHi-C Networks

For analysis of PCHi-C interaction networks we use a dataset of long-range interactions between promoters and other regulatory elements that was generated by The Babraham Institute and University of Cambridge [12]. This dataset is still largely unique because it contains genome-wide data covering a representative subset of the entire haematopoietic lineage collected using a unified protocol. The data were obtained by promoter capture Hi-C (PCHi-C) in 17 human primary haematopoietic cell types (see Fig. 1 [14]). From 31253 identified promoter interaction regions across all chromosomes, a subset of high-confidence PCHi-C interactions have been selected using CHiCAGO pipeline [3] (with interactions having score at least 5 chosen as high-confidence). These data are available from the Open Science Framework website [12].

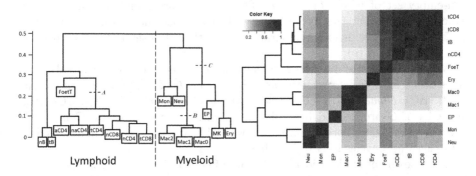

Fig. 1. (Left) Haematopoietic tree of 17 cell types [14]. The continuous distances $Dcont$ range from 0 to 1 and are proportional to distances in the tree according to the scale shown. Binary distances Db are defined to be equal to 0 for $Dcont < 0.5$ and equal to 1 otherwise. Dt is defined according to cell subtypes – it is equal to 1 between lymphoid and myeloid types and equal to 0 between cells of the same subtype. Additionally binary distances DA, DB and DC were used to test separability of subtrees 'cut' correspondingly at points A, B and C. (Right) Correlations between gene activities and hierarchical clustering for 11 cell types for which FANTOM5 expression data are also available.

The network of PCHi-C interactions we represent as a digraph (directed graph) G with a set of vertices $V = V(G)$ consisting of promoters ('baits') and detected interaction regions ('other ends'). (A vertex can also be both: a 'bait' and an 'other end'.)

The set of edges $E = E(G)$ correspond to detected high-confidence interactions and are directed from 'baits' to 'other ends' (it is possible that for some vertices $v_1, v_2 \in V$ both edges $(v_1, v_2) \in E$ and $(v_2, v_1) \in E$). Similarly as in [12] CHiCAGO score threshold of 5 or more was used to chose high-confidence interactions. However, although no comprehensive analysis was done, in a number of computational tests we used graphs that were constructed with CHiCAGO score thresholds ranging between 3 and 8. Such threshold variations had a limited impact on the stability of the results.

Such networks can be constructed either for complete interaction data set (covering all chromosomes), or separately for each of the chromosomes. Due to very few interactions between chromosomes we have adapted the latter approach as computationally more convenient and constructed 23 chromosome-specific networks (chromosome Y was omitted due to a very few interactions). In total all 23 graphs consisted of 251209 vertices (with ranges between 2904 and 23079 per chromosome) and 723165 edges.

To include information about cell-type specificity graph edges are additionally annotated with labels. By $\mathcal{T}$ we denote the set of all the available (17 for this particular dataset) cell types. For each edge $e \in E$ there is assigned a non-empty set of labels $T(e) \subseteq \mathcal{T}$. These labels correspond to cell types for which the scores for the interaction reached at least the threshold level. For $T \subseteq \mathcal{T}$ by $G(T)$ we denote a subgraph of G with vertex set $V(G)$ and edge set $\{e \in E(G) \mid T \subseteq T(e)\}$.

We will be mostly interested in the following types of topological substructures of interaction networks: *connected components* (CC), *bi-connected components* (BC), *cliques* (CL) and *strongly connected components* (SCC). CCs, BCs and CLs of G are defined by replacing G with undirected graph $\hat{G}$ in which edge directions are ignored. In addition we will be considering 'antiparallel edge' substructures – cycles in G of length 2.

For assessment of biological significance of network structural components we have used data from FANTOM5 promoter level expression atlas [18] that contains transcription start site activity data obtained by CAGE [26] protocol. The available data sets cover genome-wide information about 14 human haematopoietic cell types, 11 of these overlap with cell types for which PCHi-C interaction data are available. The expression data are available for approximately 18% vertices (corresponding to 'bait' ends) of PCHi-C interaction graphs constructed from [12] data.

Another type of more limited (restricted only to $G(\{Mon, Mac0, tB\})$ subnetwork) assessment of biological significance of network components was also performed by analysing network components for enrichment with registered transcription factor protein-protein interactions, known transcription factor binding sites, co-expressed transcription factors and binding motifs with the *Enrichr* web tool [5,13].

3   Characterisation of Structural Features of Interaction Networks

The main aim of this study is exploration of characteristic structural features of PCHi-C interaction networks and (potentially) assessment of biological significance of such features. We are also mostly focused on features that allow to distinguish between different cell types (and thus might be also indicative of different biological role or activity of the corresponding cell types).

To do this we consider (several different types of) distances between cell types based on their positions in haematopoietic tree and choose an initial set of topological features (called *metrics*) of interaction graphs. The choice of initial set of metrics is based on both: structural features that can be observed in PCHi-C networks by 'manual inspection' (and which remain comparatively stable by changing threshold for high-confidence interactions); as well as 'standard' graph structural properties that can be computed by efficient algorithms. The initial set of 57 metrics *Base57* is then analysed from the perspective of their discriminatory power in relation to the cell types. As a result we then propose a smaller subset *Base6* of 6 'characteristic' metrics that provides almost as good distance predictions as the initial *Base57* set. Since the selected metrics are mostly based on component structure of networks, we also provide some analysis of changes of component structure when only interactions for specific subsets of cell types from $\mathcal{T}$ are considered.

In broader terms this approach is similar to graphlet methods [29] that have been successfully used for analysis of different types of biological networks. These methods are based on network sampling for the presence of small subgraphs from some predefined set, however, they do not seem to be directly applicable to PCHi-C interaction graphs due to lack of precisely preserved common substructures in graphs $G(\{t\})$ for different cell types $t \in \mathcal{T}$. Some of the metrics we use could be technically regarded as graphlets, but most are based on more general structures. Somewhat similar approaches with characteristic structural features derived from typical common subgraphs we have used in our previous work on protein structure analysis [4,27].

Whilst the graph based metrics (or similar terms) have been previously used for describing analysis of several different types of biomolecular interactions (e.g. in [20] for RNA structure analysis), these metrics, however, are usually defined by vertex or edge weights or labels rather than to the topological properties of graphs.

In comparison to our previous work [14] here we have proposed a different *Base57* set of the initial metrics that provides improved predictions of distances between cell types and also allows to derive a smaller (6 instead of 11) *Base6* set of the most characteristic metrics. *Base6* set also has an improved discriminatory power and does not include any pairs of too closely related metrics.

3.1 Distances Between Cell Types

The most natural way to assign distance between different cell types would be on basis of their position in haematopoietic tree (Fig. 1). Although the molecular mechanisms underlying haematopoiesis in humans are not completely understood, the main principles of haematopoietic stem cell differentiation into erythroid, megakaryocytic, myeloid and lymphoid lineages are generally agreed upon [22]. However, whilst there is a good agreement on haematopoietic tree structure, no quantitative estimates about the length of tree branches have usually been provided (or, when some quantitative hierarchical clustering has been done, e.g. on the basis of ribosomal protein expression [11], the underlining intent is validation of the results, and the assigned quantitative distances greatly depend on the used experimental technology).

The situation with CHiCAGO based clustering of PCHi-C data from [12] is very similar – the study provides quantitative distances between cell lines, however, these are strongly related to the used PCHi-C technology. Nevertheless, since our analysis is based on the same dataset, these distances seem to be the most appropriate for comparison. It should be emphasised that we are not trying here to replicate the same results with only slightly different methods – whilst the underlining dataset is the same, the original hierarchical clustering has been based on analysis of interactions represented as weight matrix, without considering any topological features. At the same time, our analysis is based only on topological features, not taking into account weights assigned to the interactions; and the question we try to answer is whether there exists a set of specific topological properties that can be utilized to distinguish between different forms of chromatin interactions captured in Hi-C data, and whether these properties are potentially useful in describing and predicting coordinated genomic processes.

On basis of these data we consider two distance measures: $Dcont$ ranging from 0.00 to 1.00 that are proportional to distances from [12] and a binarised version Db with values 0 and 1 obtained by applying cut-off threshold 0.50 (see Fig. 1).

We also consider two distances that are based only on the relative positions in haematopoietic tree and/or biologically well-accepted cell type similarities. Dt is completely based on positions in the tree and is equal to 0 for cell types within the same (lymphoid and myeloid) subgroups and equal to 1 for cell types from different subgroups. $D4$ is based on both – the relative positions in the haematopoietic tree and (in the case of endothelial precursors EP) functional similarities. It separates cells into 5 subgroups: $G_1 = \{MK, Ery\}$, $G_{2,1} = \{Mac0, Mac1, Mac2\}$, $G_{2,2} = \{EP, Mon, Neu\}$, $G_{3,1} = \{aCD4, naCD4, tCD4, nCD4, nCD8, tCD8, FoetT\}$ and $G_{3,2} = \{nB, tB\}$ and assigns distance $D4$ equal to 0.33 between different members of the same group, distances 0.67 between pairs from groups $G_{2,1}$, $G_{2,2}$ and $G_{3,1}$, $G_{3,2}$ and distances 1.0 between pairs from other groups. For a pair of the same cell types $D4$ is 0.

In addition we also tested 3 binary distances (defined by the chosen positions of cut-points in the tree) DA, DB and DC to check the possibility to separate some closely related cell subgroups from the other cell types in the tree (see Fig. 1).

For a given distance $D \in \{Dcont, Db, Dt, D4, DA, DB, DC\}$ and pair of cell types $t_1, t_2 \in \mathcal{T}$ the distance between these cell types is denoted by $D(t_1, t_2)$, and the distance values by definition are symmetric: $D(t_1, t_2) = D(t_2, t_1)$.

3.2   Metrics for Characterisation of Structural Features of Networks

The initial set $Base57$ contains 57 different metrics. The selection of these metrics was based on manual exploration of PCHi-C networks as well as on the most often considered graph topological properties that can be computed efficiently. The currently proposed $Base57$ set is similar, but still quite different from the one we proposed initially in [14] – the types of included structural components are the same, however, the size constraints were changed to make them less inter-dependent and to cover larger range of structural features of networks.

The metrics included in the set $Base57$ are the following: $CCEr$ – the number of connected components with number of edges within range r, $CCVr$ – the number of connected components with number of vertices within range r, $BCEr$ – the number of vertex bi-connected components with number of edges within range r, $BCVr$ – the number of vertex bi-connected components with number of vertices within range r, $SCEr$ – the number of strongly connected components with number of edges within range r, $SCVr$ – the number of strongly connected components with number of vertices within range r, and $CLVn$ – a number of cliques (ignoring edge directions) of size n. The values of n range from 3 to 8. The values of r are $4, 8, 16, 32, 64$ and $+$ that correspond to the intervals $4 - 7$, $8 - 15$, $16 - 31$, $32 - 63$ and ≥ 64.

Metrics $CCVax$, $CCVver$ denote the maximal and the average numbers of vertices in connected components. $CCEmax$, $CCEaver$, $BCVmax$, $BCVaver$, $BCEmax$, $BCEaver$, $SCVmax$, $SCVaver$, $SCEmax$, $SCEaver$ are defined similarly for numbers of edges and vertices and bi-connected and strongly connected components. Finally, $CLVmax$ and $CLVaver$ denote the maximal and the average clique sizes, and $antiparallelEdges$ is the number of cycles of length 2.

Since being more based on counting rather than on network structure in addition to $Base57$ other 4 metrics closely related to the sizes of graphs were considered separately: V – the number of vertices, E – the number of edges, $E9$ – the number of edges, which are not shared by 9 or more (i.e. by no more than 50% of all) cell types and $E17$ – the number of edges, which are not shared by the all 17 cell types.

The value of a particular metric m, a chromosome represented by network G and a subset of cell types $T \subseteq \mathcal{T}$ is denoted by $m(G(T))$ and represents its value in a subgraph of G in which all edges are assigned labels from all the cell types from T. To minimise the effect of the measure of cell type distances being based simply on different numbers of particular features (which very likely will be strongly correlated to the difference in sizes of interaction graphs) the values of metrics are further normalised. These normalised values are defined only for distinct pairs of cell types: for a metric m and for a pair of two distinct cell types $t_1, t_2 \in \mathcal{T}$ its normalised value $M(\{t_1, t_2\})$ is defined as $M(\{t_1, t_2\}) = m(\{t_1, t_2\})/\sqrt{m(\{t_1\}) \times m(\{t_2\})}$. Such values $M(\{t_1, t_2\})$ were computed for all 61 metrics and all 136 distinct pairs of cell types for all 23 chromosomes as well as for network containing all the chromosomes.

One clearly expects a high correlation between the values of metrics V, E, $E9$ and $E17$; however, there are also high correlations between certain pairs from $Base57$ set, in particular, between numbers of vertices and edges in specific types of components. Only one of the metrics was kept for pairs with correlations of 0.93 and above (the main reason for choosing this threshold was very clear correlations between metrics measuring numbers of vertices and numbers of edges), leading to the removal of $CCVr$, $BCVr$, $SCVr$ for all values of r and also the removal of $CCVmax$, $CCVaver$, $BCVmax$, $BCVaver$, $SCVmax$, $SCVaver$ and (metrics based on number of edges rather than vertices were kept due to overall giving slightly better results). Also removed was $CLVmax$ that strongly correlates with $CLVaver$. For the further analysis the remaining subset $Base32$ of 32 metrics from $Base57$ was chosen.

4   Discriminatory Power of Metrics Between Different Cell Types

To estimate the discriminatory power of metrics from $Base32$ and also of 4 'counting' metrics V, E, $E9$ and $E17$ we constructed linear regression models for the prediction of cell distances on the basis of the values of these metrics. For this we computed the distances $D(t_1, t_2)$ for all distinct pairs of cell types $t_1, t_2 \in \mathcal{T}$ and for all types of $D \in \{Dcont, Db, Dt, D4, DA, DB, DC\}$ obtaining for each distance type D a vector of length 136. For the same pairs of cell types we also computed normalised values of metrics $M(\{t_1, t_2\})$ for all metrics from $Base57$ and for 4 'counting' metrics for the graph representing interaction network for all the chromosomes obtaining 61 metrics vectors of length 136. Several regression models then were constructed for prediction of the values of distance vectors from a number of subsets of the available metrics vectors.

We also applied stepwise regression using Akaike information criterion [23] and its implementation in AIC function available in language R core library to select the most discriminatory metrics from $Base32$.

The correlations between predictions of regression models and the actual distances are summarised in Table 1. They clearly show the suitability of different subsets of metrics for discrimination between cell types, although the obtained correlation values are likely somewhat influenced by over-fitting and should be treated with caution. The results are also very stable – 10 repeated bootstrapping tests with training sets containing 75% of data produced at most 2% deviations.

As statistically the most significant AIC stepwise regression identified 6 metrics: $CL3$, $antiparallelEdges$, $CCE+$, $CCEaver$, $BCEaver$ and $CCEmax$ (see Figs. 2 and 3). The set of these 6 metrics is called $Base6$.

Table 1. Pearson correlations between cell type distances and predictions of their values.

	Dcont	Db	Dt	D4	DA	DB	DC
Base57	0.82	0.68'	0.67	0.75	0.78	0.51	0.66
Base32	0.82	0.68	0.67	0.75	0.77	0.48	0.64
Base6	0.81	0.66	0.65	0.73	0.75	0.45	0.59
Base6+V	0.82	0.68	0.67	0.75	0.76	0.48	0.62
Base6+E	0.82	0.68	0.66	0.75	0.76	0.48	0.62
Base6+E17	0.82	0.68	0.66	0.75	0.76	0.48	0.62
Base6+E9	0.86	0.71	0.73	0.76	0.78	0.54	0.71
V	0.67	0.57	0.56	0.55	0.47	0.36	0.45
E	0.78	0.66	0.65	0.7	0.68	0.28	0.25
E17	0.78	0.66	0.65	0.7	0.68	0.28	0.25
E9	0.86	0.71	0.73	0.74	0.67	0.37	0.36

From these one of the most important (independently from type of distance considered) has turned out to be *CL3* – normalised number of cliques of size 3 (the presence of larger size cliques is also a good discriminator, but with smaller statistical significance due to quite small overall numbers of larger cliques). The biological significance of *CL3* at least partially could be explained by coordinated expressions of the involved genes (see Sect. 6). The second most discriminatory metrics is *antiparallelEdges* – normalised number of cycles of size 2. Its significance also potentially might be related to gene regulation, since such interactions are possible only between two 'bait' regions, which, by definition, are associated with genes.

It is not too surprising that of significant importance are numbers and sizes of connected components (see Sect. 5), although interestingly that the top 6 most significant metrics include both maximal and average sizes of CCs. The high significance of average sizes of bi-connected components, however, is quite unexpected and currently we do not have any hypothetical biological explanation for this. Of notice is the opposite sign of regression coefficient for *BCEaver*, but this appears to be a coincidence – this varies if the metrics are computed for interaction networks of individual chromosomes.

Of interest is also the comparative performance of different subsets of metrics in cell type differentiation. Good performance of 'counting' metrics *V, E, E9* and *E17* is not surprising, since one should expect that more closely related cell types will share more common PCHi-C interactions. Nevertheless, they alone do not outperform sets of *Base* metrics (apart from *E9*, which counts the interactions that are common to no more than 50% of cell types, and thus is dataset dependent). The discriminatory power of the metrics for distances *DA, DB* and *DC* (with quite arbitrarily chosen cut-points) is surprisingly varying, but it is interesting that for all of them 4 'counting' metrics perform notably worse than the topology-based ones.

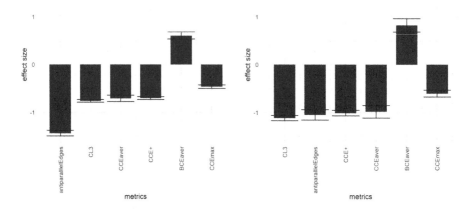

Fig. 2. The most discriminating metrics for cell type distances *Dcont* (left) and *Db* (right). The relative discriminatory power of any pair of metrics is proportional to the ratio of their absolute values of "effect size" shown on y axis. The exact ranges of "effect size" are data-dependent and are not directly comparable between different cell type distances, and (even more notably) between full genome and single chromosome metrics data.

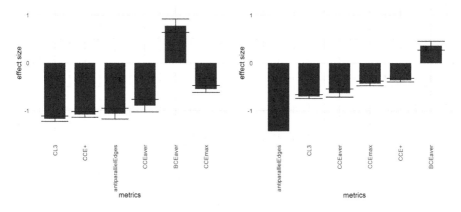

Fig. 3. The most discriminating metrics for cell type distances *Dt* (left) and *D4* (right).

In comparison with the sets of metrics we have previously proposed in [14] the current *Base57* overall provides improved discrimination between cell types for the all types of distances, *Base6* is at least comparable with the previously suggested *Base11* and contains fewer and less inter-related metrics, comparative significance of which also remains quite stable for different cell types and/or chromosomes. Overall the results confirm that topology-based metrics, and in particular even the proposed small *Base6* subset, perform well in lineage-based identification of blood cell types in chromatin interaction data.

We have also performed regression analysis at the level of individual chromosomes – in this case the values of metrics $M(\{t_1, t_2\})$ were computed separately for each of the 23 chromosomes.

An interesting feature can be observed when the performance $Base6$ is compared on different chromosomes (shown by heatmaps in Fig. 4). The chromosomes are grouped in a number of similarity clusters, which is not the case for randomised data. The clusters, however, strongly depend on the used cell type distance (although there are few stably related pairs of chromosomes as well as few persistent outliers).

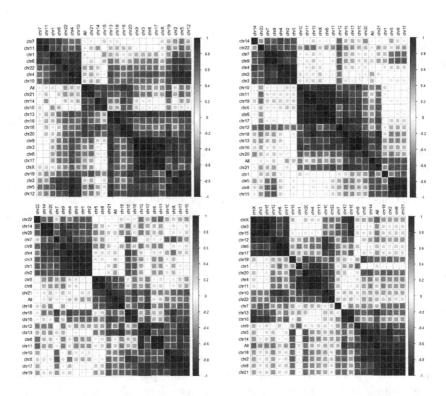

Fig. 4. Heatmaps of similarity between pairs of chromosomes using the four metrics giving the best predictions of cell type distances $Dcont$ (top left), Db (top right), Dt (bottom left) and $D4$ (bottom right).

For $Dcont$ distance Fig. 5 shows the statistical significance of $Base6$ metrics for chromosome 21 which correlates well with metrics significance for the whole chromosome set and for chromosome 1 with poor correlation with overall significances. Up to extent these results indicate that there are no strictly dominant chromosomes that could be used for cell type differentiation. At the same time the obtained distance predictions using $Base6$ on individual chromosome networks are not notably lower than predictions using the whole genome data.

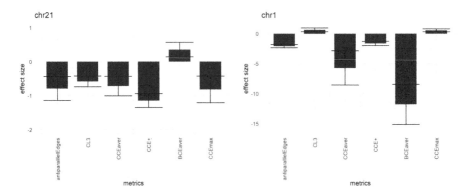

Fig. 5. Statistical significance of metrics for *Dcont* distance and chromosome 21 (left) and chromosome 1 (right), which correspondingly correlate well and poorly with metrics for the whole chromosome set.

5   Component Structure of PCHi-C Interaction Networks

In this section we more closely explore the structure of graphs describing PCHi-C interactions. The initial networks $G(T)$ (see Sect. 2) are defined separately for each of the 23 chromosomes (chromosome Y is omitted due to a very low number of interactions) and are dependent on cell type subset $T \subseteq \mathcal{T}$.

The main questions we are addressing here are: (1) what is a 'typical structure' of PCHi-C interaction graph? (2) how do the structures of graphs change if we consider common subgraphs for given sets of cell types?

Judging from the most discriminatory metrics in *Base6* set, one can expect that important role could be assigned to connected components of interaction networks, and since the interactions are related to spatial proximity, it is not unexpected that interaction networks might separate easily into connected components.

However, when we do not restrict attention to cell type specific interactions and for each of chromosomes consider its network $G(\varnothing)$ containing interactions for all 17 cell types the component structure is not particularly rich. Typically there is a single large component containing more than half of network vertices, very few components with sizes 10 or more, and also a comparatively large proportion of 2 vertex components. For example, for chromosome 1 there are only 6 components in $G(\varnothing)$ with 10 or more vertices (their sizes are 17230, 81, 73, 63, 20 and 13 vertices) and such size distribution is typical (the largest number of components is 15 for chromosome 15).

At the same time the interaction networks that are common for all 17 cell types are even surprisingly small – e.g. in $G(\mathcal{T})$ for chromosome 1 only 1289 vertices are contained in components with 2 or more vertices, there are only 38 components with 10 or more vertices and the largest component size is 66 (this again is typical for all the chromosomes).

More interesting are networks $G(\{t\})$ describing interactions for a single cell type $t \in \mathcal{T}$ with still around half of all vertices involved in interactions and already a wider range of medium-sized (between 10 and few hundreds vertices) components. The most of the connected vertices for these networks, however, still remain contained within one or two large components.

For analysis the most interesting appear to be networks $G(T)$ defined by a small subset (from 2 to 5) of (sufficiently distinct) cell types $T \subseteq \mathcal{T}$. As a (typical) example we can consider $G(T) = G(\{Mon, Mac0, tB\})$ network for chromosome 5. Approximately 40% of vertices of this network are contained in components of size 10 or more, the number of such components is around 50 with the largest component having 176 vertices. Distribution of connected component sizes for this network is shown in Fig. 6 (for comparison are included also size distributions for chromosomes 1 and 11 with the largest components correspondingly of sizes 153 and 138).

To investigate how these components change for different cell types we further consider components of 10 or more vertices (although chosen somewhat arbitrary, this threshold seems well suited to largely reduce random 'noise' in networks).

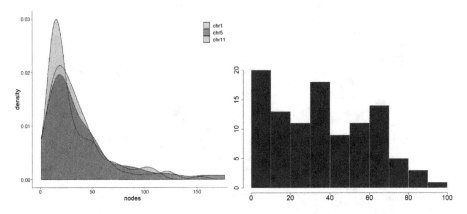

Fig. 6. (Left) The distribution of sizes of connected components in $G(\{Mon, Mac0, tB\})$ for 3 different chromosomes. Component size is shown on the horizontal axis. (Right) The reduction of sizes of connected components (with 10 or more vertices) for chromosome 5 in $G(\{Mon\})$ cell type when the component is replaced by a subgraph of $G(\{\mathcal{T}\})$ [14]. The remaining component size (in %) is shown on the horizontal axis and the percentage of components on the vertical axis.

A very interesting observation is the fact that connected components have a tendency to remain largely unchanged when shared by a number of different (component-specific) cell types and to be largely (or completely) absent in others. A typical reduction of sizes of components for chromosome and cell type-specific graph, when only parts of components shared by all cell types are considered, is shown in Fig. 6 for $G(\{Mon\})$ network for chromosome 5. The proportion of components that are shared by Mon and at least one other cell type and that

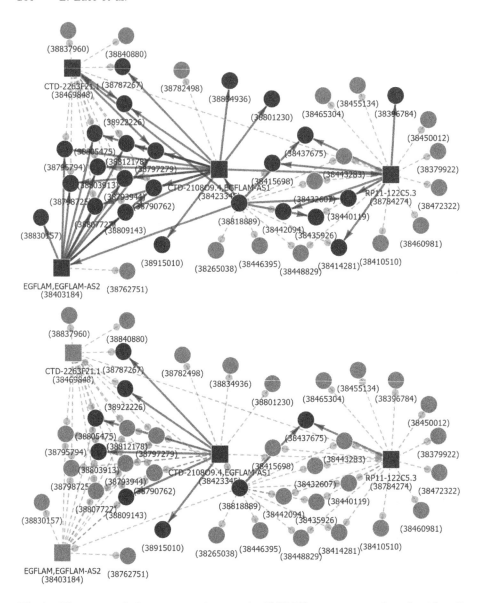

Fig. 7. The parts of chromosome 5 network $G(\{EP\})$ component shared with cell types *Mac0*, *Mac1* and *Mac2* (top) and additionally with *tCD8* (bottom). There are no common interactions shared with cell type *Neu* [14].

are almost absent in at least one other cell type is around 25%. Comparatively few (around 5%) components remain little changed in all of the cell types. The remaining 70% could be further subdivided in not very strictly separated subclasses, ranging from ones for which part of the component shows good cell type specificity, to quite noisy ones (full statistics is lacking, but manual inspections indicate that the first of these behaviours tends to be more common).

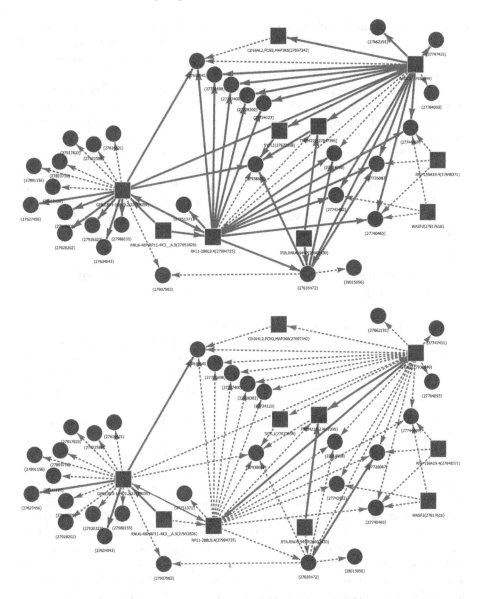

Fig. 8. The parts of chromosome 1 network $G(\{aCD4, naCD4\})$ component shared with cell types *Ery* (top) and with *Neu* (bottom).

As a concrete example, the Fig. 7 (from [14]) illustrate a connected component from $G(\{EP\})$ for chromosome 5. The initial component consists of all the vertices and all (solid and dotted) the edges. Comparatively large parts of this component remain shared with cell types *Mac0*, *Mac1* and *Mac2* – although a number of interactions and vertices are lost, the topological structure remains mostly preserved. When additionally we consider only part of the component shared also by by cell type *tCD8*, only a few vertices and interactions remain. The component is completely absent for cell type subset $\{EP, Mac0, Mac1, Mac2, tCD8, Neu\}$. (In these figures the vertices are denoted by the middle genomic coordinate of their respective segment mapped on a specific chromosome, and the gene annotations used are from the original dataset.)

As another typical example a component from $G(\{aCD4, naCD4\})$ for chromosome 1 is shown in Fig. 8 (with solid and dotted edges). With solid edges are shown parts of the component that are shared with $G(\{aCD4, naCD4, Ery\})$ and $G(\{aCD4, naCD4, Neu\})$.

This behaviour of connected components of interaction networks further strengthens the hypothesis that network component structure at least partially can be linked with certain biological roles or functionality. Up to extent this hypothesis is confirmed by biological validation (described in Sect. 6 and also in [14]) using *Enrichr* web tool for analysis of $G(T) = G(\{Mon, Mac0, tB\})$ network.

6   Assessment of Biological Significance of Network Components

An important question is whether it is possible to assign some biological interpretation of structural features of PCHi-C interaction networks. The previous analysis suggests that the structural features of the most interest could be the following: medium-sized connected components of networks $G(T)$ for some $T \subseteq \mathcal{T}$ (in particular if such components get significantly reduced in size when T is replaced by some larger superset), bi-connected components, cliques and cycles of length 2. All these features are included in *Base6* set of metrics and there is additional evidence of potential significance of medium sized CCs.

At the current stage we do not have any hypothetical biological explanation for potential significance of bi-connected components – this could require very extensive analysis of such components in the available dataset and it also seems quite possible that of importance is not bi-connectivity as such, but some related and more complex structural feature). The importance of cycles of length 2 (*antiparallelEdges* metric) could be potentially related to gene co-regulation, since such cyclic interactions are possible only between two 'bait' regions, which, by definition, are associated with genes. This could be validated with a well suited gene expression dataset; FANTOM5 data (discussed below) in principle might be suitable, but seems to have too small coverage for this purpose.

Regarding connected components, the observation that these are either largely shared by two cell types, or are present in one of them and largely absent in another, strongly suggest that they should have biological roles. These, however, might differ between the components and the very large number of these make comprehensive analysis quite infeasible. More restricted in scope analysis focusing on specific networks $G(T)$ and/or particular components, however, is possible, and we have performed such analysis for $G(T) = G(\{Mon, Mac0, tB\})$ network (quite arbitrary chosen as a typical network with large number of medium-sized components) for enrichment with registered transcription factor protein-protein interactions, known transcription factor binding sites, co-expressed transcription factors and binding motifs using the *Enrichr* web tool [5,13].

Starting from a pool of common connected components for $G(T)$ we sequentially added more cell types to the selection criteria – alternatively activated macrophages *Mac2*, neutrophils *Neu* and endothelial precursors *EP* to establish the component specificity. The majority of components found tended to be highly specific, showing 0–25% retention in the final set of linked nodes and edges (although, the most specific components also tended to have the smallest number of nodes). After collecting data about node retention, the largest components showing high (75–100%) or low (0–25%) retention from selected chromosomes (chromosomes 5, 9, 14, 15 and 19) were analysed using *Enrichr* web tool.

The analysis uncovered a variety of transcription factors that associated with different components, including an array of broadly tissue macrophage-associated factors such as STAT5, GATA6, PPARγ and MAF [16] as well as more specific factors found primarily in monocyte-derived macrophages – JUN, JUNB, MAFK, EGR3 and others [21], and even lipopolysaccharide treatment-induced transcription factors including BCL3, USF1 and SREBF2 signifying inflammatory macrophage activity or interleukin-4 and 13 activated factors such as MITF [6]. Overall the gene set enrichment analysis supported the hypothesis that the genes we have linked together into connected components may form functionally related modules, broadly fitting a loose model of specificity applied through examining the overlap between chromatin architectures of diverse cell types. In more details the analysis procedures and its outcomes are described in our paper [14].

To assess the potential biological significance of network cliques we used data from FANTOM5 promoter level expression atlas [18] that contains transcription start site activity data obtained by CAGE [26] protocol. The data covers 11 of 17 cell types of PCHi-C interaction networks and approximately 18% of network vertices. The dataset includes information about transcription start site activity data obtained by CAGE [26] protocol. For a number of genes activity levels for several different (up to 6) start sites is provided, in which case we have chosen the largest activity value. Not surprisingly, the activity profiles shown by PHANTOM5 data for different cell types are clustering in good accordance with their positions in haematopoietic tree (see Fig. 1), although an unexpected outlier is *Ery* cell type.

For validation we have chosen four different pairs of cell types: two distant pairs *Mac0*, *nCD4* and *Mac1*, *tCD4* (one of each pair lymphoid and one myeloid cell type), and two closely related pairs: *Mac0*, *Mac1* (both myeloid) and *tCD4*, *nCD4* (both lymphoid). The anticipated validation result was that gene activities within cliques in $G(\{t_1, t_2\})$ (where $\{t_1, t_2\}$ is the pair of the chosen cell types) is correlating more strongly than activities of the same number of randomly chosen gene pairs with interaction edges in $G(\{t_1, t_2\})$. To guarantee the stability of the results such random pairs were selected 100 times and the average correlation value was used for comparison.

The tests were performed for chromosome 1 interaction network (due to it being the largest). Table 2 summarises the numbers of the detected cliques, involved vertices and vertices covered by FANTOM5 data.

Table 2. Numbers of cliques in chromosome 1 and their coverage by FANTOM5 data.

	Mac0-nCD4	Mac1-tCD4	Mac0-Mac1	tCD4-nCD4
Number of cliques	715	581	1629	2246
Number of vertices	2145	1743	4887	6738
Number of vertices covered by FANTOM5 data	48	41	70	188

Although the coverage by FANTOM5 data unfortunately is rather small (especially for distant cell types for which, unsurprisingly, graphs $G(\{t_1, t_2\})$ contained fewer cliques) the results show that genes are co-expressed in cliques in networks for closely related cell types and are reasonably convincing (Fig. 9).

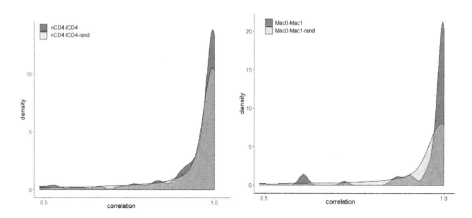

Fig. 9. Comparison of distributions of correlations of TSS activities of genes from cliques of size 3 with distributions of correlations for randomly selected gene pairs for interaction graphs of closely related cell type pairs: *nCD4* and *tCD4* (left) and *Mac0* and *Mac1* (right).

In more distant gene pairs (Fig. 10) such co-expression was not observed (for *Mac0*, *nCD4* pair being even below the random value). For distant cell types the lack of such co-expression is also not particularly surprising, although the small sizes of available datasets do not allow to conclude whether such co-expression is only weak or is completely lacking.

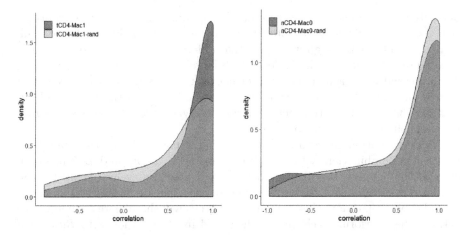

Fig. 10. Comparison of distributions of correlations of TSS activities of genes from cliques of size 3 with distributions of correlations for randomly selected gene pairs for interaction graphs of closely related cell type pairs: *tCD4* and *Mac1* (left) and *nCD4* and *Mac0* (right).

7   Conclusions

In this paper we have analysed the topological properties of Hi-C interaction networks from two related, but somewhat different perspectives: (1) are topological properties of Hi-C interaction networks alone able to distinguish between different cell types and assign biologically meaningful distances between them; (2) what is a typical structure of Hi-C interaction networks and can we assign some biological significance to structural elements or features of these networks?

In general, we think that we have obtained affirmative answers to both these questions. Regarding characterisation of interactions networks in terms of their topological properties we propose a set *Base6* of 6 metrics based on network topological features that can be used to distinguish between different cell types for 7 different distance measures that we have tested. Notably, *Base6* does not include any pairs of too closely related metrics and provide quite clear listing of network topological features of potential significance – medium-sized connected components of networks, bi-connected components, cliques and cycles of length 2.

Regarding bi-connected components, at the current stage we do not have any hypothetical biological explanation for their potential significance. For this one would need very extensive analysis of bi-connected components that can be found in the analysed dataset. Also, it seems quite possible that of importance is not bi-connectivity as such, but some related and more complex structural feature. A plausible explanation of the importance of cycles of length 2 is the co-regulation of the both involved genes. In principle such assumption could be easily tested, provided expression data fur sufficiently large number of genes involved in such cycles are available (which, unfortunately, does not yet seem to be the case). The biological role of connected components has been at least partially validated using *Enrichr* web tool, providing support for the hypothesis that the genes linked together into connected components may form functionally related modules. (Although we expect that different types of components might have quite different biological roles, which largely still need to be understood.) The potential biological significance of network cliques we have assessed using data from FANTOM5 promoter level expression atlas and the results indicate that for PCHi-C interaction networks for closely related cell types genes from the same clique tend to be co-expressed.

If discrimination between the cell types is the main priority, then *Base6* can be used in combination with 'counting metrics' *V*, *E*, *E9* and *E17* to obtain correlations between the distance-defined and predicted values of up to 0.86. Whilst the usefulness of these 'counting metrics' can be anticipated since one should expect that more closely related cell types will share more common interactions, they perform much better when used in combination with *Base6*, and a non-obvious feature is their linearity, i.e. the fact that they perform well in linear regression models.

The clustering of chromosomes according to regression coefficients that are assigned to different *Base6* metrics is an interesting observation, in particular since such clustering occurs for the all considered cell type distances D, but the clusters are different for different distances $D \in \{Dcont, Db, Dt, D4\}$. The exact reasons why such clusters of chromosomes are formed remain unclear. A probable explanation is that they could be the result of some complex (and interaction network-specific) dependencies between *Base6* metrics, or biological relations between network components that are not taken into account by the current topological approach.

Regarding further developments, it would be very important to test our approach on another genome-wide PCHi-C interaction dataset in order to assess both: (1) the applicability of *Base6* metrics for discrimination between cell types, other than haematopoietic cells studied here; and (2) to analyse the similarity of topological structure and component behaviour of interaction networks in order to assess how the properties observed for haematopoietic cells generalises to other cell types. Unfortunately, as far as we know, another appropriate PCHi-C dataset covering multiple cell types has yet to become available. Thus, the main uncertainty regarding the results that we are presenting here is whether these are quite specific to a particular dataset of PCHi-C interactions that we have analysed, or whether they at least partially applies to other PCHi-C interaction networks of similar type (i.e. are providing genome-wide coverage for a sufficiently large number of different cell types).

There is also a good potential to further extend the graph topology based approach that we have used here. The current formalism has been quite successful to show that topological properties alone could be quite informative for discrimination between different cell types and also for assigning biological meaning to specific components on interaction graphs. At the same time some useful information in the current network representation is absent, notably, an edge in an interaction network might represent an interaction that forms a well-defined loop on a chromosome (if the distance between interaction segments is limited and there are no intermediate interactions between them), or it can represent a long range interaction with a far less obvious biological role. Although we have plans to further develop the mathematical formalism for description of interaction graphs in order to incorporate and analyse such features, some additional studies are needed to determine the best way to achieve this.

Whilst significance of medium-sized connected components of interaction networks seems to be established, one of the challenges is automated identification of the components that are most likely to have certain biological role. Although search through all the networks defined by different subsets from the set of all cell types is feasible, it produces a vast number of partially overlapping components, and narrowing it down to a manageable size will require quite extensive analysis of component structure and topological relations between them.

8   Software Availability

A number of software components developed by the authors for PCHi-C network analysis and visualisation are publicly available at GitHub repository: https://github.com/IMCS-Bioinformatics/HiCGraphAnalysis.

The repository contains Python script for computing values of *Base57* and *V, E, E17, E9* metrics as well as data files describing PCHi-C interaction network and analysis results used in this study. It also contains web-based software components for visualisation and exploration of interaction networks.

References

1. Ay, F., Bailey, T., Noble, W.: Statistical confidence estimation for Hi-C data reveals regulatory chromatin contacts. Genome Res. **24**(6), 999–1011 (2014). https://doi.org/10.1101/gr.160374.113
2. Belton, J., McCord, R., et al.: Hi-C: a comprehensive technique to capture the conformation of genomes. Methods **58**(3), 268–276 (2012)
3. Cairns, J., Freire-Pritchett, P., et al.: CHiCAGO: robust detection of DNA looping interactions in capture Hi-C data. Genome Biol. **17**, 127 (2016)
4. Celms, E., et al.: Application of graph clustering and visualisation methods to analysis of biomolecular data. In: Lupeikiene, A., Vasilecas, O., Dzemyda, G. (eds.) DB&IS 2018. CCIS, vol. 838, pp. 243–257. Springer, Cham (2018). https://doi.org/10.1007/978-3-319-97571-9_20
5. Chen, E., Tan, C., et al.: Enrichr: interactive and collaborative HTML5 gene list enrichment analysis tool. BMC Bioinformatics **14**, 128 (2013)
6. Das, A., Yang, C., et al.: High-resolution mapping and dynamics of the transcriptome, transcription factors, and transcription co-factor networks in classically and alternatively activated macrophages. Front. Immunol. **9**, 22 (2018)
7. Dekker, J., Rippe, K., et al.: Capturing chromosome conformation. Science **295**(5558), 1306–1311 (2002)
8. DeMaere, M., Darling, A.: Deconvoluting simulated metagenomes: the performance of hard- and soft- clustering algorithms applied to metagenomic chromosome conformation capture (3C). PeerJ **4**, e2676 (2016)

9. Dryden, N., Broome, L., et al.: Unbiased analysis of potential targets of breast cancer susceptibility loci by capture Hi-C. Genome Res. **24**, 1854–1868 (2014)

10. Forcato, M., Nicoletti, C., et al.: Comparison of computational methods for Hi-C data analysis. Nat. Methods **14**, 679–685 (2017)

11. Guimaraes, J., Zavolan, M.: Patterns of ribosomal protein expression specify normal and malignant human cells. Genome Biol. **17**, 236 (2016)

12. Javierre, B., Burren, O., et al.: Lineage-specific genome architecture links enhancers and non-coding disease variants to target gene promoters. Cell **167**(5), 1369–1384 (2016)

13. Kuleshow, M., Jones, M., et al.: Enrichr: a comprehensive gene set enrichment analysis web server 2016 update. Nucleic Acids Res. **44**, W90–W97 (2016)

14. Lace, L., et al.: Graph-based characterisations of cell types and functionally related modules in promoter capture Hi-C data. In: Proceedings of the 12th International Joint Conference on Biomedical Engineering Systems and Technologies, vol. 3: BIOINFORMATICS, pp. 78–89 (2019)

15. Lajoie, B., Dekker, J., Kaplan, N.: The Hitchhiker's guide to Hi-C analysis: practical guidelines. Methods **72**, 65–75 (2015)

16. Lavin, Y., Mortha, A., et al.: Regulation of macrophage development and function in peripheral tissues. Nat. Rev. Immunol. **15**(12), 731–744 (2016)

17. Lieberman-Aiden, E., van Berkum, E., et al.: Comprehensive mapping of long-range interactions reveals folding principles of the human genome. Science **326**(5950), 289–293 (2009)

18. Lizio, M., Harshbarger, J., et al.: Gateways to the FANTOM5 promoter level mammalian expression atlas. Genome Biol. **16**, 22 (2015). https://doi.org/10.1186/s13059-014-0560-6

19. Mifsud, B., Tavares-Cadete, F., et al.: Mapping long-range promoter contacts in human cells with high-resolution capture Hi-C. Nat. Genet. **47**, 598–606 (2015)

20. Quadrini, R., Emanuela, M.: Loop-loop interaction metrics on RNA secondary structures with pseudoknots. In: Proceedings of the 11th International Joint Conference on Biomedical Engineering Systems and Technologies - vol. 3: BIOINFORMATICS, (BIOSTEC 2018), pp. 29–37 (2018)

21. Ramirez, R., Al-Ali, N., et al.: Dynamic gene regulatory networks of human myeloid differentiation. Cell Syst. **4**, 416–429 (2017)

22. Robb, L.: Cytokine receptors and hematopoietic differentiation. Oncogene **26**, 6715–6723 (2007)

23. Sakamoto, Y., Ishiguro, M., Kitagawa, G.: Akaike Information Criterion Statistics. D. Reidel Publishing Company, Dordrecht (1986)

24. Schulz, T., Stoye, J., Doerr, D.: GraphTeams: a method for discovering spatial gene clusters in Hi-C sequencing data. BMC Genom. **19**(5), 308 (2018). https://doi.org/10.1186/s12864-018-4622-0

25. Siahpirani, A., Ay, F., Roy, S.: A multi-task graph-clustering approach for chromosome conformation capture data sets identifies conserved modules of chromosomal interactions. Genome Biol. **17**, 114 (2016). https://doi.org/10.1186/s13059-016-0962-8

26. Takahashi, H., Sachiko, K., et al.: CAGE - cap analysis gene expression: a protocol for the detection of promoter and transcriptional networks. Methods Mol. Biol. **786**, 181–200 (2012). https://doi.org/10.1007/978-1-61779-292-2_11

27. Viksna, J., Gilbert, D., Torrance, G.: Domain discovery method for topological profile searches in protein structures. Genome Inf. **15**, 72–81 (2004)

28. Wang, H., Duggal, G., et al.: Topological properties of chromosome conformation graphs reflect spatial proximities within chromatin. In: Proceedings of the International Conference on Bioinformatics, Computational Biology and Biomedical Informatics, pp. 306–315 (2013)
29. Yaveroglu, O., Milenkovic, T., Przulj, N.: Proper evaluation of alignment-free network comparison methods. Bioinformatics **31**(16), 2697–2704 (2015)
30. Zhang, Y., An, L., et al.: Enhancing Hi-C data resolution with deep convolutional neural network HiCPlus. Nature Commun. **9**(1), 750 (2018)

Generating Reliable Genome Assemblies of Intestinal Protozoans from Clinical Samples for the Purpose of Biomarker Discovery

Arthur Morris[1]([✉]), Justin Pachebat[1], Graeme Tyson[1], Guy Robinson[2], Rachel Chalmers[2], and Martin Swain[1]

[1] IBERS, Aberystwyth University, Aberystwyth, Wales, UK
arm21@aber.ac.uk
[2] Cryptosporidium Reference Unit, Public Health Wales, Swansea, Wales, UK

Abstract. Protozoan parasites that cause diarrhoeal diseases in humans take a massive toll on global public health annually, with over 200,000 deaths in children of less than two years old in Asia and Sub-Saharan Africa being attributed to Cryptosporidium alone. They can, in particular, be a serious health risk for immuno-incompetent individuals. Genomics can be a valuable asset in helping combat these parasites, but there are still problems associated with performing whole genome sequencing from human stool samples. In particular there are issues associated with highly uneven sequence coverage of these parasite genomes, which may result in critical errors in the genome assemblies produced using a number of popular assemblers. We have developed an approach using the Gini statistic to better characterise depth of sequencing coverage. Furthermore, we have explored the sequencing biases resulting from Whole Genome Amplification approaches, and have attempted to relate those to the Gini statistic. We discuss these issues in two parasite genera: Cryptosporidium and Cyclospora, and perform an analysis of the sequencing coverage depth over these genomes. Finally we present our strategy to generate reliable genome assemblies of sufficient quality to facilitate discovery of new Variable Number Tandem Repeat (VNTR) biomarkers.

Keywords: Cryptosporidium · Genome assembly · Biomarker discovery

1 Introduction

Gastrointestinal parasitic protozoans have a significant impact on global public and veterinary health. In recent years, *Cyclospora cayetanensis* has been responsible for a number of significant outbreaks in the United Kingdom, Canada, and the United States [15,23]. The incidence of this parasite appears to be increasing [15]. In the developing world, Cryptosporidium infection alone is one of

© Springer Nature Switzerland AG 2020
A. Roque et al. (Eds.): BIOSTEC 2019, CCIS 1211, pp. 216–241, 2020.
https://doi.org/10.1007/978-3-030-46970-2_11

the main causes of childhood morbidity. A recent large-scale study identified it as contributing to approximately 202,000 deaths per year in children less than 24 months old [24]. In the UK, *C. parvum* and *C. hominis* cause most cases of cryptosporidiosis. While self-limiting after prolonged duration of symptoms (2–3 weeks) in immunocompetent hosts, severely immunocompromised patients suffer severe, sometimes life threatening disease.

The sequencing and assembly of whole or partial genomes has become an essential tool in modern science, facilitating research in every area of biology. A primary concern for parasites such as Cyclospora and Cryptosporidium is extracting from clinical samples sufficient amounts of high quality, low contaminant DNA for sequencing. Without this, sequencing may result in low coverage sequence, variable sequencing depth and poor quality genome assemblies. The impact of genomics has been limited by the fact that Cyclospora and Cryptospridium are currently unculturable *in vitro*. In 2015 this problem was overcome through an approach that now allows genomic Cryptosporidium DNA suitable for whole genome sequencing to be prepared directly from human stool samples [7]. Hadfield *et al.* [7] applied their method to the whole genome sequencing of eight *C. parvum* and *C. hominis* isolates. This method is being applied to Cyclospora, however purification still remains an issue, with no Immuno-Magnetic Seperation (IMS) kits available for this parasite. Presently, the Cryptosporidium genomics resource, CryptoDB [22], currently gives access to 13 complete genomes, with a total of 10 available from the NCBI, including a high-quality *C.parvum* reference genome [1] exhibiting a highly compact 9.1Mb genome, bearing 3,865 genes. However, there exists no such reference genome for Cyclospora, with the best quality assembly being 44.6 Mb over 865 contigs (PRJNA292682).

Currently improved understanding of Cryptosporidium epidemiology relies on conventional genotyping tests, however, such typing tools are limited for use in Cyclospora molecular investigations. The availability of whole genome sequences provides much higher resolution information for genotyping. In addition, the genomes can be used to study a wide array of aspects of pathogen biology, such as identity, taxonomy in relation to other pathogens, sensitivity or resistance to drugs, development of novel therapeutic agents, and virulence. Our interest is to develop novel genotyping approaches by identifying and evaluating variable regions around the genome of these parasites. This will allow sources of infection and routes of transmission to be characterized and compared in a cost- and time-efficient manner [6,21]. Here variable-number of tandem-repeats (VNTR) are used, with recent investigations concluding that additional loci need to be identified and validated [6]. Our work is building on that of Perez-Cordon *et al.* (2016), who used Tandem Repeats Finder [5] to identify polymorphic VNTRs around the genome of *C. parvum*, and analysed them for variation across the eight genomes sequenced by Hadfield *et al.* [7]. We aim to use whole genome sequencing of additional isolates and species to help achieve this goal, but this work is hampered by the quality of available genome sequences [21].

This paper is presented as an extension of the paper titled "Identifying and Resolving Genome Misassembly Issues Important for Biomarker Discovery in the Protozoan Parasite, Cryptosporidium" [17]. Here, we argue that the problems associated with the generation of genomes from clinical samples is seen in other gastrointestinal Apicomplexans, presenting genome assemblies of clinically isolated *Cyclospora cayetanensis*, and subjecting them to similar analysis. Furthermore we present a novel method of investigating and characterising the distribution of reads across a genome, termed Gini-granularity curves, which resolves issues associated with data granularity when calculating the Gini coefficient [16]. Finally we investigate the effect of using DNA enrichment by Whole Genome Amplification (WGA) to resolve the low DNA yields typically extracted from clinical samples of these parasites.

This paper is structured as follows. First, we explain the quality issues associated with genome sequences extracted from clinical stool samples. Then we describe our methods, including the data sets used, the novel utilisation of Gini and Gini-granularity curves to measure the distribution of read depth in a set of sequenced reads, the process of assembly with the identification of misassemblies, and the effect WGA has on coverage distribution. In the results and discussion sections, we summarise properties of the sequenced reads, show how they can lead to misassemblies, and give evidence of the types of misassembly we encounter. We also describe how using the Gini coefficient, and analysis of Gini-granularity curves can explain some of these assembly errors and characterise the distribution of reads across a genome. We then give a brief outline of the strategy we use to generate genome assemblies of sufficient quality to use for the discovery of novel VNTRs in Cryptosporidium, and extend this approach to Cyclospora, less the genome improvement (due to the lack of a reference genome). Finally we briefly discuss the value of WGA in generating high quality assemblies from low DNA yield intestinal protozoan clinical samples.

2   Sequencing and Assembly Issues in Gastrointestinal Parasitic Protozoans

Although it is possible to derive high quality DNA by culturing some parasites in donor animals [1], this is expensive, time consuming, and raises ethical concerns. It is not appropriate for clinical samples, where maintaining sequence identity is essential. Furthermore, no animal model has yet been identified for *Cyclospora cayetanensis*. Sequencing intestinal protozoan genomes directly from clinical samples suffers from three major problems:

1. The yield of oocysts from clinical samples is low.
2. The oocysts are extracted directly from faeces, necessitating extensive cleaning and purification before DNA extraction.
3. The DNA yield per oocyst is low.

These three problems commonly result in sequenced data sets with very uneven depth of coverage, see Fig. 1 for examples. The reasons for uneven depth of coverage are unclear; in this paper we have attempted to elucidate some of the issues. Uneven sequencing depth has been identified in datasets obtained from published and unpublished paired end read libraries generated by different groups, and which were prepared using the standard Nextera XT DNA sample preparation kit. Moreover, many groups use Whole Genome Amplification (WGA) to increase the quantity of extracted DNA. This may have additional impact on the depth of coverage. WGA has been touted as a potential solution to samples which yield low levels of DNA or for which little DNA exists [8,13,31]. There has, however, been limited rigorous research into coverage bias introduced by such DNA enrichment techniques. Uneven sequencing depth may lead to genome misassembly, and we have identified this an issue with a number of popular *de novo* assemblers. Poor quality genome assemblies can find their way into public repositories of genome sequence and this can confound the development of novel prevention strategies, therapeutics, and diagnostic approaches.

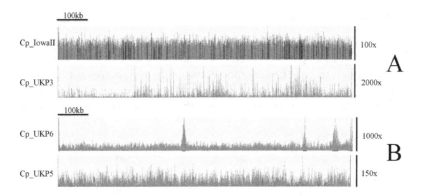

Fig. 1. A: Coverage across chromosome 7 of the *C.parvum* IowaII reference genome (top track) and *C.parvum* UKP3 (bottom track) genomes to illustrate the extreme coverage inequality of the UKP3 isolate genome (UKP3 *Gini* = 0.5489, IowaII *Gini* = 0.112). Image produced using IGV. Note that the IowaII DNA sequences were derived from an animal model, and have low or "normal" read depth variation, whereas UKP3 is more typical of DNA sequences extracted from clinical samples. **B:** The coverage over chromosome 1 for 2 genomes: Cp_UKP6 ($G \mid W_1 = 0.255$, $nAUC = 0.921$) and Ch_UKP5 ($G \mid W_1 = 0.278$, $nAUC = 0.884$) with $G \mid W_1$ across chromosome 1 alone of 0.262 and 0.264 respectively. See Sect. 4.2 for an explanation of the annotation.

3   Whole Genome Sequence Datasets Available for Analysis

As a dataset, we utilised 12 isolates of *Cyclospora cayetanensis* and 10 isolates of *Cryptosporidium spp*. There exists no high-quality Cyclospora reference genome, so reference guided scaffolding and other post-assembly processing using the PAGIT software was not undertaken for these isolates. The Cryptosporidium dataset consisted of 7 UK isolates of *C. parvum* and 3 UK isolates of *C. hominis*, presented by Hadfield *et al.* [7]. The *C. parvum* IowaII reference genome [1] was used to guide assembly and annotation of the *C. parvum* assemblies, and the *C. hominis* TU502 [9] reference genome to guide assembly and annotation of *C. hominis*. The DNA within this dataset was un-enriched by Whole Genome Amplification (WGA).

For the purpose of identifying a correlation between genes transferred to chimeric regions and Gini, and to investigate the effect of WGA on genome sequencing, unpublished isolates consisting of 29 UK *C. parvum* and 19 UK *C. hominis* isolates where also used, giving a combined total of 48 genomes. These isolates were subjected to DNA enrichment pre-sequencing, using ϕ29 Multiple Displacement Amplification (MDA) WGA.

4   Sequencing and Read Analysis Methodology

4.1   Raw Read Analysis

Raw reads were mapped to a reference genome using Burrows Wheeler Aligner (BWA) v0.7.16. [14]. Cyclospora reads were mapped back to the assemblies they were used to generate, and Cryptosporidium reads were mapped to species specific reference genomes (*C. parvum* IowaII for *C. parvum* and *C. hominis* TU502 [29] for *C. hominis*). Coverage analysis was then performed using Samtools v1.5 [14].

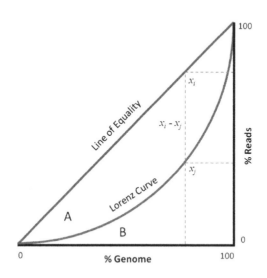

Fig. 2. Graphical representation of the Gini coefficient. In this graph, the Gini coefficient can be calculated as $A/(A + B)$, which represented area under the Lorenz curve (blue) inversely proportional to the line of equality (red). The green dotted lines denote the percentage of reads which cover 80% of a genome used to generate the Lorenz curve (unequal coverage depth) as compared to a perfectly equal distribution of reads. Taken from Morris *et al.* [17]. (Color figure online)

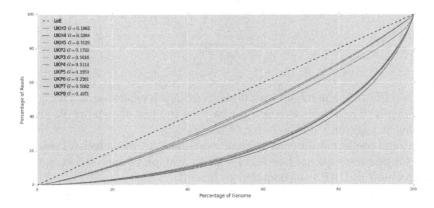

Fig. 3. Gini curves for the Hadfield *et al.* Cryptosporidium dataset. LoE refers to the Line of Equality, wherein theoretic perfect equality of the dataset it represented, achieving a Gini of 0. These Gini curves were generated using a window size of 500.

Read depth was calculated using the 'depth' tool within the samtools package [14]. The Gini coefficient is a metric used to measure the inequality within a dataset. It is commonly used in economics to measure the distribution of income within a population, where it is represented by a value between 0 and 1, with 0 representing perfectly even distribution, and higher values representing higher inequality of distribution. Here we have applied this coefficient to measure inequality of depth of coverage across a genome. For each of the genomes, we calculated the Gini coefficient of read depth. The Gini coefficient is calculated as:

$$G = A/(A + B)$$

where A is the area under the line of equality, and B the area under the Lorenz curve, on the graph of distribution inequality (see Fig. 2). The green dotted lines (marked at 80% on the x axis) in Fig. 2 gives an example of how, in the dataset used to generate the Lorenz curve, 80% of the genome is covered by only 40% of reads (the value at the position of collision of the green dotted line on the y axis), whereas in a perfect distribution it would be covered by 80% of reads.

The algorithm for calculating a genome's Gini coefficient of read depth coverage involves first calculating the mean depth of coverage of 1bp windows ($W = 1$) over the genome [17]. These windows are ordered according to their depth of coverage values, and these values rescaled between 0 and 100. This ordered set of read depth values is used to generate the Lorenz curve, L, where the value at every position i on the curve represents the sum of all values at positions $\leq i$. A line of equality, E, was generated to represent perfectly even distribution of reads across a genome. The difference between the values at each position on E and L is then calculated and the summed inverse proportional difference (the Gini coefficient) of these values calculated. This was performed using the following equation:

$$G = \frac{\sum\limits_{i=1}^{n}\sum\limits_{j=1}^{n} |x_i - x_j|}{2n \sum\limits_{i=1}^{n} x_i} \qquad (1)$$

where n refers to the number of windows (read depth values) across the genome, x_i is a depth of coverage value at position i on the line of equality E, and x_j is the value at position j on the Lorenz curve L.

The Gini coefficient for each genome represents the unevenness of read depth across the genome sequence (see Fig. 1A for an example of uneven coverage across chromosome 7 of UKP3 as compared to Iowa II).

4.2 Gini-Granularity Curves

To further investigate the read distribution throughout each assembly, the Gini coefficient was calculated across window sizes of 1–10,000 nucleotides. Furthermore, these curves were normalised such that the Gini at maximum granularity (which is obtained by calculating G at window size of 1) is adjusted to 1 for the purpose of simplified comparison. For each of these normalised and unnormalised curves, the area under the curve (AUC) was calculated. These curves are hereafter referred to as Gini-granularity curves.

More formally, consider a sequence s where the array of depth of coverage for each position in s is c. A partitioned array of c is generated using window size w, forming N partitions where $N = \frac{|c|}{w}$:

$$P_w^c = \{c_{[j,j+w]} \mid j = iw, \ 0 \le i < N\} \qquad (2)$$

The mean coverage over each partition is consequently:

$$C_w^c = \{\bar{n} \mid n \in P_w^c\} \qquad (3)$$

where $\bar{n}$ is the mean depth of coverage of partition n. Taking G_w^c as the Gini of C_w^c (see Eq. 1 for the calculation of the Gini coefficient), an array of Gini values over a range of partition sizes is, $r = [i,j]$ where $r \subset \mathbb{N}$ is:

$$G_r^c = \{G_w^c \mid w \in r\} \qquad (4)$$

A_r^c is the area under the curve generated by G_r^c. The normalised area under the curve, nA_r^c is calculated as the area under nG_r^c where:

$$nG_r^c = \{G_i^c + (1 - G_1^c) \mid 0 < i \le |G_r^c|, \ i \in \mathbb{N}\} \qquad (5)$$

4.3 DNA Enrichment Using Whole Genome Amplification

Due to the low DNA yield of Cryptosporidium, WGA was utilised to enrich the DNA for sequencing. The protocol was followed as documented in the protocol:

'Amplification of Purified Genomic DNA using the REPLI-g Mini Kit' by Qiagen. This was carried out as follows: 5 µl Buffer D1 was added to 5 µl template DNA, vortexed to mix, and briefly centrifuged. These were then incubated at room temperature for 3 min. During this time a master mix was prepared using 29 µl REPLI-g Mini Reaction Buffer and 1 µl REPLI-g Mini DNA Polymerase, to a total of 30 µl. 10µl Buffer N1 was added to the samples and mixed by vortexing, and centrifuged briefly. The master mix was then added to 20 µl of this denatured DNA, and incubated at 30 °C for 16 h. After this incubation period, the REPLI-g Mini DNA Polymerase was inactivated by heating the sample at 65 °C for 3 min.

4.4 Sequencing Bias Analysis in WGA Datasets

To investigate bias which may exist in how DNA is enriched using WGA, or sequenced, we used the depth tool within the Samtools package. Bespoke python scripts were written to analyse the relationship between coverage and GC content across windows of various sizes. Kernel density estimation was carried out on these datasets to investigate the relationship between coverage and genomic content using the SciPy package in Python [10].

5 Assembly and Post-assembly Improvement Methodology

De novo assembly was carried out in the same manner for both Cyclospora and Cryptosporidium. However, due to the lack of a reliable reference genome for Cyclospora, genome improvement and annotation using the PAGIT toolkit [25] was not possible. Consequently any statistics provided for Cyclospora assemblies are derived from the *de novo* assembly alone.

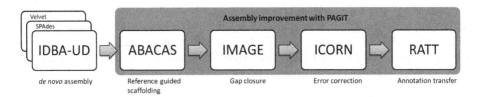

Fig. 4. The workflow for Cryptosporidium assembly, adapted from that used by Hadfield *et al.* for the assembly of genomes with high coverage depth inequality. Cyclospora genomes were assembled using only the IDBA-UD assembler. Adapted from Morris *et al.* [17].

5.1 *De novo* Assembly

First *de novo* assembly was undertaken using SPAdes v3.7.1 [3] *de novo* assembler to construct scaffolds from paired end read files. Kmer sizes of 23, 33, 55, 65, 77 & 89 were used in the assembly, with 1 iteration used for error correction, repeat resolution was enabled and the coverage cut-off set to 'off'. Various kmer sizes, coverage cut-offs, repeat masking, and a reference guided assembly approach were used in an attempt to improve assembly quality.

A second *de novo* assembly was undertaken using velvet v1.2.10 *de novo* assembler [30] on paired end read files using a maximum kmer length of 31, coverage cut-off set to auto, coverage mask set to 2, and the '-short' parameter enabled.

A third assembly was undertaken using IDBA-UD [20], to resolve low coverage regions whilst attempting to prevent generation of chimeric fragments during assembly and scaffolding.

5.2 Post Assembly Improvement

The Cryptosporidium assemblies were improved using the Post Assembly Genome Improvement toolkit (PAGIT) [25]: a pipeline consisting of four standalone tools with the aim of improving the quality of genome assemblies. The tools are, in suggested order of execution: ABACAS [2], IMAGE [28], ICORN [19], & RATT [18]. The workflow of this assembly pipeline can be found in Fig. 4. Cyclospora assemblies were not improved due to the lack of a high quality reference genome.

ABACAS: Algorithm Based Automatic Contiguation of Assembled Sequences. ABACAS is a contig-ordering and orientation tool which is driven by alignment of the draft genome against a suitable reference. Suitability of the reference is defined by amino acid similarity of at least 40%. Alignment is performed by NUCmer or PROmer from the MUMmer package [12]: a tool designed for large scale genome alignment. Contigs from the draft assembly are positioned according to alignment to the reference genome, with spaces between the contigs being filled with 'N's, generating a scaffold of the draft assembly. ABACAS was executed using the updated (All 8 chromosomes resolved) *C.parvum* IowaII [1] reference genome with default parameters.

IMAGE: Iterative Mapping and Assembly for Gap Extension. IMAGE uses Illumina paired end reads to extend contigs by closing gaps within the scaffolds of the draft genome assembly. IMAGE uses read pairs where one read aligns to the end of a contig and the other read overhangs beyond the end of the contig into the gap. This gap can then be partially closed using the overhanging sequence and by extending the contig. IMAGE was run in groups of three iterations at kmer sizes of 91, 81, 71, 61, 51, 41, & 31, totalling 21 iterations. Scaffolding was then performed with a minimum contig size of 500, joining contigs with gaps of 300 N's.

ICORN: Iterative Correction of Reference Nucleotides. ICORN was developed to identify small errors in the nucleotide sequence of the draft genome, such as those which may occur due to low base quality scores. It was designed to correct small erroneous indels, and is not suitable for, or capable of, correcting larger indels or misassemblies. ICORN was run using 8 iterations and a fragment size of 300.

RATT: Rapid Annotation Transfer Tool. RATT is an annotation transfer too used to infer orthology/homology between a reference genome and a draft assembly. This is achieved by utilising NUCmer from the MUMmer package to identify shared synteny between annotated features within the reference genome, and sequence within the draft assembly. Annotation files (EMBL format) are produced which contain regions which are inferred to be common features. The regions are filtered and transferred dependant on whether the transfer is between strains (Strain, similarity rate of 50–94%), species (Species, similarity rate of 95–99%), or different assemblies (Assembly, similarity rate of ≥99%). RATT was run using *C. parvum* IowaII annotations in EMBL format, downloaded from CryptoDB, as a reference. The Strain parameter was used to transfer feature annotations to the draft assembly.

5.3 Analysis of Draft Genomes

VNTR's around the reference and draft Cryptosporidium genomes were identified for the purpose of VNTR comparison and polymorphism analysis. Tandem Repeats Finder v4.09 [5] was used to identify VNTR's around the *C. parvum* IowaII reference genome using a matching weight of 2, mismatch and indel penalties of 5, match and indel probabilities of 80 and 10 respectively, minimum score of 50 and maximum period size of 15. The number of VNTRs per gene is included as a heat map in Fig. 8.

5.4 Identification of Misassembly

The Cryptosporidium draft genomes were analysed in two ways (1) by transferring gene annotations from the reference genome to the drafts using RATT, and (2) by aligning the contigs (from IDBA-UD) or scaffolds (from SPAdes/Velvet) from the draft assemblies to the IowaII reference genome. RATT was used to identify the number of genes which were transferred between genomes: it provided a convenient way of identifying putative chimeric regions i.e. regions on a draft chromosome that contained genes from 2 or more reference chromosomes. NUCmer was then used to investigate these putative chimeric regions by performing whole genome alignments. NUCmer (from the MUMmer package [12]) was used with a minimum length of match set to 100, preventing the report of small regions of similarity, a maximum gap of 90, and a minimum cluster length of 65.

5.5   Quality Assessment with Gini

The Gini coefficient for each isolate was calculated and plotted against the number of genes transferred to chimeric regions within the Cryptosporidium genome assemblies (detailed in Sect. 5.4). The coefficient of determination (R^2) was used to calculate the amount of variance in the number of genes transferred to chimeric regions explained by the Gini coefficient. Gini values at window size 1 were calculated and plotted against nAUC to investigate read distribution across each genome.

5.6   Data Visualisation

The *C. parvum* assemblies (UKP2-8) and VNTR annotations were visualised alongside the *C.parvum* IowaII reference genome using the Circos package v0.69 [11]. Mapped reads were visualised using Integrative Genomics Viewer v2.4.16 [26].

6   Results and Discussion for Sequencing and Read Analysis

Table 1 indicates high depth of coverage inequality throughout the genomes, represented by relatively high Gini coefficient values in comparison to that exhibited by the *C. parvum* Iowa II reference genome (0.112), which the mean depth and breadth of coverage (fraction of the reference covered) will not indicate. This appears to be a common issue when sequencing intestinal protozoans from human clinical samples. Paired end read libraries accessed from GenBank, sequenced by the Welcome Trust Sanger Institute (Bioproject PRJEB3213), and those published by Troell *et al.* (Bioproject PRJNA308172), who was attempting to generate whole genome sequences from single cells using whole genome amplification [27], also suffered from very high Gini coefficients, indicating that this problem is not restricted to a single research team. See Fig. 1 for an example of how the Gini value corresponds to actual read depth variation.

Gini granularity curves are presented here as a more complete indication of the coverage over a genome. The premise behind this is based on two shortcomings of using the Gini coefficient alone as a measure of depth of coverage inequality:

– Two genomes with identical ordered coverage arrays will produce identical Lorentz curves, and therefore an identical Gini. This does not take into account the distribution of depth of coverage across the genome.
– The Gini coefficient is known to be confounded by data granularity [16].

Curves generated from Gini granularity analysis are found in Fig. 6. These curves show a similar set of characteristics, which can be defined by two phases:

1. Decline phase: The Gini value (G) decreases quickly as the window size (W) increases.

Table 1. BWA mapping statistics for each assembly. The Gini coefficient was calculated using window size of 1. Cyclospora reads were mapped to the assemblies they were used to generate. Cryptosporidium reads were mapped to appropriate reference genomes for each species: *$C.$ parvum* IowaII, †$C.$ *hominis* TU502. Cyclospora reads were mapped back to the assembly they were used to generate. Included is the the area under the normalised gini granularity curves as an indication of read distribution (see Sect. 4.2).

Sample	Proportion of reads mapped to reference	Fraction of reference genome covered	Average coverage of reference sequence	$G \mid W_1$	nAUC
Ch_UKH3	0.903	0.98	34.71	0.237	0.888
Ch_UKH4	0.845	0.96	209.17	0.602	0.786
Ch_UKH5	0.809	0.96	201.92	0.585	0.777
Cp_UKP2	0.9251	1.00	51.8	0.224	0.892
Cp_UKP3	0.8894	0.99	166.42	0.556	0.815
Cp_UKP4	0.8906	0.99	192.48	0.566	0.806
Cp_UKP5	0.8463	0.99	26.86	0.278	0.884
Cp_UKP6	0.816	0.99	104.83	0.255	0.921
Cp_UKP7	0.8905	0.99	77.85	0.556	0.804
Cp_UKP8	0.837	0.98	174.39	0.566	0.796
Cc_7064046	N/A	N/A	51.4	0.556	0.896
Cc_7064047	N/A	N/A	82.87	0.466	0.735
Cc_7064048	N/A	N/A	69.54	0.413	0.820
Cc_7064049	N/A	N/A	49.82	0.256	0.886
Cc_7064050	N/A	N/A	94.07	0.125	0.957
Cc_7064051	N/A	N/A	49.81	0.296	0.892
Cc_7064052	N/A	N/A	18.37	0.713	0.780
Cc_7064053	N/A	N/A	61.23	0.531	0.795
Cc_7064054	N/A	N/A	73.26	0.328	0.857
Cc_7064055	N/A	N/A	55.64	0.379	0.867
Cc_7064056	N/A	N/A	77.92	0.293	0.891
Cc_21_S4	N/A	N/A	66.36	0.455	0.874
Cc_22_S5	N/A	N/A	58.69	0.514	0.904

2. Perturbation phase: The Gini value plateaus, and perturbation increases, as window size increases.

Figure 7 ($G \mid W_1$ plotted against $nAUC$) indicates that there is great variability in the read distribution throughout each sample. Samples of interest are coloured to show how placement within this plot relates to curve characteristics in Fig. 6, and therefore read distribution.

The two phases of the Gini granularity curves (Fig. 6) may be indicative of characteristics of each dataset, and the method by which were generated. The magnitude of the drop exhibited during the decline phase appears to vary considerably, with some isolates presenting a large decrease in G over smaller window size increases (e.g. Cc_7064052), and others presenting with very little drop. The initial drop in G may be as a result of the window size being less than the insert size of fragments used to generate these reads. Variation in the rate of

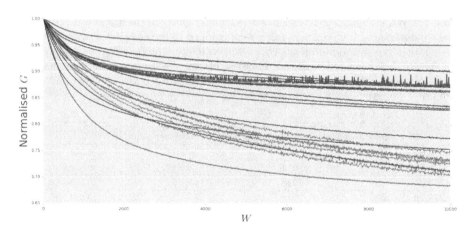

Fig. 5. Normalised Gini granularity curves generated from normalised Gini values (G) calculated using different window sizes (W) for each genome within the Cyclospora and Cryptosporidium dataset. Black samples are Cyclospora, grey samples are Cryptosporidium *spp.* Samples of interest are colourised as: blue = Cc_7064050, red = Cp_UKP5, green = Cp_UKP6, purple = Cc_7064051, and yellow = Cc_7064047. (Color figure online)

drop during the decline phase may indicate higher coverage spike granularity[1]. There appears to be some amount of variation in the characteristics of the curves generated for each species. For example, the Cryptosporidium data (seen in grey) differentiates into two discrete groups in Fig. 7, when using $G \mid W_1$ (the Gini calculated using a window size of 1, and therefore at maximum granularity). This is also seen in Fig. 3:

1. Ch_UKH4, Cp_UKP3, Cp_UKP4, Cp_UKP7, & Cp_UKP8 exhibiting $G = 0.55 - 0.60$
2. Ch_UKH3, Ch_UKH5, Cp_UKP2, Cp_UKP5, & Cp_UKP6 exhibiting $G = 0.22 - 0.28$

The magnitude and length of the decline phase appears to vary depending on the Gini value calculated over single base windows ($W = 1$ or W_1). Greater $G \mid W_1$ values appear to exhibit an extended decline phase (see Table 1). Likewise, the perturbation phase differs between the two groups, where group 1 (higher G) levels off at a much slower rate, and shows large levels of G perturbation, and group 2 (lower G) levels off at a quicker rate and shows lower levels of G perturbation. However, the Cyclospora dataset (seen in black in Fig. 7) does not appear to separate into groups. Furthermore, levels of perturbation does not appear to increase in relation to $G \mid W_1$. The variation in the characteristics of the perturbation phase may be as a result of a number of factors, such as

---

[1] Spike granularity is used here to describe the density of peaks and troughs in coverage across a sequence, wherein high spike granularity refers to a larger number of peaks and troughs within a sequence.

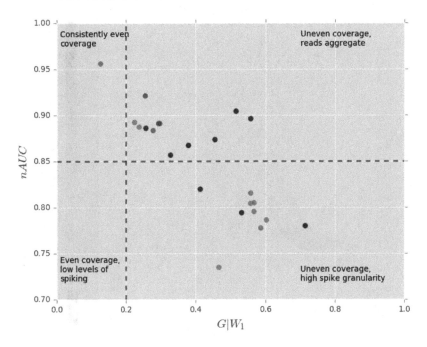

Fig. 6. $G \mid W_1$ plotted against $nAUC$. Quadrants are shown as an indication of how this graph can be interpreted. Black samples are Cyclospora, grey samples are Cryptosporidium *spp.* Samples of interest are colourised as: blue = Cc_7064050, red = Cp_UKP5, green = Cp_UKP6, purple = Cc_7064051, and yellow = Cc_7064047. (Color figure online)

the level of noise within the dataset, genome incompleteness, and the number of contigs within the final assembly. These results indicate that the analysis of these Gini curves hints at coverage features which are lost by considering a single Gini value alone.

Within high Gini isolates, a lower area under the normalised curve indicates uniformly high spike granularity, whereas a higher area under the normalised curve indicates aggregation of reads throughout the genome (see Fig. 6). Analysis of these curves allows for a more comprehensive analysis of problematic genomes with high depth of coverage inequality, wherein high spike granularity indicates a general problem with sequencing, and high read aggregation indicates problems sequencing particular regions. Colourised are curves of particular interest, such as green (Cp_UKP6) and red (Cp_UKP5) which represent the differences which may be exhibited by two genomes with similar $G \mid W_1$. These curves suggest two different distribution types, due to Cp_UKP5 bearing a more pronounced decline phase than Cp_UKP6, and therefore bearing a lower area under the normalised Gini-granularity curve, suggesting greater spike granularity. Figure 1B shows the coverage over chromosome 1 for both of these genomes to be very different in character, despite there being only a 0.002 different in Gini

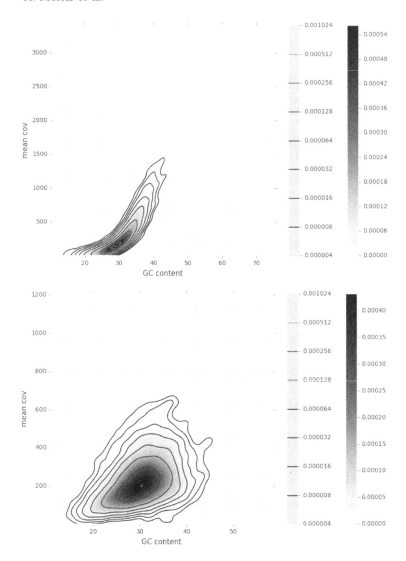

Fig. 7. Above: UKP4 $G = 0.4693$. Below: UKP94 $G = 0.2539$. Coverage vs GC contents plotted within 1000bp windows for 2 UK isolated *C. parvum* genomes. DNA of UKP4 was not subjected to enrichment by a Whole Genome Amplification (WGA) process. DNA of UKP94 was enriched by a WGA process (phi29) prior to sequencing. The plots were generated using kernel density estimation, overlaid with contour lines. The red dot marks the estimated centre of mass of the graph object. (Color figure online)

at absolute granularity. Coverage over Cp_UKP6 appears to present as relatively even, but with localised spikes of coverage reaching and exceeding 1000x (low spike-granularity). In contrast Cp_UKP5 presents with non-localised homogeneous pronounced 'spiking', with little width (high spike-granularity), and reach similar depth. This should serve as a clear example of how the difference in the nAUC of genomes which bear similar $G \mid W_1$ related to the distribution of read coverage across a genome.

In Fig. 6), the curve generated using Cc_7064050 (blue) demonstrates that this genome is very evenly covered with little inequality of read distribution or coverage, quantified by $G \mid W_1$ and $nAUC$ (0.125 and 0.957). Furthermore, Fig. 7 places this sample in the upper left quadrant, indicating high read coverage equality. Table 2 shows that the spades assembly for this sample is very good, with large mean contig size and n50 (245.5 Kb and 31.6 Kb respectively). However, as can be seen in Table 3, the IDBA assembly is highly fragmented, consisting of 32309 contigs. This indicates that IDBA performs poorly in comparison to SPAdes in instances where the coverage over a genome is even. Gini may therefore be used to indicate which assembler is most appropriate given a particular dataset. Care should be taken when attempting to predict the quality of an assembly from Gini-derived metrics, as they are a measure of the distribution of reads throughout a genome only. In particular, care should be taken as to the window size used in calculating the Gini of coverage over a genome, since the mean contig size for the Cc_7064050 IDBA assembly is 1.433 Kb, which indicates that results may be unreliable when calculating the Gini of depth of coverage over window of a greater size than this.

The curve generated from Cc_7064051 is highlighted in purple as it exhibits some unusual characteristics during the perturbation phase. The level of perturbation during this phase is unusually high, in comparison to the rest of the dataset. There appears to be a trend in the perturbation of $G \mid W_{5000<}$, wherein significant levels of perturbation are interrupted by regions of low perturbation. Furthermore the incidence of these regions of low perturbation reduces as W increases. This is very likely to be an artefact generated by behaviour influenced by the window size and the contig size distribution, since high levels of Gini-granularity curve perturbation is seen in a number of the assemblies which bear fewer contigs and a larger mean contig size.

Considering the effects of Whole Genome Amplification, Fig. 5 shows kernel density estimation plots from 2 isolates of *C. parvum*, where GC content is plotted against mean coverage over windows of 1000 nucleotides. The isolates within this dataset can be split into two cohorts:

1. Genomes which were sequenced from DNA extracted and purified from clinical isolates without any further processing to enrich DNA prior to sequencing.
2. Genomes which were sequenced from DNA extracted and purified from clinical isolates and then enriched using WGA.

The results illustrate much more dispersion in the graphs generated from enriched genomes than those generated from un-enriched genomes. This indicates that the distribution, and subsequent shape of the graph, is at least partially associated with the Gini score. There appear to be two major distinct types of distribution:

Type I. A very tight distribution with a greater than linear distribution, exhibiting a defined increase in coverage at 30% GC content. An example of this type of distribution can be seen in Cp_UKP4 in Fig. 5.

Type II. A radially dispersed distribution with no clear trend, and a centre of mass at 30% GC content. An example of this type of distribution can be seen in Cp_UKP94 in Fig. 5.

These types account for the majority of all distributions seen within the extended Cryptosporidium dataset of 45 genomes. However, there are a small number which do not clearly conform to these two distribution types.

The results detailed in Fig. 5 illustrate that the implementation of WGA as a means to enrich DNA prior to sequencing significantly alters the coverage over the genome. Rather than increasing the mean depth of coverage over the genome uniformly, however, more our analysis highlights that it selectively amplifies certain sequences. Due to the existing GC bias which has been reported within Illumina sequencing data [4] (illustrated by Type I distribution, as seen in Cp_UKP4 in Fig. 5), this has the effect of obscuring this bias, resulting in a much more radially dispersed distribution with a far less clear positive correlation between coverage and GC content. These results highlight the value of using DNA enrichment by WGA for generating high quality, reliable genome assemblies from clinically isolated samples of gastrointestinal Apicomplexan parasites. However, it also hints at a complex relationship between depth of coverage and sequence content across enriched genomes, which warrants further investigation.

7   Results and Discussion for Assembly and Post-assembly Processing

After *de novo* assembly, both the Cryptosporidium *de novo* assemblies were run through the PAGIT pipeline to make the improvements described in the methods section, including gap closing and the transfer of gene annotations. The results can be found in Tables 2 and 3. The results from assembly with Velvet were comparable to that of SPAdes, and therefore are not shown here. The SPAdes assemblies required fewer gaps to be closed by IMAGE. The mean percentage of genes transferred by RATT to the improved SPAdes assemblies is >99%. The mean percentage of genes transferred to chimeric regions is 10.6%.

Table 3 shows the results of assembly using IDBA-UD, and subsequent improvement and annotation using PAGIT. These genomes benefited greatly from gap closure by IMAGE over those produced by SPAdes (see Tables 2 and 3), since gaps in intragenic repetitive regions were much more common, potentially confounding VNTR analysis. The mean percentage of genes transferred by RATT to the improved IDBA-UD assemblies is 98%. The mean percentage of genes transferred to chimeric regions is 0.2%. In the IDBA-UD assemblies, the *C. hominis* genomes performed slightly worse, with 0, 44, and 32 genes transferred to chimeric regions respectively across UKH3, UKH4, and UKH5. Cyclospora post-PAGIT statistics are not available due to the lack of a reference genome, preventing reference guided scaffolding and improvement using PAGIT.

Table 2. The assembly statistics (SPAdes and post-PAGIT) include the number of scaffolds (No.), scaffold N50 metric, scaffold mean length (Av.), and the total size of the final assembly. The assembly size for Cryptosporidium is after improvement using PAGIT, and for Cyclospora is of the *de novo* assembly without improvement. Gene annotations were transferred to Cryptosporidium assemblies by RATT out of a total of 3805 gene annotations in the reference assembly. Genes erroneously transferred refers to genes transferred to regions which have been identified as chimeric (and therefore misassemblies). Within *C. hominis*, the erroneous transfers are putative, due to differences between *C. parvum* and *C. hominis*. Due to Cyclospora being devoid of a suitable reference genome, IMAGE and RATT were not utilised on these assemblies.

Isolate	Total length before PAGIT: No. N50 Av. (kb)	Assembly size (kb)	Gaps closed by IMAGE	Genes transferred: all (erroneously)
Ch_UKH3	168 149.9 54.0	9293	12	3792 (401)
Ch_UKH4	522 57.4 17.5	9594	95	3791 (467)
Ch_UKH5	463 54.6 19.6	9357	92	3787 (496)
Cp_UKP2	157 216.0 58.2	9254	23	3720 (356)
Cp_UKP3	270 109.8 33.7	9336	23	3688 (453)
Cp_UKP4	235 175.2 38.7	9226	22	3770 (349)
Cp_UKP5	447 70.7 20.3	9271	51	3800 (430)
Cp_UKP6	689 332.6 14.1	9826	13	3731 (96)
Cp_UKP7	521 62.6 17.3	9257	19	3797 (475)
Cp_UKP8	369 93.0 24.7	9473	26	3803 (518)
Cc_7064046	41279 4.2 2.1	86061	N/A	N/A
Cc_7064047	34386 8.0 2.2	75256	N/A	N/A
Cc_7064048	8526 10.8 5.2	44656	N/A	N/A
Cc_7064049	1846 111.1 24.3	44771	N/A	N/A
Cc_7064050	1429 245.5 31.6	45117	N/A	N/A
Cc_7064051	2753 167.4 16.6	45628	N/A	N/A
Cc_7064052	48274 1.6 1.3	64415	N/A	N/A
Cc_7064053	51427 1.6 1.3	67729	N/A	N/A
Cc_7064054	3019 34.2 14.8	44689	N/A	N/A
Cc_7064055	12577 35.8 4.2	52497	N/A	N/A
Cc_7064056	1507 94.2 29.5	44459	N/A	N/A
Cc_21_S4	17470 3.5 2.1	37339	N/A	N/A
Cc_22_S5	22122 3.5 2.0	44314	N/A	N/A

The dramatic decrease in the number of genes transferred to chimeric regions indicates significantly fewer misassemblies in improved genomes generated by IDBA-UD than in those of SPAdes, marking a significant improvement. This indicates the effectiveness of using ABACAS to identify gaps within the IDBA-UD assemblies, and IMAGE to close them, which SPAdes would resolve during assembly.

NUCmer, from the MUMMER package was used to identify misassembly, as detailed in Sect. 5.3. Figure 8 shows the extent of misassembly in the isolate genomes, denoted by coloured bars corresponding to which chromosomes regions

Table 3. Statistics for draft genomes assembled using IDBA-UD as per Table 2.

Isolate	IDBA-UD assembly statistics: No. N50 Av. (kb)	Assembly size (kb)	Gaps closed by IMAGE	Genes transferred: all (erroneously)
Ch_UKH3	419 52.9 21.5	9102.3	104	3757 (0)
Ch_UKH4	627 39.7 14.3	9212.5	229	3688 (44)
Ch_UKH5	619 38.7 14.5	9197.0	247	3699 (32)
Cp_UKP2	360 63.9 25.2	9143.7	241	3776 (0)
Cp_UKP3	563 47.8 16.0	9168.6	312	3767 (1)
Cp_UKP4	509 53.7 17.7	9154.9	292	3772 (0)
Cp_UKP5	1830 11.2 4.8	9273.8	1791	3552 (1)
Cp_UKP6	768 51.4 12.1	9135.7	105	3702 (2)
Cp_UKP7	829 32.0 10.7	9184.0	288	3775 (6)
Cp_UKP8	614 40.7 14.7	9177.8	293	3756 (0)
Cc_7064046	38758 4.0 2.1	83253	N/A	N/A
Cc_7064047	37957 6.0 2.1	79422	N/A	N/A
Cc_7064048	3233 37.0 13.7	44314	N/A	N/A
Cc_7064049	1839 111.1 24.3	44768	N/A	N/A
Cc_7064050	32309 1.9 1.4	46217	N/A	N/A
Cc_7064051	4021 52.5 11.3	45363	N/A	N/A
Cc_7064052	62780 1.2 1.2	73955	N/A	N/A
Cc_7064053	62428 1.6 1.3	80922	N/A	N/A
Cc_7064054	3859 26.9 11.5	44244	N/A	N/A
Cc_7064055	9557 26.0 5.2	49426	N/A	N/A
Cc_7064056	2757 41.5 16.0	44119	N/A	N/A
Cc_21_S4	18760 2.8 1.9	35554	N/A	N/A
Cc_22_S5	23440 2.8 1.8	42504	N/A	N/A

Table 4. The number of VNTR regions missing within the IDBA-UD assemblies pre and post gap closing with IMAGE. Taken from Morris *et al.* [17].

Isolate	VNTR regions missing before IMAGE	VNTR regions missing post-IMAGE
Cp_UKP2	48	7
Cp_UKP3	56	12
Cp_UKP4	63	10
Cp_UKP5	209	33
Cp_UKP6	62	13
Cp_UKP7	62	8
Cp_UKP8	67	13

belong to according to NUCmer. Extensive misassembly was identified in all of the genomes, to varying degrees. The most consistently misassembled chromosome is chromosome 7, with a consistent chromosome 8 misassembly. The most

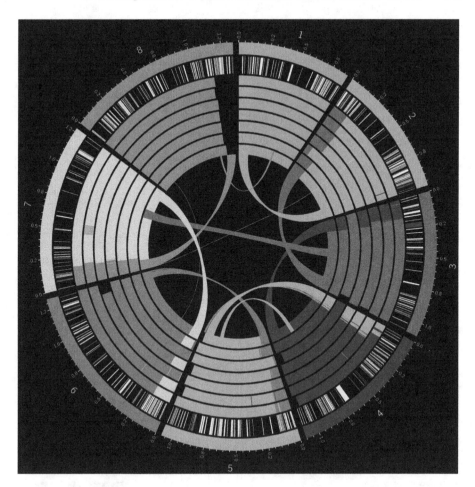

Fig. 8. Misassembled regions on each SPAdes assembled Hadfield *et al. C.parvum* genome. Regions are colour coordinated by which chromosome of the *C.parvum* IowaII reference genome (represented by the outer track) they map to. From outermost to innermost, the inner tracks represent the genomes of each isolate from UKP2-8. The innermost track (UKP8) also includes a linkage map showing precisely where the regions map to in the IowaII reference genome. The second from outer track shows a heatmap of genes bearing Tandem Repeats (TRs), from light yellow denoting a single VNTR within the gene to dark red indicating many TRs within the gene. TRs were identified using Tandem Repeats Finder (see Sect. 5.3). Taken from Morris *et al.* [17]. (Color figure online)

misassembled isolates where UKP3 and UKP8, with 8 misassemblies of larger than 10kb. These two isolates have very high Gini scores (see Table 1), of 0.550 and 0.556 respectively.

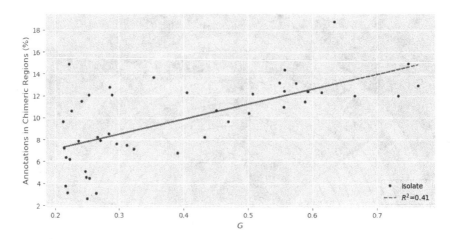

Fig. 9. The percentage of genes transferred to chimeric (misassembled) regions against Gini coefficient of coverage for 45 isolates of *C.parvum* and *C.hominis*. $R^2 = 0.41$

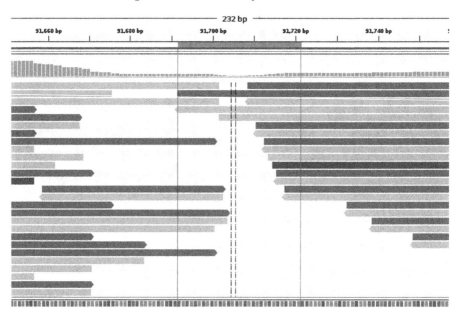

Fig. 10. The misassembly interface between fragments from chromosomes 8 and 7 on the chimeric chromosome 7 of UKP3. Single reads are shown, as is a colourised sequence track (A = Green, T = Red, C = Blue, G = Orange) at the bottom where the repeat region implicated in the formation of this chimeric contig can be seen. Image produced using IGV. Taken from Morris *et al.* [17]. (Color figure online)

Figure 9 illustrates a moderate correlation ($R^2 = 0.41$) between the Gini coefficient and number of misplaced genes within misassembled chromosomal regions across 45 isolates of the extended *C. parvum* and *C. hominis* dataset.

Table 4 shows the number of VNTR regions that were missing from the *C. parvum* IBDA-UD assemblies before and after gap closure with IMAGE. These results show that a large amount of VNTR regions were resolved using IMAGE, indicating the importance of post-assembly genome improvement in the generation of accurate and reliable genome assemblies.

Whole genome alignments were used to identify *in silico* translocation events (considered putative misassemblies), as detailed in Sect. 5.3. Figure 8 shows putatively misassembled regions (translocations) within the *C. parvum* UKP2-8 [7] PAGIT-improved SPAdes assemblies. A heatmap showing the number of VNTR's per coding sequence (CDS) is included. Every genome assembly within the dataset exhibits significant misassembly across all chromosomes, particularly at the terminal ends. Figure 8 illustrates that translocation occurred in a similar fashion throughout each of the assemblies, with the same areas being merged into similar chimeric genomes, as can be seen in chromosome 7, where the initial 120 kb region has merged into the end of chromosome 8 throughout all of the genomes. It is interesting to note that only on UKP3 was a 70 kb area from chromosome 5 seen starting at 500 kb on chromosome 7. Similarly only in UKP8 was a unique 70 kb translocated region seen in chromosome 7 from chromosome 3. These two genomes bear high Gini coefficients, as detailed in Table 1, which may contribute to this. A peculiarity of these misassemblies is the observed trend of chimeric chromosomes being a result of the native chromosome being flanked upstream by 80 kb of the downstream extreme portion of the subsequent chromosome. This is illustrated very clearly in Fig. 8.

Taxonomic evaluation carried out by Hadfield *et al.* utilising the gp60 marker show that there are five gp60 subtypes within the *C. parvum* dataset. This variation within the Hadfield *C. parvum* isolates is supported by Perez-Cordon *et al.* [21] which shows clear variation across 28 VNTR loci, suggesting a number of genetic lineages. The very low likelihood of similar translocation occurring across different populations of *C. parvum* indicates that these events are as a result of misassembly by SPAdes, rather than a biological observations.

Examination of one such chimeric contig (the chr8-chr7 chimeric region at 0-0.14Mb of UKP3 on Fig. 8) revealed that the region has very low depth of coverage, with no single read spanning the chromosomal fragments. Moreover, the sequences from different chromosomes are joined using a simple "AT" repetitive region with only three reads spanning the repeat region and no reads pairing across it (see Fig. 10). This was observed in a number of other chimeric interface regions. Due to the low complexity, high repeat rich nature of the Cryptosporidium genome, coupled with the difficulties associated with DNA extraction and sequencing of this parasite, there is insufficient evidence to suggest that this represents true biological variation. Instead, it may be attributed to a misassembly by the Spades software. This kind of assembly error was also typical of the assemblies produced by using Velvet *de novo* assembler.

Unlike SPAdes, the IDBA assembler leaves these sequence fragments unjoined, with the result that significantly less chimeric regions are seen in the IDBA assemblies. This is because IDBA is designed for the task of assembling genomes of highly uneven depth of coverage. Although IDBA-UD did not create so many chimeric contigs, the low complexity regions were often left unassembled, with the result that CDS regions contained gaps. Unfortunately, these gaps often included the VNTRs that might be suitable for incorporation into a multi-locus genotyping scheme.

Both SPAdes and Velvet (data from Velvet not shown) produced full, ungapped CDS regions (see Table 2). Thus the IDBA assemblies were not suitable for VNTR analysis and further biomarker identification without significant improvement. PAGIT was used to improve the genomes from all assemblers (see Sect. 5.2), and this improved the resolution of low complexity regions within the IDBA-UD assemblies. Within PAGIT, ABACAS performs scaffolding on the genome assemblies and introduces gaps across the unassembled regions, the IMAGE tool then performs gap closure on these regions, resulting in high quality intragenic VNTR's for biomarker analysis. The number of gaps closed within the IDBA-UD assemblies was significantly higher than within the SPAdes assemblies. This difference in gaps closed was expected, as IDBA-UD was designed for the purpose of assembling genomes which suffer from poor depth of coverage equality, and is therefore more conservative in extending reads across regions with shallow coverage.

The *C. parvum* assemblies produced by IDBA-UD and PAGIT exhibited very few misassemblies compared to the SPAdes assemblies. However, the *C. hominis* genomes suffered from a greater amount of putative misassemblies within the IDBA-UD genomes, as measured by the number of genes being transferred between chromosomes. Note that, genes are transferred from the *C. parvum* IowaII reference genome, which is as different, albeit similar species, and so some biological changes may be expected. Further analysis is required to fully eliminate assembly error as a cause of these chromosomal translocations. Table 4 shows that IMAGE is essential within this workflow for the resolution of repetitive regions which are not resolved during assembly with IDBA-UD. The results show a five to six-fold decrease in the number of VNTR regions missing within the assemblies.

8   Conclusion

In this paper we have performed a detailed analysis of genome sequencing and assembly on 23 genomes from 2 genera of gastrointestinal Apicomplexans.

To investigate sequencing depth and breadth of coverage, we have developed a novel approach that uses the Gini coefficient to determine coverage inequality. We also present a novel technique which allows for further investigation of depth of coverage inequality by generating Gini-granularity curves. We demonstrate how these curves characterise the distribution of reads across a genome and relate this to the quality of subsequent genome assemblies.

We have demonstrated that the use of WGA to enrich DNA within clinical samples is a viable way of increasing read coverage. However, these results also suggest that there is a complex relationship between the selectivity of amplified

DNA during WGA, and its sequence content, which is not explained by GC content alone. Due to the protocol required to extract DNA from clinical samples, these genome sequences often have highly uneven sequencing depth even if the coverage across the genome sequence is relatively high.

We found the SPAdes and Velvet assemblies to be problematic on our datasets. This led to misassemblies across low coverage, low complexity regions, resulting in the creation of chimeric chromosomes: up to 15% of all genes were being placed within these chimeric chromosomes. Although the assemblies generated by IDBA-UD did not suffer from the problem of chimeric sequences, they were problematic due to a different assembly approach, leading to a large number of gaps, particularly in repetitive regions. This is a significant issue because these gaps often contained the VNTR sequences that are important to us for developing new clinical genotyping strategies. However, the IMAGE gap closing tool from the genome improvement pipeline, PAGIT, was able to resolve these missing low complexity regions. Using this strategy, of assembly with IDBA followed by gap closing with IMAGE, we will be able to perform more in depth VNTR analysis with the intention of identifying biomarkers that will facilitate the development of novel prevention strategies in the fight against the diseases caused by these organisms.

References

1. Abrahamsen, M.S., et al.: Complete genome sequence of the Apicomplexan, Cryptosporidium parvum. Science **304**(5669), 441–445 (2004). https://doi.org/10.1126/science.1094786. http://www.ncbi.nlm.nih.gov/pubmed/15044751
2. Assefa, S., Keane, T.M., Otto, T.D., Newbold, C., Berriman, M.: ABACAS: algorithm-based automatic contiguation of assembled sequences. Bioinformatics **25**(15), 1968–1969 (2009). https://doi.org/10.1093/bioinformatics/btp347
3. Bankevich, A., et al.: SPAdes: a new genome assembly algorithm and its applications to single-cell sequencing. J. Comput. Biol. **19**(5), 455–477 (2012). https://doi.org/10.1089/cmb.2012.0021
4. Benjamini, Y., Speed, T.P.: Summarizing and correcting the GC content bias in high-throughput sequencing. Nucleic Acids Res. **40**(10), 1–14 (2012). https://doi.org/10.1093/nar/gks001
5. Benson, G.: Tandem repeats finder: a program to analyse DNA sequences. Nucleic Acids Res. **27**(2), 573–578 (1999)
6. Chalmers, R.M., et al.: Suitability of loci for multiple-locus variable-number of tandem-repeats analysis of Cryptosporidium parvum for inter-laboratory surveillance and outbreak investigations. Parasitology **144**(1), 37–47 (2017). https://doi.org/10.1017/S0031182015001766
7. Hadfield, S.J., et al.: Generation of whole genome sequences of new Cryptosporidium hominis and Cryptosporidium parvum isolates directly from stool samples. BMC Genom. **16**, 650 (2015). https://doi.org/10.1186/s12864-015-1805-9. https://bmcgenomics.biomedcentral.com/articles/10.1186/s12864-015-1805-9
8. Hosono, S., et al.: Unbiased whole-genome amplification directly from clinical samples. Genome Res. **13**(5), 954–964 (2003). https://doi.org/10.1101/gr.816903

9. Ifeonu, O.O., et al.: Annotated draft genome sequences of three species of Cryptosporidium: Cryptosporidium meleagridis isolate UKMEL1, C. baileyi isolate TAMU-09Q1 and C. hominis isolates TU502 2012 and UKH1. Pathogens Dis. (2016). https://doi.org/10.1093/femspd/ftw080

10. Jones, E., Oliphant, T., Peterson, P., Al, E.: SciPy: open sourcescientific tools for Python (2001)

11. Krzywinski, M., et al.: Circos. Genome Res. **19**(9), 1639–1645 (2009). https://doi.org/10.1186/1471-2105-14-244. http://genome.cshlp.org/content/19/9/1639.short

12. Kurtz, S., et al.: Versatile and open software for comparing large genomes. Genome Biol. **5**(2), R12 (2004). https://doi.org/10.1186/gb-2004-5-2-r12. http://genomebiology.com/2004/5/2/R12

13. Lasken, R.S., Egholm, M.: Whole genome amplification: abundant supplies of DNA from precious samples or clinical specimens. Trends Biotechnol. **21**(12), 531–535 (2003). https://doi.org/10.1016/j.tibtech.2003.09.010

14. Li, H., Durbin, R.: Fast and accurate short read alignment with Burrows-Wheeler transform. Bioinformatics **25**(14), 1754–1760 (2009). https://doi.org/10.1093/bioinformatics/btp324

15. Marques, D.F., et al.: Cyclosporiasis in travellers returning to the United Kingdom from Mexico in summer 2017: lessons from the recent past to inform the future. Eurosurveillance (2017). https://doi.org/10.2807/1560-7917.ES.2017.22.32.30592

16. Monfort, P.: Convergence of EU regions - measures and evolution. Eur. Union **Europa**(6), 1–32 (2008)

17. Morris, A.V., Pachebat, J., Robinson, G., Chalmers, R., Swain, M.: Identifying and resolving genome misassembly issues important for biomarker discovery in the protozoan parasite, cryptosporidium. In: Proceedings of the 12th International Joint Conference on Biomedical Engineering Systems and Technologies - Volume 3: BIOINFORMATICS, vol. 3, pp. 90–100. SciTePress (2019). https://doi.org/10.5220/0007397200900100

18. Otto, T.D., Dillon, G.P., Degrave, W.S., Berriman, M.: RATT: rapid annotation transfer tool. Nucleic Acids Res. **39**(9), 1–7 (2011). https://doi.org/10.1093/nar/gkq1268

19. Otto, T.D., Sanders, M., Berriman, M., Newbold, C.: Iterative correction of reference Nucleotides (iCORN) using second generation sequencing technology. Bioinformatics **26**(14), 1704–1707 (2010). https://doi.org/10.1093/bioinformatics/btq269

20. Peng, Y., Leung, H.C.M., Yiu, S.M., Chin, F.Y.L.: IDBA-UD: a de novo assembler for single-cell and metagenomic sequencing data with highly uneven depth. Bioinformatics **28**(11), 1420–1428 (2012). https://doi.org/10.1093/bioinformatics/bts174

21. Perez-Cordon, G., Robinson, G., Nader, J., Chalmers, R.M.: Discovery of new variable number tandem repeat loci in multiple Cryptosporidium parvum genomes for the surveillance and investigation of outbreaks of cryptosporidiosis. Exp. Parasitol. **169**(August), 119–128 (2016). https://doi.org/10.1016/j.exppara.2016.08.003

22. Puiu, D., Enomoto, S., Buck, G.A., Abrahamsen, M.S., Kissinger, J.C.: CryptoDB: the Cryptosporidium genome resource. Nucleic Acids Res. **32**(90001), 329D–331 (2004). https://doi.org/10.1093/nar/gkh050. https://academic.oup.com/nar/article-lookup/doi/10.1093/nar/gkh050

23. Qvarnstrom, Y., et al.: Draft genome sequences from Cyclospora cayetanensis oocysts purified from a human stool sample. Genome Announc. (2015). https://doi.org/10.1128/genomeA.01324-15

24. Sow, S.O., et al.: The Burden of Cryptosporidium diarrheal disease among children <24 months of age in moderate/high mortality regions of Sub-Saharan Africa and South Asia, utilizing data from the Global Enteric Multicenter Study (GEMS). PLoS Negl. Trop. Dis. **10**(5), 1–20 (2016). https://doi.org/10.1371/journal.pntd.0004729

25. Swain, M.T., Tsai, I.J., Assefa, S.A., Newbold, C., Berriman, M., Otto, T.D.: A post-assembly genome-improvement toolkit (PAGIT) to obtain annotated genomes from contigs. Nat. Protocols **7**(7), 1260–84 (2012). https://doi.org/10.1038/nprot.2012.068. http://www.nature.com/doifinder/10.1038/nprot.2012.068%5Cn

26. Thorvaldsdóttir, H., Robinson, J.T., Mesirov, J.P.: Integrative genomics viewer (IGV): high-performance genomics data visualization and exploration. Brief. Bioinf. **14**(2), 178–192 (2013). https://doi.org/10.1093/bib/bbs017

27. Troell, K., et al.: Cryptosporidium as a testbed for single cell genome characterization of unicellular eukaryotes. BMC Genom. **17**(1), 1–12 (2016). https://doi.org/10.1186/s12864-016-2815-y. http://dx.doi.org/10.1186/s12864-016-2815-y

28. Tsai, I.J., Otto, T.D., Berriman, M.: Improving draft assemblies by iterative mapping and assembly of short reads to eliminate gaps. Genome Biol. **11**(4), R41 (2010). https://doi.org/10.1186/gb-2010-11-4-r41

29. Xu, P., et al.: The Genome of Cryptosporidium hominis. Lett. Nat. **431**(October), 1107–1112 (2004). https://doi.org/10.1038/nature02990

30. Zerbino, D.R., Birney, E.: Velvet: algorithms for de novo short read assembly using de Bruijn graphs. Genome Res. **18**(5), 821–829 (2008). https://doi.org/10.1101/gr.074492.107

31. Zhang, L., Cui, X., Schmitt, K., Hubert, R., Navidi, W., Arnheim, N.: Whole genome amplification from a single cell: implications for genetic analysis. Proc. Natl. Acad. Sci. **89**(13), 5847–5851 (2006). https://doi.org/10.1073/pnas.89.13.5847

Analysis of Discrete Models for Ecosystem Ecology

Cinzia Di Giusto[1]([✉]), Cédric Gaucherel[2], Hanna Klaudel[3], and Franck Pommereau[3]

[1] Université Côte d'Azur, CNRS, I3S, Sophia Antipolis, France
cinzia.digiusto@gmail.com
[2] AMAP - INRA, CIRAD, CNRS, IRD, Université Montpellier, Montpellier, France
[3] IBISC, Univ Evry, Université Paris-Saclay, Evry, France

Abstract. We consider discrete qualitative models of ecosystems viewed as collections of interacting living (animals, plants ...) and nonliving entities (air, water, soil ...), whose conditions of appearance/disappearance are controlled by a set of formal rules (i.e., processes). We present here two methods to statically analyze models. The first one is used to simplify models removing redundant information. The second one is a rule-based method allowing to compare ecosystems. This method relies on a measure of similarity and on an optimization algorithm. In addition, the proposed method allows detecting patterns (i.e., ecological processes or sets of processes) in ecosystems. We have validated the method by applying it against a set of models and patterns provided by research projects of ecologists.

Keywords: Rewriting systems · Similarity rate · Pattern matching · Ecosystem models

1 Introduction

Ecosystems are understood as complex processes of highly different nature: e.g., bio-ecological, physico-chemical and socio-economical. The dynamics of such systems is difficult to grasp as it is the result of an intricate interplay between a large number of processes: the functioning of living species (e.g., fauna and flora) and of inert components (e.g., dynamics of soil and climate).

On top of this, human activities influences and highly impacts a setting that is already complex in its own. Hence, understanding the functioning of ecosystems becomes crucial for a more sustainable management of the environment. Indeed, we face today fast and dangerous changes of most ecosystems (due to climate change, to uncontrolled human activities, etc.) that we are compelled to discern so to appropriately and promptly react. Unfortunately the development of ecosystems models and their analysis remains a challenge and constitutes a critical bottleneck. In practice, ecosystems are modeled on a case-by-case basis with few generalizations.

One relevant way of improving our understanding of ecosystem functioning is to provide more formal frameworks, as they can speed up and reinforce the decision procedures. The dominant modeling methodology for ecosystems is based on ordinary differential equations (ODEs) [23,24]. The drawbacks of such models are that:

© Springer Nature Switzerland AG 2020
A. Roque et al. (Eds.): BIOSTEC 2019, CCIS 1211, pp. 242–264, 2020.
https://doi.org/10.1007/978-3-030-46970-2_12

i) They usually require to quantify various parameters (mostly unknown) and variables.

ii) They are not able to faithfully represent the time scale required for observation of ecological processes, which is usually large. In addition, traditional models are no able to grasp the possible asynchronous behaviour of ecosystem components.

iii) On top of this, analytic solutions usually do not exist and models often represent averaged and sometimes unrealistic behaviors of ecosystems.

In contrast, discrete qualitative models are high level abstractions of observed processes and they allow unraveling the tangled causal relationships between system's entities. The success of discrete qualitative approaches is witnessed, for instance, in systems biology with formalisms like Petri nets [5], Boolean networks [33], process algebras [6] and rewriting systems [18], to cite a few.

In ecology, discrete qualitative modelling is still pioneering and under exploited. Approaches such as those by Gaucherel et al. [16,17], where the authors study the driving rules needed to change agricultural mosaics and model contrasted landscapes, are promising. However, much more may be obtained by developing original solutions based on the suitable application of existing theory and associated (automated) tools. One of the goals of this paper is to contribute in this regard.

As a starting point of our developments we take a general discrete qualitative formalism proposed by Gaucherel and Pommereau in [15]. Ecosystems are modeled as a set of (living and nonliving) entities together with a set of rewriting rules expressing the conditions of their appearance/disappearance (i.e., the ecosystem component responses). These rules may be interpreted as the functioning bricks of landscape modelling. Each rule is, thus, part of a broader process contributing to the overall behavior of the whole ecosystem.

In this paper, we propose two techniques to study ecosystems modeled as in [15] without fully developing their semantics. In the first part we consider single ecosystems and we want to remove redundant information that could have been (unintentionally) introduced during the modelling process and that could greatly lengthen computations.

The second part, intends to compare models by focusing on their syntax. Indeed, many processes are common to most ecosystems: e.g., for species interactions: predation, competition, symbiosis etc. and it is crucial to be able to identify them to better describe the ecosystem under study. In this paper, we propose a method to detect whether a given process is present in an ecosystem. This can help to understand if the introduction of a new entity could cause the appearance of a known process, and to understand the real nature of a new process. Indeed, to detect wanted or unwanted interaction patterns would guide decisions for taking actions according to the management objectives, such as preventing or reinforcing some ecosystemic processes or components. Identify certain ecological processes or *interaction patterns* –in a more computer science oriented terminology– by employing classical graph-theoretical methods on the state space is ineffective. Indeed, in realistic ecosystem models, the modeled dynamics usually leads to huge state spaces (often hundreds of thousands of states). It is more efficient to search for patterns by referring only to the (limited) syntactical system specification as similar processes look similar at the (upstream) rule level.

Generalizing the reasoning, a pattern search corresponds to a variant of the problem of assessing the similarity between models of ecosystems. In order to compare two models of ecosystems, we introduce a pair of mappings, the first identifying entities and the latter rules, and a similarity measure expressed as a scoring function. This scoring majors the number of matched entities and rules, and penalizes those that do not perfectly match. Similarity is then defined as an optimization problem through the scoring function. Indeed, the scoring function with optimal value uniquely determines the mappings of entities and rules. The definition of the scoring function is used to search for interaction patterns in the rule-based models of ecosystems. As the complexity of this kind of search is exponential, it is not always possible in realistic cases to find optimal solutions in a reasonable time. Nevertheless, optimization tools generally allow obtaining a sub-optimal solution quite efficiently, solutions that can then be then refined.

We implemented a prototype that allows encoding the matching of two models into a pseudo-Boolean optimization problem and invoked tool Sat4j [22] to solve it. We applied this prototype to systematically match a collection of predefined interaction patterns against a set of models of realistic ecosystems.

Structure of the Paper. Section 2 introduces the formal modeling of ecosystems we have used and presents a couple of examples. Section 3 introduces four strategies to simplify ecosystem models and remove redundant information. Then Sect. 4 defines similarity measures used to compare ecosystems and discusses possible extensions of them. Several comparisons between ecosystems are used as illustrations for the scoring function. In Sect. 5, we present the results of our main case study: a search of interaction patterns in realistic ecosystems. Finally, some concluding remarks and perspectives are presented in Sect. 6, as well as an overview on related works. This paper is the extended and revised version of the conference article [9]. The improvements with respect to the original paper have been collected in Sect. 3.

2 Ecosystems, Syntax and Semantics

In this section, we recall the formal definition of a model of an ecosystem as given in [15]. An ecosystem consists of a set of *entities* E that can be present (On) or absent (Off). We assume that no entity may be simultaneously On and Off. The status (the presence) of an entity a is called polarity, we use $a+$ to denote that a is On, $a-$ to denote that a is Off. The set of entities E with polarities $p \in \{+, -\}$ is $E^p = \{a+, a- \mid a \in E\}$. The (functional) presence of those entities in the ecosystem is regulated by a sets of rewriting *rules* R. More formally:

Definition 1 (Ecosystem). *An ecosystem $\mathcal{E}$ is a tuple (E, R) such that:*

– E *is a set of entities,*
– R *is a set of rewriting rules of the form $r : \alpha^+, \alpha^- \gg \omega^+, \omega^-$, where r is the name of the rule, α^+ and ω^+ are sets of entities that are On, and α^- and ω^- are sets of entities that are Off.*

We denote by lhs(r) (respectively rhs(r)) the set of entities in the left (respectively right) hand side of the rule r.

An ecosystem state s is defined by the information about the presence or absence of all its entities. It is described as the set of entities that are currently On: thus $s \subseteq E$, and we assume that the remaining entities $E \setminus s$ are Off.

The dynamics of an ecosystem (E, R) is parametric over its initial state s_0. It comprises all reachable states obtained by asynchronously applying the rules in R, in a non-deterministic way. A rule r is enabled at a state s if the rule's left hand side, i.e., (α^+, α^-), matches the entities defining s. It means that $\alpha^+ \subseteq s$ and $\alpha^- \cap s = \emptyset$. If it is the case, the rule may apply and a new state s' is generated by updating s according to the rule's right hand side: $s' = (s \setminus \omega^-) \cup \omega^+$.

Example 1 (Pond). We consider a toy-model of a pond (aquatic ecosystem) populated with two species of fish, piscivorous and insectivorous ones. The pond behavior is described by the following rules:

1. *if the pond disappears, all fish species disappear too,*
2. *in summer the pond dries and disappears,*
3. *if the pond is not dried, both species of fish may live in it,*
4. *if the piscivorous fish are present, insectivorous fish disappear,*
5. *if insectivorous fish disappear, piscivorous fish disappear too.*

It consists of four entities: the summer, the pond, and two kinds of fish (piscivorous and insectivorous); and seven rules (see Table 1): Rules 1–5 correspond to items 1–5 above, and rules 6 and 7 are used to simulate the alternation of seasons.

Table 1. Entities and Rules for Example 1. (Table 1 in [9]).

rules:

entities:

Su:	Summer
P:	Pond
PF:	Piscivorous Fish
IF:	Insectivorous Fish

1: P− ≫ PF−, IF−
2: Su+ ≫ P−
3: P+ ≫ PF+, IF+
4: PF+ ≫ IF−
5: IF− ≫ PF−
6: Su+ ≫ Su−
7: Su− ≫ Su+

As an example of the dynamics, let $s_0 = \{P\}$ be the initial state. Then rule 3 is enabled and its application gives $s' = \{P, IF, PF\}$. The whole dynamics is then a directed graph whose vertices are the reachable states and whose edges correspond to the application of rules.   ◇

Example 2 (Pesticides). As a second small example useful for the following, consider a fragment of another (terrestrial) ecosystem with four entities: birds, insects, pesticides and rain.

Table 2. Entities and Rules for Example 2. (Table 2 in [9]).

rules :

entities:		
	B: Birds	1': B+ $\gg$ I−
	I: Insects	2': I− $\gg$ B−
	Pe: Pesticide	3': Pe−, R+ $\gg$ I+
	R: Rain	4': Pe+ $\gg$ I−
		5': R+ $\gg$ Pe−
		6': B−, Pe− $\gg$ I+

The ecosystem is governed by the following principles: birds eat insects and if insects disappear, birds will vanish as well. As a disturbing factor we add pesticides that may kill insects. Pesticides are washed away by the rain and when there are no pesticides and it is still raining, insects proliferate. Similarly insect proliferation happens when there are no pesticides and no birds. We do not take into account in this example, all the rules (and possibly entities) that are necessary to regulate the presence/absence of rain. Entities and rules are given in Table 2.   ◇

3   Static Analysis

In this section, we aim at simplifying models so that they are smaller and their analysis can be faster. We propose four strategies that may be divided into two groups: First those that look for and remove redundant information, which could have been unintentionally introduced during the modelling process:

1. Immutable entities,
2. Correlations and

and second, those that are intended to find and hide some local behaviour in a controlled way:

3. Cascading,
4. Spontaneous production.

The first two (Immutable entities and Correlations) are conservative in the sense they do not modify the state space of the model but remove redundancy in entities and rules. The second two (Cascading and Spontaneous production) slightly modify the state space but always in a controlled way. As the effect, for example, some entities or unwanted oscillations may become non-observable, which may contribute to better understand other phenomena, which are not modified.

Example 3. As running example, we take previous Example 1 and modify it, by adding redundant information. Table 3 gives the sets of entities and rules.   □

In the rest of this section, we consider fixed an ecosystem $\mathcal{E} = (\mathsf{E}, \mathsf{R})$ with its initial state s_o.

Table 3. Entities and Rules for Example 3.

rules:

entities:

Su:	Summer	
P:	Pond	
PF:	Piscivorous Fish	
IF:	Insectivorous Fish	
W:	Water	
Air:	Air	
Pred:	Predation	
FM:	Fisherman	

1: P−, W− ≫ PF−, IF−
2: Su+   ≫ P−, W−
3: P+, W+ ≫ PF+, IF+
4: PF+   ≫ Pred+
5: IF−   ≫ PF−
6: Su+   ≫ Su−
7: Su−   ≫ Su+
8: Su−   ≫ P+ , W+
9: −   ≫ Air+
10: Air−   ≫ PF−, IF−
11: Pred+ ≫ IF−
12: FM+   ≫ PF−

3.1 Immutable Entities

We consider entities that cannot change their state along the evolution of a system. Those entities are never produced or consumed by a rule, i.e., they are never on the right hand side. Thus if they are included in the initial state, they will always be present and conversely if they do not belong to s_0 they will never appear in the ecosystem. As a consequence, we can simplify the model by removing occurrences of those entities or entire rules depending on the initial state and whether the rule requires the presence or the absence of such an entity.

$$s_0 = \{P, W\}$$

We proceed in the following way: take an entity $X \in E$ that does not appear on the right hand side of any rule in R. Then depending on whether X is On or Off, we modify rules $r : \alpha^+, \alpha^- \gg \omega^+, \omega^-$ in R according to the following strategies:

1. If X^+ appears on the left side of a rule ($X^+ \in \alpha^+$)
   (a) if X belongs to the initial state (meaning that X^+ is true) then we can remove X from the entities set and we can remove X^+ from the rule ($\alpha'^+ := \alpha^+ \setminus \{X^+\}$);
   (b) if X does not belong to the initial state (meaning that X^- is true) then remove the rule (as the rule has no chance to be used).
2. If X^- appears on the left side of a rule ($X^- \in \alpha^-$)
   (a) if X belongs to the initial state then remove the rule (as the rule has no chance to be used);
   (b) if X does not belong to the initial state then we can remove X from the entities set and we can remove X^- from the rule ($\alpha'^- := \alpha^- \setminus \{X^-\}$).

Example 4. Take the ecosystem of Table 3, and apply "Immutable entities" strategy. It is easy to see that entity FM does not appear on the right hand side on any rule. Moreover FM $\notin s_0$. Whence by applying point 1(b) above we can safely remove rule 12 as it will never be used.   □

3.2 Correlations

Correlation is another source of simplification. We look for sets of entities (compounds) that appear in rules always together (i.e., no entity appears separated from the compound) and with consistent polarity (i.e., if the compound is the set of entities $\{A^+, B^-\}$ then it appears in rules as it is or with flipped polarities $\{A^-, B^+\}$). To find such compounds we build a lattice whose infima represent the searched correlations.

We first introduce some notation, let $e \in \mathsf{E}$ be an entity, we denote by $\mathsf{Flip}(e^+) = e^-$ and $\mathsf{Flip}(e^-) = e^+$ the flip of sign of entity e. With a slight abuse of notation, we extend Flip also to sets of entities. Note that $\mathsf{Flip}(\mathsf{Flip}(\alpha)) = \alpha$ for any set of entities α.

Then, let $(L, \subseteq)$ be the *correlation lattice*, ordered by inclusion, where $L \subseteq 2^{\mathsf{E}^+ \cup \mathsf{E}^-}$ is the smallest set of nodes, i.e., sets of entities with their polarities satisfying:

- L contains a node corresponding to the initial state and one with its flip: $Init = \{e^+ \mid e \in s_0\} \cup \{e^- \mid e \in \mathsf{E} \setminus s_0\} \in L$ and $\mathsf{Flip}(Init) \in L$;
- all premises and conclusions of rules with respective flips are in L: for each rule $\alpha \gg \omega$, $\alpha, \omega, \mathsf{Flip}(\alpha), \mathsf{Flip}(\omega) \in L$;
- all non-empty intersections of sets in L are also in L: $X \cap Y \in L$, for all $X, Y \in L$ such that $X \cap Y \neq \emptyset$.

Now, observe that each infima of L that is not a singleton represents a set of entities that are present consistently together in possibly more than one rule. This is a direct consequence of the fact that the lattice is closed by intersection. Let $\mathsf{Sink}(L)$ be the set of infima, each element of $\mathsf{Sink}(L)$ with at least two elements represents a correlation.

Notice that for all $S \in \mathsf{Sink}(L)$ there exist $T \in \mathsf{Sink}(L)$ such that $S = \mathsf{Flip}(T)$. It is always possible to take a fresh name Z and fix $Z^+ = S$ and $Z^- = T$ (the choice of sign is arbitrary). The idea is that such new compound Z replaces[1] its constituents in E and the rules are modified according to the following:

- if S appears in a rule (on the left side or on the right, or both), it is replaced by Z^+,
- if it appears in its flipped form, it is replaced by Z^-.

Example 5. Take the following ecosystem $\mathcal{E} = (\mathsf{E}, \mathsf{R})$, with $\mathsf{E} = \{A, B, C, D, E\}$ and rules $\mathsf{R} = \{A^+, D^+, B^-, C^- \gg B^-, B^+, E^+, A^- \gg B^+, D^+, C^-\}$ The initial state is $s_0 = \{A, B, D\}$ Fig. 1 depicts the lattice and its sinks. Lattice nodes are:

$$L : \{(A^+, B^-, C^-, D^+, E^-), (A^-, B^+, C^+, D^-, E^+),\ \text{Init and its flip}$$
$$(A^+, B^-, C^-, D^+), (B^+), (B^-), (A^-, B^+, C^+, D^-),\ \text{First rule and its flip}$$
$$(B^+, C^-, D^+), (B^-, C^+, D^-), (A^-, B^+, E^+), (A^+, B^-, E^-)\ \text{Second rule}$$
$$(C^-, D^+), (C^+, D^-), (A^-, B^+), (A^+, B^-)\}\ \text{Intersections}$$

We see one correlation: (C^+, D^-) that we rename with Z. We, thus, remove entities C and D and add the new compound Z to set E. The initial state thus becomes $\{A, B\}$ and the effect of this simplification on the rules is:

$$A^+, B^-, Z^- \gg B^-$$
$$B^+, E^+, A^- \gg B^+, Z^-$$

$\square$

---

[1] Of course the substitution is saved and may be recovered if necessary.

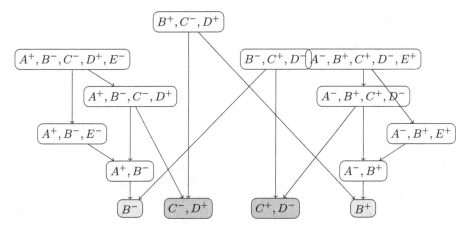

Fig. 1. Example of a lattice for correlation research. Blue nodes are the sinks. (Color figure online)

The procedure is sound and complete, it eliminates all correlations and it does not introduce correlation that were not present.

Theorem 1. *Let* $\mathcal{E} = (\mathsf{E}, \mathsf{R})$ *be an ecosystem and* $(L, \subseteq)$ *the correlation lattice. All* $S \in \mathrm{Sink}(L)$ *such that* $|S| \geq 2$ *are correlations and there exists no correlation* $S' \notin \mathrm{Sink}(L)$.

Proof. We first prove that for all $S \in \mathrm{Sink}(L)$ such that $|S| \geq 2$, S is a correlation. The proof proceeds by contradiction. Let $S \in \mathrm{Sink}(L)$ with $|S| \geq 2$ but S is not a correlation. Since $S \in \mathrm{Sink}(L)$ we have two possible scenarios:

1. if S appears (possibly in its flipped form) in a single rule either on the right or on the left side and none of the entities in S appears in any other rule (otherwise S would not be an infimum). Then this is a degenerative case of correlation, thus reaching a contradiction.
2. if S appears (possibly in its flipped form) in several rules either on the right or on the left side, then since S is an infimum, there are no other rules that use part of the entities in S. Then S has to be a correlation, concluding this side of the proof.

Now we show that there exists no correlation $S' \notin \mathrm{Sink}(L)$. We proceed again by contradiction. Suppose the existence of a correlation $S' \notin \mathrm{Sink}(L)$ and such that S' is not included in any of the sets in $\mathrm{Sink}(L)$. Nonetheless if S' is a correlation then it appears as it is or in its flipped form in several rules and there exists no subset of entities in S' that appears in other rules. Thus by construction S' has to be an infimum of L, reaching a contradiction and concluding the proof. □

Example 6. Take the ecosystem in Table 3 and apply the correlations algorithm. It is easy to see that the set {P+, W+} represents a correlation and it can be substituted with a new entity Z, obtaining the following set of rules:

$$1: Z- \gg PF-, \quad IF-$$
$$2: Su+ \gg Z-$$
$$3: Z+ \gg PF+, \quad IF+$$
$$4: PF+ \gg Pred+$$
$$5: IF- \gg PF-$$
$$6: Su+ \gg Su-$$
$$7: Su- \gg Su+$$
$$8: Su- \gg Z+$$
$$9: -- \gg Air+$$
$$10: Air- \gg PF-, \quad IF-$$
$$11: Pred+ \gg IF-$$
$$12: FM+ \gg PF-$$

$\square$

3.3 Cascading

With this strategy we remove rules which may be reduced as an effect of transitivity. Intuitively, if we have rules $r_1 : \alpha \gg \omega$, $r_2 : \omega \gg \gamma$ and entities in ω are not used in any other rule, then we may remove rules r_1 and r_2 and introduce a new rule $r_3 : \alpha \gg \gamma$. This way we can remove stuttering and the introduction of intermediate states that are not used.

To this aim, we construct a graph that shows to how many rules an entity is participating in, distinguishing whether the entity is on the right hand side or on the left hand side. Thus, let $G = (V, A)$ be a graph where:

- the set of nodes is composed of all entities with their polarity and all rule names: $V = \mathsf{E}^+ \cup \mathsf{E}^- \cup \mathsf{R}$
- the edges connect entities with rule names and vice-versa depending on whether the entity appears or not in the rule. We have an edge from the entity to the rule, if the entity appears in the premises; from the rule to the entity if it is in the conclusions. More precisely:

$$A = \{(v_1, v_2) \mid v_1 \in \mathsf{E}^+ \cup \mathsf{E}^-, v_2 : \alpha \gg \omega \in \mathsf{R}, v_1 \in \alpha\} \cup$$
$$\{(v_1, v_2) \mid v_1 : \alpha \gg \omega \in \mathsf{R}, v_2 \in \mathsf{E}^+ \cup \mathsf{E}^-, v_2 \in \omega\}$$

Then for each entity with polarity $e \in \mathsf{E}^+ \cup \mathsf{E}^-$, we build two sets that record in which rules the entity is participating: $\mathsf{In}(e) = \{r \mid (r, e) \in A\}$ if e appears in the premises, $\mathsf{Out}(e) = \{r \mid (e, r) \in A\}$ if it appears in the consequences. Moreover, let $\mathsf{In}(\alpha)$ and $\mathsf{Out}(\alpha)$ be the point-wise extensions of $\mathsf{In}(e)$ and $\mathsf{Out}(e)$, respectively. Next, let set Ω collect all $\omega \in 2^{\mathsf{E}^+ \cup \mathsf{E}^-}$ that satisfy all the following constraints:

1. entities in ω appear either in the premises or in the conclusion of rules but never in both at the same time: $\mathsf{In}(e) \cap \mathsf{Out}(e) = \emptyset$ for all $e \in \omega$;
2. all entities in ω participate to the same rules: $\mathsf{In}(e_i) = \mathsf{In}(e_j)$ and $\mathsf{Out}(e_i) = \mathsf{Out}(e_j)$ for all pairwise distinct $e_i, e_j \in \omega$.

Finally, we can simplify our model by taking all $\omega \in \Omega$ and i) removing all rules in $\mathsf{In}(\omega)$ and $\mathsf{Out}(\omega)$ ii) adding the following set of rules:

$$\{\alpha \gg \gamma \mid r_1 : \alpha \gg \omega \in \mathsf{In}(\omega), r_2 : \omega \gg \gamma \in \mathsf{Out}(\omega)\},$$

and iii) removing entities in ω from E.

Example 7. Take Example 3 and apply "Cascading" strategy. Notice that the strategy is not applicable to rules 7 and 8 and both entities Su+ and Su- are used in other rules. Instead, the strategy can be applied to rules 4 and 11, replacing those rules by $PF+ \gg IF-$ and removing Pred from the set of entities. $\square$

3.4 Spontaneous Production

Here we tackle rules that are of the kind: $\emptyset \gg \omega$. Such rules entail that all entities in ω are always present. In this case we raise an alert and leave the choice to the user:

Table 4. Interaction pattern for predation pattern. (Table 3 in [9]).

entities:	rules:
Pred: Predator population	$1''$: Pred+ $\gg$ Prey−
Prey: Prey population	$2''$: Prey− $\gg$ Pred−

1. if the user is interested in the asymptotic behaviour (the entity should not disappear from the system) then it is better to add entities in ω to the initial state and simplify the model by eliminating all the effects of those entities on rules. For all $X \in \omega$:
   - remove all rules $\alpha, X^- \gg \gamma$ as they will never be used;
   - Remove X^+ from all rules where it appears on the left hand side, as the entity cannot be eliminated from the system, its presence in the rule is redundant. Thus: $\alpha, X^+ \gg \gamma$ becomes: $\alpha \gg \gamma$;
   - Finally, as the entity cannot disappear from the system, remove all occurrences of X^- from rules where it appears on the right hand side: $\alpha \gg \gamma, X^-$ becomes $\alpha \gg \gamma$.
2. if the user is interested in observing possibly "oscillating" behaviours then leave the system as it is. This means that components in ω will appear non-deterministically when the rule $\emptyset \gg \omega$ is used. They can disappear as an effect of other rules to reappear back when the rule is used again.

Example 8. Take the example in Table 3, previous strategy is applicable to rule 9: $\emptyset \gg$ Air+. We choose to adopt the first solution. We add Air to the initial state s_0 and we remove rule 10.

4 Similarity Between Ecosystems

As mentioned in the introduction, our objective is to identify interaction patterns. An interaction pattern can be considered as a "tiny" ecosystem restricted to few entities and rules. Thus it may be formalized in the same syntax as the one for the whole ecosystem. For example, the "habitat" interaction pattern is composed of one entity featuring a specific environment (aquatic, terrestrial, pond, ...) and several entities inhabiting this environment:

1. *if the environment disappears, all inhabitants disappear as well.*

Similarly, an interaction pattern for the "predation" process is composed of two populations of entities and two rules only:

1. *if predators are present, then preys disappear,*
2. *if preys disappear, then predators disappear too.*

In the example of the pond ecosystem, instances of both above patterns are present. The predation instance is composed of piscivorous and insectivorous species, and of rules 4 and 5; while the habitat instance is composed of entities pond, piscivorous and insectivorous species and of rule 1. Table 4 shows a formal representation of the predation pattern. We may observe that there is a syntactical "similarity" between rules 4 and 5 in the pond ecosystems and rules 1 and 2 in the predation pattern.

The concept of similarity will be the basis of our investigation. Similarity is discussed in theory (see for instance the philosophical work in [34]) and also used in practice: in law [26], in natural sciences [21] and in various branches of computer science. Intuitively, we express it in terms of how many groups of components with the same roles are present in both ecosystems. This means that, given two mappings, between entities and rules respectively, the similarity rate is defined as the number of mapped entities plus how many mapped entities the rules have in common. More formally, let $\mathcal{E}_1 = (E_1, R_1)$ and $\mathcal{E}_2 = (E_2, R_2)$ be two ecosystems, and μ and ρ be two mappings between entities and rules respectively. The first one is $\mu : E_1^p \to E_2^p$. The mapping μ is injective but not necessarily total and polarities are consistent: i.e., if $a+$ is matched with $b-$ then $b+$ is matched with $a-$. It is encoded as a rectangular matrix X of size $(|E_1^p| \times |E_2^p|)$ of Boolean values defined for each pair of entities with polarities $(m, n) \in E_1^p \times E_2^p$ as[2]

$$X_{m,n} = 1 \text{ if } \mu(m) = n, 0 \text{ otherwise.}$$

In order to implement injectivity and the correspondence between polarities we introduce three restrictions (see Fig. 2a):

1. There is at most one "1" in each line:

$$\forall m \in E^p{}_1 : \quad \sum_{n \in E^p{}_2} X_{m,n} \leq 1;$$

2. There is at most one "1" in each column:

$$\forall n \in E^p{}_2 : \quad \sum_{m \in E^p{}_1} X_{m,n} \leq 1;$$

3. Polarities are consistently matched:

$$\forall a \in E_1, b \in E_2 : \quad X_{a+,b-} = X_{a-,b+} \wedge X_{a+,b+} = X_{a-,b-}.$$

Likewise, the mapping $\rho : R_1 \to R_2$ maps the rules. Similarly as for entities, it is encoded as a rectangular matrix Y of size $(|R_1| \times |R_2|)$ of Boolean values defined for each pair of rules $(u, v) \in R_1 \times R_2$ as

$$Y_{u,v} = 1 \text{ if } \rho(u) = v, 0 \text{ otherwise.}$$

It is subjected to the following restrictions that implements injectivity (see Fig. 2b):

---

[2] This formula and all the following ones were also present in [9].

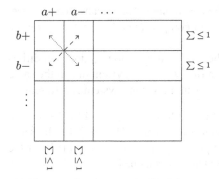

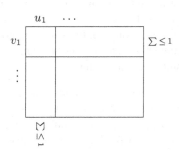

(a) The encoding into matrix X of the mapping μ for entities and the illustration of corresponding restrictions.

(b) The encoding of matrix Y of the mapping ρ for the rules and the corresponding restrictions.

Fig. 2. Encoding of mappings μ and ρ. (Figure 1 in [9]).

1. There is at most one "1" in each line:

$$\forall u \in \mathsf{R}_1 : \quad \sum_{v \in \mathsf{R}_2} Y_{u,v} \leq 1;$$

2. There is at most one "1" in each column:

$$\forall v \in \mathsf{R}_2 : \quad \sum_{u \in \mathsf{R}_1} Y_{u,v} \leq 1.$$

For each pair of mappings (μ, ρ) between ecosystems $\mathcal{E}_1$ and $\mathcal{E}_2$ we define a *scoring* function S. The function assesses the quality of the matching rules with respect to the number of matching entities. The simplest way to express the score is to count, for each pair of matching rules $\rho(u) = v$ (i.e., $Y_{u,v} = 1$), the number of matching entities through function μ on both the left and right hand side (i.e., for each pair of entities n and m in rules u and v respectively, we count the sum of all $X_{n,m} = 1$). The scoring function is a ratio between previous sum and a constant that counts the number of rules times the maximal number of entities in a rule. More precisely:

$$S_0(X,Y) = \frac{1}{\mathbf{T} \cdot \mathbf{r}} \cdot \sum_{\substack{u \in \mathsf{R}_1, \\ v \in \mathsf{R}_2}} \left(Y_{u,v} \cdot \sum_{n \in u, m \in v} X_{n,m} \right)$$

where $\mathbf{r} = \min(|\mathsf{R}_1|, |\mathsf{R}_2|)$ is the cardinality of the set of rules in the ecosystem having the smallest number of them, and $\mathbf{T} = \max_{u \in \mathsf{R}_1 \cup \mathsf{R}_2}(|\mathsf{lhs}(u)| + |\mathsf{rhs}(u)|)$ is the maximal number of entities in a rule in both ecosystems, considering at the same time the left (lhs($\cdot$)) and right (rhs($\cdot$)) hand side. However this simple scoring does not take into account:

1. the different contribution of the left and right hand side. This means, for instance, that a good matching on the left hand side can compensate a bad matching on the right hand one;
2. the proportion of entities that are not matched. Scoring function S_0 does not differentiate between two rule mappings that for a rule in one ecosystem match the same number of entities but the size of matched rules in the second system is different.

Example 9. For example, take the ecosystems R_1 with one rule $r_1 : A+, B+ \gg C+$ and R_2 with two rules $r_2 : A+, B+ \gg C+$ and $r_3 : A+, B+, D- \gg C+$. The score for ρ_1 mapping r_1 to r_2 should be greater than ρ_2 mapping r_1 to r_3 as in the latter the mapping is less perfect and there are entities that are not matched. ◇

We thus propose a better formulation for the scoring function that takes into account these remarks. The scoring function is now the sum of the scores of the left hand side and the right hand side and can be summarized as follows:

$$S(X,Y) \overset{\text{df}}{=} \frac{1}{\mathbf{r} \cdot (\mathbf{L} + \mathbf{R})} \cdot \sum_{u \in R_1, v \in R_2} Y_{u,v}(\mathit{left}(u,v) + \mathit{right}(u,v))$$

where $\mathbf{r} = \min(|R_1|, |R_2|)$ as above,

$$\mathbf{L} = \max_{u \in R_1 \cup R_2} (\|\mathsf{lhs}(u)\|)$$

and

$$\mathbf{R} = \max_{u \in R_1 \cup R_2} (|\mathsf{rhs}(u)|)$$

are the maximal numbers of entities occurring in the left (respectively right) hand side of the rules from both ecosystems, and $\mathit{left}(u,v)$ and $\mathit{right}(u,v)$ are the scores for each pair of matching rules $u \in R_1$ and $v \in R_2$:

$$
\begin{aligned}
\mathit{left}(u,v) = & \sum_{\substack{n \in \mathsf{lhs}(u), \\ m \in \mathsf{lhs}(v)}} X_{n,m} - \left(\min(\|\mathsf{lhs}(u)\|, \|\mathsf{lhs}(v)\|) - \sum_{\substack{n \in \mathsf{lhs}(u), \\ m \in \mathsf{lhs}(v)}} X_{n,m} \right) \\
& - \mathrm{abs}(\|\mathsf{lhs}(u)\| - \|\mathsf{lhs}(v)\|) \\
= & \ 2 \cdot \sum_{\substack{n \in \mathsf{lhs}(u), \\ m \in \mathsf{lhs}(v)}} X_{n,m} - \min(\|\mathsf{lhs}(u)\|, \|\mathsf{lhs}(v)\|) - \mathrm{abs}(\|\mathsf{lhs}(u)\| - \|\mathsf{lhs}(v)\|)
\end{aligned}
$$

$$
\mathit{right}(u,v) = \ 2 \cdot \sum_{\substack{n \in \mathsf{rhs}(u), \\ m \in \mathsf{rhs}(v)}} X_{n,m} - \min(|\mathsf{rhs}(u)|, |\mathsf{rhs}(v)|) - \mathrm{abs}(|\mathsf{rhs}(u)| - |\mathsf{rhs}(v)|)
$$

The construction of this scoring function is depicted in Fig. 3 below. The part $\mathit{left}(u,v)$ takes the number of matching entities

$$M_L = \sum_{n \in \mathsf{lhs}(u), m \in \mathsf{lhs}(v)} X_{n,m}$$

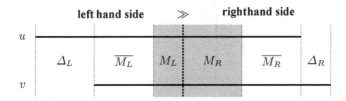

Fig. 3. Schema of the scoring function for rules u and v represented as two horizontal lines; M_L and M_R are the matching parts of u and v; $\overline{M_L}$ and $\overline{M_R}$ are the parts which do not match while the length of the rules would allow to do so, and Δ_L and Δ_R are the parts which cannot match because of the different length of the rules. (Figure 2 in [9])

and subtracts two penalties. The first one: $\min(\|\text{lhs}(u)\|, \|\text{lhs}(v)\|) - M_L$ corresponds to the maximum number of entities, which could be matched minus those that are actually matched. The second one: $\text{abs}(\|\text{lhs}(u)\| - \|\text{lhs}(v)\|)$ expresses the number of entities which could never be matched because of the difference in the length of the left hand sides of the two rules. This score is maximal when $left(u, v) = \min(\|\text{lhs}(u)\|, \|\text{lhs}(v)\|)$ and $\|\text{lhs}(u)\| = \|\text{lhs}(v)\|$, i.e., the left hand sides of u and v have the same length, and all their entities match. The part for the right hand sides is defined analogously. The overall score is normalized with respect to the number of rules **r** times **L** plus **R**. As an effect of penalties, the score can be negative but it is always between -1 and 1.

Similarity is then defined with respect to the scoring function, as the maximal value it can have with respect to all the possible mappings μ and ρ. It is possible to enumerate all solutions having a score greater than a given threshold.

Also, depending on the specific objective, coefficients may be introduced in the scoring function to weight preferences: the matching of entities and rules can be guided adding additional restrictions or regulating the importance of penalties for not matching parts of the rules.

Example 10 (Similarity). Let us consider the following pairs of mappings between the ecosystems from Examples 1 and 2:

$$
1. \quad \mu_1 = \begin{cases} PF+ \rightarrow Pe+ \\ IF+ \rightarrow R+ \\ Su+ \rightarrow B+ \\ P+ \rightarrow I+ \end{cases} \qquad \rho_1 = \begin{cases} 1 \rightarrow 1' \\ 2 \rightarrow 2' \\ 3 \rightarrow 3' \\ 4 \rightarrow 4' \\ 5 \rightarrow 5' \\ 6 \rightarrow 6' \end{cases}
$$

$$
S(\mu_1, \rho_1) = -12/24
$$

$$
2. \quad \mu_2 = \begin{cases} PF+ \rightarrow Pe+ \\ IF+ \rightarrow I+ \\ Su+ \rightarrow R+ \\ P+ \rightarrow B+ \end{cases} \qquad \rho_2 = \begin{cases} 1 \rightarrow 3' \\ 2 \rightarrow 5' \\ 3 \rightarrow 1' \\ 4 \rightarrow 4' \\ 5 \rightarrow 2' \end{cases}
$$

$$
S(\mu_2, \rho_2) = -3/24
$$

3. $\mu_3 = \begin{cases} PF+ \to B+ \\ IF+ \to I+ \\ Su+ \to R+ \\ P+ \to Pe- \end{cases}$ $\rho_3 = \begin{cases} 1 \to 4' \\ 2 \to 5' \\ 3 \to 3' \\ 4 \to 1' \\ 5 \to 2' \end{cases}$

$$S(\mu_3, \rho_3) = 5/24$$

The first pair of mappings is the trivial one, where we match entities and rules in the same order as they appear. In this case and as expected, the similarity score is rather low as there are only hazardous correspondences. The second and the third one have better scores and they are closer to the optimal solution that is discussed in the next section. The third matching suggests that birds and insects have the same role as piscivorous and insectivorous fish respectively, while the presence of the pond can be assimilated to the absence of pesticides.   ◇

Ecosystems may be compared through the scoring function. In particular, if one of the ecosystems represents an interaction pattern we can search for it using the same method, as shown in Example 11.

Example 11. Take the interaction pattern of predation in Table 4.
The scores that we obtain for some mappings between the pattern above and the ecosystems from Examples 1 and 2 are given below.

1.

$$\mu_1 = \begin{cases} Pred+ \to Pe+ \\ Prey+ \to R+ \end{cases} \qquad \rho_1 = \begin{cases} 1'' \to 1' \\ 2'' \to 2' \end{cases}$$

$$S(\mu_1, \rho_1) = -4/6$$

2.

$$\mu_2 = \begin{cases} Pred+ \to Pe+ \\ Prey+ \to I+ \end{cases} \qquad \rho_2 = \begin{cases} 1'' \to 4' \\ 2'' \to 2' \end{cases}$$

$$S(\mu_2, \rho_2) = 2/6$$

3.

$$\mu_3 = \begin{cases} Pred+ \to B+ \\ Prey+ \to I+ \end{cases} \qquad \rho_3 = \begin{cases} 1'' \to 1' \\ 2'' \to 2' \end{cases}$$

$$S(\mu_1, \rho_1) = 4/6$$

One may observe that the third pair of mappings, having also the best score among the three matches, matches perfectly the entities and the rules, i.e., we may easily identify that B plays the role of the predator and I the role of the prey. It turns out that this is indeed an optimal solution, i.e., a pair of mappings that maximizes the scoring function. The second match also gives a good but less perfect score as rule $2''$ and 2 do not match on their outputs. Nevertheless, this second mapping suggests that pesticides, even if they are not living entities, may also be interpreted as predators. The first match is more arbitrary and as expected its score is also the lowest among the three matches.   ◇

5   Experiment: Searching Patterns into Models of Ecosystems

In order to evaluate how practical our matching method is, we have implemented a prototype tool and used it to search patterns into various models of ecosystems. Both patterns and models are originated from previous works involving realistic ecosystem modeling. This tool performs the following steps that use the definition of scoring function given above:

1. Read models $\mathcal{E}_1$ of the pattern and $\mathcal{E}_2$ of the ecosystem in which the pattern is searched for.
2. Build the variables in matrices X and Y, and the scoring function $S(X, Y)$ as explained in the previous section.
3. Encode $S(X, Y)$ into a pseudo-Boolean optimization (PBO) problem following the requirements of the *competitions of pseudo-Boolean solvers* [28, 29].
4. Call a PBO solver and extract its solution. The solution can be interpreted back as the mappings of entities and rules that gives the best score.

```
### reading 'pond.rr'
### 4 variables / 7 rules / 0 constraints
### reading 'pest.rr'
### 4 variables / 6 rules / 0 constraints
### building model
### running sat4j
... satisfiable [0:00:00.637612]
... objective function=2/24 [0:00:00.639101]
... objective function=4/24 [0:00:01.144709]
... objective function=6/24 [0:00:01.649645]
... optimum found
=== done running sat4j in 0:00:03.193784
*** OPTIMAL SAT => 6/24
### states
P+    ==>   Pe+
IF+   ==>   I+
Su+   ==>   R+
PF+   ==>   B+
### rules
R5: IF- >> PF-    ==>   R2: I- >> B-
R4: PF+ >> IF-    ==>   R1: B+ >> I-
R2: Su+ >> P-     ==>   R5: R+ >> Pe-
### normal exit
```

Fig. 4. A sample run of our prototype searching matches between the Pond and Pesticides models presented in Examples 1 and 2. (Figure 3 in [9]).

As PBO solver, we have used Sat4j that appears to be quite fast and can be interrupted during its computation, in which case it proposes the best solution found so far.

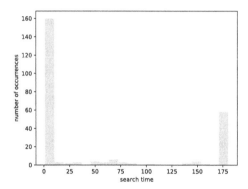

Fig. 5. Histogram of search times (in seconds) in the benchmark. (Figure 4 in [9]).

This is a very nice feature considering that searching for an optimal solution may be very long while non-optimal solutions may already correspond to interesting matches for the modeler. The prototype itself was implemented in Python using SymPy [31] to build the scoring function as defined above and simplified to match the constraints of the PBO format.

This is illustrated in Fig. 4 where we see how our prototype executes on the ecosystems from Examples 1 and 2: it prints the values of the scoring function as soon as Sat4j finds them. At any time, it is possible to kill Sat4j which interrupts its computation and force it to print the best solution it has discovered so far. It is interesting to note that this solution corresponds to none of those proposed in Example 10 which are all matches that have been crafted manually and corresponded to our intuition about the two models. So, this shows that our method is able to propose something new, i.e., something that a modeler would not necessarily imagine even on small examples.

5.1 Benchmark

Using this prototype, we have systematically searched for 12 patterns into 21 realistic models of ecosystems. These patterns and models are all originated from various works performed by ecologists, in particular master students who have modeled contrasted ecosystems. The models are representation of ecosystems from the south of France (Camargue, aquatic socio-ecosystem), the Alpes (Chamrousse, terrestrial socio-ecosystem) and ecosystems in Africa (Uganda, Karamoja, tropical socio-ecosystem). The patterns searched are mainly species interactions such as predation, competition, symbiosis, etc. It is out of the scope of this paper to describe these interactions, but we would like to pinpoint that they are all patterns and models that ecologists are actually interested in and not arbitrary examples. In particular, we did not include the "pond" and "pesticides" models in this benchmark, because they have been designed to illustrate this paper and have no ecological relevance. For each search, we have defined a timeout

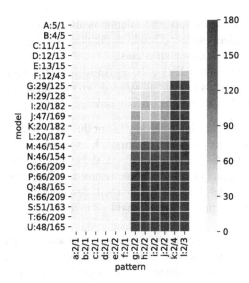

Fig. 6. Search times (in seconds) with respect to models and patterns. Models are indicated with an upper-case letter, patterns with a lower-case letter. Model and pattern names are followed by pairs of numbers e/r: e is the number of entities and r the number of rules. (Figure 5 in [9]).

of 3 min (180 s)[3] after which Sat4j was interrupted. Among the 252 searches resulting from this benchmark[4], 194 (77%) returned an optimal solution before the timeout, and 58 (23%) have been interrupted resulting in a non-optimal solution, as summarized in Fig. 5. Even if the search time is short, we can observe that an optimal solution is found in most cases. For the other ones a solution, even if not optimal, is found anyway.

A more detailed view of this benchmark is provided in the "heat-map" depicted in Fig. 6 that shows for each pattern and each model a color corresponding to the search time. In this heat-map, models are named with an upper-case letter, and patterns with a lower-case letter; names are followed by pairs of numbers e/r where e is the number of entities and r the number of rules in the model or pattern. For instance, the "prey-predator" and "live-in" patterns we have presented in the introduction are e and d respectively. Columns and rows have been sorted with respect to the sum of the values in the column and row, which allows to group larger search times in the lower-right corner. From this plot we can draw the following observations:

- neither patterns nor models size seem to be the key factor that lead to the significant search time increase. For instance, models S and J have very similar sizes but do not yield similar search times. The same remark applies to patterns e and g to j;
- however, the shape of the heat-map shows that a key factor lies in patterns as pattern choice may yield a significant increase of search time, while increasing is more progressive with respect to model choice;

---

[3] The choice of 3 min is arbitrary.

[4] The machine used is: Intel Core i7 64 bits quad-core at 2.9 GHz with 32G RAM, running Linux 4.4, SAT4J version NIGHTLY.v20171122 OpenJDK 25/Java 1.8.

- for toy models (A to F at the top), the solution is always quickly found;
- for large, more detailed, models (O to U at the bottom), the pattern structure is the key factor to determine if a timeout occurs;
- this is confirmed on intermediary models (G to N in the middle) where we can observe that more searches timeout as we go down the plot and, patterns all have the same size while models are not necessarily ordered by size.

So far, we have not identified what is the key factor that forbids a quick search. For sure pattern size is a factor as we can see for patterns k and l (or models O to U), but what we observe from patterns g—j and models F—L shows that this is not the only aspect. Considering our scoring function, search time is probably linked to the size of rules in the pattern and in the model, but this question will deserve further work to examine in more details the characteristics of patterns that lead to the observed increasing of search times.

As a conclusion of this benchmark, we observe that searching a pattern in a model is always possible, often in a very short time. Moreover, in every case, a solution has been found quickly, which allows the user to interrupt the search very soon and yet get a match that is not optimal with respect to the scoring function but may yet be interesting.

A future extension of the implementation would be to enable re-injecting found matches in the PBO problem as negative constraints, in order to forbid the search to find them again. In addition, this would give a way to enumerate matches. It is indeed particularly relevant for ecologists to (automatically) identify several instances of the same interaction pattern (ecological processes) in the ecosystem dynamics under study.

6   Concluding Remarks and Related Works

In this paper, we have worked on a modelling proposal for ecosystems and we have proposed two ways of studying such systems without fully developing (computing) their semantics. Firstly, we have proposed a method to isolate and remove redundant information from models. Secondly, we have introduced a method for automatically comparing and assessing similarity between ecosystems defined as specific kinds of rewriting systems. We have defined a scoring function that takes into account not only the number of matching entities and rules, but also the quality of partial mappings between the left and right hand sides of rules. The approach has been successfully applied to the search of known interaction patterns (i.e., ecological processes) in realistic models of ecosystems.

The results we have obtained in our benchmark are promising: we quickly obtain optimal solutions for the vast majority of the studied cases. For the remaining ones, we obtain a solution that is not optimal in a short time, but we have no assessment of how far from optimal it is. A possible option to solve this issue could be to add ecological information to assess the quality of a match (with a relevance score) closer to the modeler's expectations. In other words, a bigger match is not necessarily a better match. So far, our method searches for bigger matches only. When the search is interrupted and yields to a sub-optimal solution, a relevance score may help deciding whether it is already a "good" match or not. In practice, the matching of entities (here, ecosystemic entities) and rules (ecological processes) can be guided by adding additional constraints, such as to:

- enforce the matching/identity between subsets of entities or rules. For example, if the model allows different categories of rules (each category possibly having a different semantics), the scoring function could be adapted to take into account this extension;
- enforce the matching between entities/rules of the same category (for example match carnivores among them);
- diminish the importance of some entities/rules (i.e., set a different weight for each matching up to forget some, if necessary).

Finally, as a long term perspective, we may use our method to discover invariant patterns that are not known in advance, thus increasing the understanding about ecosystem functioning. This could account for using our concept of similarity to identify matching parts of ecosystems and extract from those the new patterns. The experiments we have conducted so far in this direction showed poor performances (as if we would have used patterns whose sizes are close to the studied models' sizes). This entails that additional constraints, as those mentioned above, are necessary to deal with this kind of problem. However, sub-optimal patterns may provide interesting matches (which remains to be studied), or we may find a way to guide the search with respect to additional constraints (related to the previous idea of a relevance score).

6.1 Related Work

The model of ecosystems developed in this paper is an instance of the more general family of rewriting systems [32]. Such systems have been shown convenient in formalizing models, in particular for systems biology and chemistry. In these domains, we thus find formalizations that are reminiscent of ours: the Biocham [13], the κ-calculus [7], reaction systems [11], activity networks [8], P-systems [27], cellular automata [1, 14] that describe the evolution of cells and/or molecules applying rewriting rules.

The strategies of Sect. 3 are specific to the application domain, it is therefore complex to find some related works. On the contrary, to our knowledge, the question of similarity here appears novel in rewriting systems. In a broader context, it is usually associated to the notion of equivalence. In concurrent systems like ours, equivalences are usually semantics based, notable examples are partial ordering equivalences, trace equivalence [19], bisimulation [30], principal transition sequences [35], etc. These notions are usually explored in theory and tailored to highly abstracted languages, moreover computed with a few existing tools. In practice, we cannot expect to use such approaches on the huge state spaces generated from detailed and realistic (qualitative) models of ecosystems.

Works that are closer to ours can therefore be found in domains in which models use structural aspects rather than their behaviors. For instance in systems biology, several similarity measures can be found (a good survey summarizing the used techniques may be found in [21]). Technically speaking, these methods include the analysis of similar pathways through a structural approach, namely the search of t-invariants in Petri net models [3,4,20]. They also define a similarity score, but our goal and underlying modelling are considerably different.

Another domain that focuses on similarity rates is business process modeling. For instance in [36], the authors evaluate the similarity of Petri nets by comparing the set of structural elements such as places and transition arcs. Similarity is based on rates of identical elements. Instead, our approach is finer-grained and more flexible: the mappings allow different names of entities and rules, and we allow partially matched rules. In [2], process-based models are studied and similarity is defined on sets of nodes as the proportion of matched ones. Yet, these authors do not deal with relations between them. Likewise, in [10], other similarities are explored. In this context the authors still compare structural elements of workflows (e.g., sets of nodes), but they allow different kinds of distance measures: string-edit distance, labels synonyms and contextual similarity. The latter measure is the closest to ours, as we consider separately the input (or conditions, the left hand side of a rule) and the output (realization, the right hand side of a rule) of a node. Conversely, here, we take into consideration penalties for elements that are not matched. The work in [10] shows how similarities in business process model are linked to the semantic web domain, a survey of which on corresponding metrics can be found in [12].

Finally, concerning the pattern search, the work in [25] has analogous goals. These authors search for patterns by counting the number of occurrences of a given sub-graph in specific networks (world wide web, electronic circuits, ...) and comparing it to the number of occurrences in random generated networks. This approach is completely different to ours, as their method applies to graphs while ours applies to "hyper-graphs". Moreover, they use techniques from statistics while we do not.

Acknowledgments. We would like to thank David Monniaux for his suggestions on MAXSAT and PBO solvers, and Daniel Le Berre who has recommended Sat4j and has been very helpful concerning its installation and use. We would also like to thanks the anonymous reviewers for their precious work.

References

1. Agnihotri, K., Sharma, N.: Developments in ecological modeling based on cellular automata. Innov. Syst. Des. Eng. **6**, 75–78 (2015)
2. Bae, J., Liu, L., Caverlee, J., Rouse, W.B.: Process mining, discovery, and integration using distance measures. In: 2006 IEEE International Conference on Web Services (ICWS 2006), pp. 479–488, September 2006
3. Baldan, P., Bocci, M., Cocco, N., Simeoni, M.: Comparing metabolic pathways through potential fluxes: a selective opening approach. In: BioPPN@Petri Nets (2013)
4. Baldan, P., Cocco, N., Giummolè, F., Simeoni, M.: Comparing metabolic pathways through reactions and potential fluxes. Trans. Petri Nets Other Models Concurr. **8**, 1–23 (2013). https://doi.org/10.1007/978-3-642-40465-8
5. Baldan, P., Cocco, N., Marin, A., Simeoni, M.: Petri nets for modelling metabolic pathways: a survey. Nat. Comput. **9**(4), 955–989 (2010)
6. Cardelli, L.: Abstract machines of systems biology. Trans. Comput. Syst. Biol. **3737**, 145–168 (2005)
7. Danos, V., Laneve, C.: Formal molecular biology. TCS **325**(1), 69–110 (2004)
8. Delaplace, F., Di Giusto, C., Giavitto, J., Klaudel, H.: Activity networks with delays an application to toxicity analysis. Fundamenta Informaticae (2018, to appear)
9. Di Giusto, C., Gaucherel, C., Klaudel, H., Pommereau, F.: Pattern matching in discrete models for ecosystem ecology. In: Maria, E.D., Fred, A.L.N., Gamboa, H. (eds.) Proceedings

of the 12th International Joint Conference on Biomedical Engineering Systems and Technologies (BIOSTEC 2019), BIOINFORMATICS, Prague, Czech Republic, 22–24 February 2019, vol. 3, pp. 101–111. SciTePress (2019). https://doi.org/10.5220/0007485801010111

10. Dijkman, R., Dumas, M., van Dongen, B., Käärik, R., Mendling, J.: Similarity of business process models: metrics and evaluation. Inf. Syst. **36**(2), 498–516 (2011). http://www.sciencedirect.com/science/article/pii/S0306437910001006, Special Issue: Semantic Integration of Data, Multimedia, and Services

11. Ehrenfeucht, A., Rozenberg, G.: Reaction systems. Fund. Inform. **75**(1–4), 263–280 (2007)

12. Euzenat, J., Shvaiko, P.: Ontology Matching. Springer, Heidelberg (2007). https://doi.org/10.1007/978-3-540-49612-0

13. Fages, F., Soliman, S.: Formal cell biology in biocham. In: Bernardo, M., Degano, P., Zavattaro, G. (eds.) SFM 2008. LNCS, vol. 5016, pp. 54–80. Springer, Heidelberg (2008). https://doi.org/10.1007/978-3-540-68894-5_3. http://dl.acm.org/citation.cfm?id=1786698.1786702

14. Gaucherel, C.: Influence of spatial patterns on ecological applications of extremal principles. Ecol. Model. **193**, 531–542 (2006). https://doi.org/10.1016/j.ecolmodel.2005.08.035

15. Gaucherel, C., Pommereau, F.: Using discrete systems to exhaustively characterize the dynamics of an integrated ecosystem. Methods Ecol. Evol. 1–13 (2019). https://doi.org/10.1111/2041-210X.13242

16. Gaucherel, C., Boudon, F., Houet, T., Castets, M., Godin, C.: Understanding patchy landscape dynamics: towards a landscape language. PLoS ONE **7**(9), 16 (2012). https://doi.org/10.1371/journal.pone.0046064. https://halshs.archives-ouvertes.fr/halshs-00750971

17. Gaucherel, C., Houllier, F., Auclair, D., Houet, T.: Dynamic landscape modelling: the quest for a unifying theory. Living Rev. Landscape Res. **8**(2), 5–31 (2014). https://hal.archives-ouvertes.fr/hal-01211675

18. Giavitto, J.L., Malcolm, G., Michel, O.: Rewriting systems and the modelling of biological systems. Comp. Funct. Genomics **5**, 95–99 (2004)

19. van Glabbeek, R., Goltz, U.: Equivalence notions for concurrent systems and refinement of actions. In: Kreczmar, A., Mirkowska, G. (eds.) MFCS 1989. LNCS, vol. 379, pp. 237–248. Springer, Heidelberg (1989). https://doi.org/10.1007/3-540-51486-4_71

20. Grafahrend-Belau, E., et al.: Modularization of biochemical networks based on classification of Petri net t-invariants. BMC Bioinform. **9**(1), 90 (2008). https://doi.org/10.1186/1471-2105-9-90

21. Henkel, R., Hoehndorf, R., Kacprowski, T., Knüpfer, C., Liebermeister, W., Waltemath, D.: Notions of similarity for systems biology models. Briefings Bioinform. **19**(1), 77–88 (2018). https://doi.org/10.1093/bib/bbw090

22. Le Berre, D., Parrain, A.: The Sat4j library, release 2.2. J. Satisfiability Boolean Model. Comput. **7**, 59–64 (2010)

23. Lotka, A.J.: Elements of Physical Biology. Williams & Wilkins Company, Baltimore (1925). http://library.wur.nl/WebQuery/clc/529141

24. May, R.M.: Will a large complex system be stable? Nature **238**, 413–414 (1972). https://doi.org/10.1038/238413a0

25. Milo, R., Shen-Orr, S., Itzkovitz, S., Kashtan, N., Chklovskii, D., Alon, U.: Network motifs: simple building blocks of complex networks. Science **298**(5594), 824–827 (2002). http://science.sciencemag.org/content/298/5594/824

26. Mooiman, L.: Comparing stories with the use of Petri nets. Technical report, University of Amsterdam (2015)

27. Paun, A., Paun, M., Rodríguez-Patón, A., Sidoroff, M.: P systems with proteins on membranes: a survey. Int. J. Found. Comput. Sci. **22**(1), 39–53 (2011)

28. PB16: Pseudo-Boolean competition 2016. Satellite Event of SAT 2016 (2016). http://www.cril.univ-artois.fr/PB16

29. Roussel, O., Manquinho, V.: Input/output format and solver requirements for the competitions of pseudo-Boolean solvers (2012). http://www.cril.univ-artois.fr/PB12/format.pdf
30. Sangiorgi, D.: Introduction to Bisimulation and Coinduction. Cambridge University Press, New York (2011)
31. SymPy development team: SymPy (2016). http://www.sympy.org
32. Terese: Term Rewriting Systems, Cambridge Tracts in Theoretical Computer Science, vol. 55. Cambridge University Press (2003)
33. Thomas, R.: Boolean formalisation of genetic control circuits. J. Theor. Biol. **42**, 565–583 (1973)
34. Tversky, A.: Features of similarity. Psychol. Rev. **84**(4), 327–352 (1977)
35. Wang, J., He, T., Wen, L.; Wu, N., ter Hofstede, A.H.M., Su, J.: A behavioral similarity measure between labeled Petri nets based on principal transition sequences. In: Meersman, R., Dillon, T., Herrero, P. (eds.) OTM 2010. LNCS, vol. 6426, pp. 394–401. Springer, Heidelberg (2010). https://doi.org/10.1007/978-3-642-16934-2_27
36. Xiao, L., Zheng, L., Xiao, J., Huang, Y.: A graphical query language for querying Petri nets. In: Yang, J., Ginige, A., Mayr, H.C., Kutsche, R.-D. (eds.) UNISCON 2009. LNBIP, vol. 20, pp. 514–525. Springer, Heidelberg (2009). https://doi.org/10.1007/978-3-642-01112-2_52

Application of Data Mining and Machine Learning in Microwave Radiometry (MWR)

Vladislav Levshinskii[1], Christoforos Galazis[2], Lev Ovchinnikov[3,4], Sergey Vesnin[3], Alexander Losev[1], and Igor Goryanin[2,4(✉)]

[1] Volgograd State University, Volgograd, Russia
{v.levshinskii,alexander.losev}@volsu.ru
[2] University of Edinburgh, Edinburgh, UK
{s1747971,goryanin}@inf.edu.ac.uk
[3] Medical Microwave Radiometry Ltd., Edinburgh, UK
vesnin47@gmail.com
[4] Okinawa Institute of Science and Technology, Okinawa, Japan

Abstract. Microwave radiometry has seen its way in successful usage in medical applications. The focus here is its applicability in cancer detection and monitoring, specifically for breast cancer, as an additional and alternative tool. This is done by capturing the temperature of the skin and the internal tissue. However, the amount of data required by clinical specialist to process in a short time to reach to a confident decision is becoming insurmountable. This can be tackled by developing a diagnostic system that will help pinpoint irregularities associated with pathologies. The key factors of a successful diagnostic system is the accuracy of the predictions and its informativeness and interpretability. The core component of such a system is a machine learning algorithm. Models that were explored were random forest, k-nearest neighbors, support vector machines, variants of cascade correlation neural networks, deep neural network and convolution neural network. From all these models evaluated, the best performing on the test set was the deep neural network. Also, we proposed a method for forming the space of thermometric features, which at the same time ensures a sufficiently high efficiency of the classification algorithms. More importantly, the model is inherently able to provide an explanation of the diagnostic solution.

Keywords: Microwave radiometry · Breast cancer · Diagnostic system · Machine learning · Neural network · Rule-based classification · Cascade Correlation Neural Network · Convolutional Neural Network · Random Forest · Support Vector Machine

1 Introduction

Microwave radiometry is being rapidly developed as for it has generated a lot of interest for its medical applications, more so in recent years [66]. One of its applications is

AL and VL are grateful to Russian Foundation for Basic Research (grant No RFBR 19-01-00358) for the financial support of the development of mathematical models for early diagnosis of breast cancer.

A. Roque et al. (Eds.): BIOSTEC 2019, CCIS 1211, pp. 265–288, 2020.
https://doi.org/10.1007/978-3-030-46970-2_13

for cancer detection and monitoring, such as breast cancer which will be the focus here. These devices are able to measure temperatures of internal tissues noninvasively. In turn, this makes them ideal for detecting malignant tumors due to the fact that their released temperature is closely associated with their growth rate.

It is a fairly new approach that is gradually being utilized. However, its novelty creates a learning curve barrier for practitioners hindering its adaption rate. Usually one would prefer to use approaches and methods that they are more familiar with and experienced. Additionally, by taking advantage of another device it requires more effort and time to analyse and extract information from. But this is not always possible with the requirement in making faster and more accurate diagnosis in conjunction with the increased number of patients per doctor.

For the reasons stated above, it is crucial to introduce an accurate automated diagnostic system to tackle the current issues. Its intention will be to extract useful information from the reading and suggest and justify the diagnostic prognosis in terms that doctors understand. Hence, the focus will be in evaluating how effective such data alone can be used for diagnosis of cancer, using data collected from mammary glands. In turn, as a classification problem, it is also important to determine if a machine learning algorithm is able to offer an accurate prediction of diagnosis. In addition, there will be a proposed method for constructing spaces of thermometric features that ensure high efficiency of the classification algorithm. At the same time, this approach will make it possible to substantiate the proposed diagnostic solution in an understandable way for doctors.

This chapter is an extended version of the paper [26]. The base paper focused on proposing a model that improved the sensitivity and specificity of the classification problem. However, here we shift focus towards the importance of interpretability of a machine learning algorithm that is used as part of an automated diagnostic system. The additional contribution is with the introduction of a rule based classification algorithm. It incorporates user-friendly interpretability in the model itself while still maintaining high accuracy. Also, it is compared against an already established model-agnostic approach for neural network interpretability, named shapely additive explanations [45].

In this chapter, we will start with some brief information about microwave radiometry devices, how they are able to capture temperature readings in biological tissues and why they are important for detecting malignant tumors. Next, we give details about the dataset used and how we distributed it to three subsets in preparation for training and evaluation. In addition, we will present two preprocessing steps that were employed, temperature normalization and oversampling. After the setup information has been provided, the description and results of various machine learning models will be presented for the task of classifying low or high risk presence of cancer. Further, on the basis of mathematical models of the behavior of thermal fields inside the mammary glands and the currently existing medical knowledge, a new method for constructing spaces of thermometric features will be proposed. At the same time, two problems are solved simultaneously. First, it provides high sensitivity and specificity, built on the basis of these feature spaces, classification algorithms. Secondly, the possibility of consciousness of the mechanisms for substantiating the proposed diagnostic prediction is provided. This approach is then compared against techniques used to interpret complex models such as neural networks.

Finally, we end with some conclusions derived from our work and paving out possible future work.

2 Microwave Radiometry for Breast Cancer Detection

Tissues omit electromagnetic radiation in the microwave range [66]. Various type of tissues have different biological properties which in turn impact the levels of electromagnetic radiation [57]. These properties of the tissues depend significantly on the levels of water in each due to their dielectric constant at a given temperature [24, 25]. For example, muscle has much higher concentration of water compared to fat and bone tissues and thus can be differentiated by the levels of microwave emissivity. In addition, various physiological and pathological conditions can interfere with the normal dielectric properties of the affected tissues [57].

Capturing such radiometric measurements can be used to acquire temperature values for both the skin's surface and also internal tissues. Due to this factor is where microwave radiometry can be utilized to detect and monitor various pathological conditions. Naturally, it has found its way in various medical applications such as detecting breast cancer [66], thermal denaturation of albumin [33], carotid artery diseases [22], drown adipose tissue activity [20], rheumatoid arthritis [49], inflammation levels in joints [39], brain temperature levels [53], lung transcapillary water exchange [9] and varicose of a vein [62].

Here we will focus on capturing temperature data through microwave radiometry for breast cancer detection. Cell replication requires energy in which some of that energy is lost as heat during metabolic reactions. This is no different for tumors which they emit heat in relation to their growth rate [27]. During the rapid growth stage of the tumorous cells, the cells replicate themselves at a faster pace which is contributed by an increase in glycolytic flux. At this stage, tumorous cells are easily distinguishable from neighboring healthy cells. Hence, using microwave radiometry it is able to detect pathologies at an early stage more effectively than other methods. However, once it reaches its maximum volume the growth rate is reduced to match that of the cell death rate [55]. This state of the cell will result in near normal temperature readings making their detection more difficult [66].

During the past years, significant improvements have been made to the sensitivity and specificity for cancer detection, by narrowing the reading error at low growth stages of the tumor [66]. Over and above accuracy improvements, it is a noninvasive, nonionizing and safe method for the patient which also offer the benefit of high throughput of results at a low cost [57, 66]. Hence, this can be used more frequently, without any age restrictions and is suitable for someone during pregnancy or lactation. In addition to detecting the presence of malignant tumors, it is able to return information about the thermal activity of the tissue, the rate in which cancerous cells multiply and the risk level for mutagenesis [66]. Overall, this makes it a viable approach for cancer detection and can be added as an additional tool set to existing approaches, such as mammography or biopsy.

The dataset consists of temperature readings of mammary glands during regular monitoring or suspicion of pathology, which will be used to evaluate the models and determine potential feasibility of a diagnostic system. The data were captured using the RTM-01-RES (www.mmwr.co.uk) device from across multiple clinical centers. The device captures microwave emissions with an accuracy of up to ±0.2 °C of the actual values and a detection depth between 3–7 cm. For the cases in the dataset, the temperature detection depth of the internal tissue was fixed to 5 cm while also measuring the skin values at the same point.

For each mammary gland, the device captures the temperature at the nipple (denoted as point 0) and eight symmetrical points around the nipple (points 1–8). In addition, another point is measured at the axillary region (point 9). Because of the ambient temperature variations another two pointer were captured at the lower chest (points T1 and T2), so the values can be normalized. In total, there are 44 captured points for both measurements at the skin and at a depth. A graphical representation of the previously listed points can be seen in Fig. 1.

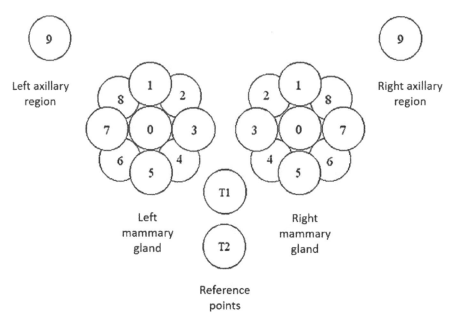

Fig. 1. Sampling points on each mammary gland (0–8) including the axillary point (9). Points T1 and T2 are used as reference values when normalizing the values against ambient temperature [26].

The dataset consists of 363 pairs of mammary glands of which 77 are classified as healthy or low risk (labeled as class 0) and 286 classified as potentially cancerous or high risk (labeled as class 1). Statistical analysis of this data was conducted under a previous research scope [46]. For each sample, to be classified as low risk both glands must be considered as healthy and for it to be considered as high risk then at least one must be of high risk. Individual glands compromise of 319 low risk and 407 high risk samples. In detail, it consists of 13 diffused cancer, 185 nodal cancer, 119 diffuse changes with no presence of cancer and 90 nodal changes with no presence of cancer. The following experiments, unless specified otherwise, will have the data class balanced split into three sets. The training set with allocated 60% (low risk: 46 and high risk: 171), validation set 20% (low risk: 15 and high risk: 57) and test set with the remaining 20% (low risk: 16 and high risk: 58).

3 Preprocessing

3.1 Ambient Temperature Normalization

When analyzing temperature values for prediction systems breast size, age and external conditions that can impact the results must be taken into account [2, 63]. One such external condition is the environmental temperature which ideally needs to be normalized so they are comparable. Typically, the measurements were taken under temperatures ranging from 20 to 27 °C. A previous research [8, 26] that used the same dataset proposed and evaluated a normalization algorithm to overcome this issue, which is defined as following:

For every point $t_{d,i,j}$ captured, plot their values against one of the control temperature points $T_{c,d,j}$, where $i = 0, ..., 9, c \in \{1, 2\}, j \in \{skin, depth\}$ and $d = 0, ..., n - 1$, with n the total number of samples:

1. On the plotted graph between temperature points and one of the reference values, we use linear regression to find a and b such that the error is minimized through least square fit method on the function:

$$T_{d,i,j} = a * T_{c,d,j} + b \qquad (1)$$

2. Calculate the average value of the temperature point such that:

$$T_{avg_{c,j}} = \frac{1}{n} \sum_{d=0}^{n-1} T_{c,d,j} \qquad (2)$$

3. Update the temperature points:

$$t_{d,i,j} = t_{d,i,j} + a * \left(T_{avg_{c,j}} - T_{c,d,j} \right) \qquad (3)$$

4. Replace the control points with the average value found:

$$T_{c,d,j} = T_{avg_{c,j}}, \qquad (4)$$

for $d = 0, ..., n - 1$.

Bochkarev et al. showed that when applying their proposed algorithm it improved the specificity and sensitivity of a regression prediction model. There was a strong linear correlation coefficient between points 0–9 against either of the two reference points as the temperature increased. However, using reference point T2 obtained slightly better performance with an improvement of 4%. Therefore, this same approach was applied against reference point T2 as a preprocessing step for the experiments. As a result, this allowed the removal of the two reference points because they would be the same value across all samples.

3.2 Class Balancing Through Oversampling

As described in Sect. 2, the dataset is heavily imbalanced towards the high risk class with a total of 286 against 77 samples of the low risk. Consequently, this introduces a classification bias in favor of the majority class [37]. Some algorithms can handle this imbalance by introducing loss function weights to give more importance to the least represented class during training or by introducing an appropriate metric [31]. While both of these techniques were used in the experiments where applicable, applying oversampling allows for a uniformly approach to various models.

The techniques explored were random resampling, Synthetic Minority Over-Sampling Technique (SMOTE) with regular, borderline 1, borderline 2 and Support Vector Machine (SVM) variations [13, 29] and Adaptive Synthetic (ADASYN) [30]. The oversampling techniques were compared using a random forest [11] from the scikit-learn library [48] having set a sample weight importance to handle imbalance. Additionally, for each case the tree was optimized using the hyperopt [6] library with tree of Parzen (TPE) [5] optimizer and weighted Geometric mean (G-mean) loss [4, 38] as the function to minimize on.

Using both weight balance and G-Mean loss means that it eliminates the need for oversampling. However, we want to evaluate whether oversampling is equivalent and interchangeable with these techniques and does not negatively impact the results. The results of the various oversampling techniques are summarized in Table 1. The main metric used for comparison is G-mean loss then sensitivity and specificity and lastly accuracy. Improvements against no oversampling based on the loss function is observed for SMOTE with all variations but SVM. However, with borderline 1 variation one can observe a significant improvement in regards to specificity without hampering to an excessive degree its specificity. It obtained a G-mean loss value of 0.3268, sensitivity of 0.8621, specificity of 0.5 and accuracy of 0.7838. Hence, for the model evaluations the low risk class from the training set was oversampled using SMOTE borderline 1. It was sampled until the total number matched that of the high risk being 286.

Table 1. Summary of the results on the test set of a random forest classifier when using oversampling on the least represented class (low risk) in the dataset so it becomes balanced [26].

Oversampling	G-mean loss	Accuracy	Sensitivity	Specificity
No oversampling	0.3894	0.7702	0.8793	0.375
Random	0.3994	0.6622	0.7069	0.5
SMOTE regular	0.3749	0.6622	0.6897	0.5625
SMOTE borderline1	0.3268	0.7838	0.8621	0.5
SMOTE borderline2	0.3693	0.7568	0.8448	0.4375
SMOTE SVM	0.4126	0.7297	0.8276	0.375
ADASYN	0.401	0.7027	0.7759	0.4375

4 Model Evaluations

4.1 Non-neural Network Models

Non-neural network models are still a vital alternative to neural network ones and can set a good baseline for future models [41, 61]. Non-neural network models usually can train their weights with much less time than compared to their counterparts. Also, this leads to requiring fewer computational resources, allowing them to be trained on personal machines. In addition, they require less hyperparameter tuning and setup time and do not require an architecture to be designed specifically for the problem, making them production-ready sooner. Lastly, a subset of such algorithms offer inherently interpretability on why a decision was made and are easier to understand how a change in a feature will affect the results of the model. While having all these benefits, the results can also be in par with what is obtained from neural networks but depends on the complexity of the problem in hand. Additionally, the best non-neural network model can act as a base line for comparison of various network architectures.

The models evaluated were Random Forest (RF), XGBoost [14], K-Nearest Neighbors (K-NN) [19], Support Vector Machine (SVM) with linear kernel and radial basis function (RBF) [12, 18]. The algorithms were obtained from the scikit-learn library, apart from XGBoost which was obtained from its own library [14]. Each of these models, their optimal hyperparameters were determined through the usage of the hyperopt library with the TPE optimizer. Additionally, the loss function used to minimize the error on was the weighted G-mean loss.

From the models evaluated, the top performer based on the lowest achieved weighted G-mean loss value is XGBoost with a value of 0.3994. It also obtained a decent sensitivity of 0.7069 but just 0.5 on specificity and a biased accuracy of 0.6622. Following came SVM with linear kernel obtaining a weighted G-mean loss of 0.4241 and closely in third RF with 0.4281. K-NN and SVM with RBF obtained significantly worse results with a weighted G-mean loss of 0.4829 and 0.5687 respectively. The full summary of the results on the test set are shown in Table 2.

Table 2. Summary of the results on the test set for the non-neural network models [26].

Oversampling	G-mean loss	Accuracy	Sensitivity	Specificity
RF	0.4281	0.7027	0.7931	0.375
XGBoost	0.3994	0.6622	0.7069	0.5
K-NN	0.4829	0.527	0.5345	0.5
SVM Linear Kernel	0.4241	0.6216	0.6551	0.5
SVM RBF Kernel	0.5687	0.7432	0.7826	0.0625

4.2 Rule Based Classification

Practical analysis of microwave thermometry identified the problem of developing methods, algorithms and software for processing, qualitative and quantitative analysis of thermometric data and other medical information about the patient. Currently, for the purpose of biomedical research, data mining methods are commonly used to solve problems of classification and forecasting. However, most popular machine learning algorithms (neural networks, etc.) are not able to effectively provide a qualitative justification of the result to the doctor-diagnostician. The development of advisory intelligent systems, i.e. expert systems, which contain a mechanism for explaining and justifying the proposed solutions in user-friendly language, is aimed to address this problem [36].

At first, it seemed quite natural to use the feature space of vectors $T_{c,d,j}$ as points, i.e. temperature values only. It is easy to identify that the location of points contributing to the diagnosis are rather chaotic and there is no clear separation between one class from another. However, during medical examinations conducted over the past two decades, as well as analysis of microwave thermometry data, specialists identified a number of qualitative features of breast cancer (see, for example, [36, 44, 66]). For patients with pathology we can note the following: an increased value of thermal asymmetry between the corresponding points of mammary glands; a high temperature variance between individual points in the affected breast; a high difference between nipple temperatures; an increased temperature of the nipple in comparison with the mean breast temperature considering age-related temperature changes; the difference between surface and inner temperatures and some others. Initial work appeared on the range analysis of functions, which describe the presence of anomalies in temperature fields of human organs [43, 44]. The first studies also appeared on the application of data mining methods and the development of classification algorithms in this field [26, 44, 54, 65, 67]. At the same time, there were proposed several mathematical models that describe temperature fields of mammary glands in terms of solutions of partial differential equations [50, 52].

It is important to determine the most significant characteristics of temperature fields for anomaly detection, analysis and interpretation of patient temperature data. This is achieved by studying the most recently available mathematical modeling of the dynamics of thermal and radiation fields in biological tissues, in conjunction with biological and medical knowledge, which is based on the physiological structure of the human body.

We formulate the core hypotheses of the behavior of the temperature fields, on the basis of which it is supposed to perform an analysis of the obtained data. First, there is the hypothesis of the "mirror" symmetry of the right and left mammary glands' temperature fields of healthy patients. It is confirmed both by existing experience of microwave thermometry application and by analyzing existing mathematical models of the temperature fields' behavior. As a consequence, the temperature values at mirror-symmetric points of healthy patients should differ slightly. Naturally, the temperature values at symmetrical points of patients with pathologies may differ significantly. This hypothesis is applicable not only in the analysis of thermometric data of mammary glands, but also in the analysis of almost all paired organs of humans. At the same time, we note that in some cases the temperature difference at symmetrical points of healthy patients can be quite large: up to 2.5° in microwave and 3.5° in infrared range. However, the difference can reach up to 6° for patients with pathologies. In addition to the above, not all patients with pathologies have significant thermal asymmetry.

To test the hypothesis, we propose functionals of the form:

$$T_{as} = \|T_1(\vec{r}) - T_r(\vec{r})\|, \tag{5}$$

where $T_1(\vec{r})$ and $T_r(\vec{r})$ are temperatures of the left and right mammary glands. It is supposed to apply different types of functionals, including various norms $(C(\Omega), C^1(\Omega), C^2(\Omega),$ etc.$)$, seminorms and similar, calculated both over the entire range and over its various subranges. Following are some examples of functionals that determine the "proximity" of temperature fields:

$$f_1(T_1, T_r) = \max_{\vec{r} \in M} |T_1(\vec{r}) - T_r(\vec{r})|, \tag{6}$$

$$f_2(T_1, T_r) = \max_{\vec{r} \in M} |\nabla(T_1(\vec{r}) - T_r(\vec{r}))|, \tag{7}$$

$$f_3(T_1, T_r) = \max_{\vec{r} \in M} \left| D^2(T_1(\vec{r}) - T_r(\vec{r})) \right|, \tag{8}$$

where $D^2(f)$ is the Hessian matrix of the corresponding function, and $\|.\|$ is a certain matrix norm;

$$f_4(T_1, T_r) = \int_M |T_1(\vec{r}) - T_r(\vec{r})| dr, \tag{9}$$

$$f_5(T_1, T_r) = \sup_{\Omega \subset M} \frac{1}{|\Omega|} \int_\Omega |T_1(\vec{r}) - T_r(\vec{r})| dr, \tag{10}$$

as well as various Steklov averages, variations of Hardy and Arzela, and other functionals.

It is also supposed to apply the hypothesis of low temperature variance in a healthy breast. It is based on the absence of heat sources in healthy breasts, which would otherwise be caused by metabolic processes and cancers, and on the symmetry of heat sources produced by blood flow and adequate boundary conditions. To test the hypothesis, we propose functionals of the form:

$$T_D = \|T(\vec{r}) - T_{st}(\vec{r})\|, \tag{11}$$

where, as above, it is supposed to use different types of functionals, including various norms $(C(\Omega), C^1(\Omega), C^2(\Omega), L^2(\Omega),$ etc.$)$, seminorms and similar, calculated both over the entire range and over its various subranges. $T_{st}(\vec{r})$ is a function, that describes the "standard" temperature distribution of the breast. Some versions of this approach are described in [45].

Formally, we denote a set of thermometric data as:

$$X = \begin{pmatrix} x_1^1 & \cdots & x_n^1 \\ \vdots & \ddots & \vdots \\ x_1^m & \cdots & x_n^m \end{pmatrix}, y = \begin{pmatrix} y_1 \\ y_2 \\ \vdots \\ y_m \end{pmatrix}, Y = \{0, 1, \ldots, C\}, \tag{12}$$

where m is the number of objects, n is the number of features, $x^i = \left(x_1^i, \ldots, x_n^i\right)$ is the feature vector of object i, and $y_i \in Y$ is the class label.

Considering that the initial dataset contains 44 temperature values for each patient: 10 inner and 10 surface temperatures for the left and right mammary glands and temperature values at pivot points, the initial feature vector can be represented as the following:

$$
\begin{aligned}
x^i = (&T_{0,r}^{i,mw}, \ldots, T_{9,r}^{i,mw}, T_{0,r}^{i,ir}, \ldots, T_{9,r}^{i,ir}, T_{0,l}^{i,mw}, \ldots, \\
&T_{9,l}^{i,mw}, T_{0,l}^{i,ir}, \ldots, T_{9,l}^{i,ir}, T_{0,p}^{i,mw}, T_{1,p}^{i,mw}, T_{0,p}^{i,ir}, T_{1,p}^{i,ir}),
\end{aligned} \tag{13}
$$

where $T_r^{i,mw} = \left(T_{0,r}^{i,mw}, \ldots, T_{9,r}^{i,mw}\right)$ and $T_r^{i,ir} = \left(T_{0,r}^{i,ir}, \ldots, T_{9,r}^{i,ir}\right)$ are values of the inner and surface temperatures respectively at the points $0, \ldots, 9$ of the right breast, similarly, but with the index 1, we denote temperature values of the left breast, and $T_{0,p}^{i,mw}, T_{1,p}^{i,mw}, T_{0,p}^{i,ir}, T_{1,p}^{i,ir}$ are inner and surface temperature values at the pivot points T1 and T2 respectively. We also denote $T_r^{i,g} = T_r^{i,mw} - T_r^{i,ir}$.

At the next stage, we define the quantitative characteristics of these functionals, that are specific for different classes of patients. The rule is a triple (f, V, X), where f is a functional, which describes the behavior of temperature fields, $V = I(S, f, X)$ is a rule informativeness, X is a subrange of f. Informativeness is a quantitative characteristic, that determines how well a rule can distinguish objects of one class from another. As $I(S, f, X)$ we applied the statistical informativeness, that is calculated by the formula:

$$
ST(S, f, X) = -\ln\left(\frac{C_k^h C_{(n-k)}^s}{C_{k+(n-k)}^{h+s}}\right), \tag{14}
$$

where h is the number of healthy patients for which $f \in X$, and s is the number of patients with pathologies for which $f \in X$. Examples of the most informative rules are presented in the Table 3. The following notation is used: I is the statistical informativeness, $\frac{C_h}{\bar{C}_h}$ и $\frac{C_s}{\bar{C}_s}$ - are proportions of healthy and sick patients covered by the rule, and $\bar{A}$ is an average value of A.

We analyzed two sets of thermometric data, which were split by sensor type:

- A set of temperature data of 175 patients measured by the noise-proof sensor (A), among which 90 patients do not have pathologies and 85 have breast cancer;
- A set of temperature data of 185 patients measured by the combined sensor (B), among which 102 patients do not have pathologies and 83 have breast cancer.

The main reason for splitting the dataset is due to the sensor type of the device, which was used for measurements, in which it has a direct effect on the temperature values of both healthy patients and patients with pathologies. As a result the sensor type itself is an important feature. This is partly due to the fact that during consecutive measurements with noise-proof sensors the overall temperature decreases, since temperature measurements in different ranges are performed separately and the examination takes longer. On the other hand, the combined sensor allows to measure temperatures in two ranges at once. Thus, there is a notable difference in the variance, mean and median values

Table 3. Examples of rules for the dataset B.

Rule	I	$\frac{C_h}{\bar{C}_h}$	$\frac{C_s}{\bar{C}_s}$
$\sqrt{\sum_{j=0}^{8} \left(T_{j,r}^{i,ir} - T_{j,1}^{i,ir}\right)^2} \in (2.53, \infty)$	32.4	0.09	0.61
$\max_{t \in T_r^{i,g}} \{t\} \in (-\infty, 1.35)$	32.1	0.53	0.04
$\max_{t \in T_l^{i,g}} \left\{\overline{T_l^{i,g}} - t\right\} \in (-\infty, 0.63)$	28.3	0.76	0.24
$\max_{t \in T_l^{i,g} \setminus \left\{T_{0,l}^{i,g}\right\}} \left\{T_{0,l}^{i,g} - t\right\} \in (-\infty, 0.25)$	24.4	0.01	0.33
$\sqrt{\dfrac{\sum_{t \in T_r^{i,g}} \left\|\left(t - \overline{T_r^{i,g}}\right)\right\|^2}{\left\|T_r^{i,g}\right\| - 1}}$	23.9	0.46	0.05
$\sqrt{\sum_{j=0}^{8} \left(T_{j,r}^{i,ir} - T_{j,1}^{i,ir}\right)^2} \in (2.53, \infty)$	32.4	0.09	0.61

of temperatures measured by devices with different sensor types, which is important to consider when learning classification rules.

In total, we propose 48 generic features which can be used to form a new feature space for each object $x \in X$: $\tilde{x} = (f_1(x), \ldots, f_8(x))$, where $f_i(x)$ is a value of i-th functional for object x. Subsequently, various classification models can be built. For example, we built a weighted voting classifier based on the defined set of rules.

To evaluate the model, we applied nested cross validation with stratified shuffle split at each step:

- A dataset was randomly split 10 times into tuning and test sets with ratio of 80:20;
- A tuning set was also randomly split 10 times into training and validation sets with ratio of 80:20;
- For each set of hyperparameters and each pair of training and validation sets a model was built and evaluated. At the end of the tuning process there was one set of hyperparameters, which allowed to achieve the best average score on the validation sets. The model was trained with the selected hyperparameters on the entire tuning set and evaluated on the test set;
- The final score of the model is the average score on the test sets.

The results are presented in Tables 4 and 5. It is seen that the proposed features can be used for building sufficiently efficient classification models, which can provide an explanation of results.

Table 4. Weighted voting scores (dataset A).

Metric	Mean	Stdev
G-mean	0.637	0.067
Sensitivity	0.659	0.105
Specificity	0.622	0.085

Table 5. Weighted voting scores (dataset B).

Metric	Mean	Stdev
G-mean	0.858	0.081
Sensitivity	0.841	0.091
Specificity	0.88	0.103

4.3 Neural Network Models

Here the neural networks will no longer directly use the weighted G-mean loss function to optimize the parameters on but instead use a categorical cross entropy function [21] to measure the error of the network. The weighted G-mean loss was not used because it is not possible to obtain a differentiable global G-mean loss on batch operations. However, to be able to compare the results to that obtained in the non-neural networks a non-weighted G-mean batch-wise loss function was applied. Also, to be able to obtain a respective weighted loss value from the batch-wise loss function class weight balancing was preferred over oversampling. Additionally, it was used as an early stopping criteria on the validation set. Its implementation is the same as that of a normal G-mean loss function and was executed at the end of each batch, which was set to a size of 50 samples, during training and obtained the average at the end of each epoch.

By using categorical cross entropy, the class labels were transformed to binary values by applying one-hot encoding. Hence, the classes were represented as vectors with the low risk class (0) as (1, 0) and the high risk (1) as (0, 1). Additionally, the loss function assumes that the passed input represents the probability for each encoding to be true. That is, it expects a vector which sums to 1 and each individual value is within [0, 1]. For the network to oblige by this constraint, the output layer's activation function used was a softmax function [7] which from a vector of real numbers outputs a probability distribution. The optimal hyperparameters were found through the usage of grid search based on the validation results of the G-mean loss. Additionally, the architecture which includes the number of layers and neurons, activation functions, optimizers and regularization methods were determined through experimentation with a variety of combinations. All the networks were implemented using Keras [16] with Tensorflow [1] backend.

Cascade Correlation Neural Network. On this specific dataset, the best performing diagnostic model concluded from a variety of models from a previous research [64] was a Cascade Correlation Neural Network (CCNN) [23]. Subsequent goal here is to further explore and improve the CCNN. For the evaluation, the previous network will be reimplemented so results are comparable. This model will be distinguished as the base CCNN model. Further, taking advantage of the previously positive results, another two variations are being proposed in this paper and are defined as improved and extended CCNN models, in an attempt to further refine the results.

The CCNN was proposed by Fahlman and Lebiere (1990) as an approach that is not only limited to tuning the parameters of the network but also dynamically determining the optimal architecture, constraint to the number of hidden layers. The network initially consists of a fully connected input and output layers, which their size is defined by the problem. Then the algorithm executes repeatedly these following steps until convergence:

- All weights of units connected to the output layer are trained until the minimum error is reached;
- A pool of candidate units is generated which have as input the output of all previously added layers excluding the output layer;
- These candidate units are trained such that their output maximizes the correlation coefficient between the residual error of the network;
- The candidate that has the maximum correlation is selected to be added to the network. Its input weights are frozen and its output is connected with the output layer.

The network continues this iterative process until the addition of a unit does not lead to a smaller error than the previous execution.

The base CCNN model reflects closely to the initially proposed algorithm [23] with some minor changes over and above those mentioned in Sect. 4.3. The hidden and candidate units used the sigmoid function as their activation function. Additionally, the weights were initialized randomly from a normal distribution which had a mean of 0 and standard deviation of 0.5 and the bias was set to 0. After every loop the weights of the output layer were reinitialized to avoid being stuck at bad local minimums. Furthermore, the optimization function used was Stochastic Gradient Descent (SGD) [10]. Its learning rate was set to 0.00001 and 0.000005 for the output and hidden candidate layers respectively. Noting that in the previous research [64] the authors used Simulated Annealing, but SGD was preferred in expectation of better generalization. Finally, the candidate pool size was set to 16 and each candidate layer had two units, the same as the output layer.

For the proposed improved model, only the differences from the base one will be noted. The focus of this CCNN model is to utilize more recent techniques to improve performance. Firstly, the weight initialization scheme was changed from random distribution to Xavier [28] sampling from a normal distribution. Also, the optimizer was changed to Adam [34] as a further improvement to SGD. Its learning rate was set to 0.00001 and 0.000005 for the output and candidate layers respectively. For both cases, the decay of first-order gradient to 0.9, decay of second-order gradient to 0.99 and a small epsilon of 1e−08. Additionally, the activation functions of the hidden layers were changed to Rectified Linear Units (ReLUs) [47]. Lastly, for the output layer warm-start weight initialization was added to carry over weights that contributed the most to lowering the loss value.

The extended model, building from the improved model, focused on further expanding the capabilities of dynamically constructing the architecture by also introducing regularization layers to the pool in an attempt to improve generalization. The hidden candidate layer was changed to have the following format and order:

- Gaussian noise layer with a mean of 0 and a standard deviation of 0.5;
- Dense layer (original unit);
- Batch normalization layer [32] with momentum at 0.99, epsilon at 0.00001 and a trainable beta value;
- Dropout layer [59], which randomly drops one of the two units.

The candidate pool consisted twice of all possible combinations of the regularization layers, while strictly maintaining the order presented. Thus, the total pool size was maintained to 16 with only two candidate layers being the same in comparison to all 16 in the two previous models.

Based on the G-mean loss value on the test set the best performer from the CCNNs was the improved variation with a value of 0.5417, accuracy of 0.5541, sensitivity of 0.6207 and specificity of 0.375. A marginal difference followed the extended model with G-mean loss of 0.5495 and lastly the base model with a value of 0.5889. The full summary of the results on the test set can be found in Table 6.

On the validation results there is a significant point to note out. The G-mean loss value obtained by the models on the validation set were 0.3512, 0.2677, 0.1578 for the base, improved and extended models respectively. The extended model was able to extract more information from the training set to improve its score on that of the validation. However, having nearly the same score as the top performer, there was at least no loss of information compared to the improved model, but the recognition of patterns that were useful on the validation set were not carried over for the test set. This is possibly due to the fact that the dataset contains considerable number of unique cases in such a small sample. This in turn prevents separation of the data in such a way that each set samples from the possible distribution of the problem. Also, it is highly likely that with each proposed variation they suffered more from overfitting on the validation set.

Table 6. Summary of the results on the test set for the neural network models [26].

Model	G-mean loss	Accuracy	Sensitivity	Specificity
Base CCNN	0.5889	0.4324	0.4483	0.375
Improved CCNN	0.5417	0.5541	0.6207	0.3125
Extended CCNN	0.5495	0.5405	0.6034	0.3125
Deep Neural Network	0.2843	0.7703	0.8103	0.625
Convolutional Neural Network	0.3637	0.6081	0.5862	0.6875

Deep Neural Network. A Deep Neural Network (DNN) was also constructed to compare the performance of the cascade networks. Specifically, it was used to evaluate the results, training speed and memory usage between the models. The design of the DNN was based on the results obtained previously in Sect. 4.3. Thus, the network will also focus on using various generalization methods.

The DNN's hidden layers used ReLU for their activation function and their weights were initialized used Xavier's method. Also, the optimizer used was Adam with a learning rate of 0.00005, the decay of first-order gradient at 0.9, decay of second-order gradient at 0.999 and an epsilon value at $1e-8$. For regularization, Gaussian noise layers, with a standard deviation of 0.2 and mean of 0, and dropout layers, with 20% dropout rate, were included in the model. Additionally, batch normalization layers were added with momentum set to 0.99, epsilon to 0.00001 and a trainable beta value. Lastly, details described in Sect. 4.3 still apply here. The final layout of the network consists of five hidden layers, excluding the input and output layers. The network's architecture is described in a previous publication [26].

The DNN was able to obtain a G-mean loss of 0.2843, accuracy of 0.7703, sensitivity of 0.8103 and specificity of 0.625 on the test set, as shown in Table 6. The results obtained are significantly better than that obtained from the improved CCNN, which had a G-mean loss of 0.5417. It was also able to achieve this with a noticeably faster training time. However, the CCNN model was able to obtain its results requiring less memory, as for it constructed a network with a total of 47 hidden layers with 2 units each based

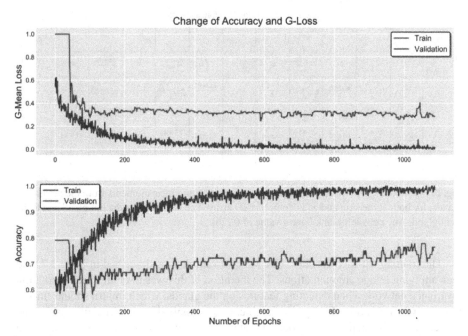

Fig. 2. The average batch-wise G-mean loss and accuracy of the deep neural network as it is trained [26].

on the improved variant. But with today's state of available hardware the memory usage from the DNN is not of a concern.

As seen in Fig. 2, the regularization techniques prevented overfitting the training data against the validation. While the network has extracted all possible information from the training set needed to classify those samples, it does not cover all possible cases in the validation set. The limitation of the model is derived again from the limited available data in expressing an accurate distribution of the problem within the three sets.

Convolutional Neural Network. Convolutional Neural Networks (CNNs) have shown great results for detecting breast cancer using various imaging data [3, 17, 58]. In an attempt to further improve the results of the DNN, a CNN model was also explored. Its design was based on the previously obtained results with higher focus around its ability to generalize.

Building a CNN implies that the input will be a 2D image with one or more channels. Thus, the input vector was transformed to a 2D image with two channels. The channels were used to represent the measured data at the skin and at a depth. The image itself will be of size 13×6 containing the normalized measurements from both glands and axillary points. The positioning on the image resembles closely to that of Fig. 1, while also obtaining the average of neighboring positions to better represent the overlap as depicted in Fig. 3. The values, before being formed to an image representation, they were centered using a robust scaler based on the interquartile range to maintain outliers.

Image Transformation Calculations

$L9$											$R9$
$L8$	$\frac{L8+L1}{2}$	$L1$	$\frac{L1+L2}{2}$	$L2$		$R2$	$\frac{R2+R1}{2}$	$R1$	$\frac{R1+R8}{2}$	$R8$	
$\frac{L7+L8}{2}$	$\frac{L0+L1+L7+L8}{4}$	$\frac{L0+L1}{2}$	$\frac{L0+L1+L2+L3}{4}$	$\frac{L2+L3}{2}$		$\frac{R3+R2}{2}$	$\frac{R0+R1+R2+R3}{4}$	$\frac{R0+R1}{2}$	$\frac{R0+R1+R7+R8}{4}$	$\frac{R8+R7}{2}$	
$L7$	$\frac{L0+L7}{2}$	$L0$	$\frac{L0+L3}{2}$	$L3$		$R3$	$\frac{R0+R3}{2}$	$R0$	$\frac{R0+R4}{2}$	$R7$	
$\frac{L6+L7}{2}$	$\frac{L0+L5+L6+L7}{4}$	$\frac{L0+L5}{2}$	$\frac{L0+L3+L4+L5}{4}$	$L3+L4 \over 2$		$\frac{R4+R3}{2}$	$\frac{R0+R3+R4+R5}{4}$	$\frac{R0+R5}{2}$	$\frac{R0+R5+R6+R7}{4}$	$\frac{R7+R6}{2}$	
$L6$	$\frac{L5+L6}{2}$	$L5$	$\frac{L4+L5}{2}$	$L4$		$R4$	$\frac{R5+R4}{2}$	$R5$	$\frac{R6+R5}{2}$	$R6$	

Fig. 3. Methodology in transforming a vector of temperature measurements from the mammary glands, for both at the skin and at a depth, to a 2D array. The L represents the left gland and R the right gland. Any cells left blank have a value of 0 [26].

The training set used for the CNN was oversampled, as described in Sect. 3.2, and then applying image augmentations. The intention of this was to obtain a more rotation invariance network when detecting features on the glands, which in turn should further improve generalization. The type of augmentations applied were image flipping on the vertical axis and rotations of the outer pointer of the mammary glands. The result was a total of 5472 samples split equally between low and high risk for the training set.

The hidden layers of the network used ReLU activation functions and Adam optimizer with a learning rate of 0.0000005, decay of first-order gradient at 0.9, decay of second-order gradient at 0.999 and epsilon at 1e−8. Additionally, the weights of all the layers were initialized using the Xavier method from a uniform distribution. The type of layers used were dense, convolutional [40], separable convolution [15], max pooling [40], global average pooling [42], dropout, spatial dropout [60], batch normalization and Gaussian noise. The convolution and pooling layers used a kernel of size 3 × 3, stride of 1 with the exception of spatial which used 2, padding set to same and no bias value. Lastly, all dropout layers had a dropout percentage of 20%. The full network architecture in defined in a previous paper [26].

The CNN obtained a G-mean loss value of 0.3637, accuracy of 0.681, sensitivity of 0.5862 and specificity of 0.6875, which are included in Table 6. The network was not able to outperform that of the DNN based on the G-mean loss but did obtain the highest specificity rate from all other models. Additionally, the Fig. 4 shows the training and validation G-mean loss and accuracy as the training of the network progresses. With the addition of augmentation it should of helped with generalization, but there was still some slight overfitting of the training set against the validation. Finally, there is a similar pattern as before where limited information from the training set can be generalized to the validation.

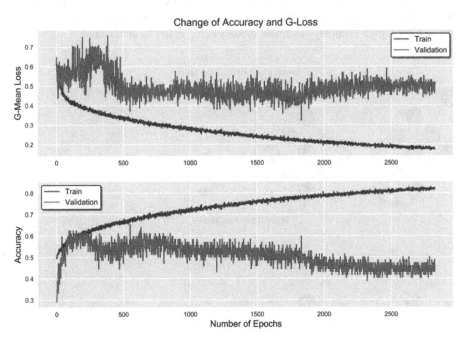

Fig. 4. The average batch-wise G-mean loss and accuracy of the convolutional neural network as it is trained [26].

5   Model Interpretation

Statistical results on the test set are useful for evaluating the generalizability and future capabilities of the model selected. However, the dataset used during development will highly likely not represent the whole population and thus limits the confidence on relying on such results alone. Such cases can take the form of lack of data on pathologies/conditions and not fully representing the diversity of people. These are over and above the expected inaccuracies of the model. In addition, the 'black-box' usage of machine learning algorithms brings a lot of concerns on the legality of their usage and what ethical implications they might have [56]. Understanding what a model does is being for the most part limited during development. Hence, such results on their own are insufficient to offer significant levels of confidence when making critical decisions for a patient.

Developing a diagnostic system is not only crucial in making accurate predictions but also give a reason to why such an output was given. In recent years, there have been made some steps to improve the interpretability of complex models such as local interpretable model-agnostic explanations (LIME) [51] and shapley additive explanations (SHAP) [45]. Before such approaches were developed, the options were either sacrifice predictive performance or interpretability, with more complex models like deep neural networks usually offer higher accuracy but linear models being easier to understand.

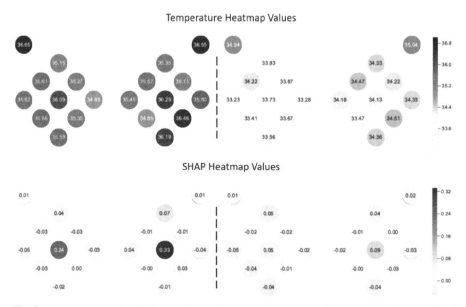

Fig. 5. Temperature and SHAP values for a single sample represented as heatmaps. The positional representation is as depicted in Fig. 1. The top figure indicates the temperature values, while the lower the SHAP values obtained using deepSHAP. For each of the figures, the left side represents the inner values and the right side the surface values obtained. This specific case is labeled as high risk and was predicted as such.

Such an explanation model was used for this application and specifically the deepSHAP approach available from the SHAP library [45]. An example of results from deepSHAP are shown in Fig. 5, in which the base model used is that of the proposed deep neural network. The results indicate which of the input features contributed positively or negatively to the final decision, which for this case it is correctly predicted as high risk.

The interpretability approaches mentioned require the creation of an addition model, the explanation model, which is an approximation of the model used to create the predictions. It is limited to indicating which features contributed to the prediction but not the relationship between the features. However, as described in Sect. 4.2, this is not the case for the rule based classification approach. The model determines a new set of highly informative features, which either capture key individual points or the relationship between points that contribute to the final decision. In addition, it is a self-explanatory model in its decision making.

6 Conclusions and Future Work

The top performing models introduced in this paper is the rule based classification (4.2) and the DNN (4.5). The DNN obtained a weighted G-mean loss of 0.2843 on the test set. On the other hand, the rule based approach obtained 0.363 and 0.142 G-mean loss on the dataset A and B respectively. Following in third was the CNN with a loss value of 0.3637. These two approaches are not directly comparable because the dataset was handle differently, but offer a strong indication of their capabilities.

While the results obtained show potential for the models to be included as part of a diagnostic system, they utilized only information from readings from microwave radiometry. For implementing a complete diagnostic system, it will benefit from developing a model that incorporates a broader range of information. Including information from other devices or systems and data directly inputted from clinical professionals about the physiological condition of the patient [61], can potentially further improve model accuracy.

Out of the models presented, the rule based classification method offers the most reasoning into its decisions. While for the other models an external ad hoc solution was used which is limited to showing which feature, temperature point for this case, have contributed positively to the final prediction. The informativeness for both cases can be further improved by expanding the classification problem. As more descriptive and broader data becomes available it can be expanded from a binary to a multi-class task. Some possible labels are benign and malignant tumors, noncancerous tumors, inflammation, infection and healthy patients. Additionally, it will be interesting to investigate additional interpretability methods that focus on high level concepts, such as Testing with Concept Activation Vectors (TCAV) [35], and evaluate if they are capable of extracting similar information to the rule based approach.

Despite the fact that thermometric data are objective, the diagnosis based on data substantially depends on experience of doctor and is largely subjective. The latter significantly restricts unique capabilities of microwave radiometry in early diagnosis. This problem is not a specific feature of microwave radiometry. In many cases an appliance of modern medical equipment, while solving some problems, can give rise to the others. Often, difficulties of diagnostics arise not because of a lack of information, but because of insufficient methods for processing it. To some extent, a solution of these problems can be provided by the development of systems for the interpretation and analysis of medical data. At the same time, the greatest interest is aroused by the development of diagnostic advisory systems, i.e. expert systems, which contain a mechanism for explaining and justifying proposed solutions in a user-friendly language. Thus, the urgent task is a development of an expert system that provides high sensitivity and specificity of diagnostics and, at the same time, has the ability to justify a proposed solution. A particular complexity of this problem is caused by the finding of highly informative features of diseases. As noted by most experts, the performance of classification algorithms is affected by the qualitative and quantitative composition of the informational feature space. In this paper, a new method is proposed for constructing a feature space, that is based on validated and tested hypotheses about the behavior of temperature fields of mammary glands. An obtained set of thermometric features allows to simultaneously propose a diagnostic solution based on artificial intelligence algorithms, as well as justify it in terms that are understandable to a doctor.

References

1. Abadi, M., et al.: TensorFlow: a system for large-scale machine learning. In: Proceedings of the 12th USENIX Conference on Operating Systems Design and Implementation, OSDI 2016, pp. 265–283. USENIX Association, Berkeley (2016)
2. Anisimova, E.V., Zamechnik, T.V., Larin, S.I., Losev, A.G.: Teoreticheskie issledovaniya otdelnih fizicheskih i fiziologicheskih faktorov vliyayuschih na kachestvo obsledovaniya pacientov s varikoznoi boleznyu ven nijnih konechnostei metodom kombinirovannoi termografii [the theoretical research of separate physical and physiological factors influencing the quality of checking up patients with venous varicosity of lower extremities by the method of combined thermography]. Vestnik novih medicinskih tehnologii [J. New Med. Technol.] **18**(4), 280–282 (2011)
3. Arajo, T., et al.: Classification of breast cancer histology images using convolutional neural networks. PLoS ONE **12**(6), 1–14 (2017)
4. Barandela, R., Sanchez, J., Garca, V., Rangel, E.: Strategies for learning in class imbalance problems. Pattern Recogn. **36**, 849–851 (2003)
5. Bergstra, J., Bardenet, R., Bengio, Y., Kégl, B.: Algorithms for hyper-parameter optimization. In: Proceedings of the 24th International Conference on Neural Information Processing Systems, NIPS 2011, pp. 2546–2554. Curran Associates Inc., USA (2011)
6. Bergstra, J., Yamins, D., Cox, D.D.: Hyperopt: a python library for optimizing the hyperparameters of machine learning algorithms (2015)
7. Bishop, C.M.: Pattern Recognition and Machine Learning. Information Science and Statistics. Springer, Heidelberg (2006)
8. Bochkarev, O.A., Zenovich, A.V., Losev, A.G.: Regressionnaya model diagnostiky patologiy molochnykh zhelez po dannym mikrovolnovoy radiotermometrii [regression model for diagnosis of breast pathology according to microwaves radiometry data]. Vestnik Volgogradskogo gosudarstvennogo universiteta. Seriya 1. Mathematica. Physica [Sci. J. Volgograd State Uni. Math. Phy.] **6**(31), 72–82 (2015)
9. Bondar, S.S., Terekhov, I.V., Voevodin, A.A., Leonov, B.I., Khadartsev, A.A.: Assessment of transcapillary water exchange in the lungs by active radiometry. Biomed. Eng. **51**(3), 211–214 (2017)

10. Bottou, L.: Large-scale machine learning with stochastic gradient descent. In: Lechevallier, Y., Saporta, G. (eds.) Proceedings of COMPSTAT 2010, pp. 177–186. Physica-Verlag, Heidelberg (2010). https://doi.org/10.1007/978-3-7908-2604-3_16

11. Breiman, L.: Random forests. Mach. Learn. **45**(1), 5–32 (2001)

12. Burges, C.J.C.: A tutorial on support vector machines for pattern recognition. Data Min. Knowl. Disc. **2**, 121–167 (1998)

13. Chawla, N.V., Bowyer, K.W., Hall, L.O., Kegelmeyer, W.P.: SMOTE: synthetic minority oversampling technique. J. Artif. Int. Res. **16**(1), 321–357 (2002)

14. Chen, T., Guestrin, C.: XGBoost: a scalable tree boosting system. In: Proceedings of the 22nd ACM SIGKDD International Conference on Knowledge Discovery and Data Mining, KDD 2016, pp. 785–794. ACM, New York (2016)

15. Chollet, F.: Xception: Deep learning with depthwise separable convolutions. CoRR, abs/1610.02357 (2016)

16. Chollet, F., et al.: Keras (2015). https://keras.io

17. Cireşan, D.C., Giusti, A., Gambardella, L.M., Schmidhuber, J.: Mitosis detection in breast cancer histology images with deep neural networks. In: Mori, K., Sakuma, I., Sato, Y., Barillot, C., Navab, N. (eds.) MICCAI 2013. LNCS, vol. 8150, pp. 411–418. Springer, Heidelberg (2013). https://doi.org/10.1007/978-3-642-40763-5_51

18. Cortes, C., Vapnik, V.: Support-vector networks. Mach. Learn. **20**(3), 273–297 (1995)

19. Cover, T., Hart, P.: Nearest neighbor pattern classification. IEEE Trans. Inf. Theor. **13**(1), 21–27 (2006)

20. Crandall, J.P., et al.: Measurement of brown adipose tissue activity using microwave radiometry and 18F-FDG PET/CT. J. Nucl. Med. **59**(8), 1243–1248 (2018)

21. de Boer, P.-T., Kroese, D.P., Mannor, S., Rubinstein, R.Y.: A tutorial on the cross-entropy method. Ann. Oper. Res. **134**(1), 19–67 (2005)

22. Drakopoulou, M., Moldovan, C., Toutouzas, K., Tousoulis, D.: The role of microwave radiometry in carotid artery disease diagnostic and clinical prospective. Curr. Opin. Pharmacol. **39**, 99–104 (2018)

23. Fahlman, S.E., Lebiere, C.: The cascade-correlation learning architecture. In: Advances in Neural Information Processing Systems 2, pp. 524–532. Morgan Kaufmann Publishers Inc., San Francisco (1990)

24. Gabriel, S., Lau, R.W., Gabriel, C.: The dielectric properties of biological tissues: II. Measurements in the frequency range 10 Hz to 20 GHz. Phys. Med. Biol. **41**(11), 2251 (1996)

25. Gabriel, S., Lau, R.W., Gabriel, C.: The dielectric properties of biological tissues: III. Parametric models for the dielectric spectrum of tissues. Phys. Med. Biol. **41**(11), 2271 (1996)

26. Galazis, C., Vesnin, S., Goryanin, I.: Application of artificial intelligence in microwave radiometry (MWR). In: Proceedings of the 12th International Joint Conference on Biomedical Engineering Systems and Technologies, vol. 3, pp. 112–122 (2019). https://doi.org/10.5220/0007567901120122

27. Gautherie, M.: Thermopathology of breast cancer: measurement and analysis of in vivo temperature and blood flow. Ann. N. Y. Acad. Sci. **335**(1), 383–415 (1980)

28. Glorot, X., Bengio, Y.: Understanding the difficulty of training deep feedforward neural networks. In: Teh, Y.W., Titterington, M. (eds.) Proceedings of the Thirteenth International Conference on Artificial Intelligence and Statistics. Proceedings of Machine Learning Research, vol. 9, pp. 249–256. PMLR, Sardinia (2010)

29. Han, H., Wang, W.-Y., Mao, B.-H.: Borderline-SMOTE: a new over-sampling method in imbalanced data sets learning. In: Huang, D.-S., Zhang, X.-P., Huang, G.-B. (eds.) ICIC 2005. LNCS, vol. 3644, pp. 878–887. Springer, Heidelberg (2005). https://doi.org/10.1007/11538059_91

30. He, H., Bai, Y., Garcia, E.A., Li, S.: ADASYN: adaptive synthetic sampling approach for imbalanced learning. In: 2008 IEEE International Joint Conference on Neural Networks (IEEE World Congress on Computational Intelligence), pp. 1322–1328 (2008)
31. He, H., Ma, Y.: Imbalanced Learning: Foundations, Algorithms, and Applications, 1st edn. Wiley-IEEE Press (2013)
32. Ioffe, S., Szegedy, C.: Batch normalization: accelerating deep network training by reducing internal covariate shift. CoRR, abs/1502.03167 (2015)
33. Ivanov, Y., et al.: Use of microwave radiometry to monitor thermal denaturation of albumin. Front. Physiol. **9**, 956 (2018)
34. Kingma, D.P., Ba, J.: Adam: a method for stochastic optimization. CoRR, abs/1412.6980 (2014)
35. Kim, B., et al.: Interpretability beyond feature attribution: quantitative testing with concept activation vectors (TCAV). In: International Conference on Machine Learning (2018)
36. Kobrinskii, B.A.: Konsul'tativnye intellektual'nye medicinskie sistemy: klassifikaciya, principy postroeniya, effektivnost' [Advisory intelligent medical systems: classification, principles of construction, efficiency]. Vrach i informacionnye tekhnologii [Inf. Technol. Phys.] **2**, 38–47 (2008)
37. Krawczyk, B.: Learning from imbalanced data: open challenges and future directions. Prog. Artif. Intell. **5**(4), 221–232 (2016)
38. Kubat, M., Matwin, S.: Addressing the curse of imbalanced training sets: one-sided selection. In: Proceedings of the Fourteenth International Conference on Machine Learning, pp. 179–186. Morgan Kaufmann (1997)
39. Laskari, K., Pitsilka, D., Pentazos, G., Siores, E., Tektonidou, M., Sfikakis, P.: SAT0657 microwave radiometry-derived thermal changes of sacroiliac joints as a biomarker of sacroiliitis in patients with spondyloarthropathy. Ann. Rheum. Dis. **77**(Suppl. 2), 1178 (2018)
40. Lecun, Y., Bengio, Y., Hinton, G.: Deep learning. Nature **521**(7553), 436–444 (2015)
41. Lim, T.-S., Loh, W.-Y., Shih, Y.-S.: A comparison of prediction accuracy, complexity, and training time of thirty-three old and new classification algorithms. Mach. Learn. **40**(3), 203–228 (2000)
42. Lin, M., Chen, Q., Yan, S.: Network in network. CoRR, abs/1312.4400 (2013)
43. Losev, A.G., Mazepa, E.A., Suleymanova, Kh.M.: O vzaimosvyazi nekotorykh priznakov RTM-diagnostiki zabolevaniy molochnykh zhelez [on interrelation of some signs of RTM diagnostics of mammary glands deseases]. Vestnik Volgogradskogo gosudarstvennogo universiteta. Seriya 1. Mathematica. Physica [Sci. J. Volgograd State Univ. Math. Phy.] **4**(229), 35–44 (2015)
44. Losev, A.G., Levshinskii, V.V.: Intellektual'nyj analiz dannyh mikrovolnovoj radiotermometrii v diagnostike raka molochnoj zhelezy [Data mining of microwave radiometry data in the diagnosis of breast cancer]. Matematicheskaya fizika i komp'yuternoe modelirovanie [Math. Phys. Comput. Simul.] **20**(5), 49–62 (2017)
45. Lundberg, S., Lee, S.-I.: A unified approach to interpreting model predictions. CoRR, abs/1705.07874 (2017)
46. Mazepa, E.A., Suleymanova, Kh.M.: Ob optimizacii chisla diagnosticheskih priznakov zabolevanii molochnih jelez na osnove termometricheskih dannih [On optimization of the number of diagnostic signs for breast diseases through thermometric data]. Vestnik Volgogradskogo gosudarstvennogo universiteta. Seriya 1. Mathematica. Physica [Sci. J. Volgograd State Univ. Math. Phys.] **6**(37), 128–140 (2016)
47. Nair, V., Hinton, G.E.: Rectified linear units improve restricted boltzmann machines. In: Proceedings of the 27th International Conference on International Conference on Machine Learning, ICML 2010, pp. 807–814. Omnipress, USA (2010)
48. Pedregosa, F., et al.: Scikit-learn: machine learning in python. J. Mach. Learn. Res. **12**, 2825–2830 (2011)

49. Pentazos, G., Laskari, K., Prekas, K., Raftakis, J., Sfikakis, P., Siores, E.: Microwave radiometry-derived thermal changes of small joints as additional potential biomarker in rheumatoid arthritis: a prospective pilot study. J. Clin. Rheumatol. **24**(1), 259–263 (2018)

50. Polyakov, M.V., Khoperskov, A.V., Zamechnic, T.V.: Numerical modeling of the internal temperature in the mammary gland. In: Siuly, S., et al. (eds.) HIS 2017. LNCS, vol. 10594, pp. 128–135. Springer, Cham (2017). https://doi.org/10.1007/978-3-319-69182-4_14

51. Ribeiro, M.T., Singh, S., Guestrin, C.: "Why Should I Trust You?": explaining the predictions of any classifier. In: Proceedings of the 22nd ACM SIGKDD International Conference on Knowledge Discovery and Data Mining (KDD 2016), pp. 1135–1144. ACM, New York (2016). https://doi.org/10.1145/2939672.2939778

52. Rodrigues, D.B., et al.: Numerical 3D modeling of heat transfer in human tissues for microwave radiometry monitoring of brown fat metabolism. In: Proceeding of SPIE, vol. 8584 (2013)

53. Rodrigues, D.B., Stauffer, P.R., Pereira, P.J.S., Maccarini, P.F.: Microwave radiometry for noninvasive monitoring of brain temperature. In: Crocco, L., Karanasiou, I., James, M.L., Conceição, R.C. (eds.) Emerging Electromagnetic Technologies for Brain Diseases Diagnostics, Monitoring and Therapy, pp. 87–127. Springer, Cham (2018). https://doi.org/10.1007/978-3-319-75007-1_5

54. Saniei, E., Setayeshi, S., Akbari, M.E., Navid, M.: Parameter estimation of breast tumour using dynamic neural network from thermal pattern. J. Adv. Res. **7**(6), 1045–1055 (2016)

55. Schneider, B.P., Miller, K.D.: Angiogenesis of breast cancer. J. Clin. Oncol. **23**(8), 1782–1790 (2005). PMID: 15755986

56. Schönberger, D.: Artificial intelligence in healthcare: a critical analysis of the legal and ethical implications. Int. J. Law Inf. Technol. **27**(2), 171–203 (2019). https://doi.org/10.1093/ijlit/eaz004

57. Semenov, S.: Microwave tomography: review of the progress towards clinical applications. Philos. Trans. Math. Phys. Eng. Sci. **367**(1900), 3021–3042 (2009)

58. Spanhol, F.A., Oliveira, L.S., Petitjean, C., Heutte, L.: Breast cancer histopathological image classification using convolutional neural networks. In: 2016 International Joint Conference on Neural Networks (IJCNN), pp. 2560–2567 (2016)

59. Srivastava, N., Hinton, G., Krizhevsky, A., Sutskever, I., Salakhutdinov, R.: Dropout: a simple way to prevent neural networks from overfitting. J. Mach. Learn. Res. **15**, 1929–1958 (2014)

60. Tompson, J., Goroshin, R., Jain, A., LeCun, Y., Bregler, C.: Efficient object localization using convolutional networks. CoRR, abs/1411.4280 (2014)

61. Wilkins, M.F., Boddy, L., Morris, C.W., Jonker, R.: A comparison of some neural and non-neural methods for identification of phytoplankton from flow cytometry data. Bioinformatics **12**(1), 9–18 (1996)

62. Zamechnik, T.V., Larin, S.I., Losev, A.G.: Kombinirovannaya radiotermometriya kak metod issledovaniya venoznogo krovoobrascheniya nijnih konechnostei [Combined radiothermometry as a method for the study of venous circulation of the lower extremities] Volgograd. 252 p. (2015)

63. Zamechnik, T.V., Mazepa, E.A., Cherkesova, S.I., Pankova, J.V.: K voprosu ob optimizacii skriningovogo obsledovaniya molochnih jelez metodom mikrovolnovoi radiotermometrii [About the optimization of breast screening by means of microwave radiothermometry]. J. New Med. Technol. **21**(4), 34–38 (2014)

64. Zenovich, A.V., Glazunov, V.A., Oparin, A.S., Primachenko, F.G.: Algoritmy prinyatiya resheniy v konsultativnoy intellektualnoy sisteme diagnostiki molochnykh zhelez [Algorithms of decision-making in the advisory intellectual system of diagnostics of mammary glands]. Math. Phys. Comput. Model. **6**, 129–142 (2016)

65. Zenovich, A.V., Grebnev, V.I., Primachenko, F.G.: Algoritmy klassifikacii zabolevanij parnyh organov na osnove nejrosetej i nechetkih mnozhestv [Algorithms for the classification of diseases of paired organs on the basis of neural networks and fuzzy sets]. Matematicheskaya fizika i komp'yuternoe modelirovanie [Math. Phys. Comput. Simul.] **20**(6), 26–37 (2017)
66. Vesnin, S., Turnbull, A.K., Dixon, J.M., Goryanin, I.: Modern microwave thermometry for breast cancer. J. Mol. Imaging Dyn. **7**(2) (2017). https://doi.org/10.4172/2155-9937.1000136
67. Zadeh, H.G., Montazeri, A., Kazerouni, I.A., Haddadnia, J.: Clustering and screening for breast cancer on thermal images using a combination of SOM and MLP. Comput. Methods Biomech. Biomed. Eng. Imaging Vis. **5**(1), 68–76 (2017)

Bio-inspired Systems and Signal Processing

Special Techniques in Applying Continuous Wavelet Transform to Non-stationary Signals of Heart Rate Variability

Sergey Bozhokin⬤, Irina Suslova$^{(\boxtimes)}$ ⬤, and Daniil Tarakanov

Peter the Great Polytechnic University, Polytechnicheskaya str. 29, Saint-Petersburg, Russia
bsvjob@mail.ru, ibsus@mail.ru, daniil.tarakanov@gmail.com

Abstract. The analysis of heart rate variability (HRV) is central for cardiac diagnostics, but the essential non-stationarity of heart rate has started to gain attention only recently. The aim of this work is to develop a set of special new techniques for calculating mathematical indicators of HRV spectral properties associated with non-stationarity in frequency. The analysis is done both for the new model of a tachogram taking into account frequency modulation and for the true tachogram record during head up tilt test. Continuous wavelet transformation of the frequency-modulated signal (CWT) has been derived in analytical form. The local frequency of heart rhythm giving the maximum of CWT has been determined. Treated as another non-stationary signal, this frequency has been subjected to CWT following double CWT procedure (DCWT). The special algorithm for eliminating boundary effects at the computing CWT is used. The transient periods for local frequency, the frequencies of local frequency fluctuation against the main trend and the periods of emergence and attenuation of such fluctuations have been defined by estimating the spectral integrals in the ranges {ULF, VLF, LF, HF}. The combined use of several new techniques taking into account the non-stationary character of heart rate can provide reliable diagnostic results.

Keywords: Continuous wavelet transform · Boundary effects · Non-stationary heart tachogram

1 Introduction

A great number of signals $Z(t)$ depending on time t and encountered in various branches of science (astrophysics, nuclear physics, electrodynamics, hydrodynamics, solid state physics, radio-physics, biology and medicine) are non-stationary. This means that spectral and statistical properties of such signals vary with time. The traditional Fourier transform (FT) calculating the Fourier component $Z(f)$ of such signals as a function of the frequency f has a serious drawback. The Fourier transform makes it possible to detect the presence of various harmonics in signal $Z(t)$, but does not allow us to trace the time evolution in the emergence and disappearance of local frequencies.

If it is necessary to detect the time variation in the spectral composition of the signal, a certain local interval $[t - W/2, t + W/2]$ is considered instead of the entire

© Springer Nature Switzerland AG 2020
A. Roque et al. (Eds.): BIOSTEC 2019, CCIS 1211, pp. 291–310, 2020.
https://doi.org/10.1007/978-3-030-46970-2_14

time interval $-\infty < t < +\infty$ of integration. The interval (window) is centred at the instant time point t and has duration W. Such a transform is known as the Short Time Fourier transform (STFT). It is known that the rectangular window has a significant drawback. The function of the rectangular window is discontinuous at the borders of this window. Consequently, the Fourier transform with this type of window function oscillates strongly. With increasing frequency, it decreases rather slowly. This leads to the appearance of many side maxima on the graphs of STFT. Such false maxima for a complex signal can distort the frequency localization of the spectral components of the signal. Unlike the rectangular window, the use of the Gaussian window does not lead to the appearance of spurious harmonics (side maxima). For the Gaussian shape window, such a windowed Fourier transform was developed by Gabor (Gabor transform, GT). The disadvantage of the GT is that the success of its application depends on the size W of the window. The choice of the optimal window duration W requires knowledge of the characteristic time scales in which the rearrangement of spectral properties of the signal takes place. Choosing a window with large duration W, it is possible to obtain a high frequency resolution, but the time resolution is poor in this case. A wide window is useful for detecting low frequency components of the signal, but its width is excessive for detecting high frequency harmonics.

A new approach developed for studying non-stationary signals was the wavelet theory that has found wide application in many fields of science [1–6]. The discrete wavelet transform (DWT) with thoroughly elaborated numerical algorithms has been developed comprehensively. Another trend in the wavelet theory is the continuous wavelet transform (CWT), which makes it possible to obtain analytic expressions describing the time variation of spectral properties for many time dependent signals $Z(t)$. The explicit form of the CWT depends on the choice of the mother wavelet function, which plays the role of an adaptive window ensuring a certain resolution both in time and in frequency. The self-adjusted character of the CWT makes it possible to determine automatically the changes in frequency properties, which may appear or disappear at certain time instants t.

The window used for calculating the CWT has a larger width for signals with low frequency components and short time duration, – for high frequency components. It should be noted that in contrast to DWT, the CWT makes it possible to consider any continuous shifts of the center of the mother wavelet both in terms of time t and of frequency ν.

The technique of CWT (continuous wavelet transform) allows us to develop a system of quantitative parameters for analysing non-stationary (NS) signals, with statistical and spectral properties changing in time. The first important operation in the wavelet theory is the scaling procedure, in which we change the region of wavelet function localization in frequency. The second step is the shift operation, in which we change the localization of wavelet function in time. In this way, we can clearly reveal the amplitude-frequency properties of the signals under study. CWT represents three-dimensional surface $V(\nu, t)$ depending on frequency ν and time t. Analytical CWT calculations using the Morlet mother wavelet function show that for harmonic signal $Z(t) = \cos(2\pi f_0 t)$ (f_0 is the frequency), the maximum of $|V(\nu, t)|$ is reached at $\nu = f_0$, and this maximal value does not depend on t. In the case of two infinite harmonic signals with frequencies f_1, f_2 and the same amplitude, we observe the peaks of ridges with the same amplitude $|V(v, t)|$ at points $v = f_1$ and $v = f_2$ [7–11].

The majority of CWT studies use numerical calculations. In this case, the question arises of how accurately CWT reproduces the properties of $Z(t)$ given in the finite interval $t = [0, T]$ (T is the time of observation). The shortcoming of CWT is the finite temporal resolution of the mother wavelet function. This causes boundary effects near the initial and final moments of time, where we can observe significant differences in the amplitude-frequency properties of the original signal $Z(t)$ and its CWT image $V(v, t)$. To correct this drawback and improve the resolution of low frequency signal components in the case of short signal duration, the authors of [12–15] undertook a modification of CWT algorithm. The work [16] presents a discussion of boundary effects depending on the type of the mother wavelet function. The numerical estimation of boundary effects at CWT for real experimental non-stationary signals was carried out in [12–15, 17].

When analysing non-stationary signals in medicine, the development of quantitative parameters to describe heart rate variability is of great importance. Heart rate variability (HRV) inferred from the analysis of the tachogram – a series of RR intervals between heart contractions – is known as an important index in cardio-vascular system assessment (CVS) [5, 18–21]. However, the statistical parameters of HRV (*RRNN, SDNN, RMSSD*), the spectral characteristics of cardio intervals employing the Fourier transform (*ULF, VLF, LF, HF*), and the histogram methods given in the Standards can be used only in stationary situations. The condition of stationarity, meaning the repetition of statistical and spectral characteristics of the cardio signal taken arbitrarily over any time segment, is not fulfilled in the majority of cardiac situations. In particular, it is true of the passive tilt test used in complex assessment of the cardiovascular system (CVS) to elucidate the mechanisms of its autonomous regulation. This test allows good standardization. The passive tilt test is performed on a special automated tilt table, which brings the body from the horizontal into the vertical position. There are two types of orthostatic tests, in which the human head rises (HUT – head up table) and in which the human head falls (HDT – head down table). Tilt tests are used to determine the tolerance of the organism to abrupt changes of a body position in occupational selection (pilots and cosmonauts), prescription of drugs that affect blood redistribution in diagnosing neuro-circulatory disorders, and elucidation of the mechanisms of functional impairment of the autonomous system (ANS), in particular, detecting patients with neuro-cardiac fainting spells (syncope).

The heart rhythm results from the activity of atypical cardiomyocytes of the sinoauricular node, and its rhythmic character is determined by the effect of the autonomic nervous system (ANS), which consists of two subdivisions: the sympathetic nervous system (SNS) accelerates the heart rate and increases the strength of heart beats, while the parasympathetic nervous system (PSNS) exerts the opposite effects.

In respiratory sinus arrhythmia, the heart rate increases during inhalation and decreases during exhalation. The phenomenon is explained by the fact that activity of the vagus nerve, which belongs to the PSNS, falls during inhalation and rises during exhalation. An effect on sinus arrhythmia is additionally exerted by reflexes from baroreceptors, which respond to the blood pressure and contribute to regulating the heart rate and blood pressure. The reactivity of the PSNS is evaluated in a controlled deep breath test with a continuous recording of the cardiogram. A subject lying in a horizontal position is instructed by the researcher to start breathing deeply and regularly at a certain constant rate for several minutes. Deep breath tests make it possible to evaluate the interplay of the heart function and the function of the bulbar respiratory center, which is located in the medulla oblongata, and to assess the function of PSNS regulatory mechanisms. Thus, the heart and breathing rates are synchronized.

In recent years, there has been significant progress in the development of diagnostic methods of arrhythmology and creation of compact antiarrhythmic implantable devices: implantable pacemakers, ICDs (implantable cardioverter defibrillators) and devices for cardiac therapy. The production of artificial pacemakers and devices restoring sinus rhythm in the case of life-threatening arrhythmias requires the development of automated medical diagnostic complexes MCPS, performing the analysis and wireless automatic transfer of the information on myocardial electric instability.

Traditional implantable cardiac pacemakers require systematic visits to the doctor for monitoring and optimizing the functions of implants, long-term ECG scanning for the detection of symptomatic cases in the ECG recording.

Unfortunately, the consequences of late detection of such events can be the progressive arrhythmia, increased risk of stroke, and progressive heart failure.

Permanent remote monitoring can in some cases save the patient's life. In case computer ECG diagnostic techniques are used, it is necessary to develop a system for automatic monitoring and control (correction) of heart rate in real time.

The usual scheme of automated cardio complex consists of the following components:

1) Implantable devices (pacemaker, cardioverter defibrillator, the device for cardiac resynchronization therapy).
2) Internet server, which provides receiving an unlimited number of ECGs, processing, storage and access to the stored data. Information is sent via GPRS, which involves identification and access rights of each remote user.
3) Cardiological experts, who have computers connected to the server, which processes the information.

Thus, the system of information transfer is formed the chain: patient-service center-doctor. The decisions pass the feedback chain: doctor-service center-patient. Automated complex should include a system of permanent analysis of heart rate variability by calculating the characteristic markers in spectral parameters of the tachogram. This type of signal processing requires a correct mathematical model of non-stationary tachogram and a set of quantitative parameters related to the heart rhythm disorders.

The wavelet theory has been successfully applied in HRV studies [5, 22, 23]. Most HRV studies based on the wavelet theory use the models of amplitude-modulated signals, i.e., when the regular sampling interval Δt coincides with the mean RR interval ($\Delta t =$ RRNN). However, in many actual situations, where it is necessary to analyze the cardiac arrhythmia accurately, the time points of heartbeats are spaced very irregularly. Thus, developing of new models to study the transitional processes in the heart rhythm, which occur very often, for example, at tilt tests, remains a pressing problem.

We propose here that the HRV signal is a superposition of the Gaussian peaks of the same amplitude. The centres of heart beats separated by RR_n time intervals are located on a very irregular grid, which is characterized by time points t_n, where $t_n = t_{n-1} + RR_n$, $n = 1, 2, 3, \ldots, N-1$, and $t_0 = RR_0$. These time points strictly correspond to the time points of the actual RR intervals. The advantage of the approach is that the new tachogram model considers frequency modulated signals and provides an analytical solution using CWT with the Morlet mother wavelet function. The maximal CWT value corresponds to the value of local frequency function $F_{\max}(t)$. Applying the second CWT (DCWT) for the signal $F_{\max}(t)$ allows us to study both aperiodic and oscillatory movements of the local frequency in *ULF, VLF, LF, HF* spectral ranges.

In this work we use a new model of the heart tachogram [7], the double wavelet transform method with the Morlet mother wavelet function [24], the analysis of spectral integrals [9], and a special technique of removing edge effects [17]. We focused on the combined use of several new techniques (DCWT, frequency modulated model, spectral integrals, STS), which provides a reliable assessment of heart rate variability. All these methods together provide an opportunity to describe accurately non-stationary heart rate during real diagnostic manipulations. In this paper, the main attention is paid to the quantitative description of the unsteady tachogram. The quantitative parameters of real tachograms, which describe the violations in heart rhythm, are introduced and analyzed in detail. The article discusses the use of the proposed methods as a part of automated medical complexes (MCPS-Medical Cyber-Physical Systems).

2 Methods

2.1 Mathematical Model of Non-stationary Signal

We consider nonstationary signal $Z(t)$ with the amplitude varying strongly in time. The characteristic feature of the proposed model is the complex behavior of the signal amplitude at the edges of time interval. We represent $Z(t)$ as a superposition of N elementary nonstationary signals (ENS)

$$Z(t) = \sum_{L=0}^{N-1} z_L(t - t_L). \tag{1}$$

centered in the points $t = t_L$ and determined by the system of L parameters. The signal $z_L(t - t_L)$ in (1) has the shape of the Gaussian envelope of oscillating function [7]

$$z_L(t - t_L) = \frac{b_L}{2\sqrt{\pi}\tau_L} \exp\left[-\frac{(t - t_L)^2}{4\tau_L^2}\right] \cos[2\pi f_L(t - t_L) + \alpha_L]. \tag{2}$$

Five parameters

$$L = (b_L; f_L; t_L; \tau_L; \alpha_L), \tag{3}$$

which determine the ENS, are: the amplitude b_L having the dimensions (*volt* × *second*); the frequency of oscillations f_L in (*Hz*); the characteristic size τ_L of signal time local-ization in (*s*); the initial phase α_L in radians. Hereinafter, we assume that the condition

$f_L \tau_L \gg 1$ holds for all ENS considered in the present paper. This means that time interval τ_L, which equals to the characteristic scale of amplitude decreasing, covers many oscillation periods $T_L = 1/f_L$.

As an example, we consider the signal $Z(t)$ (1) represented by four ENS (2) at $L = 0, 1, 2, 3$. Suppose the frequencies of all signals equal $f_L = 2$ Hz, and their phases have zero values.

Table 1 [17] displays all other parameters of the ENS. The parameters in Table 1 are chosen in such a way that the total signal has the form

$$Z(t) = B(t) \cos(2\pi f_0 t), \tag{4}$$

where $f_0 = 2$ Hz.

Table 1. The parameters of four *ENS* in (1).

L	b_L (s)	t_L (s)	τ_L (s)
0	-0.3	3	0.75
1	$10\sqrt{\pi}$	25	5
2	$-10\sqrt{\pi}$	25	4.5
3	-0.3	47	0.75

The value of $B(t)$ can be represented in the form

$$B(t) = \frac{1}{2\sqrt{\pi}} \sum_{L=0}^{N-1} \frac{b_L}{\tau_L} \exp\left[-\frac{(t - t_L)^2}{4\tau_L^2}\right] \tag{5}$$

Let us introduce the notations

$$A(t) = |B(t)|, \quad A(t)/A_m, \tag{6}$$

where A_m is the maximal value of the amplitude.

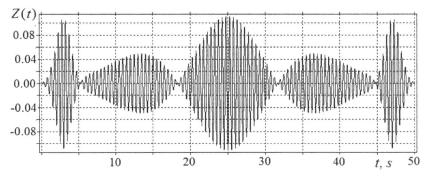

Fig. 1. Time dependence of the signal $Z(t)$ (1) with the parameters given in Table 1 [17].

Figure 1 shows the proposed model (1) of the signal. It is essential that the signal has the points of zero amplitude. Besides, the graph shows two high peaks with narrow localization $\tau_0 = 0.75$ s and $\tau_3 = 0.75$ s at the beginning $t = 3$ s, and at the end $t = 47$ s of the process.

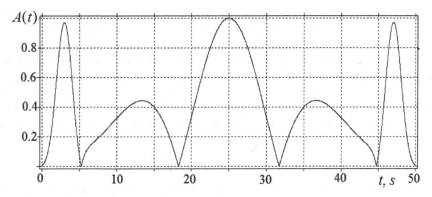

Fig. 2. Dependence of $A(t)/A_m$ in time [17].

Figure 2 shows the behavior of $A(t)/A_m$ within the interval $0 \leq A(t)/A_m \leq 1$.

It is important to emphasize that the proposed model allows us to set the amplitude exactly. Hereupon, the model gives the analytical solution for CWT.

Further study will focus on computing CWT, formulating the criteria for determining how correctly CWT shows the time behavior of the amplitude $A(t)$, and eliminating boundary effects in CWT implementation.

2.2 Continuous Wavelet Transform

The continuous wavelet transform $V(v, t)$ (CWT) maps non-stationary signal $Z(t)$ with varying time-frequency structure on time-frequency plane [5, 25]:

$$V(v, t) = v \int_{-\infty}^{\infty} Z(t')\psi^*\big(v(t' - t)\big)dt', \tag{7}$$

where $\psi(x)$ is the mother wavelet function, and symbol * means complex conjugation. The mother wavelet $\psi(x)$ should be localized near the point $x = 0$, have the unit norm value and zero mean value calculated over the interval $-\infty < x < \infty$. The adaptive Morlet mother wavelet function (AWM), which we introduced in [11], satisfies all these properties. The formulas for AMW and its Fourier image are

$$\psi(x) = D_m \exp\left(-\frac{x^2}{2m^2}\right)\left[\exp(2\pi i x) - \exp\left(-\Omega_m^2\right)\right], \tag{8}$$

$$\psi(F) = \frac{D_m \Omega_m}{\sqrt{\pi}} \exp\left[-\Omega_m^2 (F - 1)^2\right]\left[1 - \exp\left(-2\Omega_m^2 F\right)\right], \tag{9}$$

$$D_m = \frac{(2\pi)^{1/4}}{\sqrt{\Omega_m \left(1 - 2\exp\left(-\frac{3\Omega_m^2}{2}\right) + \exp\left(-2\Omega_m^2\right)\right)}}. \tag{10}$$

The value m in (8)–(10) plays the role of a control parameter, while $\Omega_m = m\pi\sqrt{2}$. The parameter of localization Δ_x, which indicates the extension of $\psi(x)$ along x-axis, and Δ_F, which corresponds to the extension of Fourier spectrum $\psi(F)$ [1, 4] along the frequency axis, have the values $\Delta_x \approx m/\sqrt{2}$, and $\Delta_F \approx 1/(\sqrt{8}\pi\, m)$. Their product is close to the lowest value $\Delta_x \Delta_F = 1/(4\pi)$. The values of Δ_x and Δ_F vary with the change in m. Thus, we get the opportunity to vary the time and spectral resolution of the signals under study. At $m = 1$ we obtain the formula for the ordinary Morlet mother wavelet function. If the characteristic length of $\psi(x)$ is $\Delta_x \approx m/\sqrt{2}$, the characteristic time moments, which make the main contribution to the integral (7), satisfy the relation

$$t - \frac{\Delta_x}{\nu} < t' < t + \frac{\Delta_x}{\nu}. \tag{11}$$

Thus, AMW (8) behaves like a varying window depending on the control parameter. The window width automatically becomes large for small frequencies and small for the large ones.

The ratio of Fourier components at negative and positive frequencies is $\psi(-|F|)/\psi(|F|) = -\exp\left[-2\Omega_m^2|F|\right]$. Note that such a quantity can be neglected at the characteristic frequencies of F ≈ 1.

The condition for C_ψ to be finite: $C_\psi = \int\limits_{-\infty}^{\infty} \frac{\left|\hat{\psi}(F)\right|^2 dF}{|F|}$ makes it possible to reconstruct signal $Z(t)$ using its CWT image $V(\nu, t)$ (7). The method that enables to calculate the corrections to the saddle-point method can be used to show the asymptotic expression $C_\psi = 1 + 1/(4\Omega_m^2)$. It differs from exact value C_ψ by less than 0.05% at $\Omega_m \gg 1$ and m > 1. The constant C_ψ for the Morlet mother wavelet (8) is approximately 1.013 ($m = 1$).

The following expression is valid for AMW [11]:

$$\frac{2}{C_\psi} \int\limits_0^{\infty} d\nu\, \nu \int\limits_{-\infty}^{\infty} dt_0 \mathrm{Re}\{\psi^*\left[\nu(t' - t_0)\right]\psi[\nu(t - t_0)]\} = \delta(t - t'),$$

where $\delta(t - t')$ is the Dirac delta function.

CWT (7) can be obtained using the Fourier images of all functions in (7):

$$V(\nu, t) = \int\limits_{-\infty}^{\infty} Z(f)\psi^*\left(\frac{f}{\nu}\right)\exp(2\pi\, i\, f\, t)df,$$

where $Z(f)$ and $\psi^*(f/\nu)$ are the Fourier components of signal $Z(t)$ and mother wavelet $\psi(x)$ (8).

We note, that the wavelet transform (7) with the mother wavelet (8) for elementary non-stationary signals (2), with the amplitude varying in time and constant frequency, can be calculated analytically [11].

2.3 Wavelet Analysis of Mathematical Model of Non-stationary Signal

After applying CWT with $m = 1$ to (1), we can observe that at $v = f_L$ the time behavior $|V_L(f_L, t)|^2 \approx \exp[-(t - t_L)^2/(2\tau_L^2)]$ exactly reproduces the time behavior of $A^2(t)$. If the control parameter $m \gg f_L\tau_L$, then the behavior of $|V_L(v, t = t_L)|^2$ exactly repeats the behavior of power spectrum $P(v) = |z_L(v)|^2$, and $\Delta_v^{(CWT)}$ exactly coincides with $\Delta_v^{(0)}$, which characterizes the width of ENS (2) power spectrum, i.e. $\Delta_v^{(CWT)} \approx \Delta_v^{(0)} = 1/(4\pi\tau_L)$.

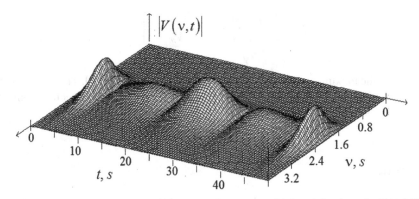

Fig. 3. Analytical dependence of $|V(v, t)|$ on frequency $v(Hz)$ and time $t(s)$ for $Z(t)$ [17].

Figure 3 shows the complex amplitude and frequency properties of the signal. At $t_L = 3\,s\,(L = 0)$ and $t_L = 47\,s\,(L = 3)$ corresponding to the sharp peaks, we have wide frequency distribution. It is due to the fact that the length $\tau_L = 0.75\,s$ of these peaks $(L = 0, L = 3)$ is much smaller than the lengths of two other peaks $\tau_L = 5\,s\,(L = 1)$ and $\tau_L = 4.5\,s\,(L = 2)$. To find out how $|V(v, t)|$ reproduces the behavior of the signal amplitude $A(t)$, we make a cross-section of the surface at $v = f_0$ along the time axis. Figure 4 shows the cross-section of $|V(f_0, t)|$ in comparison with $A(t)$.

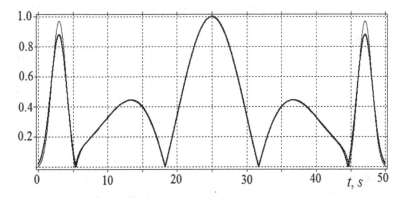

Fig. 4. Comparison of time behavior for $A(t)$ (thin line) and cross section of $|V(f_0, t)|$ (bold line) at $m = 1$ [17].

In Fig. 4 we can see that the curves diverging only in a close neighborhood of peaks $t_L = 3\,\text{s}\,(L = 0)$ and $t_L = 47\,\text{s}\,(L = 3)$. It is because these two peaks are located at the beginning and at the end of the interval $[0, T]$, where the condition $f_L \tau_L \gg 1$ is violated ($f_0 = 2\,\text{Hz}$; $\tau_0 = \tau_3 = 0.75\,\text{s}$). The curves nearly coincide at all other points of the interval $[0, T]$, where $T = 50\,\text{s}$. We conclude that for $f_L \tau_L \gg 1$, the curves $A(t)$ and $|V(f_0, t)|$ are similar. To characterize the deviation of $|V(f_0, t)|$ from $A(t)$, we introduce the parameter of mean square deviation by the formula

$$\sigma_t^2 = \frac{1}{T} \int_0^T \left[\frac{A(t)}{A_m} - \frac{|V(f_0; t)|}{V_m} \right]^2 dt, \tag{12}$$

where V_m is the maximal value of $|V(f_0, t)|$ within the interval $[0, T]$. Thus, CWT with $m = 1$ is well suited to describe the time variation of $A(t)$ for some specific moments near the points, where $A(t) = 0$ (Fig. 2).

3 Results

3.1 Boundary Effects in the Analysis of Spectral Properties

The foregoing results are based on the analytical expressions for $|V(\nu, t)|$ and $A(t)$ for the proposed mathematical model of non-stationary signal. For real signals, we are to carry out numerical calculations to find $|V(\nu, t)|$. In this case, we face the problem of boundary effects. Let us determine the influence of boundary effects in calculating $|V(\nu, t)|$ [9]. Boundary effects can appear at both the left ($0 < t < t_{off}$) and the right ($T - t_{off} < t < T$) ends of the observation interval T. The value of t_{off} will be determined later. The reason of edge effects corresponds to the finite value of wavelet's length Δ_x, which leads to significant errors in numerical CWT calculation. To eliminate the errors, we use to take the values of $V(\nu, t)$ in these intervals equal to zero. Naturally, we lose the valuable information on the time-frequency behavior of the signal near the edges. How can you keep this information?

Let us formulate the problem of finding the minimal value $\nu_{\min}$ of frequency that will allow us to determine CWT correctly. Analyzing (11), we conclude that in the initial interval $[0, t_{off}]$, the minimal frequency $\nu_{\min}$ relates to t_{off} as

$$t_{off} = 2\Delta_x / \nu_{\min}. \tag{13}$$

A similar formula can be obtained near the right-hand boundary $\left[T - t_{off}; T \right]$ of the signal. To determine $\nu_{\min}$ correctly, we need n ($n \gg 1$) periods of frequency oscillations with the duration of $1/\nu_{\min}$ that can be placed within the remaining time interval $\left[T - 2t_{off} \right]$. The observation interval T consists of two boundary sections with the lengths $4\Delta_x/\nu_{min}$ and n/ν_{min} (the interval to determine CWT correctly). Then we have

$$\nu_{min} = (n + 4\Delta_x)/T. \tag{14}$$

Taking into account the boundary effects leads to the value of ν_{min} approximately $n + 4\Delta_x$ times larger than $f_{min} = 1/T$ used in the Fourier analysis. After determining ν_{min} (14), we can calculate the value of t_{off} (13).

To eliminate boundary effects, we propose an algorithm, which we call Signal Time Shift (STS) [17] (Fig. 5).

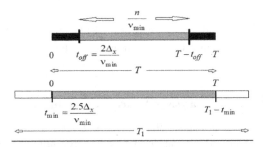

Fig. 5. The upper drawing corresponds to the interval T with two boundary sections marked in black; the lower drawing corresponds to T_1 [17].

Let us compare the analytical behavior of $A(t)$ (Fig. 2) with that of $|V(f_0, t)|$ (Fig. 4), numerical implementation $|V^{(num)}(f_0, t)|$ of CWT without the procedure of Signal Time Shift (STS), and the numerical implementation $|V^{(sts)}(f_0, t)|$ of CWT with the use of STS. All calculations are carried out for the model (1)–(2) and the parameters given in Table 1. Numerical calculations are made for the Morlet wavelet with $m = 1$, the characteristic length $\Delta_x = 1$, the number of oscillation periods $n = 10$. In this case, $T = 50\,\text{s}$, $\nu_{min} = 0.28\,\text{Hz}$, $t_{off} = 7.14\,\text{s}$, $t_{min} = 8.93\,\text{s}$, $T_1 = 61.76\,\text{s}$.

Figure 6 represents a small fragment of the signal near the beginning to demonstrate the boundary effects. The duration is 5 s. In Fig. 6 the dash-dot line shows CWT calculated numerically $|V^{(num)}(f_0, t)|$, in which the boundary effects appear. For the frequencies $\nu \approx 1\,\text{Hz}$, the cut-off time is $t_{off} \approx 2\,\text{s}$. We observe strong differences between $|V^{(num)}(f_0, t)|$ and $A(t)$ at times $0 < t < t_{off}$. This requires us to take as zeros the wrong values of $|V^{(num)}(f_0, t)|$ in the interval $0 < t < 2\,\text{s}$. The dot line represents the result $|V^{(sts)}(f_0, t)|$ of applying STS method. This line reproduces the analytical behavior of $|V(f_0, t)|$ quite well.

Thus, the numerical implementation together with STS method allows us to save the important information about the amplitude–frequency behavior of the signal near the beginning and the end of the observation interval. The signal time shift allows us to consider all the time points of the signal under study.

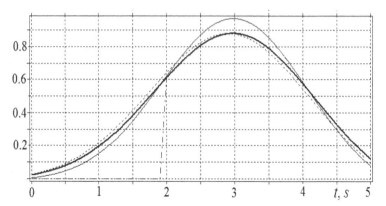

Fig. 6. Thin line – $A(t)$; bold line – analytical $|V(f_0, t)|$; dash-dot line – numerical $\left|V^{(\text{num})}(f_0, t)\right|$, which takes zero values at small times; dot line – numerical with the use of signal time shift [17].

3.2 STS Algorithm in the Analysis of Heart Tachogram

The method of eliminating boundary effects (STS), developed in the previous section, can be applied in the study of non-stationary signal representing the heart tachogram.

In the framework of frequency modulated model, we represent the heart tachogram signal as a set of identical Gaussian peaks. Let the centers of RR_n heart peaks be located at non-uniform grid characterized by time points t_n. In reality it is the heartbeat with the number n and the amount of time between n and $n - 1$ heartbeat equal to RR_n:

$$t_n = \sum_{m=0}^{n} RR_m$$

Following [26], let us introduce the average duration $RRNN$ of cardiac intervals RR_n during the entire observation period T as:

$$RRNN = \frac{1}{N} \sum_{n=0}^{N-1} RR_n$$

where N is the total number of beats. If $RRNN$ is measured in ms, the heart rate (HR – heart rate), measured in $1/\min$, is expressed by relation $HR = 60 \cdot 1000/RRNN$. If the frequency of cardiac contractions ν_{HR} is measured in Hz and $RRNN$ – in s, then $\nu_{HR} = 1/RRNN$. The time of the last beat t_{N-1} is related to $RRNN$ (1) by the ratio $t_{N-1} = N \cdot RRNN$.

Assume that all the peaks R of the heart complex P-QRS-T have the same amplitude, measured in mV, and the form approximated by Gaussian peak. In this case, the tachogram signal $Z(t)$ is the superposition of N Gaussian peaks of the same unit amplitude with the centers located on a non-uniform time scale t_n:

$$Z(t) = \sum_{n=0}^{N-1} z_0(t - t_n), \quad z_0(t - t_n) = \frac{1}{2\tau_0 \sqrt{\pi}} \exp\left[-\frac{(t - t_n)^2}{4\tau_0^2}\right] \tag{15}$$

The width $\tau_0 = 20$ ms of each Gaussian peak is equal to the width of the QRS complex. Such a model makes it possible to obtain the analytic expression for $V(v, t)$ (7). Let us write this expression for the usual Morlet wavelet ($m = 1$):

$$V(v, t - t_n) = \frac{D_1 v}{a_0(v)} \exp\left[-\frac{x^2 + 4\pi^2(a_0^2 - 1)}{2a_0^2(v)}\right] \cdot \left[\exp\left(\frac{2\pi i x}{a_0^2(v)}\right) - \exp\left(-\frac{2\pi^2}{a_0^2(v)}\right)\right]$$

where $x = v(t - t_n)$ and function $a_0(v) = \sqrt{1 + 2v^2\tau_0^2}$.

The analytical expression for CWT of the complex model signal (15) can be calculated due to the principle of superposition

$$V(v, t) = \sum_{n=0}^{N-1} V(v, t - t_n).$$

Figure 7 shows human heart tachogram registered during Head Down Tilt Test. It consists of three stages: A, B, C. Stages A, C correspond to the horizontal position of the table. Stage B is the lowering of the table with a turn of $30°$, which leads to the transients in the frequency of heart beats.

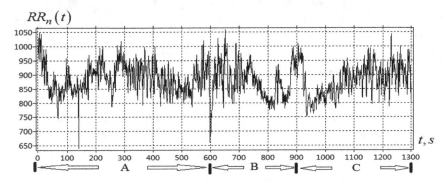

Fig. 7. Dependence of heart beat interval RR_n on time $t\,(ms)$ [17].

Let us consider the experimental tachogram (Fig. 7) registered during head-down tilt test (HDT) The duration of intervals RR_n between the centers of heartbeats changes. Stage B, when the HDT takes place, lasts 300 s ($600 \leq t \leq 900$ s). For the proposed model of the tachogram (15), the Gaussian peaks (15) are centered at the times t_n when heartbeats occur: $t_n = t_{n-1} + RR_n$, $n = 1, 2, 3, \ldots N-1$, and $t_0 = RR_0$. Substituting these t_n into (15), we obtain the frequency-modulated tachogram signal $Z(t)$. The analytical expressions for the signal (15) and the mother wavelet function $\psi(x)$ (8) allow us to find the analytical expression for CWT (7). The value $F_{max}(t)$ shown in Fig. 8 corresponds to the maximum value of $|V(v, t)|$ for each point in time t. The function $F_{max}(t)$ varies in the range 0.4 Hz $\leq F_{max}(t) \leq 2.5$ Hz.

The study of $F_{max}(t)$ during HDT (stage B, 600 s $\leq t \leq 900$ s) shows the appearance of low-frequency oscillations. The characteristic period t_F of such oscillations approximately equals 100 s. In Fig. 7 the graph for $RR_n(t)$ shows two heartbeats at the time $t \approx 600$ s separated by the interval $RR_n(t) \approx 650$ ms. Therefore, at the same moment $t \approx 600$ s, the value of $F_{max}(t) \approx 1.54$ Hz (Fig. 8). Thus, for the model of frequency-modulated signal (17), we can calculate the maximum local frequency $F_{max}(t)$ at any time t.

Another wavelet transform applied to $F_{max}(t)$ (double continuous wavelet transform DCWT [9]) makes it possible to study transients in the variation of frequency. When calculating the DCWT defined as $V_{DCWT}(v, t)$ signal $Z(t)$ in the expression (7) is replaced by $F_{max}(t)$.

Applying double continuous wavelet transform to the signal $F_{max}(t)$ allows us to detect both aperiodic and oscillatory movements of the local frequency relative to the trend.

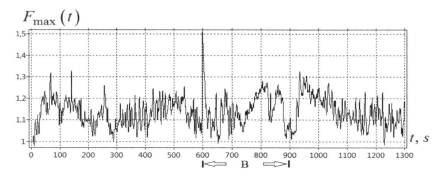

Fig. 8. Dependence $F_{max}(t)$ on time $t\,(ms)$ [17].

Figure 9 displays the result of DCWT with the procedure of STS, which shows a sharp change in the spectral structure of the signal at stage B. Figure 9 shows that the tachogram is an alternation of bursts of spectral activity in different spectral ranges:

$$ULF = (v_{min}; 0.015\,\text{Hz}); \ (VLF = (0.015; 0.04\,\text{Hz}); \ LF = (0.04; 0.15\,\text{Hz}); \ HF = (0.15; 0.4\,\text{Hz}).$$

The value of v_{min} is determined by the Eq. (16), with the number of periods $n = 5$, $\Delta_x = 2$.

To analyze the heart rate, we introduced quantitative characteristics describing the dynamics of changes in spectral properties of $F_{max}(t)$. Such characteristics are the instantaneous spectral integrals $E_\mu(t)$, and the mean values of the spectral integrals $<E_\mu(S)>$ at the stages $S = \{A, B, C\}$ in different spectral ranges $\mu = \{ULF, VLF; LF; HF\}$. To study the appearance and disappearance of low-frequency oscillations $F_{max}(t)$, we can calculate the skeletons of DCWT showing the extreme line of $|V_{DCWT}(t)|$ on the plane v and t. The value $\varepsilon(v, t)$ illustrates instantaneous frequency distribution of the signal energy (local density of energy spectrum of the signal)

$$\varepsilon(v, t) = \frac{2}{C_\psi} \frac{|V_{DCWT}(v, t)|^2}{v} \tag{16}$$

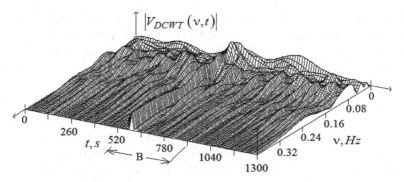

Fig. 9. Dependence of $|V_{DCWT}(t)|$ on frequency $v(Hz)$ and time $t(ms)$ [17].

The dynamics of time variation for different frequencies is determined by spectral integral $E_\mu(t)$:

$$E_\mu(t) = \frac{1}{\Delta v} \int_{v_\mu-\Delta v/2}^{v_\mu-\Delta v/2} \varepsilon(v,t)\,dv \qquad (17)$$

Spectral integral $E_\mu(t)$ represents the average value of the local density of the signal energy spectrum integrated over a certain frequency range $\mu = [v_\mu-\Delta v/2;\ v_\mu+\Delta v/2]$, where v_μ denotes the middle of the interval, Δv – its width. The time-variation of $E_\mu(t)$ performs a kind of signal filtration summing the contributions from the local density of the spectrum $\varepsilon(v,t)$ only in a certain range of frequencies $\mu = \{ULF, VLF, LF, HF\}$. By studying DCWT of the signal and calculating $E_\mu(t)$ in μ-range one can follow the dynamics of appearance and disappearance of low-frequency spectral components $F_{\max}(t)$.

The quantitative characteristics that describe the average dynamics of the spectral properties of a tachogram during the test have average values of the spectral integrals at the stages S = {A, B, C} in the ranges μ. Assuming that stage S starts at $t_I(S)$ and ends at $t_F(S)$, the average spectral integrals at stage S are

$$<E_\mu(S)> = \frac{1}{[t_F(S) - t_I(S)]} \int_{t_I(S)}^{t_F(S)} E_\mu(t)\,dt. \qquad (16)$$

We introduce the function, which shows the instantaneous value of the spectral integral in μ range at t as compared to its average value at rest (Stage A):

$$d_\mu(t) = \frac{E_\mu(t)}{<E_\mu(A)>}, \qquad (19)$$

and the function, which shows how the instantaneous ratio $E_\mu(t)/E_v(t)$ varies over the ratio of average spectral integrals $<E_\mu(A)>/<E_v(A)>$ calculated at the stage of rest (Stage A):

$$d_{\mu/v}(t) = \frac{E_\mu(t)<E_v(A)>}{E_v(t)<E_\mu(A)>}. \qquad (20)$$

The functions $d_\mu(t)$ and $d_{\mu/\nu}(t)$ represent the variation of spectral characteristics during the total tachogram period as compared with the respective average values observed at Stage A ($\mu = \{ULF, VLF, LF, HF\}$; $\nu = \{ULF, VLF, LF, HF\}$)
The heart rhythm assimilation coefficient in the spectral range μ:

$$D_\mu(B/A) = \frac{<E_\mu(B)>}{<E_\mu(A)>} \tag{21}$$

It reports the fold increase in the average spectral integral $<E_\mu(B)>$ for the μ-range at Stage B relative to the average value $<E_\mu(A)>$ of spectral integral for the same μ-range at rest (Stage A). Figures 10, 11, 12 and 13 represent the results of DCWT analysis of nonstationary heart rhythm using the STS technique.

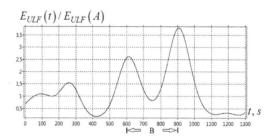

Fig. 10. Spectral integral $E_{ULF}(t)$ divided by its average value in the stage A [17].

Figure 10 gives the plot of time behavior for $d_{ULF}(t)$ (19). The heart rhythm assimilation coefficient $D_{ULF}(B/A)$ (21) in the $\mu = ULF$ spectral range is 1.92. The coefficient $d_{ULF}(t)$ (19) reaches the maximal value ≈ 3.8 at $t \approx 900$ s. This means that the instantaneous value of $E_{ULF}(t)$ at Stage B (test phase) is approximately 3.8 times greater than the average value of $E_{ULF}(A)$ at Stage A (at rest). In this spectral range (ULF) during the time period $600 \leq t \leq 900$ s a strong trend in $F_{max}(t)$ is noticeable (Fig. 8).

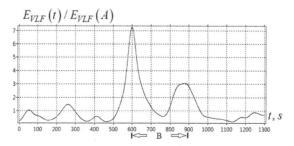

Fig. 11. Spectral integral $E_{VLF}(t)$ divided by its average value $E_{VLF}(A)$ at the stage A [17].

When HDT is completed ($t > 900$ s), there occurs a slow relaxation of the heart rate to the equilibrium state, which takes about 300 s. The characteristic time of frequency changes is equal to 100 s.

Figure 11 shows the behavior of $d_{VLF}(t)$ (19). The heart rhythm assimilation coefficient $D_{VLF}(B/A)$ in the $\mu = VLF$ spectral range equals 2.32 (21). The maximum of $d_{ULF}(t) \approx 7.4$ (19) takes place at $t \approx 600$ s. Figure 11 shows rapid VLF rhythm activation at Stage B ($600 \leq t \leq 900$ s) in comparison to Stage A ($0 \leq t \leq 600$ s).

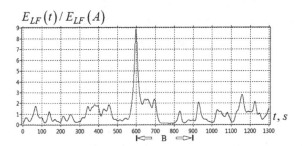

$E_{LF}(t)/E_{LF}(A)$

Fig. 12. Spectral interval $E_{LF}(t)$ divided by its average value $E_{VLF}(A)$ at the stage A [17].

Figure 12 represents the coefficient $d_{LF}(t)$ as a function of time. Note that at Stage B in the range $\mu = LF$, the rhythm is also noticeably higher than at stage A. The heart rhythm assimilation coefficient $D_{LF}(B/A) = 1.15$. Considering the oscillatory motion of the maximal frequency $F_{max}(t)$, we detect flashes of vibrational activity in this spectral range $LF = (0.04; 0.15$ Hz). For such flashes, the magnitudes of spectral integrals can many times exceed the background signal activity.

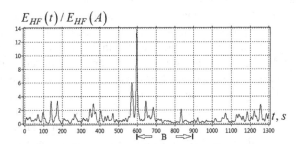

$E_{HF}(t)/E_{HF}(A)$

Fig. 13. Spectral interval $E_{HF}(t)$ divided by its average value $E_{HF}(A)$ at the stage A [17].

In the range $HF = (0.15; 0.4$ Hz), we can also observe short flashes of activity in spectral integrals. The maximum of $d_{HF}(t)$ is approximately 14 times greater than the background, but $D_{HF}(B/A) = 0.67$. This means that the average activity at Stage B is less than the average activity at Stage A.

Figure 14 demonstrates the temporal behavior of $d_{LF/HF}(t)$ (20), which characterizes the instantaneous ratio of $E_{LF}(t)/E_{HF}(t)$ to the average value $<E_{LF}(A)>/<E_{HF}(A)>$ calculated at stage A. The graph shows that at some time points the instantaneous value $d_{LF/HF}(t)$ becomes significantly large. This indicates the moments of tension in the physiological state of the patient and can be used for diagnostic purposes.

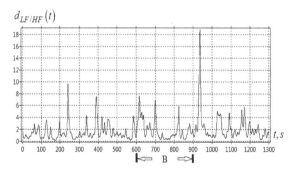

Fig. 14. Temporal dependence of $d_{LF/HF}(t)$ [17].

Analysis of an unsteady tachogram, performed using the spectral integral technique $E_\mu(t)$ (Figs. 10, 11, 12, 13 and 14), shows that the characteristic times τ_μ of flashes of heart rate activity in the corresponding ranges $\mu = (ULF, VLF, LF, HF)$ are $\tau_{ULF} \approx 180$ s, $\tau_{VLF} \approx 90$ s, $\tau_{LF} \approx 25$ s, $\tau_{HF} \approx 10$ s.

4   Conclusion

The combination of several new techniques (DCWT, frequency modulated model, spectral integrals, STS) allows us to detect various scenarios of oscillatory rearrangement in the real heart tachogram record during diagnostic procedures.

We have obtained such characteristics of non-stationarity in the HRV signal as the time periods, when the oscillations against the main trend appear or disappear, as well as the durations of transient processes. In our opinion, this is just the main feature and the advantage of DCWT method, when comparing it with the others. The calculations have been done both for the mathematical model of a frequency modulated signal and for the record during the real head up tilt test and deep breath test. The analysis indicates a strong non-stationarity in the spectral properties of the tachogram signal during the head up tilt table test and deep breath test. We should add that in medical practice this approach allows avoiding long-lasting visual evaluation of the tachogram at Holter monitoring.

We compared spectral characteristics of non-stationary heart rate variability (NHRV) calculated using the traditional amplitude-modulated signal of cardiac tachogram (AMS model) and the frequency modulates signal (FMR model). The latter model is proposed by the authors. The analysis shows that Fourier spectrum of NHRV signal calculated by AMS approach differs from that based on FMS model, which accurately reproduces the relationship $RR_n(t)$. These deviations are especially noticeable, when the signal of the tachogtam has a significant trend throughout the period of observation. Thus, the authors can conclude that true characteristic frequencies of NHRV signal and real rearrangements in heart rhythm are most accurately described by FMS model and DCWT method.

The algorithm STS (Signal Time Shift), which allows us to eliminate boundary effects in the numerical implementation of CWT, becomes especially important in the case of signals with the predominant influence of low frequencies, when the observation period for such signals is not too large. If the signal shows significant variations, the information on the behavior of the signal at the initial and final observation stages becomes very important for the correct conclusion about its amplitude-frequency properties.

The accuracy in revealing the heart rate violations over time during the performance of functional tests makes it possible to:

1) identify the early stages of the disease, manifested in violations of rhythm;
2) test the adaptive abilities of a person, which is an important task of training in many areas;
3) study the dynamics of interaction between sympathetic and parasympathetic divisions of the autonomic nervous system (ANS);
4) analyze tachograms during the biofeedback session.

Using DCWT with the STS procedure of boundary effect correction while calculating the diagnostic parameters helps to solve the problem of the correct evaluation of the physiological state of patients, to reveal the interaction between parasympathetic and sympathetic parts of the human autonomic nervous system and to test the adaptive capabilities of the human organism during various physical, orthostatic, respiratory, psycho-emotional and medicated tests.

The proposed algorithms can be included into Medical Cyber-Physical Systems (MCPS) for online estimation of quantitative parameters related to cardiac arrhythmias and also for the analysis of cardiac rhythm turbulence associated with ectopic beats.

Acknowledgments. The work has been supported by the Russian Science Foundation (Grant of the RSF 17-12-01085).

References

1. Mallat, S.: A Wavelet Tour of Signal Processing, 3rd edn. Academic Press, New York (2008)
2. Cohen, A.: Numerical Analysis of Wavelet Method. Elsevier Science, North-Holland (2003)
3. Baleanu, D.: Advances in Wavelet Theory and Their Applications in Engineering, Physics and Technology (2012)
4. Chui, C.K., Jiang, O.: Applied Mathematics. Data Compression, Spectral Methods, Fourier Analysis, Wavelets and Applications. Mathematics Textbooks for Science and Engineering, vol. 2. Atlantis Press, Paris (2013)
5. Addison, P.S.: The Illustrated Wavelet Transform Handbook. Introductory Theory and Application in Science, Engineering, Medicine and Finance, 2nd edn. CRC Press, Boca Raton (2017)
6. Hramov, A.E., Koronovskii, A.A., Makarov, V.A., Pavlov, A.N., Sitnikova, E.: Wavelets in Neuroscience. SSS. Springer, Heidelberg (2015). https://doi.org/10.1007/978-3-662-43850-3
7. Bozhokin, S.V.: Continuous wavelet transform and exactly solvable model of nonstationary signals. Tech. Phys. **57**(7), 900–906 (2012)
8. Andreev, D.A., Bozhokin, S.V., Venevtsev, I.D., Zhunusov, K.T.: Gabor transform and continuous wavelet transform for model pulsed signals. Tech. Phys. **59**(10), 1428–1433 (2014)
9. Bozhokin, S.V., Suslova, I.M.: Double wavelet transform of frequency-modulated nonstationary signal. Tech. Phys. **58**(12), 1730–1736 (2013)
10. Bozhokin, S.V., Suslova, I.B.: Wavelet-based analysis of spectral rearrangements of EEG patterns and of non-stationary correlations. Phys. A **421**, 151–160 (2015)

11. Bozhokin, S.V., Zharko, S.V., Larionov, N.V., Litvinov, A.N., Sokolov, I.M.: Wavelet correlation of nonstationary signals. Tech. Phys. **62**(6), 837–845 (2017)
12. Tankanag, A.V., Chemeris, N.K.: Adaptive wavelet analysis of oscillations in the human peripherical blood flow. Biophysics **4**(3), 375–380 (2009)
13. Podtaev, S., Morozov, M., Frick, P.: Wavelet-based corrections of skin temperature and blood flow oscillations. Cardiovasc. Eng. **8**(3), 185–189 (2008)
14. Boltezar, M., Slavic, J.: Enhancements to the continuous wavelet transform for damping identification on short signals. Mech. Syst. Signal Process. **18**, 1065–1076 (2004)
15. Ulker-Kaustell, M., Karoumi, R.: Application of the continuous wavelet transform on the free vibration of a steel-concrete composite railway bridge. Eng. Struct. **33**, 911–919 (2011)
16. Cazelles, B., et al.: Wavelet analysis of ecological time series. Oecologia **156**, 297–304 (2008)
17. Bozhokin, S., Suslova, I., Tarakanov, D.: Elimination of boundary effects at the numerical implementation of continuous wavelet transform to nonstationary biomedical signals. In: Proceedings of the 12th International Joint Conference on Biomedical Engineering Systems and Technologies (BIOSTEC 2019), vol. 4, pp. 22–24. BIOSIGNALS, Prague, Czech-Republic (2019)
18. Baevskii, R.M., Ivanov, G.G., Chireikin, L.V., et al.: Analysis of heart rate variability using different cardiological systems: methodological recommendations. Vestnik Arrhythm. **24**, 65–91 (2002)
19. Anderson, R., Jonsson, P., Sandsten, M.: Effects of age, BMI, anxiety and stress on the parameters of a stochastic model for heart rate variability including respiratory information. In: Proceedings of the 11th International Joint Conference on Biomedical Engineering Systems and Technologies (BIOSTEC 2018), vol. 4, pp. 17–25. BIOSIGNALS, Lisbon, Portugal (2018)
20. Bhavsar, R., Daveya, N., Sun, Y., Helian, N.: An investigation of how wavelet transform can affect the correlation performance of biomedical signals. In: Proceedings of the 11th International Joint Conference on Biomedical Engineering Systems and Technologies (BIOSTEC 2018), vol. 4, pp. 139–146. BIOSIGNALS, Lisbon, Portugal (2018)
21. Hammad, M., Maher, A., Adil, K., Jiang, F., Wang, K.: Detection of abnormal heart conditions from the analysis of ECG signals. In: Proceedings of the 11th International Joint Conference on Biomedical Engineering Systems and Technologies (BIOSTEC 2018), vol. 4, pp. 240–247. BIOSIGNALS, Lisbon, Portugal (2018)
22. Keissar, K., Davrath, L.R., Akselrod, S.: Coherence analysis between respiration and heart rate variability using continuous wavelet transform. Philos. Trans. R. Soc. A. **367**(1892), 1393–1406 (2009)
23. Ducla-Soares, J.L., Santos-Bento, M., Laranjo, S., et al.: Wavelet analysis of autonomic outflow of normal subjects on head-up tilt, cold pressor test, Valsalva manoeuvre and deep breathing. Exp. Physiol. **92**(4), 677–686 (2007)
24. Bozhokin, S.V., Suslova, I.B.: Analysis of non-stationary HRV as a frequency modulated signal by double continuous wavelet transformation method. Biomed. Signal Process. Control **10**, 34–40 (2014)
25. Van den Berg, J.C.: Wavelets in Physics. Cambridge University Press, Cambridge (2004)
26. Guidelines: Heart rate variability, standards of measurement, physiological interpretation, and clinical use. Task Force of the European Society of Cardiology and the North American Society of Pacing and Electrophysiology. Eur. Heart J. **17**, 354–381 (1996)

Cardiac Arrhythmia Detection from ECG with Convolutional Recurrent Neural Networks

Jérôme Van Zaen[✉], Ricard Delgado-Gonzalo, Damien Ferrario, and Mathieu Lemay

Swiss Center for Electronics and Microtechnology (CSEM), Neuchâtel, Switzerland
jerome.vanzaen@csem.ch

Abstract. Except for a few specific types, cardiac arrhythmias are not immediately life-threatening. However, if not treated appropriately, they can cause serious complications. In particular, atrial fibrillation, which is characterized by fast and irregular heart beats, increases the risk of stroke. We propose three neural network architectures to detect abnormal rhythms from single-lead ECG signals. These architectures combine convolutional layers to extract high-level features pertinent for arrhythmia detection from sliding windows and recurrent layers to aggregate these features over signals of varying durations. We applied the neural networks to the dataset used for the challenge of Computing in Cardiology 2017 and a dataset built by joining three databases available on PhysioNet. Our architectures achieved an accuracy of 86.23% on the first dataset, similar to the winning entries of the challenge, and an accuracy of 92.02% on the second dataset.

Keywords: Cardiac arrhythmia · Machine learning · Neural networks · ECG

1 Introduction

Irregular electrical conduction in cardiac tissue often causes heart arrhythmia. Atrial fibrillation is the most prevalent arrhythmia as it affects 1–2% of the population [1]. Its prevalence increases with age, from <0.5% at 40–50 years to 5–15% at 80 years. Despite not being a life-threatening condition from the start, it can lead to serious complications [15]. In particular, atrial fibrillation is associated with a 3–5 fold increased risk of stroke and a 2-fold increased risk of mortality [16]. It was also shown to be linked with a 3-fold risk of heart failure [29]. Heart palpitations, shortness of breath, and fainting are common symptoms. However, around one third of the cases are asymptomatic, which prevents early diagnosis. This, in turn, delays early treatment which might protect the patient from the consequences of atrial fibrillation and stop its progression. Indeed, atrial fibrillation causes electrical and structural remodeling of the atria which

© Springer Nature Switzerland AG 2020
A. Roque et al. (Eds.): BIOSTEC 2019, CCIS 1211, pp. 311–327, 2020.
https://doi.org/10.1007/978-3-030-46970-2_15

facilitates its further development, i.e. atrial fibrillation begets atrial fibrillation [7,22,30].

The 12-lead ECG is the gold standard to diagnose abnormal heart rhythms. A trained electrophysiologist can select the most appropriate therapy after reviewing ECG signals and the patient history. This is a time-consuming task, especially for long recordings such as the ones collected with Holter monitors. Several approaches have been proposed to make this task easier and less time-consuming [6,23]. Indeed, even without perfect accuracy, these approaches are helpful to quickly select relevant ECG segments for in-depth analysis by a specialist.

Recently, neural networks have shown remarkable performance in numerous domains compared to other methods. In particular, image processing was the first field where deep neural networks surpassed existing approaches by a large margin [18]. Since then they have also been applied to multiple signal processing classification and regression tasks with time series as inputs. In particular, several neural networks have been proposed to detect and classify cardiac arrhythmia from ECG signals.

In the context of the challenge of Computing in Cardiology 2017 [3], a few approaches based on neural networks were proposed to classify single-lead ECG signals into one of the following classes: normal rhythm, atrial fibrillation, other rhythm, and noise. One of these approaches applies two-dimensional convolutional layers to spectrograms computed over sliding windows [36]. Aggregation of the features extracted from the spectrograms was done either with a simple averaging over time or a recurrent layer. However, due to convergence issues, convolutional and recurrent layers were trained separately. A similar approach used a 16-layer convolutional network to classify arrhythmia from ECG records [33]. Each layer includes batch normalization, ReLU activation, dropout, one-dimensional convolution, and global averaging.

Cardiologist-level arrhythmia detection was reached recently by a convolutional neural network [25]. This network with 34 layers was trained on a very large dataset of 64,121 single-lead ECG signals collected from 29,163 unique patients. It can detect 12 different types of cardiac arrhythmia, including atrial fibrillation, atrial flutter, and ventricular tachycardia. Another approach applied convolutional neural networks to time-frequency representations of ECG data in order to classify arrhythmia [31]. Two types of time-frequency representations were compared: the short-time Fourier transform and the stationary wavelet transform. In this study, the second transform led to a neural network yielding higher performance.

Thus, several neural network architectures achieved good classification performance for the detection of abnormal heart rhythms from ECG signals. These results are promising as they prefigure detection systems that will quickly process long ECG records to extract pertinent segments for further analysis by an electrophysiologist. Hopefully, this will reduce the time needed to achieve a diagnosis and thus to select the most appropriate therapy as early as possible. We recently proposed an approach to tackle this issue [28]. This approach combined a smart vest to record a single-lead ECG over long periods of time and a convolutional recurrent neural network to detect abnormal rhythms. In this paper, we consider variations of the neural network architecture proposed previously and apply them to two datasets for the classification of cardiac arrhythmia. This paper is structured as follows. First, the datasets of ECG data and the considered neural network architectures are presented in Sect. 2. Then, the results are reported in Sect. 3 and discussed in Sect. 4. Finally, a brief conclusion ends this paper in Sect. 5.

2   Materials and Methods

2.1   Datasets

We trained neural networks to classify cardiac arrhythmia from ECG data with two datasets. The first one is the dataset used for the challenge of Computing in Cardiology 2017 [3]. It includes 8528 single-lead ECG signals recorded with an AlivCor device. The signals are sampled at 300 Hz with durations ranging from 9 to 60 s. Each record was acquired when the subject placed their hands on the two electrodes. This resulted in a lead I (left arm – right arm) ECG. However, many signals are inverted (right arm – left arm) as the device has no specific orientation.

All ECG records were labeled with one of the following four classes: *normal sinus rhythm, atrial fibrillation, other rhythm,* and *noise*. No additional information was available about the heart rhythms included in the *other rhythm* class. The class proportions are not balanced and vary from 3.27% for *noise* to 59.52% for *normal sinus rhythm*. For training and evaluation, we split the dataset into a training set with 6000 signals (70.4%), a validation set with 1264 signals (14.8%), and a test set with 1264 signals (14.8%) while approximately preserving class proportions. The full breakdown for each class and each subset is reported in Table 1.

Table 1. Breakdown of training, validation, and test sets for the dataset of the challenge of Computing in Cardiology 2017.

Class	Training		Validation		Test	
Normal rhythm	3571	(59.5%)	752	(59.5%)	753	(59.6%)
Atrial fibrillation	534	(8.9%)	112	(8.9%)	112	(8.9%)
Other rhythm	1699	(28.3%)	358	(28.3%)	358	(28.3%)
Noise	196	(3.3%)	42	(3.3%)	41	(3.2%)
Total	6000	(100%)	1264	(100%)	1264	(100%)

The participants of the challenge of Computing in Cardiology 2017 were ranked according to the following score evaluated on a private test set [3]:

$$S_{\text{CinC}} = \frac{F_{1n} + F_{1a} + F_{1o}}{3} \tag{1}$$

where F_{1n}, F_{1a}, and F_{1o} are the F_1 scores for *normal rhythm*, *atrial fibrillation*, and *other rhythm*. The four winners [4,13,27,34] reached a score of 0.83. It is worth mentioning that the private test set used during the challenge was not released yet and thus could not be used for evaluation purposes.

A number of features make this dataset challenging for cardiac arrhythmia classification. First, as mentioned previously, many ECG signals are inverted since the recording device lacks a clear usage orientation. Second, the classes are not balanced. There are few records labeled *atrial fibrillation* and *noise compared* to the ones labeled *normal rhythm* and *other rhythm*. Third, the record durations are not identical but instead vary between 9 and 60 s. These variations are illustrated in Fig. 1. Most ECG signals last around 30 s but a significant number have shorter or longer durations. Furthermore, labeling is relatively coarse as there is a single label for each ECG record. Using more than a single label would have been more appropriate as the cardiac rhythm seems to change over the course of the several signals. Finally, the signal quality of a non-negligible part of the records is quite poor. Four examples are shown in Fig. 2 to illustrate some of these issues. The first two examples are labeled *normal rhythm* and *atrial fibrillation* and their overall quality is good. The third example is labeled *normal rhythm* and has good quality as well. However, it is inverted (R peaks are negative) compared to the first example. In this case, the device was most likely held in the wrong orientation. The last example is an example of *atrial fibrillation* with poor quality and very short duration. Indeed, the ECG signal is very noisy at the end and seems to miss some heart beats. It also illustrates that the records do not share the same duration. This dataset will be referred to as the CinC 2017 dataset in the rest of the manuscript.

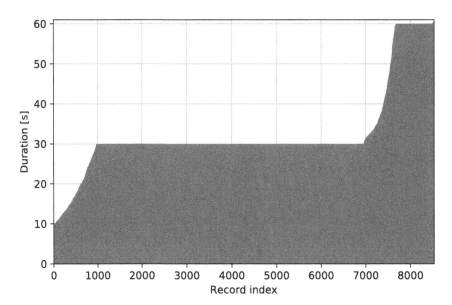

Fig. 1. Durations of ECG records from the dataset of the challenge of Computing in Cardiology 2017 sorted in ascending order [28].

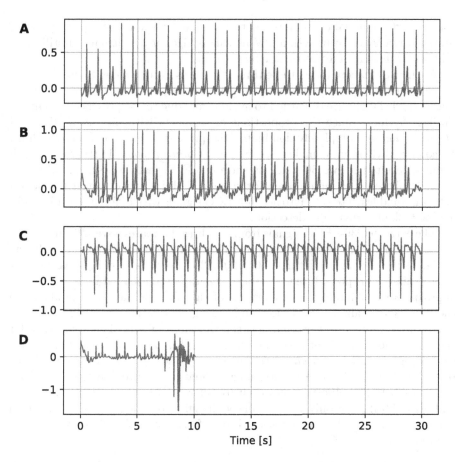

Fig. 2. Examples of ECG records from the dataset of the challenge of Computing in Cardiology 2017: (A) normal rhythm from record A00026, (B) atrial fibrillation from record A00102, (C) normal rhythm from record A00007, (D) atrial fibrillation from record A00405.

The second dataset we considered was built by combining three databases from PhysioNet [9]: the MIT-BIH Atrial Fibrillation Database [20], the MIT-BIH Arrhythmia Database [21], and the Long-Term Atrial Fibrillation Database [24]. The MIT-BIH Atrial Fibrillation Database includes 23 two-lead ECG records sampled at 250 Hz that last 10 h. The MIT-BIH Arrhythmia Database is composed of 48 half-hour ECG records with two leads collected from 47 subjects. The signals were sampled at 360 Hz. The Long-Term Atrial Fibrillation Database includes 84 two-lead ECG records sampled at 128 Hz. These records were collected from subjects with paroxysmal or sustained atrial fibrillation and their durations varied but were typically between 24 and 25 h. These three databases were annotated with several different cardiac rhythms: atrial bigeminy, atrial fibrillation, atrial flutter, ventricular bigeminy, heart block, idioventricular rhythm, normal rhythm, nodal rhythm, paced rhythm, pre-excitation, sinus bradycardia, supraventricular tachyarrhythmia, ventricular trigeminy, ventricular fibrillation, ventricular flutter, and ventricular tachycardia.

As the ECG records from these three databases were too long to use as inputs for neural networks, we extracted 30-s segments. Segments annotated with more than a single label were discarded to avoid errors due to the presence of multiple cardiac rhythms. Since the proportions of segments with *normal rhythm* and *atrial fibrillation* completely dominated the proportions for the other rhythms, we combined them in a single class labeled as *other rhythm*. Furthermore, each segment resulted in two 30-s signals since two ECG leads were recorded in the three databases. The main reason for keeping both leads was to test if a neural network could learn to take into account ECG signals with different morphologies for the task of arrhythmia detection.

The extracted 30-s ECG signals from the three databases were split into training, validation, and test sets. We applied an iterative procedure to assign subjects to these subsets while targeting a 60%/20%/20% split and keeping class proportions similar. This procedure was applied separately to each database in order to approximately maintain the proportions of signals from the three databases in the subsets for training, validation, and testing. The rationale for this approach was to avoid any subject overlap between the three subsets. The breakdown for each class and each subset is summarized in Table 2. In addition, as the proportion of signals labeled as *other rhythm* was very low (<2%), we repeated the procedure to split the data into training, validation, and test sets while excluding this label. The objective was then to differentiate between normal rhythm and atrial fibrillation only with a binary classifier. In this case, the breakdown is reported in Table 3. This dataset will be referred to as the PhysioNet dataset from now on.

Table 2. Breakdown of training, validation, and test sets for the dataset combining three databases from PhysioNet with three classes.

Class	Training	Validation	Test
Normal rhythm	132474 (44.7%)	43828 (44.0%)	44080 (44.7%)
Atrial fibrillation	158832 (53.6%)	53972 (54.2%)	52028 (52.8%)
Other rhythm	4816 (1.6%)	1862 (1.9%)	2420 (2.5%)
Total	296122 (100%)	99662 (100%)	98528 (100%)

Table 3. Breakdown of training, validation, and test sets for the dataset combining three databases from PhysioNet with two classes.

Class	Training	Validation	Test
Normal rhythm	133150 (45.5%)	43132 (44.8%)	44100 (45.7%)
Atrial fibrillation	159180 (54.5%)	53250 (55.2%)	52402 (54.3%)
Total	292330 (100%)	96382 (100%)	96502 (100%)

2.2   Pre-processing

After splitting both datasets into training, validation, and test sets, the signals were pre-processed before using them as inputs to the neural networks. The first step was to apply a digital Butterworth band-pass filter between 0.5 and 40 Hz. The filter was applied twice, once forward and once backward, to avoid phase distortion. The specifications were chosen based on the analog filter included in the device used to record the CinC 2017 dataset. Then, the signals were resampled to 200 Hz in order to standardize the sampling frequency across datasets. Finally, the signals were scaled by the mean of the standard deviations estimated over the training set. Scaling was shown to be helpful to accelerate training [19]. It is worth mentioning that the scaling operation was performed separately for each database in the PhysioNet dataset to take into account potential differences in ECG amplitude.

2.3   Network Architectures

Special care must be taken to handle signals with different lengths like the ones in the first dataset. A simple solution would be to truncate all signals to the length of the shortest one. This would make it possible to use a convolutional network to automatically extract high-level features for classification. However, it is not clear which part (beginning, middle, or end) of longer signals to keep. More importantly, it would waste a huge amount of data, especially for the first dataset where the shortest signal is around 9 s and the longest around 60 s.

A more appropriate approach is to use recurrent networks. Indeed, this class of neural networks are well-suited to take into account sequences with different lengths as they can, by design, remember past values for long periods of time. However, they are not as efficient for extracting high-level features compared to convolutional networks.

We recently proposed a neural network architecture combining convolutional and recurrent layers to classify cardiac arrhythmia [28]. It was selected as it uses the strong points of both types of layers: convolutional layers to extract high-level features and recurrent layers to handle signals with different lengths. In this paper, we extend this architecture and test different variations.

Each ECG signal is divided into sliding windows with 50% overlap. We selected two windows sizes: 512 and 1024 samples corresponding approximately to 2.5 and 5 s as the signals are sampled at 200 Hz. The number of windows extracted from each signal depended on its duration. For 30-s signals, the most common duration, this resulted in 22 windows with 512 samples and 10 windows with 1024 samples. Convolutional layers were then applied to all windows of a signal. Each convolutional layer is composed of a one-dimensional convolution and a max pooling operation [35]. The convolution used a kernel of size 5, zero padding, and a ReLU activation function [10]. The max pooling operation used a pool size of 2. The first convolutional layer has 8 output channels and the subsequent layers double the number of output channels. Therefore, the number of channels is doubled at each layer while the window size is halved since the

Table 4. Neural network architectures. The output size of convolutional layers is given as $N \times W \times C$ where N is the number of windows, W is the window size, and C is the number of channels. The number of classes is denoted by K and the number of convolutional layers by L.

Layer	$W = 512, L = 7$ Output size	$W = 1024, L = 7$ Output size	$W = 1024, L = 8$ Output size
Input windows	$N \times 512 \times 1$	$N \times 1024 \times 1$	$N \times 1024 \times 1$
Convolutional layer 1	$N \times 256 \times 8$	$N \times 512 \times 8$	$N \times 512 \times 8$
Convolutional layer 2	$N \times 128 \times 16$	$N \times 256 \times 16$	$N \times 256 \times 16$
Convolutional layer 3	$N \times 64 \times 32$	$N \times 128 \times 32$	$N \times 128 \times 32$
Convolutional layer 4	$N \times 32 \times 64$	$N \times 64 \times 64$	$N \times 64 \times 64$
Convolutional layer 5	$N \times 16 \times 128$	$N \times 32 \times 128$	$N \times 32 \times 128$
Convolutional layer 6	$N \times 8 \times 256$	$N \times 16 \times 256$	$N \times 16 \times 256$
Convolutional layer 7	$N \times 4 \times 512$	$N \times 8 \times 512$	$N \times 8 \times 512$
Convolutional layer 8			$N \times 4 \times 1024$
Global average pooling	$N \times 512$	$N \times 512$	$N \times 1024$
LSTM layer	128	128	128
Softmax (or logistic) layer	K (1)	K (1)	K (1)
Number of parameters	1.2 M	1.2 M	4.1 M

max pooling operation downsamples windows by two. We tested using 7 and 8 of these convolutional layers. Then, a global average pooling layer is applied to prepare features for the next step. The features are fed to a long short-term memory (LSTM) layer [12] with 128 units. Finally, a softmax layer outputs the probability of each class for the input ECG windows. When training a neural network with the second dataset without the *other rhythm* class, the softmax layer is replaced by a logistic layer since there are only two classes. The three considered architectures are summarized in Table 4 with the approximate numbers of parameters. It is worth mentioning that we did not try to apply an eighth convolutional layer when using a window size of 512. The reason is that after the seventh layer, the window size is reduced to 4. Thus, it does not make sense to apply an additional convolutional layer with a kernel of size 5 to such short windows.

2.4 Data Augmentation

The CinC 2017 dataset is relatively small for fitting a neural network with only 6000 signals in the training set. Therefore, we applied two strategies to synthetically augment the number of ECG signals available. The first strategy is to simply flip the sign of each signal with probability 0.5. This strategy is particularly useful for the CinC 2017 dataset where, as mentioned previously, many signals are inverted since the recording device lacks a clear usage orientation.

Indeed, we found it easier to let the neural networks learn to take into account inverted signals than developing an approach for detecting and rectifying such signals before training. There is no clear justification to apply this strategy to the PhysioNet dataset. Therefore, we trained the neural networks for this dataset with and without random sign flipping.

The second strategy for data augmentation uses the fact that, when extracting sliding windows, it is not possible to use all samples for the large majority of ECG signals. Indeed, the maximum number N of sliding windows of size W with 50% overlap in a signal with M samples is given by

$$N = \left\lfloor \frac{2(M - W)}{W} \right\rfloor + 1 \qquad (2)$$

assuming $M \geq W$. In the previous expression, $\lfloor \cdot \rfloor$ denotes the floor function. We took advantage of this observation to place the first window at a random offset from the start of the signal. This random offset is drawn uniformly from

$$\{0, 1, 2, \ldots, M - (N - 1) \cdot W/2 - W\} \qquad (3)$$

for each signal at each epoch. The rationale behind this strategy is to prevent the neural network from learning the precise positions of the QRS complexes in the signals from the training set. However, to avoid wasting ECG samples, we always used the maximum possible number of sliding windows for each signal. Finally, it is also important to mention that these data augmentation strategies were only applied during training and not during evaluation.

2.5   Training

We implemented our neural networks and the associated training pipeline with data augmentation in Python with the Keras package [2]. We trained the different neural network architectures for 100 epochs by minimizing the cross-entropy with the Adam algorithm [17]. We set the initial learning rate to 0.0005. The learning rate was divided by two if the cross-entropy evaluated on the validation set did not decrease for 5 consecutive epochs with a lower limit at 10^{-5}.

The batch size was set to 50 signals. We applied zero padding to ensure that all signals in a batch had the same number of samples. Specifically, signals that were too short were prepended with all-zero windows. To limit zero padding as much as possible, we sorted the signals by duration and grouped them in batches of similar lengths. This resulted in batches with varying number of windows.

The LSTM layer was regularized by applying dropout with a rate of 0.5 to both the input and recurrent parts [8,26]. We monitored the accuracy on the validation set and selected the weights at the best epoch as the parameters for evaluation for each dataset and neural network architecture.

3   Results

We evaluated the three neural network architectures described in Table 4 on the CinC 2017 and PhysioNet datasets. The PhysioNet dataset was used with all

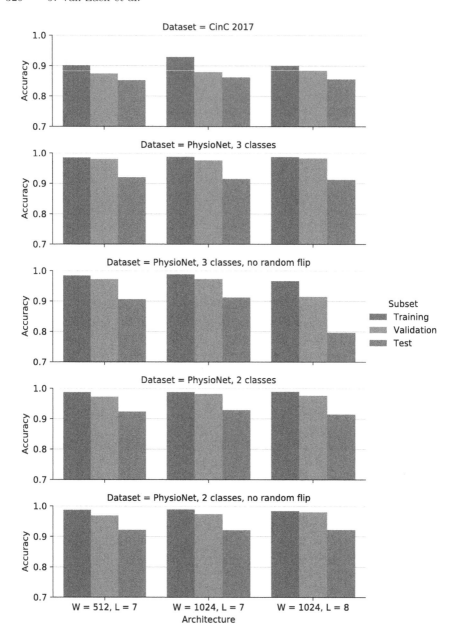

Fig. 3. Cardiac rhythm classification accuracy evaluated on training, validation, and test sets for each dataset and each architecture. The window size is denoted by W and the number of convolutional layers by L.

Table 5. Cardiac rhythm classification accuracy evaluated on the test set for each dataset and each architecture. The window size is denoted by W and the number of convolutional layers by L. The best accuracy for each dataset is shown in bold.

Dataset	$W = 512, L = 7$	$W = 1024, L = 7$	$W = 1024, L = 8$
CinC 2017 dataset	0.8521	**0.8623**	0.8560
PhysioNet dataset			
3 classes	**0.9202**	0.9147	0.9121
3 classes, no random flip	0.9056	0.9117	0.7967
2 classes	0.9234	**0.9289**	0.9149
2 classes, no random flip	0.9216	0.9211	0.9221

three classes and after discarding the *other rhythm* class due its low proportion. Furthermore, we tried training neural networks on this dataset with and without the data augmentation strategy consisting in random flipping the sign of ECG signals. Indeed, flipping signal signs might be detrimental to classification accuracy since the PhysioNet dataset should not include inverted ECG records. After selecting the best neural networks for all cases, we evaluated them without zero padding by selecting a batch size of 1. The classification accuracy measured on the training, validation, and test sets are shown in Fig. 3. In addition, the accuracy measured on the test set is reported in Table 5.

The best results on the CinC 2017 dataset were obtained with a neural network taking sliding windows with 1024 samples as input and extracting features with 7 convolutional layers. The accuracy on the test set was 86.23%. Despite applying dropout, there was overfitting as shown by the difference in accuracy between the training, validation, and test sets. It also appears that using an additional convolutional layer did not help to improve generalization performance. By contrast, using a window size of 1024 instead of 512 was beneficial in terms of classification accuracy. However, the performance difference between the three considered architectures was limited to around 1% on the test set. We also computed the score used to evaluate the participants of the challenge of Computing in Cardiology 2017 (1) for our best network. It achieved a score of 0.829 on our test set which is comparable to the winning entries (0.83 [4,13,27,34]). However, it is important to note that we could not evaluate the score on the test set used during the challenge as it remains private at the time of writing this paper. Instead, we had to split the official training set into smaller sets for training, validation, and testing which reduced the available data.

We considered two cases on the PhysioNet dataset: training with three classes (*normal rhythm*, *atrial fibrillation*, and *other rhythm*) and training with two classes (by discarding the class for *other rhythm*). In the first case, the best architecture used a window size of 512 and 7 convolutional layers for feature extraction and achieved an accuracy of 92.02%. Using a larger window size or an additional convolutional layer did not help to increase classification accuracy. In the second case, a window size of 1024 and 7 convolutional layers led to the best performance on the test set with an accuracy of 92.89%. This is an expected improvement compared to the first case since we dropped the class with the least number of signals.

A few observations can be made after reviewing the results obtained on the PhysioNet dataset. First, it appears that randomly flipping the sign of ECG signals during training helped to improve classification accuracy. Indeed, the performance on the test was better for both two and three classes when this data augmentation strategy was used during training. This result is unexpected as the PhysioNet dataset should not include inverted ECG signals. It is possible that this strategy, by introducing more diversity during training, led to slightly better generalization performance.

The second observation is that there is little difference in terms of classification accuracy between the three considered neural network architectures. Indeed, the maximum difference was less than 2% in all cases on the test set. In particular, a window size of 512 was better for the case with three classes while, in the binary case, a window size of 1024 yielded a better classification accuracy. However, it seems that using more than 7 convolutional layers to extract high-level features is not advantageous.

The third observation that comes to mind is the large gap in accuracy due to overfitting between training and validation sets on the one hand and test set on the other hand. Indeed, training set accuracy was usually above 98% and validation set accuracy decrease only slightly while test set accuracy was 6 or 7% lower. The small difference between the first two subsets can be explained by the fact that we monitored performance on the validation set to select the best weights for the neural networks. A possible explanation for the drop in performance observed on the test set is the approach used for splitting the original dataset. Indeed, we ensured that data for one subject was used either for training or for evaluation (but never for both). In other words, there is no overlap between subjects in the training, validation, and test sets. Thus, it is possible that the ECG signals recorded from subjects assigned to the test set are sufficiently different to cause this performance gap. It can also be partly explained by the presence of ECG signals with poor quality in the test set. An example of such signals is shown in Fig. 4. Due to the poor signal quality, this signal was misclassified as *atrial fibrillation* instead of *normal rhythm*. We were also unable to reliably extract the RR intervals. Figure 5 shows another example of misclassification. However, the signal quality is good in the case. It seems the neural network predicted *atrial fibrillation* instead of *normal rhythm* due to relatively large variations in RR intervals. Indeed, atrial fibrillation is not associated with heart rates below 60 bpm.

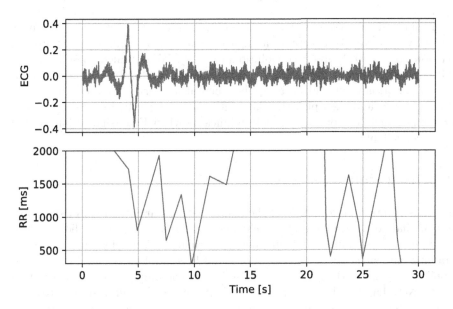

Fig. 4. Example of ECG signal with poor quality labeled as *normal rhythm* (top) and corresponding RR intervals (bottom) from the PhysioNet dataset. Due to poor signal quality, the RR intervals could not be extracted reliably.

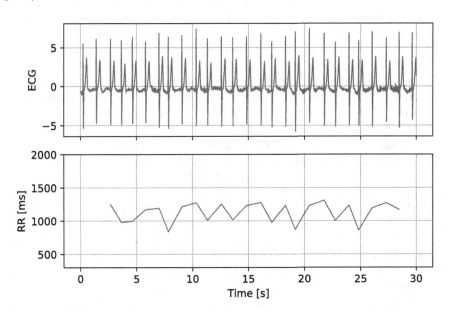

Fig. 5. Example of ECG signal labeled as *normal rhythm* (top) and corresponding RR intervals (bottom) from the PhysioNet dataset.

Despite the observed overfitting, the classification accuracy measured on the test set was above 90% except for a single case (3 classes, no random sign flipping, window size of 1024, and 8 convolutional layers). We obtained these results on 30-s signals. A simple yet effective post-processing method to improve classification performance would be to apply a neural network on several consecutive 30-s segments and then pick the class with the most predictions as the output. Of course, such an approach is only applicable when ECG signals longer than 30 s are available.

4   Discussion

The classification performance of the neural network architectures we developed was similar to the winners of the challenge of Computing in Cardiology 2017. However, we could only evaluate their performance on a subset of the original training data since the official test set has not been publicly released yet. We also applied these network architectures to a dataset combining three databases from PhysioNet. The classification accuracy was above 92% when grouping together or discarding rhythms that were neither *normal rhythm* nor *atrial fibrillation*.

The three neural network architectures we considered combined convolutional and recurrent layers. The convolutional layers were used to extract high-level features from signal windows. Indeed, there is no need for feature engineering with this approach as these layers learn features relevant for arrhythmia classification during training directly from ECG data. Consequently, we applied only a band-pass filter and scaling during pre-processing to make training faster. The recurrent layer was used to take into account signals with different lengths as the CinC 2017 dataset includes ECG records ranging from 9 to 60 s. As all signals had a duration of 30 s in the PhysioNet dataset, it might have been more appropriate to avoid using recurrent layers. However, we were interested in estimating the performance of same architectures on a different dataset. Using only convolutional layers in this case might lead to better performance.

We also applied two strategies for data augmentation. The first one was to randomly flip the sign of each ECG signal during training. The main reason for using such a strategy was to let the neural networks learn to take into account inverted signals included in the CinC 2017 dataset. Surprisingly, this strategy also proved to be effective for the PhysioNet dataset which should not include inverted signals. Random sign flipping most likely helped to increase diversity during training. The second strategy for data augmentation was to apply random offsets from the start of each signal during training to prevent the neural networks from learning the exact locations of QRS complexes.

Collectively, these results demonstrate that detecting cardiac arrhythmia with neural networks from raw ECG signals is feasible. And even if classification accuracy is imperfect, they can help to select and extract segments with potential abnormal rhythms from long ECG recordings for further analysis by a trained specialist. If needed, a 12-lead ECG can then be performed to confirm or refine the diagnosis.

Despite these promising results, there is room for improvements. First, the CinC 2017 dataset is relatively small with only 8528 records. Comparatively, the PhysioNet dataset is much larger. However, it only includes records from 154 subjects and thus lacks diversity. In addition, several abnormal rhythms were either grouped together or simply discarded due to the limited number of available examples. The number of different subjects with these rhythms is even lower. Therefore, there is a need for datasets including ECG records from a large number of subjects with many examples of each rhythm. Obviously, this is a difficult task as building such a dataset would be costly and time-consuming. It is also important to note that we decided to use each lead of the PhysioNet dataset independently in order to use the same architectures for both datasets. Using both leads as two input channels might help to better identify abnormal heart rhythms. In addition, as the field of neural networks is rapidly evolving, several modifications are possible for the neural network architectures we considered in this paper. In particular, residual connections [11,32] as well as dense connections [14] have shown impressive results in the context of image processing. These approaches might also be useful for processing time series in general and ECG signals in particular.

5 Conclusion

We applied three neural network architectures combining convolutional and recurrent layers to two datasets of ECG data for the detection and classification of cardiac arrhythmia. However, in the considered datasets, several rhythms with only a few available examples had to be grouped together. Future developments will need to tackle this issue by either using additional data from other databases or by learning to recognize arrhythmia with few examples. Furthermore, several modifications to our network architecture, such as skip connections, might help to improve generalization performance. We are also investigating approaches to embed these neural network architectures into low-power wearable devices [5].

Acknowledgements. We would like to thank Clémentine Aguet and João Jorge for their helpful comments and suggestions.

References

1. Camm, A.J., et al.: Guidelines for the management of atrial fibrillation. Eur. Heart J. **31**(19), 2369–2429 (2010)
2. Chollet, F., et al.: Keras (2015). https://keras.io
3. Clifford, G.D., et al.: AF classification from a short single lead ECG recording: the PhysioNet/computing in cardiology challenge 2017. In: Proceedings of Computing in Cardiology, vol. 44, p. 1 (2017)
4. Datta, S., et al.: Identifying normal, AF and other abnormal ECG rhythms using a cascaded binary classifier. In: 2017 Computing in Cardiology (CinC), pp. 1–4 (2017)

5. Faraone, A., Delgado-Gonzalo, R.: Convolutional-recurrent neural networks on low-power wearable platforms for cardiac arrhythmia detection. In: Proceedings of the 2nd IEEE International Conference on Artificial Intelligence Circuits and Systems (AICAS 2020) (2020)

6. De Chazal, P., O'Dwyer, M., Reilly, R.B.: Automatic classification of heartbeats using ECG morphology and heartbeat interval features. IEEE Trans. Biomed. Eng. **51**(7), 1196–1206 (2004)

7. Frick, M., Frykman, V., Jensen-Urstad, M., Östergren, J.: Factors predicting success rate and recurrence of atrial fibrillation after first electrical cardioversion in patients with persistent atrial fibrillation. Clin. Cardiol. **24**(3), 238–244 (2001)

8. Gal, Y., Ghahramani, Z.: A theoretically grounded application of dropout in recurrent neural networks. In: Advances in Neural Information Processing Systems, pp. 1019–1027 (2016)

9. Goldberger, A.L., et al.: PhysioBank, PhysioToolkit, and PhysioNet: components of a new research resource for complex physiologic signals. Circulation **101**(23), e215–e220 (2000)

10. Hahnloser, R.H.R., Sarpeshkar, R., Mahowald, M.A., Douglas, R.J., Seung, H.S.: Digital selection and analogue amplification coexist in a cortex-inspired silicon circuit. Nature **405**(6789), 947 (2000)

11. He, K., Zhang, X., Ren, S., Sun, J.: Deep residual learning for image recognition. arXiv e-prints arXiv:1512.03385 (2015)

12. Hochreiter, S., Schmidhuber, J.: Long short-term memory. Neural Comput. **9**(8), 1735–1780 (1997)

13. Hong, S., et al.: ENCASE: an ENsemble ClASsifiEr for ECG classification using expert features and deep neural networks. In: 2017 Computing in Cardiology (CinC), pp. 1–4 (2017)

14. Huang, G., Liu, Z., van der Maaten, L., Weinberger, K.Q.: Densely connected convolutional networks. In: The IEEE Conference on Computer Vision and Pattern Recognition (CVPR) (2017)

15. January, C.T., et al.: 2014 AHA/ACC/HRS guideline for the management of patients with atrial fibrillation: a report of the American College of Cardiology/American Heart Association task force on practice guidelines and the Heart Rhythm Society. J. Am. Coll. Cardiol. **64**(21), e1–e76 (2014)

16. Kannel, W.B., Wolf, P.A., Benjamin, E.J., Levy, D.: Prevalence, incidence, prognosis, and predisposing conditions for atrial fibrillation: population-based estimates. Am. J. Cardiol. **82**(7), 2N–9N (1998)

17. Kingma, D.P., Ba, J.: Adam: a method for stochastic optimization. arXiv e-prints arXiv:1412.6980 (2014)

18. Krizhevsky, A., Sutskever, I., Hinton, G.E.: ImageNet classification with deep convolutional neural networks. Adv. Neural Inf. Process. Syst. **25**, 1097–1105 (2012)

19. LeCun, Y.A., Bottou, L., Orr, G.B., Müller, K.-R.: Efficient backprop. In: Montavon, G., Orr, G.B., Müller, K.-R. (eds.) Neural Networks: Tricks of the Trade. LNCS, vol. 7700, pp. 9–48. Springer, Heidelberg (2012). https://doi.org/10.1007/978-3-642-35289-8_3

20. Moody, G.B., Mark, R.G.: A new method for detecting atrial fibrillation using RR intervals. In: Computers in Cardiology, pp. 227–230 (1983)

21. Moody, G.B., Mark, R.G.: The impact of the MIT-BIH arrhythmia database. IEEE Eng. Med. Biol. Mag. **20**(3), 45–50 (2001)

22. Nattel, S., Burstein, B., Dobrev, D.: Atrial remodeling and atrial fibrillation mechanisms and implications. Circ. Arrhythm. Electrophysiol. **1**(1), 62–73 (2008)

23. Owis, M.I., Abou-Zied, A.H., Youssef, A.B.M., Kadah, Y.M.: Study of features based on nonlinear dynamical modeling in ECG arrhythmia detection and classification. IEEE Trans. Biomed. Eng. **49**(7), 733–736 (2002)

24. Petrutiu, S., Sahakian, A.V., Swiryn, S.: Abrupt changes in fibrillatory wave characteristics at the termination of paroxysmal atrial fibrillation in humans. Europace **9**(7), 466–470 (2007)

25. Rajpurkar, P., Hannun, A.Y., Haghpanahi, M., Bourn, C., Ng, A.Y.: Cardiologist-level arrhythmia detection with convolutional neural networks. arXiv e-prints arXiv:1707.01836 (2017)

26. Srivastava, N., Hinton, G., Krizhevsky, A., Sutskever, I., Salakhutdinov, R.: Dropout: a simple way to prevent neural networks from overfitting. J. Mach. Learn. Res. **15**(1), 1929–1958 (2014)

27. Teijeiro, T., Garcí, C.A., Castro, D., Félix, P.: Arrhythmia classification from the abductive interpretation of short single-lead ECG records. In: 2017 Computing in Cardiology (CinC), pp. 1–4 (2017)

28. Van Zaen, J., Chételat, O., Lemay, M., Calvo, E.M., Delgado-Gonzalo, R.: Classification of cardiac arrhythmias from single lead ecg with a convolutional recurrent neural network. In: Proceedings of the 12th International Joint Conference on Biomedical Engineering Systems and Technologies - Volume 4 BIOSIGNALS, pp. 33–41 (2019). https://doi.org/10.5220/0007347900330041

29. Wang, T.J., et al.: Temporal relations of atrial fibrillation and congestive heart failure and their joint influence on mortality: the Framingham Heart Study. Circulation **107**(23), 2920–2925 (2003)

30. Wijffels, M.C.E.F., Kirchhof, C.J.H.J., Dorland, R., Allessie, M.A.: Atrial fibrillation begets atrial fibrillation. Circulation **92**(7), 1954–1968 (1995)

31. Xia, Y., Wulan, N., Wang, K., Zhang, H.: Detecting atrial fibrillation by deep convolutional neural networks. Comput. Biol. Med. **93**, 84–92 (2018)

32. Xie, S., Girshick, R., Dollár, P., Tu, Z., He, K.: Aggregated residual transformations for deep neural networks. arXiv e-prints arXiv:1611.05431 (2016)

33. Xiong, Z., Stiles, M.K., Zhao, J.: Robust ECG signal classification for detection of atrial fibrillation using a novel neural network. In: 2017 Computing in Cardiology (CinC), pp. 1–4 (2017)

34. Zabihi, M., Rad, A.B., Katsaggelos, A.K., Kiranyaz, S., Narkilahti, S., Gabbouj, M.: Detection of atrial fibrillation in ECG hand-held devices using a random forest classifier. In: 2017 Computing in Cardiology (CinC), pp. 1–4 (2017)

35. Zhou, Y.T., Chellappa, R.: Computation of optical flow using a neural network. In: IEEE International Conference on Neural Networks, pp. 71–78 (1988)

36. Zihlmann, M., Perekrestenko, D., Tschannen, M.: Convolutional recurrent neural networks for electrocardiogram classification. In: 2017 Computing in Cardiology (CinC), pp. 1–4 (2017)

Heart Rate Variability and Electrodermal Activity Biosignal Processing: Predicting the Autonomous Nervous System Response in Mental Stress

Rodrigo Lima[1,2]([email]) , Daniel Osório[1,3] , and Hugo Gamboa[1,2,3]

[1] Plux-Wireless Biosignals S.A, Avenida 5 de Outubro 70, 1050-59 Lisbon, Portugal
[2] Department of Physics, Faculdade de Ciências e Tecnologia da Universidade Nova de Lisboa, Monte de Caparica, 2892-516 Caparica, Portugal
r.lima@campus.fct.unl.pt
[3] Laboratório de Instrumentação, Engenharia Biomédica e Física da Radiação (LIBPhys-UNL), Faculdade de Ciências e Tecnologia da Universidade Nova de Lisboa, Monte de Caparica, 2892-516 Caparica, Portugal

Abstract. The study of the autonomous nervous system (ANS) has played an important role, over the last years, in prognostic and diagnostic of cardiac diseases, as well as, in the assessment of psychological stress. The most common techniques to evelute the balance of the ANS are invasive and unable to provide a continuous monitoring of the patients. The advances in technology and the development of wearable sensors have provided new alternative methods to study the ANS. The analysis of Heart Rate Variability (HRV) and Electrodermal Activity (EDA) are nonivasive methods to assess the ANS with wearables devices. The wearable device used provides information about HRV with the acquisition of photoplethysmography signals from the wrist and EDA from the fingers. The processing of the biosignals was performed by submitting the participants to a mental arithmetic stress test. The results showed that the participants exhibited two distinct response during stress - "Flight or Fight". These responses were classified using machine-learning techniques. The constructed models were able to predict how the subjects will respond in a situation of stress, based only on baseline features. The accuracy of the models using only HRV baseline features was of approximately 80% and the accuracy using simultaneously HRV and EDA baseline features was of 77%, when assigning the correct response during stress to the participant.

Keywords: Heart rate variability · Electrodermal activity ·
Photoplethysmography · Autonomous nervous system · Wearable
device · Biosignals · Machine-learning · Classification

© Springer Nature Switzerland AG 2020
A. Roque et al. (Eds.): BIOSTEC 2019, CCIS 1211, pp. 328–351, 2020.
https://doi.org/10.1007/978-3-030-46970-2_16

1   Introduction

For the past few years, the study of the autonomous nervous system (ANS) has been associated with cardiovascular research. The assessment of the changes in the sympathetic and parasympathetic activity of the ANS with certain diseases and pathologies, such as myocardial infarction, cardiac transplantation, diabetic neuropathy and depression, has been demonstrated to have important prognostic and diagnostic value [31].

The ANS is regulated by the central autonomous network in the brain, comprised of multiple neuroanatomical structures. These brain related structures influence heart activity, responding and adapting to environmental challenges, through the adjustment of physiological arousal by transmitting output to the sinoatrial node of the heart [13].

The ANS transmits its signals to the body through the sympathetic nervous system (SNS) and the parasympathetic nervous system (PNS). The SNS terminal endings secrete a synaptic transmitter, epinephrine. These fibers that secrete epinephrine are also called adrenergic fibers, a term derived from adrenaline, thus the influence of the SNS in the heart is mediated through the release of epinephrine, increasing the force of contraction and the heart rate [12]. On the other hand, the PNS fibers secrete acetylcholine, being also denominated as cholinergic fibers, thus its influence on the heart is to decrease the force of contraction and the heart rate [13]. In a situation of stress, usually, vagal activity withdraws, decreasing the control and influence on the heart by the vagus nerve, facilitating the activation of the SNS, with excitatory influences to the heart [37].

Methods to directly measure the SNS and PNS systems activity are invasive and unable to provide a continuous monitoring of the ANS, leading to inaccurate measurements of the ANS [32]. Recently, wearable sensors have become an active area of research in biomedical science, allowing continuous monitoring of physiological signals of the patients, thus being a useful asset in remote-health monitoring. Additionally, with the improvements in machine learning, these signals acquired with wearable devices, are also good indicators for early prognosis and diagnosis of diseases [22].

A non-invasive method to assess the ANS is to analyze Heart Rate Variability (HRV) [3,15,31,32,45]. HRV is the study of the differences between consecutive heart beats, obtained from the time series of consecutive heart beats intervals, from an electrocardiogram (ECG) [46]. HRV can also be obtained by acquiring photoplethysmography signals (PPG).

PPG is an optical technique, with widespread clinical application, used to detect blood volume changes in the microvascular bed of tissue. PPG signals are a source of HRV, due to the synchronization in time between the R-wave in the ECG and the systolic peak in the PPG signals, making PPG a reliable signal to be applied in clinical settings, such as ambulatory patient monitoring [2].

Spectral Analysis of HRV has been used to assess the level of unbalance between the SNS and the PNS. The high-frequency (HF) component (0.15–0.40 Hz) is influenced only by the parasympathetic system, while the low-frequency (LF) component (0.04–0.15 Hz) is considered to be a marker for sympathetic modulation, despite being influenced by both the parasympathetic and sympathetic systems [7,24,46]. The LF/HF ratio reflects the level of balance between the SNS and PNS, although it has not been accepted as an accurate measure of the level of balance of the ANS, since the LF component is also influenced by the parasympathetic system [30,31,40].

Several studies have analyzed the results concerning the reproducibility of HRV in both time-domain and frequency-domain. Some studies verified that HRV has low reproducibility, even in controlled experiments [21,26], while other studies concluded that HRV is a reliable measurement, when performed in controlled settings [27,35].

Electrodermal Activity (EDA) is an alternative method to directly assess the SNS, being widely used in psychological research [29,40]. The human skin is innervated by numerous efferent fibers, including sympathetic fibers, such as eccrine sweat glands, which produce sweat when the acetylcholine transmitter passes from sudomotor fibers to these glands, changing the skin's electrical characteristics [5]. Eccrine glands are mostly involved in emotional responses to external stimulus and reflect only activity from the SNS, because there is no innervation of the PNS in these glands [33].

EDA signals can be divided into two different components, related to the time-domain: a phasic component - Skin Conductance Response (SCR), that is the result of the activation of the SNS, to an external stimuli presentation, and a tonic component - Skin Conductance Level (SCL), which is a slow changing signal, related to the baseline level of EDA [4,10].

In order to acquire both of these signals and determine the level of balance between the SNS and PNS, the participants were submitted to a mental arithmetic stress test, the Paced Visual Serial Addition Test (PVSAT). This test is the visual version of the PASAT, a test in which participants are presented with a series of digits that must be summed in a defined time interval. The participants must respond aloud the correct answer, prior to the presentation of the next digit [25,34,41].

This work is an extended version of the conference paper "Heart Rate Variability and Electrodermal Activity in Mental Stress Aloud: Predicting the Outcome" [19], presented at the Proceedings of the 12th International Joint Conference on Biomedical Engineering Systems and Technologies - Volume 4: BIOSIGNALS. This version has new state of the art content in the introduction, algorithms that were used in Session 3 - Data Processing, and a more detailed view on the results obtained in Session 4, with the visualization of the boxplots obtained.

2   Materials and Protocol

2.1   Study Population

Data was acquired from a group of volunteer subjects. Fifteen participants (9 females and 6 males) of ages from 21 to 55 years old (31 ± 11), height from

1.57 to 1.85 m (1.73 ± 0.09) and weight from 52 to 94 kg (72 ± 13) signed an informed consent. Table 1 gives the statistics for the study population.

Table 1. Study population statistics. Adapted from [19].

	Mean	SE	Min	Max
Age (years)	31	11	21	55
Height (m)	1.72	0.09	1.57	1.85
Weight (kg)	72	13	52	94

SE - Standard Error

2.2 Materials

The acquisition of the biosignals was made with a BITalino (PLUX - Wireless Biosignals) wearable wrist device prototype (see Fig. 1) composed of six different sensors: EDA wrist sensor with dry electrodes (two stainless steel stubs), PPG, Spare sensor, Total Volatile Organic Compounds (TVOC), Carbon Dioxide (CO_2) and Temperature (TEMP), developed by PLUX - Wireless Biosignals (see Table 2).

For this experiment only the PPG (Channel 2) and an EDA spare sensor (Channel 3) were used. Both the PPG and EDA signals were acquired, simultaneously, with a sampling rate of 1000 Hz and 10-bit resolution. The PPG sensor is a green LED with a photo-detector in reflection mode while the EDA sensor uses Ag/Cl gelled electrodes.

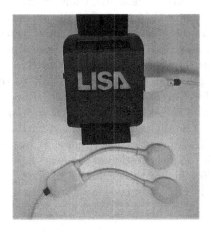

Fig. 1. Wearable device.

Table 2. Description of the wearable wrist device specifications. Adapted from [19].

Sensor	Channel	Resolution (bit)	Sampling rate
EDA wrist	1	10	10 Hz
PPG	2	10	100 Hz
Spare	3	10	1000 Hz
TVOC	4	10	
CO2	5	6	
TEMP	6	6	

2.3 Protocol

This study was performed in controlled conditions. The participants were seated in a comfortable chair, in a quiet room, in order to avoid any external interference that would distract them, while performing the PVSAT, due to the fact that the PVSAT requires several cognitive functions, such as attention and working memory [41]. The experiment's duration was 12 min, divided in two consecutive segments: a 6 min segment in baseline, followed by a 6 min segment in stress, without any break between segments. The baseline status is the segment, in which the participants are seated without performing any task, and without speaking. On the other hand, the stress status is defined by the changes in physiological signals, derived by the complexity and difficulty while performing the PVSAT, in comparison with the baseline status.

The physiological signals (PPG and EDA) were acquired simultaneously using the wearable device described in Sect. 2.2. The PPG signals were recorded on the posterior distal left wrist (Fig. 2(b)), while the EDA signals were acquired by attaching the electrodes to the anterior middle phalanges of the 2nd and 3rd finger (Position 1 and 2 in Fig. 2(a)) of the left hand. During the entire experiment, the participants were asked to avoid any type of movement, specially on the left arm, to avoid artifacts on the signals recorded.

The experiment began by explaining the PVSAT to the participants. This test was chosen to induce stress in the last 6-min segment of the experiment. A 12.2″ tablet with white singles numbers from 1 to 9, on a black background was used in the study. The digits were presented with a 3 s rate for the first 2 min, decreasing half a second every two minutes (2.5 s and 2 s). The subjects had to respond prior to the presentation of the next digit, and speak aloud each response. A warning 30 s before the beginning of the PVSAT was given to all participants (Blue line in Fig. 3). In baseline status, the subjects were asked not to speak.

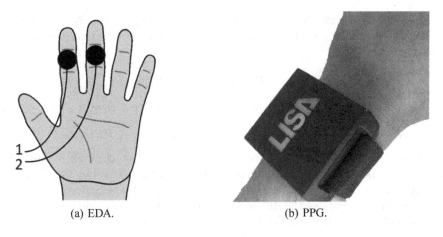

(a) EDA.   (b) PPG.

Fig. 2. Recording sites for the biosignals [19].

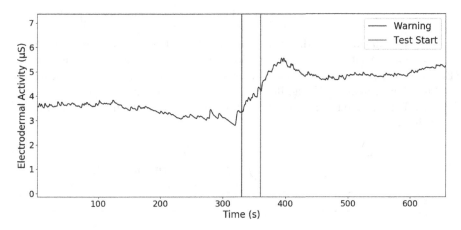

Fig. 3. Representation of the warning and start of the PVSAT. EDA signal increases at the warning 30 s before the PVSAT starts (Blue line - 330 s). The start of the PVSAT is represented by the Red line - 360 s [19]. (Color figure online)

3 Data Processing

3.1 Heart Rate Variability

PPG Peak Detection. HRV features were acquired with PPG signals. The algorithm implemented to detect a peak in a PPG wave is based on the algorithm used in [17]. First, it is necessary to filter the signal in order to remove noise. The signal was filtered with a 2nd order lowpass Butterworth filter at 2 Hz, followed by a 2nd order highpass Butterworth filter at 0.1 Hz. Then, the algorithm detects all the peaks and valleys of the signal, as well as their locations.

Being the PPG signal a time series represented by Eq. 1, where N is the length of the PPG signal, the peaks and the valleys are those points that satisfies the following criteria:

$$PPG(i) = \{PPG_1, PPG_2, ..., PPG_N\} \tag{1}$$

$$\text{Peaks PPG} = PPG(i) : PPG(i-1) < PPG(i) > PPG(i+1) \tag{2}$$

$$\text{Valleys PPG} = PPG(i) : PPG(i-1) > PPG(i) < PPG(i+1) \tag{3}$$

This step assumes that the processing of the signal starts with a valley. In case the first peak location comes first compared to the first valley location, the first peak location is discarded and the processing of the signal starts with a valley. Then, it calculates the difference in amplitude between the peaks (Eq. 2) and the valleys (Eq. 3) using Eq. 4.

$$\text{Peaks to Valleys Difference (i)} = \text{Peaks PPG (i)} - \text{Valleys PPG (i)} \tag{4}$$
$$i = 1, 2, ..., k; \quad k = \text{number of peaks}$$

After calculating these differences in amplitude, the algorithm will search for the differences that are greater than 50% of a 5-point window moving average (Eq. 5), discarding the lower points that do not verify this criteria, getting the final number of peaks with significance for heart rate computation (Fig. 4). This last step is performed iteratively until the number of peaks from two iterations stays the same.

$$PVD(i) > 0.5 * [PVD(i-2) + PVD(i-1) + PVD(i) \tag{5}$$
$$+ PVD(i+1) + PVD(i+2)]/5$$

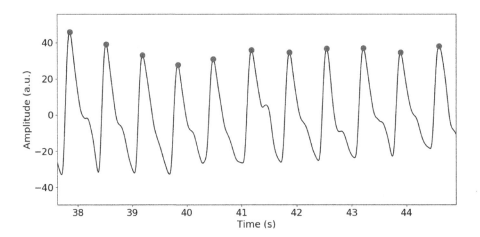

Fig. 4. Peaks detected (Red dots) with the algorithm implemented. Adapted from [19]. (Color figure online)

Heart Rate Computation. Heart rate is obtained by calculating the interval between two consecutive systolic peaks, detected with the algorithm in Sect. 3.1. In order to remove artifacts influence or errors in the detection of the peaks, RR intervals lower than 380 ms were removed due to physiological conditioning, as a normal heart cycle lasts at least 380 ms. The instantaneous heart rate (IHR) in beats per minute (Bpm) is given by Eq. 6.

$$\text{IHR (Bpm)} = \frac{60}{\Delta RR}; \quad \Delta RR = RR_i - RR_{i-1}; \tag{6}$$

RR-interval Series Filtering. RR-interval series recorded from a wearable device PPG sensor are subject to different kinds of artifacts [16], as the most common are motion artifact, breathing artifact and ectopic beats, leading to a wrong detection of the R-peak [20].

To correct the miscalculated peak, a 7-point moving average window was computed. If a RR-interval differs more than 20% of the moving average, or if the RR_{i+1} is smaller than 75% of the value RR_{i-1}, those points are considered as a wrong detection [20]. Then, a linear interpolation is computed to replace each interval considered as a wrong detection. Finally the corrected heart rate is calculated using the new interpolated RR-interval series with Eq. 6 in Sect. 3.1.

Time-Domain Features. Time-domain features were calculated to analyze HRV, in segments of 5-min for baseline status (at rest) and stress status (performing the PVSAT). The time between the 5th and 7th minute of each signal was considered to be the transition band, where heart rate significantly varies from baseline status to stress status. The first (start to 5th min) and last (7th to 12th min) 5-min segments of the acquisition were selected for analysis as the heart rate is more stable during those segments (Fig. 5).

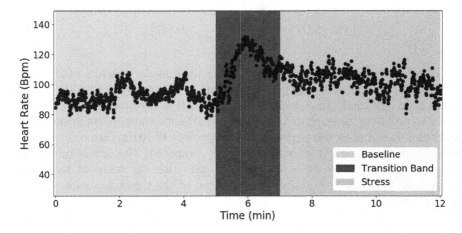

Fig. 5. HRV data division in 5-min segments. Baseline status - 0-min to 5-min (Green band), Stress status - 7-min to 12-min (Yellow band). The Red band corresponds to the excluded Transition band. Adapted from [19]. (Color figure online)

From Eq. 6 in Sect. 3.1, the mean heart rate was calculated for each signal, as well as statistical variables and non-linear variables.

HRV statistical variables are related to the variance of the RR-intervals. These variables are given by the following equations (Eq. 7 to Eq. 10), where RR_i is the ith interval between peaks, $\overline{RR}$ is the average RR-interval and n is the total number of intervals [43].

$$SDNN = \sqrt{\frac{1}{n-1} \sum_{i=1}^{n} (RR_i - \overline{RR})^2} \tag{7}$$

$$RMSSD = \sqrt{\frac{1}{n-1} \sum_{i=1}^{n-1} (RR_{i+1} - RR_i)^2} \tag{8}$$

$$NN50 = \#(|RR_i - RR_{i-1}|) > 50\,\text{ms} \tag{9}$$

$$pNN50 = \frac{NN50}{n} * 100\% \tag{10}$$

HRV non-linear variables are derived from the 5-min Poincaré plot, which represents the diagram in which each RR-interval is plotted against the previous RR-interval. From this plot, it is possible to extract the non-linear variables SD1 and SD2, given by Eqs. 11 and 12, where SDRR is the standard deviation of the RR-intervals and SDSD is the standard deviation of the successive differences of RR-intervals. The ratio SD2/SD1 was also computed, reflecting the balance between the SNS and PNS [15].

$$SD1^2 = \frac{1}{2}Var(RR_n - RR_{n+1}) = \frac{1}{2}SDSD^2 \tag{11}$$

$$SD2^2 = 2SDRR^2 - \frac{1}{2}SDSD^2 \tag{12}$$

Frequency-Domain Features. The frequency-domain variables of HRV can be obtained by computing the power spectrum of RR-intervals. The RR-interval series is an irregularly time-samples series, thus it is necessary to resample the series to avoid the appearance of additional harmonic components in the power spectrum. Resampling was performed at a frequency of 10 Hz, then a cubic spline representation of the RR-interval series was computed. The new regular time-sampled RR-interval series is obtained by evaluating the spline at the points in the new time array. Additionally, the mean of the signal was subtracted to remove any trend.

The power spectrum for baseline and stress status (Fig. 6), was computed using a periodogram, applying to each segment, a Hanning window. Then, the Fast Fourier Transform (FFT) was calculated for each windowed segment. Very-low (VLF), Low (LF), High (HF) frequency components and total power were obtained by integrating the power in each frequency band. The normalized frequency components were calculated by dividing the LF power (Eq. 13) and HF power (Eq. 14), by the total power minus the power of the VLF band. The ratio between the LF and HF components is calculated in Eq. 15 [11].

$$LF(n.u) = \frac{LF}{\text{Total Power} - VLF} * 100 \tag{13}$$

$$HF(n.u) = \frac{HF}{\text{Total Power} - VLF} * 100 \tag{14}$$

$$\text{LF/HF ratio} = \frac{LF(n.u)}{HF(n.u)} \tag{15}$$

3.2   Electrodermal Activity

Time-Domain Features. Time-domain features were also calculated to analyze EDA recordings, by dividing the data in five segments, each with 2 min duration: two bands in baseline (Baseline 1, Baseline 2), two bands in stress (Stress 1, Stress 2) and a transition band (4th to 6th minute), where EDA level changes significantly, due to the warning of the start of the PVSAT test, 30 s before the start of the test. These bands are shown in Fig. 7.

Time-domain features were extracted for each band, by applying a 4th order lowpass Butterworth filter at 1 Hz. In order to compute the SCR and SCL components, the model proposed by [10] was applied.

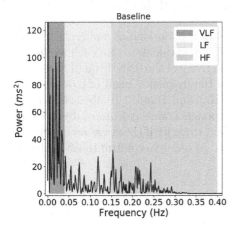
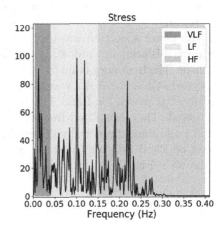

Fig. 6. RV power spectrum. The left spectrum corresponds to a Baseline status and the rigth spectrum corresponds to the Stress status. VLF (0.0033-0.04 Hz) - Red band, LF (0.04-0.15 Hz) - Green band, HF (0.15-0.4 Hz) - Yellow band. Adapted from [19]. (Color figure online)

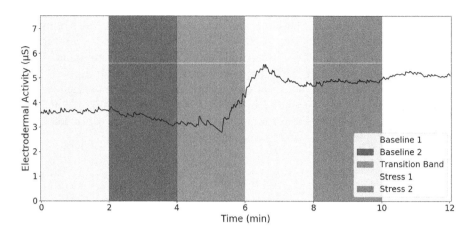

Fig. 7. EDA data division in 2-min segments. Baseline 1 - 0-min to 2-min (Green Band), Baseline 2 - 2-min to 4-min (Blue band), Stress 1 - 6-min to 8 min (Yellow band), Stress 2 - 8-min to 10-min (Purple band). The Red band corresponds to the Transition band. Adapted from [19]. (Color figure online)

From the SCR waveform, features such as SCR amplitude, Rise time, Recovery Time 50% (Rec.t 50%) and Recovery Time 63% (Rec.t 63%) were obtained. A threshold of 0.005 μs was applied. The tonic component was obtained by subtracting the total EDA signal by the phasic component.

Frequency-Domain Features. Frequency-domain analysis was also performed [28]. After filtering, the signal was downsampled. The downsampling process was performed from 1000 Hz to 1 Hz in three consecutive factor of 1/10. Finally, a 8th order Butterworth highpass filter at 0.01 Hz was applied, to remove any trend.

The power spectrum was computed using a periodogram, applying to each segment, a Blackman window. Then, the FFT was calculated for each windowed segment. The frequency band to assess the activity of the SNS through EDA used by Posada-Quintero et al., was modified to the frequency band of 0.04–0.35 Hz. Finally, the power for Band 1 (0.04–0.35 Hz) and Band 2 (0.35–0.50 Hz) was computed. The normalized frequency components were calculated by dividing Band 1 and Band 2 power, by the total power, to verify if there was an increase in power on Band 1 during the stress situation, in order to confirm the stimulation of the SNS (Fig. 8).

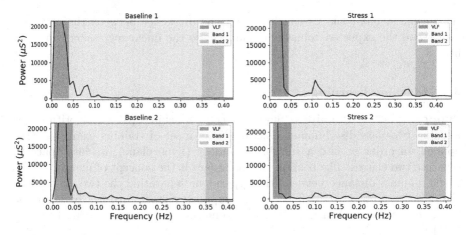

Fig. 8. EDA power spectrum. VLF (0–0.045 Hz) - Red band, Band 1 (0.045–0.35 Hz) - Green band, Band 2 (0.35–0.5 Hz) - Yellow band. Adapted from [19]. (Color figure online)

3.3 Statistical Analysis

Statistical tests were performed in order to assess the significance of the results obtained, between the baseline and stress features extracted.

Kruskal-Wallis Test. The Kruskal-Wallis 1-way analysis of variance by ranks is a non-parametric alternative test to the 1-way ANOVA test, so it does not assume the normality of the data nor the homoscedaticity (standard deviation are equal). The 1-way ANOVA is used to assess whether there is any significant difference between the means of two independent groups, while the 1-way Kruskal-Wallis searches for any significant difference between the ranked means of two independent groups. Ranked values, means that the observed values are converted to their ranks in the dataset: the smallest value gets a rank 1, the next smallest gets rank 2, and so on. The Kruskal-Wallis null-hypothesis is that the mean ranks of the different groups are equal [23]. Probabilities lower than the significance level of 5% ($p\text{-}value < 0.05$) were considered significant, concluding that the null hypothesis may not adequately explain the observation - there is in fact variation between the ranked means of the groups.

Chi-Square Test. Chi-square test χ^2 was applied to test the goodness of fit in Sect. 4.4. This test is applied to determine whether a categorical variable from a single population is consistent with a hypothesized distribution. The null hypothesis is that the categorical data has the given frequencies [8]. In the context of this paper, the χ^2 test will be applied to determine the goodness of the fit of the linear regression line performed, by comparing the values observed calculated using the regression line obtained, with the expected values.

A (*p-value* < 0.05) lets us conclude that the difference between the observed values and the expected values is minimized, so the linear regression is a good fit.

3.4 Machine-Learning

Support Vector Machines. Support Vector Machines (SVM) algorithms for learning two-class discriminant functions from a set of training examples were applied, in order to find a suitable boundary (hyperplane), in data space to separate two classes. The basis of this boundary is the concept of margin, which is the minimal distance between the hyperplane separating the two classes and the closest points to it, defined as the support vectors. In linearly separable data, the kernel of SVM used is the maximal margin classifier or hard margin SVM [42].

Random Forest Classifier. Random Forest classifiers are based on the Decision Tree algorithm. Decision Trees are a supervised method of classification in machine learning, using pre-classified data. The division of the data is based on the values of features of the given data, by deciding which features, best divide ir, creating a set of rules for the values of each feature. The Random Forest classifier is a combination of multiple decision trees, where each decision tree is made by randomly selecting portions of the data, reducing the correlation between trees, improving the prediction power and results with a higher efficiency [6,9].

4 Results

4.1 EDA

The results obtained for both EDA and HRV showed that the PVSAT induced stress to the participants, reflected by the increase in heart rate and in EDA features, such as SCR and SCL, during stress (Fig. 9).

Concerning EDA time-domain features, significant between the median results were found for SCR and SCL. A *p-value* of 0.05 was used to test the significance. For both these features a significant increase in the median was obtained, as the major difference can be seen between the second segment of baseline status (Baseline 2) and the two segments of the stress status (Stress 1 and 2). These results can be observed in Fig. 10.

Frequency-domain analysis of EDA, also confirmed that the PVSAT induced stress in the participants, leading to the activation of the sympathetic nervous system. There was a significant increase in Band 1 power (nu) during stress, especially in the second segment of stress (Stress 2), compared to the baseline segments (Fig. 10(a)). In band 2, there was also a significant increase in Stress 2 compared to the other segments (Fig. 10(b)).

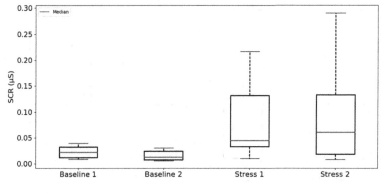

(a) SCR component.

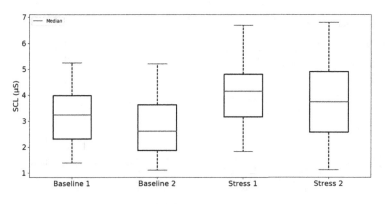

(b) SCL component.

Fig. 9. EDA time-domain boxplots: SCR and SCL.

4.2 HRV

As mentioned in Sect. 4.1, the PVSAT induced stress to the participants. This statement is supported by Fig. 11, in which is possible to verify the significant increase in heart rate between the baseline and stress segments.

Concerning to the frequency-domain analysis, the results obtained for spectral measures were opposite to the expected. It was expected to verify an increase in LF(nu) and LF/HF ratio during stress, but no significant result was found for frequency-domain features (Fig. 12).

Despite no significance was obtained in frequency-domain features for HRV, a thorough analysis of these spectral characteristics, revealed that in some subjects the LF(nu) decreased in stress, while in other subjects there was an increase in stress. Actually, within the 15 subjects that were analyzed, there was a division of 8 subjects in which LF(nu) decreased during stress, and 7 subjects that LF(nu) increased during stress. So, when analyzing the group as a whole, it is possible

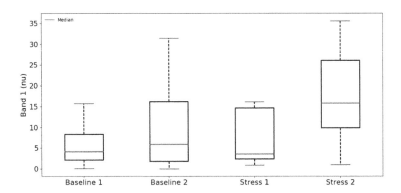

(a) Band 1 (0.04 - 0.35 Hz) power in normalized units.

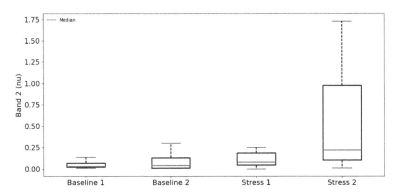

(b) Band 2 (0.35 - 0.50 Hz) power in normalized units.

Fig. 10. EDA frequency-domain boxplots: Band 1 and Band 2.

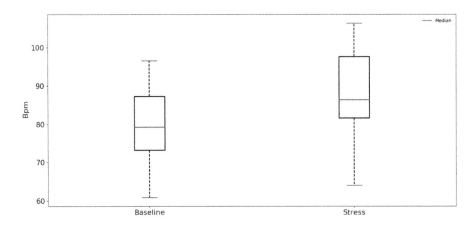

Fig. 11. HRV time-domain boxplot: heart rate (Bpm).

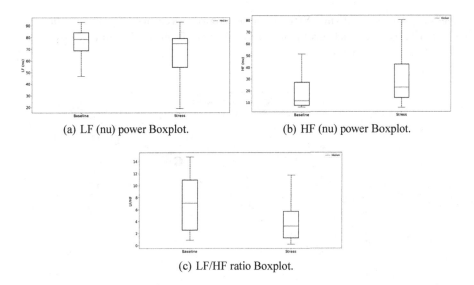

(a) LF (nu) power Boxplot.

(b) HF (nu) power Boxplot.

(c) LF/HF ratio Boxplot.

Fig. 12. HRV frequency-domain boxplots: LF(nu), HF(nu) and LF/HF.

that the opposite responses cancels out the LF(nu) results. Therefore, two distinct groups were formed: group 1 consisted of subjects which LF(nu) decreased during stress, and group 2 consisted of subjects which LF(nu) increased during stress. Then, all features for HRV were analyzed for each group.

For group 1, the results showed a significant increase in HF(nu) power, LF(nu) power and LF/HF ratio. For group 2, the results showed significant effect only for Bpm and RR interval .

4.3 SVM

SVM were applied in this section in order to verify if the two different responses (decrease in LF(nu) and increase in LF(nu) (see Fig. 13) could be separated by a hyperplane. This separation is based on the work of Vuksanovic et al. [44], that verified this distinct response to stress, but in respect to HF power.

A binary classification was assigned to each group: Group 1 - Decrease in LF(nu) was classified as $Y = -1$ and Group 2 - Increase in LF(nu) was classified as $Y = 1$. The hyperplane that separates the two groups is given by a decision function defined by Eq. 16, where w_1 and w_2 represents, respectively, the weights for groups 1 and 2, $\boldsymbol{x_1}$ and $\boldsymbol{x_2}$ represents, respectively, a point for group 1 (Blue circles in Fig. 13) and group 2 (Red circles in Fig. 13).

$$w_1.\boldsymbol{x_1} + w_2.\boldsymbol{x_2} + b = 0 \qquad (16)$$

The results obtained for the weights and the b parameter were: $w_1 = -0.31$, $w_2 = 0.25$ and $b = 4.85$. The number of support vectors for each group were: Group 1 - 1 support vector, Group 2 - 2 support vectors. The coordinates

([LF(nu) Baseline, LF(nu) Stress]) of the support vectors (Black not filled circles in Fig. 13) for each group were: Group 1 - [78.48,74.64] and in Group 2 - [77.35,81.25];[63.08,63.41].

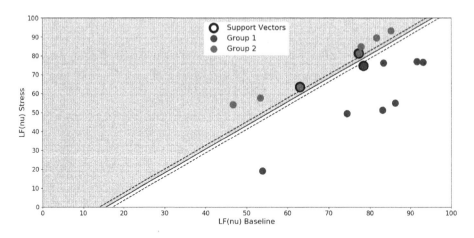

Fig. 13. SVM group separation by the hyperplane: $-0.31.x_1 + 0.25.x_2 + 4.85 = 0$. Blue circles - Group 1. Red circles - Group 2. The support vectors are the points with black border. (Color figure online)

4.4   Linear Regression

In Sect. 4.3, the results showed that the responses of the groups were parallel, so it was possible to predict the LF (nu) values during stress based on the baseline values for each group separately. A linear regression was then computed for each group (Fig. 14). For Group 1 regression (Red line in Fig. 14), the following regression line was obtained: LF(nu) Stress $= 1.40 \times$ LF(nu) Baseline $- 53.15, r^2 = 0.728$. For Group 2 regression (Blue line in Fig. 14), the regression line obtained was LF(nu) Stress $= 1.06 \times$ LF(nu) Baseline $+ 1.48, r^2 = 0.972$.

Finally, a chi-squared test for goodness of fit was applied to the regression lines, comparing the expected values with the observed values using the regression line obtained. For group 1 the chi-square result was $\chi^2(6) = 12.785; p = 0.047$ and for group 2 was $\chi^2(5) = 0.674; p = 0.984$. With the results obtained for the χ^2 statistic, it is possible to reject at a significance level of 5%, the null hypothesis for group 1, concluding that the fit of the regression line is not adequate, while for group 2, with a *p-value*=0.984 it is possible to accept the null hypothesis, concluding that the fit of the regression line is suitable.

4.5   Random Forest Classifier

In Sect. 4.3, it was possible to separate the subjects into two groups, by evaluating their response to stress, with an increase or a decrease in LF(nu) during stress. As this separation is based on a frequency-domain feature, requiring the recording

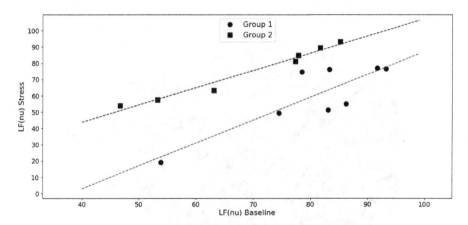

Fig. 14. Linear regression for each group. Group 1 regression line (Red line): LF(nu) Stress $= 1.40 \times$ LF(nu) Baseline $- 53.15, r^2 = 0.728$; Group 2 regression line (Blue line): LF(nu) Stress $= 1.06 \times$ LF(nu) Baseline $+ 1.48, r^2 = 0.972$. (Color figure online)

of the data for at least 10 min (5-min in baseline, 5-min in stress), in order to predict the subject's response to a situation of stress in a shorter recording time, a classification of the subjects using only time-domain features for both HRV and EDA, was performed, to classify the subjects into the two different groups obtained in the previous section.

This classification was performed with a random forest classifier, with 10 decision trees, and a Gini criteria to assess the impurity and the quality of the split. Training of the classifier was performed with a cross validation method, using 6 different random splits and a test sample of 30% of the subjects. This process was repeated 100 times, so that it was possible to choose the model that best classifies the data, that is, the model with a higher accuracy score for the cross validation training method.

First, a random forest classifier using only the following time-domain features for HRV was performed: Bpm, RR-interval and SD2/SD1 ratio. The RR-interval is the most important feature in this model, followed by the SD2/SD1 ratio and the Bpm. The accuracy score for this model to classify correctly each subject to the corresponding group was approximately 80%.

In order to obtain a better visualization of the regions defined by the random forest classifier, the features boundaries are shown in a 3D graph (Fig. 15). A subject with features coordinates that belong to the blue region will be assigned to group 1 - decrease in LF(nu), and subjects that belong to the red region will be assigned to group 2 - Increase in LF(nu).

Information related to EDA was added to the classifier. Similarly to the previous classifier, in order to reduce the recording time, only time-domain features for EDA were added to the classifier. The following features for EDA were selected: SCR, SCL and Rise Time. The more accurate estimators were selected, with the corresponding decision trees. The accuracy score for this model was approximately 77%.

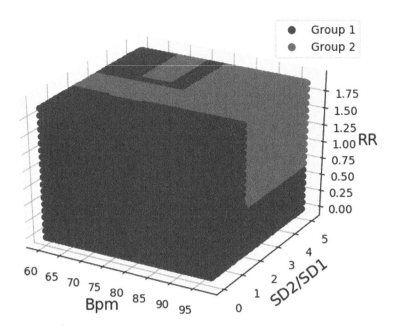

Fig. 15. 3D decision surface for the random forest classifier. Features selected: Bpm, SD2/SD1 and RR-interval (s). Blue region - Group 1 and Red region - Group 2. (Color figure online)

5 Discussion

This was a pilot study to see the influence of stress induction on the autonomous nervous system, by processing HRV and EDA from a wearable device.

The results obtained in Sect. 4, showed that the arithmetic test (PVSAT) induced stress to the subjects, reflected by the increase in heart rate (Bpm) and in EDA features, such as, SCR and SCL, during stress.

For EDA features, SCR, SCL, Rise time, Rec.t 50% and Rec.t 63%, revealed to be good markers of stress, with the increase of values during all the segments studied during stress compared to the baseline segments. In Sect. 3.2, the frequency analysis of EDA signals was performed to confirm the activation of the sympathetic nervous system with an increase in power for low frequency bands. The results obtained showed that there was a significant increase in Band 1 power. This confirms that the dynamics of the sympathetic nervous system are confined to low frequencies, in agreement with the work performed by Posada et al., although in this paper the frequency band studied was extended more 0.10 Hz, the increase in power was also verified, making frequency analysis of EDA a potential marker of quantitative assessment of the level of stress and sympathetic nervous system impairments [30,31].

For HRV, the results obtained for spectral measures were opposite to the expected. The inducement of stress in subjects was expected to increase LF(nu) and LF/HF ratio [14,44]. Contrarily to the expectation, the results obtained showed that there was a decrease in LF(nu) and LF/HF ratio during stress, results also reported by [14,39,44]. Vuksanovic et al. reported that vocalization of the answers, assigned to parasympathetic activity, during the PVSAT interfered with the spectral analysis and concealed out the changes in spectral measures of HRV [44]. Langewitz et al. showed that the breathing pattern for some subjects during vocalization affects the low frequency band power, as the breathing frequency falls in the 0.1 Hz frequency band, the resonance phenomenon will not increase the power in the LF band [18], concluding that the fact subjects answered the PVSAT aloud might have influenced the spectral measures of HRV. These facts also show that the LF band does not reflect purely the cardiac response to the activation of the sympathetic nervous system, but a mixture of the sympathetic and parasympathetic systems, with counteracting effects of activation of the sympathetic system and withdrawal of the parasympathetic system [36]. From the point of view of humoral mechanisms, these results can be explained, as, during a situation of stress, the sympathetic nervous system affects the heart through release of catecholamines [38], such as epinephrine, leading to an increase in heart rate without changing heart rate variability measures, as the release of epinephrine does not affect spectral measures [1].

In Sect. 4.3, despite the results for HRV were concealed out when analyzing the subjects as a whole, it was possible to verify significant changes in spectral measures for HRV after separating the subjects into the two different groups, based on the work performed by Vuksanovic et al., and as an exploratory method in order to find a pattern, taking into account that subjects can exhibit distinct response when submitted to stress ("Flight or Fight"). From Fig. 14, it is possible to see that the slopes for each group do not intercept with one another, so the two responses are parallel. For group 2, the results obtained were in agreement with the expectations that during stress, the LF(nu) and the LF/HF ratio increased with a small decrease in HF(nu) power with no significance. This group responds to stress with the withdrawal of the parasympathetic nervous system and the activation of the sympathetic nervous system. For group 1, the results showed significant decrease in LF(nu) and LF/HF ratio during stress and significant increase in HF(nu) power. The simultaneous increase in HF(nu) and heart rate is more difficult to explain, although it could be an influence of complex respiratory pattern [44], or it could be the effect of different co-activation humoral mechanims, caused by compensatory sympatho-adrenal activation with catecholamine release into the circulation [38].

In terms of EDA, both groups showed an increase in Band 1 power, although significance was only found in group 2 between baseline 2 and stress 1 segments. It is possible to conclude that even if there is a distinct response to stress in terms of HRV, there is activation of the sympathetic nervous system during the stress situation, due to the fact that the sympathetic nervous system influences the heart and sweat through distinct hormones, respectively, epinephrine and acetylcholine.

Finally, the classification model implemented in Sect. 4.5, showed that it was possible to predict the type of response for each subject during stress, using only their baseline features for both HRV and EDA features, making it possible to classify the subjects into the two different groups, with an accuracy of approximately 80% for HRV features in baseline and an accuracy of approximately 77% for HRV and EDA simultaneous features. This model could to be a good asset for future assessment of the type of response when the subjects are under a stress situation, albeit an extended study should be done to confirm the results of this pilot project.

References

1. Ahmed, M.W., Kadish, A.H., Parker, M.A., Goldberger, J.J.: Effect of physiologic and pharmacologic adrenergic stimulation on heart rate variability. J. Am. Coll. Cardiol. **24**(4), 1082–1090 (1994). https://doi.org/10.1016/0735-1097(94)90874-5
2. Allen, J.: Photoplethysmography and its application in clinical physiological measurement. Physiol. Meas. **28**(3), R1 (2007). https://doi.org/10.1088/0967-3334/28/3/R01
3. Bansal, D., Khan, M., Salhan, A.: A review of measurement and analysis of heart rate variability. In: 2009 International Conference on Computer and Automation Engineering, pp. 243–246 (2009). https://doi.org/10.1109/ICCAE.2009.70. http://ieeexplore.ieee.org/document/4804526/
4. Benedek, M., Kaernbach, C.: A continuous measure of phasic electrodermal activity. J. Neurosci. Methods **190**(1), 80–91 (2010). https://doi.org/10.1016/j.jneumeth.2010.04.028, http://dx.doi.org/10.1016/j.jneumeth.2010.04.028
5. Boucsein, W.: Electodermal Activity. 2 edn. (2012). https://doi.org/10.1007/978-1-4614-1126-0
6. Breiman, L.: Random forests. Mach. Learn. **45**(1), 5–32 (2001). https://doi.org/10.1023/A:1010933404324
7. Bussmann, B.: Differentiation of autonomic nervous activity in different stages of coma displayed by power spectrum analysis of heart rate variability. Eur. Arch. Psychiatry Clin. Neurosci. **248**, 46–52 (1998). https://doi.org/10.1007/s004060050016
8. Cochran, W.G.: The $\chi 2$ test of goodness of fit. Ann. Math. Stat. **23**(3), 315–345 (2013)
9. Donges, N.: The random forest algorithm (2018). https://machinelearning-blog.com/2018/02/06/the-random-forest-algorithm/. https://towardsdatascience.com/the-random-forest-algorithm-d457d499ffcd
10. Gamboa, H., Fred, A.: Electrodermal activity model. Psychophysiology (April), 30 (2008)
11. Guidelines: Guidelines heart rate variability. Eur. Heart J. **17**, 354–381 (1996). https://doi.org/10.1161/01.CIR.93.5.1043. http://www.mendeley.com/research/guidelines-heart-rate-variability-2/
12. Guyton, A.C., Hall, J.E.: Textbook of Medical Physiology (2011)
13. Hamilton, J.L., Alloy, L.B.: Atypical reactivity of heart rate variability to stress and depression across development: systematic review of the literature and directions for future research (2016). https://doi.org/10.1016/j.cpr.2016.09.003, http://dx.doi.org/10.1016/j.cpr.2016.09.003
14. Hjortskov, N., Rissén, D., Blangsted, A.K., Fallentin, N., Lundberg, U., Søgaard, K.: The effect of mental stress on heart rate variability and blood pressure during computer work. Eur. J. Appl. Physiol. **92**(1–2), 84–89 (2004). https://doi.org/10.1007/s00421-004-1055-z

15. Hsu, C.H., et al.: Poincaré plot indexes of heart rate variability detect dynamic autonomic modulation during general anesthesia induction. Acta Anaesthesiol. Taiwanica **50**(1), 12–18 (2012). https://doi.org/10.1016/j.aat.2012.03.002, http://dx.doi.org/10.1016/j.aat.2012.03.002

16. Jang, D.G., Park, S., Hahn, M., Park, S.H.: A real-time pulse peak detection algorithm for the photoplethysmogram. Int. J. Electron. Electr. Eng. **2**(1), 45–49 (2014). https://doi.org/10.12720/ijeee.2.1.45-49

17. Kuntamalla, S., Ram, L., Reddy, G.: An efficient and automatic systolic peak detection algorithm for photoplethysmographic signals. Int. J. Comput. Appl. **97**(19), 975–8887 (2014)

18. Langewitz, W., Ruddel, H.: Spectral analysis of heart rate variability under mental stress. J. Hypertens Suppl. **7**(6), S32-3 (1989). https://doi.org/NLM; 19900511. http://www.ncbi.nlm.nih.gov/pubmed/2632731

19. Lima., R., Osório., D., Gamboa., H.: Heart rate variability and electrodermal activity in mental stress aloud: predicting the outcome. In: Proceedings of the 12th International Joint Conference on Biomedical Engineering Systems and Technologies - Volume 4: BIOSIGNALS, pp. 42–51. INSTICC, SciTePress (2019). https://doi.org/10.5220/0007355200420051

20. Logier, R., De Jonckheere, J., Dassonneville, A.: An efficient algorithm for R-R intervals series filtering. In: Conference proceedings: ... Annual International Conference of the IEEE Engineering in Medicine and Biology Society, vol. 6, pp. 3937–3940. IEEE Engineering in Medicine and Biology Society (2004). https://doi.org/10.1109/IEMBS.2004.1404100

21. Lord, S.W., Senior, R.R., Das, M., Whittam, A.M., Murray, A., McComb, J.M.: Low-frequency heart rate variability: reproducibility in cardiac transplant recipients and normal subjects. Clin. Sci. **100**(1), 43 (2001). https://doi.org/10.1042/cs20000111

22. Mahmud, M.S., Fang, H., Wang, H.: An integrated wearable sensor for unobtrusive continuous measurement of autonomic nervous system. IEEE Internet Things J. **6**(1), 1104–1113 (2019). https://doi.org/10.1109/JIOT.2018.2868235

23. McDonald, J.H.: Kruskal–Wallis test - Handbook of Biological Statistics (2014). http://www.biostathandbook.com/kruskalwallis.html

24. Miranda Dantas, E., et al.: Spectral analysis of heart rate variability with the autoregressive method: what model order to choose? Comput. Biol. Med. **42**(2), 164–170 (2012). https://doi.org/10.1016/j.compbiomed.2011.11.004

25. Parsons, T.D., Courtney, C.G.: An initial validation of the virtual reality paced auditory serial addition test in a college sample. J. Neurosci. Methods **222**, 15–23 (2014). https://doi.org/10.1016/j.jneumeth.2013.10.006, http://dx.doi.org/10.1016/j.jneumeth.2013.10.006

26. Piepoli, M., et al.: Reproducibility of heart rate variability indices daring exercise stress testing and inotrope infusion in chronic heart failure patients. Clin. Sci. **91**(s1), 87–88 (1996). https://doi.org/10.1042/cs0910087supp

27. Pinna, G.D., et al.: Heart rate variability measures: a fresh look at reliability. Clin. Sci. **113**(3), 131–140 (2007). https://doi.org/10.1042/cs20070055

28. Posada-Quintero, H., Florian, J., Orjuela-Cañón, A., Chon, K.: Electrodermal activity is sensitive to cognitive stress under water. Front. Physiol. **8**(JAN), 1–8 (2018). https://doi.org/10.3389/fphys.2017.01128

29. Posada-Quintero, H.F., Bolkhovsky, J.B.: Machine learning models for the identification of cognitive tasks using autonomic reactions from heart rate variability and electrodermal activity. Behav. Sci. **9**(4), 45 (2019). https://doi.org/10.3390/bs9040045

30. Posada-Quintero, H.F., Dimitrov, T., Moutran, A., Park, S., Chon, K.H.: Analysis of reproducibility of noninvasive measures of sympathetic autonomic control based on electrodermal activity and heart rate variability. IEEE Access **7**, 22523–22531 (2019). https://doi.org/10.1109/ACCESS.2019.2899485

31. Posada-Quintero, H.F., Florian, J.P., Orjuela-Cañón, A.D., Aljama-Corrales, T., Charleston-Villalobos, S., Chon, K.H.: Power spectral density analysis of electrodermal activity for sympathetic function assessment. Ann. Biomed. Eng. **44**(10), 3124–3135 (2016). https://doi.org/10.1007/s10439-016-1606-6

32. Posada-Quintero, H.F., Florian, J.P., Orjuela-Cañón, Á.D., Chon, K.H.: Highly sensitive index of sympathetic activity based on time-frequency spectral analysis of electrodermal activity. Am. J. Physiol. - Regul. Integr. Comparat. Physiol. **311**(3), R582–R591 (2016). https://doi.org/10.1152/ajpregu.00180.2016. http://ajpregu.physiology.org/lookup/doi/10.1152/ajpregu.00180.2016

33. Posada-quintero, H.F., Member, S., Chon, K.H., Member, S.: Frequency - domain electrodermal activity index of sympathetic function, pp. 497–500 (2016)

34. Royan, J., Tombaugh, T.N., Rees, L., Francis, M.: The adjusting-paced serial addition test (adjusting-PSAT): thresholds for speed of information processing as a function of stimulus modality and problem complexity. Arch. Clin. Neuropsychol. **19**(1), 131–143 (2004). https://doi.org/10.1016/S0887-6177(02)00216-0

35. Sandercock, G.R., Bromley, P.D., Brodie, D.A.: The reliability of short-term measurements of heart rate variability (2005). https://doi.org/10.1016/j.ijcard.2004.09.013

36. Sloan, R.P., Korten, J.B., Myers, M.M.: Components of heart rate reactivity during mental arithmetic with and without speaking. Physiol. Behav. **50**(5), 1039–1045 (1991). https://doi.org/10.1016/0031-9384(91)90434-P

37. Taelman, J., Vandeput, S., Vlemincx, E., Spaepen, A., Van Huffel, S.: Instantaneous changes in heart rate regulation due to mental load in simulated office work. Eur. J. Appl. Physiol. **111**(7), 1497–1505 (2011). https://doi.org/10.1007/s00421-010-1776-0

38. Terkelsen, A.J., Mølgaard, H., Hansen, J., Andersen, O.K., Jensen, T.S.: Acute pain increases heart rate: differential mechanisms during rest and mental stress. Auton. Neurosci.: Basic Clin. **121**(1–2), 101–109 (2005). https://doi.org/10.1016/j.autneu.2005.07.001

39. Tharion, E., Parthasarathy, S., Neelakantan, N.: Short-term heart rate variability measures in students during examinations. Natl Med. J. India **22**(2), 63–66 (2009)

40. Thomas, B.L., Claassen, N., Becker, P., Viljoen, M.: Validity of commonly used heart rate variability markers of autonomic nervous system function. Neuropsychobiology **1508** (2019). https://doi.org/10.1159/000495519

41. Tombaugh, T.N.: A comprehensive review of the Paced Auditory Serial Addition Test (PASAT). Arch. Clin. Neuropsychol. **21**(1), 53–76 (2006). https://doi.org/10.1016/j.acn.2005.07.006

42. Vapnik, V.N.: An overview of statistical learning theory. IEEE Trans. Neural Netw./Publ. IEEE Neural Netw. Counc. **10**(5), 988–99 (1999). https://doi.org/10.1109/72.788640. http://www.ncbi.nlm.nih.gov/pubmed/18252602

43. Vollmer, M.: A robust, simple and reliable measure of heart rate variability using relative RR intervals. Comput. Cardiol. **42**(6), 609–612 (2015). https://doi.org/10.1109/CIC.2015.7410984

44. Vuksanović, V., Gal, V.: Heart rate variability in mental stress aloud. Med. Eng. Phys. **29**(3), 344–349 (2007). https://doi.org/10.1016/j.medengphy.2006.05.011

45. Wachowiak, M.P., Hay, D.C., Johnson, M.J.: Assessing heart rate variability through wavelet-based statistical measures. Comput. Biol. Med. **77**, 222–230 (2016). https://doi.org/10.1016/j.compbiomed.2016.07.008, http://dx.doi.org/10.1016/j.compbiomed.2016.07.008
46. Zoltan, G.S.: Wavelet transform based HRV analysis. In: The 7th International Conference Interdisciplinarity in Engineering (INTER-ENG 2013), vol. 12, pp. 105–111 (2013). https://doi.org/10.1016/j.protcy.2013.12.462

ECGpp: A Framework for Selecting the Pre-processing Parameters of ECG Signals Used for Blood Pressure Classification

Monika Simjanoska[1], Gregor Papa[2], Barbara Koroušić Seljak[2],
and Tome Eftimov[2(✉)]

[1] Faculty of Computer Science and Engineering, Ss. Cyril and Methodius University,
Rugjer Boshkovikj 16, 1000 Skopje, North Macedonia
monika.simjanoska@finki.ukim.mk
[2] Computer Systems Department, Jožef Stefan Institute,
Jamova cesta 39, 1000 Ljubljana, Slovenia
{gregor.papa,barbara.korousic,tome.eftimov}@ijs.si

Abstract. There are many commercially available sensors for acquiring electrocardiogram (ECG) signals, and the predictive analyses are extremely welcome for real-time monitoring in public healthcare. One crucial task of such analysis is the selection of the pre-processing parameters for the ECG signals that carry the most valuable information. For this reason, we extended our previous work by proposing a framework, known as ECGpp, which can be used for selecting the best pre-processing parameters for ECG signals (like signal length and cut-off frequency) that will be involved in predictive analysis. The novelty of the framework is in the evaluation methodology that is used, where an ensemble of performance measures are used to rank and select the most promising parameters. Thirty different combinations of a signal length and a cut-off frequency were evaluated using a data set that contains data from five commercially available ECG sensors in the case of blood pressure classification. Evaluation results show that a signal length of 30 s carries the most valuable information, while it was demonstrated that lower cut-off frequencies, where the ECG components overlap with the baseline wander noise, can also provide promising results. Additionally, the results were tested according to the selection of the performance measures, and it was shown that they are robust to inclusion and exclusion of correlated measures.

Keywords: Biomedical signal analysis · Blood pressure classification · ECG · Pre-processing

1 Introduction

In the field of healthcare many sensors exist and a large amount of people have access to early warning diagnoses through the use of commercially available wear-

A. Roque et al. (Eds.): BIOSTEC 2019, CCIS 1211, pp. 352–377, 2020.
https://doi.org/10.1007/978-3-030-46970-2_17

able sensors. There are different ECG sensors, sweating-rate sensors, respiration-rate body sensors. The data collected with these sensors can be further used for development of mobile applications for real-time diagnosis that are based on machine learning (ML) methods [13]. Currently, several systems for non-invasive blood pressure (BP) monitoring exist, such as: i) the Superficial Temporal Artery Tonometry-based device [40], ii) the PPG optical sensor [9], iii) the ARTSENS (ARTerial Stiffness Evaluation for Non-invasive Screening) for brachial arterial pressure [33], iv) the electronic system based on the oscillometric method [41], v) the BP estimation device based on the principle of volume compensation [29], vi) the Modulated Magnetic Signature of Blood mechanism [49], and vii) the portable equipment that includes a cuff-based BP sensing system [26]. However, most of them are stand-alone devices that cannot be easily incorporated into the commercial sensors that usually estimate the vital parameters from ECG. In [46], the relation between the complexity features of the ECG signals and the BP were explored.

One of the crucial tasks when building such relation models is pre-processing of the ECG signal in order to extract valuable information for further usage. Different parameters can be involved with different values, and the question is how one can find a good parameters that will lead to promising results in a predictive analysis. Some of the significant parameters are signal length used for signal segmentation and cut-off frequency for baseline removal.

Most of the state-of-the-art systems for ECG measuring usually use signal length of 30 s and cut-off frequency for baseline removal of 0.30 Hz. However, in real-life scenarios (e.g., civil and military emergency situations) there is no guaranty that there will be always enough time to measure such long ECG samples.

For this reason, in our previous study [47], we compared different configurations of parameters for signal length and frequency used for baseline removal (i.e., different ECG signal analysis) and their influence to the problem of BP classification. We considered signal lengths of 10 s, 20 s, and 30 s, and cut-off frequencies starting from 0.05 Hz up to 0.50 Hz, with a step length of 0.05 Hz. The novelty of the approach presented in that paper is in the evaluation, where a set of performance measures are used with a data-driven approach in order to make a general conclusion.

In this paper, we extended this approach by explaining it in a more general way, by presenting an ECGpp framework, which can be used to select the best configuration of pre-processing parameters of ECG signals. Since the main benefit is the evaluation methodology that is used, we additionally investigate the influence of different preference functions that can be used during the evaluation methodology. We need to point out that our previous work was done only with one selected preference function, which linearly takes into account the preference with regard to the difference. Also the evaluation is made using an ensemble of performance measures. In our previous work we used a set of 17 performance measures, however in this paper we also explored the influence of the selection of these performance measures in the process of selecting the best pre-processing parameters. We investigate these by removing the correlated measures with regard to some threshold values. We look at linear (Pearson) [4] or monotonic (Spearman) [34] correlations that exist between the performance measures.

The remainder of the paper is organized as follows: in Sect. 2 an overview of the related work is presented. Section 3 explains the ECGpp framework for selecting the best pre-processing parameters of ECG signals. In Sect. 4 we present the experimental results and discussion. Finally, the conclusions are presented followed by directions for future work.

2   Related Work

Most of the recently published studies on the BP estimation use a combination of data from ECG and photoplethysmogram (PPG) sensors [22,42,51]. The common techniques for obtaining measurements on BP mainly rely on Pulse Wave Velocity (PWV), Pulse Arrival Time (PAT), or Pulse Transit Time (PTT) [12,18,35,44]. These all require an accurate PPG measurement, which is not simple to get unobtrusively yet, and no clear proof on the PPG measurement's relation to the BP has been provided [10,37,54].

The relationship between the ECG signal and BP estimation has been discussed in [2,11]. Both methods used an additional PPG sensor with an ECG sensor. The results from studies that address the ECG-BP relationship [20,43] confirm that no strong relationship exists between hypertension occurrence and morphological changes in ECG. For this reason, in [46], instead of using morphological changes in ECG, complexity analysis was used to detect bio-system complexity. For this reason, the ECG signals were segmented using signal length of 30 s, and cut-off frequency of 0.30 Hz was applied for baseline removal.

3   ECGpp Framework

To select the most promising pre-processing parameters of ECG signals that will be further involved in more complex predictive analysis, we propose a new framework named ECGpp. It consists of four levels, which in general can be described as: pre-processing, learning signal representations, predictive analysis, and evaluation of results.

Pre-processing. In this step, pre-processing parameters of ECG signals that are of interest should be selected. Then, for each one its range should be defined specifying the lowest and the highest value, together with the incremental step to change it. Having all of them, all different combinations can be generated and tested for selecting the best configuration. For example, if we are interested in a number of parameters, and each one can have one from a set of values x_i, $i = 1, \ldots, a$, the number of configurations that should be tested is a product combination without repetition for each parameter $\prod_{i=1}^{a} C_{x_i}^1$.

Learning Signal Representation. After the pre-processing step is performed, the next step is to find a representation of the raw signal data that will be further used in the predictive analysis. These means finding features that will represent each signal segment.

Predictive Analysis. To select the most promising configuration (i.e. combination of pre-processing parameters), the learning representations for each configuration (i.e. the datasets where each signal segment is described by a set of features) are further involved in some predictive analysis for which ML model is learned for a specific application scenario.

Evaluation of Results. Having the results from the same ML model that is learned on each configuration, the most promising configuration is selected by ranking the configurations based on the results obtained by the ML model using an ensemble of performance measures.

The pipeline of the ECGpp framework is presented in Fig. 1.

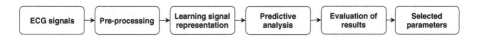

Fig. 1. The ECGpp framework pipeline.

Next, we explain each level in detail focusing on our study for BP classification.

3.1 Pre-processing

In our study, the focus is on two pre-processing parameters, the length used for ECG signal segmentation and the frequency for baseline removal. For the signal length three different values were considered 10 s, 20 s, and 30 s, while the cut-off frequency for baseline removal was in the range [0.05 Hz, 0.50 Hz], with a step length of 0.05 Hz. Baseline removal is needed to remove the noise from the ECG signal and to keep only the part that contains useful information. Using these two parameters, the number of configurations (i.e pairs of signal length and cut-off frequency for baseline removal) is 30. We should mention here that in the pre-processing step each signal segment was also labeled with the appropriate BP class.

3.2 Learning Signal Representation

After the pre-processing, each configuration is a data set that consists of raw signal segments. The next step is to find signal segment representation in order to describe the segments for the BP classification.

Most of the related works used features that described morphological properties of the ECG signal [15, 30, 32], however in our study complexity analysis is used to describe signal segments. By applying it, five complexity metrics are extracted: signal mobility, signal complexity, fractal dimension, auto-correlation, and entropy.

Signal Mobility. It measures the level of variation in the signal [47]. It is calculated as a ratio between the first-order factors S_1 and S_0 of the signal:

$$Mobility = \frac{S_1}{S_0},$$ (1)

where

$$S_0 = \sqrt{\frac{\sum_{i=1}^{N} x_i^2}{N}},$$ (2)

$$S_1 = \sqrt{\frac{\sum_{j=2}^{N-1} d_j^2}{N-1}},$$ (3)

where x_i, $i = 1, \ldots, N$ is the ECG signal of length N and $d_j = x_{j+1} - x_j$ is the first-order variation presented in the signal.

Signal Complexity. It is defined as the second-order factor of the signal [47]. Having the first-order variation of the ECG signal d_j, $j = 1, \ldots, N-1$, the second-order variation of the signal can be calculated as $g_k = d_{k+1} - d_k$. Then, the signal second-order factor is calculated as:

$$S_2 = \sqrt{\frac{\sum_{k=3}^{N-2} g_k^2}{N-2}},$$ (4)

Hereupon, the complexity is calculated by using the first-order and the second-order factors:

$$Complexity = \sqrt{\frac{S_2^2}{S_1^2} - \frac{S_1^2}{S_0^2}}$$ (5)

We need to mention here that for calculating the signal mobility and signal complexity the Hjorth parameters method is used [25].

Fractal Dimension. It measures the self-similarity of the signal by describing fundamental patterns that are hidden in the signal [47]. It can be calculated by the Higuchi algorithm [31]. For a set of k subseries with different resolutions, the algorithm creates a new time series X_k, for $m = 1, \ldots, k$:

$$X_k^m : x(m), x(m+k), x(m+2k), \ldots, x(m + \lfloor \frac{N-m}{k} \rfloor k).$$ (6)

The length of the curve X_k^m, $l(k)$ is calculated as:

$$l(k) = \frac{(\sum_{i=1}^{\lfloor N-m/k \rfloor} |x(m+ik) - x(m+(i-1)k)|(N-1))}{(\lfloor \frac{N-m}{k} \rfloor)k}. \tag{7}$$

Then, for each k in range 1 to k_{max}, the average length is calculated as the mean of the k lengths $l(k)$ for $m = 1, ..., k$. The fractal dimension is the estimation of the slope of the plot $ln(l(k))$ vs. $ln(1/k)$.

Autocorrelation. It is a measure for the similarity between the signal and its shifted version [47]. For an amount of shift τ, the autocorrelation can be calculated as:

$$r_{xx}(\tau) = \int_{-\inf}^{+\inf} x(t)x(t-\tau)p_{xx}(x(t), x(t-\tau))dt, \tag{8}$$

where $p_{xx}(x(t), x(t-\tau))$ presents the joint probability density of $x(t)$ and $x(t-\tau)$.

Entropy. It refers to disorder or uncertainty [47]. Let p_i be the probability of each outcome x_i within the ECG signal X for $i = 1, ..., N-1$. The entropy is calculated as:

$$Entropy = \sum_{i=0}^{N-1} p_i \log(\frac{1}{p_i}). \tag{9}$$

3.3 Predictive Analysis

After we represent the signal segments for each configuration by describing them using the complexity analysis features, we can use them with the same ML methodology for predictive analysis, which in our case is BP classification. This way, comparing the obtained results for the same ML methodology applied on different configurations, we can estimate which configuration (i.e. pre-processing parameters) conveys the most useful information.

In our case, for blood pressure classification, we applied previously developed ML methodology, where meta-classifier is learned for a segment length 30 s and cut-off frequency of 30 Hz [46]. The meta-classifier is based on a stacking design and seven classifiers are used:

- Bagging [8],
- Boosting [16],
- SVM [21],
- K-means [27],
- Random Forest [28],
- Naive Bayes [39],
- J48 [36].

Each of these classifiers provides probabilities for each signal segment to belong in each class. Next for each signal segment, the probabilities that are returned from each classifier are concatenated and, as a consequence, for each signal segment in each configuration we have a new learned representation (i.e. feature vector). Then Random Forest meta-classifier is trained in order to predict the BP class.

3.4   Selecting the Pre-processing Configuration

After learning the meta-classifier for each configuration, the most promising configuration is selected based on the evaluation results.

Since we are working with multiple **independent measurement** for each subject (i.e. participant) and as the **number of measurements varies for each subject**, each data set is m-times split into training and validation set. We also need to mention that if a subject is included in one of the sets, none of its measurements may occur in another set. This way, for each configuration, m different meta-classifiers are learned.

To perform evaluation of the results, a multi-criteria decision approach is used, i.e., PROMOTHEE II method [6]. This comes from the fact that we are not interested in evaluation of the results with regard to one performance measure, but using an ensemble of performance measures. Using an ensemble of performance measures helps us to make a more general conclusion and avoids the bias to the selection of the performance measure used. If we would use one performance measure only, it could happen that the results using different measures can give different results.

In our study, we use an ensemble of 17 performance measures that can be used for multi-class classification such as: accuracy (ACC), Cohen'a kappa (KAPPA), precision (PR), recall (RC), F-measure (F), area under precision-recall curve (PRC), area under the receiver operating characteristic curve (ROC), Matthews correlation (COR), relative absolute error (RAE), root relative squared error (RRSE), root mean squared error (RMSE), informedness (INF), markedness (MAR), micro F-measure (MF), log likelihood (LL), mutual information (MI), and Pearson's chi-squared test (PRS). More explanation about the measures can be find in [47]. The selected set includes the most relevant performance measures for multi-class classification that can be found in the literature.

The relative absolute error (RAE), root relative squared error (RRSE), and root mean squared error (RMSE), require minimization when the preference function is considered, or lower value is better, while all other require maximization, or higher value is better.

After the performance measures are calculated for each meta-classifier learned for each combination, the PROMOTHEE II method compare the results on three levels:

– Pairwise comparisons between pairs of meta-classifiers with regard to one performance measure;

- Pairwise comparisons between pairs of meta-classifiers with regard to all performance measures;
- Multiple comparison between all meta-classifiers, where the influence of all measures are considered.

The results from the three levels are hierarchically connected, which means that the output of one level is the input to the next level.

The PROMOTHEE method requires a decision matrix as an input, which consists of the results for the performance measures obtained by the meta-classifiers for each configuration. The decision matrix is presented in Table 1. The rows of the decision matrix correspond to different meta-classifier, one per each configuration, and the columns correspond to the values obtained for the performance measures.

Table 1. Decision matrix [47].

	q_1	q_2	$\cdots$	q_{17}
C_1	$q_1(C_1)$	$q_2(C_1)$	$\cdots$	$q_{17}(C_1)$
C_2	$q_1(C_2)$	$q_2(C_2)$	$\cdots$	$q_{17}(C_2)$
$\vdots$	$\vdots$	$\vdots$	$\vdots$	$\vdots$
C_{30}	$q_1(C_{30})$	$q_2(C_{30})$	$\cdots$	$q_{17}(C_{30})$

Pairwise Comparisons Between Pairs of Classifiers with Regard to One Performance Measure. Here all pairwise comparisons within all methods are calculated with regard to one performance measure. For this reason a preference function for each performance measure should be defined. This function takes into account the difference between the values of the performance measure between two meta-classifiers (i.e. C_{i_1} and C_{i_2}, $i_1, i_2 = 1, \ldots, 30$, $i_1 \neq i_2$), and it is defined as:

$$P_j(C_{i_1}, C_{i_2}) = \begin{cases} p_j(d_j(C_{i_1}, C_{i_2})), & maximization \ q_j \\ p_j(-d_j(C_{i_1}, C_{i_2})), & minimization \ q_j \end{cases}, \qquad (10)$$

where $d_j(C_{i_1}, C_{i_2}) = q_j(C_{i_1}) - q_j(C_{i_2})$ is the difference between the values of the meta-classifiers for the performance measure q_j, $j = 1, \ldots, 17$.

The most important step in this level is the selection of the function $p_j(\cdot)$, which is a generalized preference function that should be defined for each performance measure. This function defines the preference of the decision-maker for a meta-classifier C_{i_1} with regard to meta-classifier C_{i_2}, and it can be one of six generalized preference functions that exist [7].

Pairwise Comparisons Between Pairs of Classifiers with Regard to All Performance Measures. Here the results from the first level of comparison are used as inputs in order to calculate the pairwise comparisons between pairs of meta-classifiers with regard to all measures. To do this, the average preference index should be calculated, which aggregated the information obtained for each performance measure separately, and provides information of global comparison between the pair of meta-classifiers with regard to all performance measures. It is defined as:

$$\pi(C_{i_1}, C_{i_2}) = \frac{1}{n} \sum_{j=1}^{n} w_j P_j(C_{i_1}, C_{i_2}), \tag{11}$$

where w_j represents the weight of the jth performance measure. The weight defines the significance of the measure, where higher value means higher significance. The weights can be specified by the user or learned by a data-driven method. In our study, the weights are learned using the Shannon entropy weighted method [14].

Multiple Comparison Between All Meta-classifiers, Where the Influence of All Measures are Considered. The last level of comparison aggregates the information from the second one, where the pairwise comparisons between all pairs of meta-classifiers are made with regard to all measures. The aggregation is made with regard to all methods, so the best meta-classifier that indicated also the best configuration can be selected. For this reason, the positive, the negative, and the net flow should be calculated. The positive preference flow gives information how a given meta-classifier is globally better than the other, while the negative preference flow gives the information about how a given meta-classifier is outranked by all others. The net flow of a meta-classifier is the difference of its positive and negative flow.

The positive preference flow is defined as:

$$\phi(C_i^+) = \frac{1}{(n-1)} \sum_{x \in C} \pi(C_i, x), \tag{12}$$

while the negative preference flow is defined as:

$$\phi(C_i^-) = \frac{1}{(n-1)} \sum_{x \in C} \pi(x, C_i). \tag{13}$$

The net flow of a meta-classifier is defined as:

$$\phi(C_i) = \phi(C_i^+) - \phi(C_i^-). \tag{14}$$

After calculating the net flows, the meta-classifiers are ranked by ordering them with regard to decreasing values of the net flows.

The flowchart of the evaluation methodology is presented in Fig. 2.

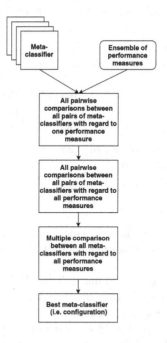

Fig. 2. The evaluation methodology flowchart.

More details can be found in [14].

4   Results and Discussion

This section presents the data that is used for evaluation of the proposed ECGpp framework, as well as the relevant experiments and their corresponding results.

4.1   Data

Data used for evaluation of the ECGpp framework were acquired by five different ECG sensors. Four data sets are based on commercially available sensors [5,19,50,52] and the fifth set is from the online available Physionet database [17]. Each ECG signal is also equipped with reference values for the systolic and diastolic blood pressure that were measured in parallel, using electronic sphygmomanometer. In addition, Table 2 summarizes information on each sensor's reliability, the number of measured participants, and their age.

Following the standards and data protection policies, we need to mention that all participants involved in the research signed an agreement on allowing their ECG data to be used for research purposes. They were of different age and health status, and the measurements were performed under different conditions, in moving and sitting positions. Among the available data in the Physionet database only those were explicitly selected to include patients that suffer brain injuries.

Table 2. Sensors summary information [47].

Dataset	Reliability	Participants	Age
Cooking hacks [19]	[53]	16	16–72
180° eMotion FAROS [5]	[3]	3	25–27
Zephyr Bioharness module [50]	[23]	14	20–73
Savvy sensor platform [52]	[52]	21	15–54
Charis Physionet database [17]	[24]	7	20–74

Since we are interested in BP classification, we labeled each ECG signal using the BP class. This was done using a publicly available scheme presented in Table 3 [1,38].

As BP classes do not seem to be mutually exclusive more priority was given to more severe BP conditions, by checking the AND conditions at the end of the ECG samples mapping procedure. To imbalanced-class data issue was solved by grouping the BP classes into three main categories: hypotension (HPTN) and normal (N) as Normal class (denoted as 0); prehypertension (PHTN) as Pre-hypertension class (denoted as 1); and stage 1 hypertension (S1HTN), stage 2 hypertension (S2HTN), isolated systolic hypertension (ISHTN), and hypertensive crisis (HTNC) as Hypertension class (denoted as 2) [1,38].

Table 3. Rules and categorization [47].

Joined class	Class	SBP (mmHg)	Logical	DBP (mmHg)
Normal	HPTN	<=90	OR	<=60
	N	90–119	AND	60–79
Prehypertension	PHTN	120–139	OR	80–89
Hypertension	S1HTN	140–159	OR	90–99
	S2HTN	>=160	OR	>=100
	ISHTN	>=140	AND	<90
	HTNC	>=180	OR	>=110

4.2   Experiments

To evaluate the ECGpp framework, the data was pre-processed with regard to the segment length and cut-off frequency of baseline removal and it ended up with 30 different data sets (i.e. configurations), one data set per each pre-processing pair of parameters. This data sets were further processed to describe them using the complexity analysis features. After that, the next step was to learn and evaluate a meta-classifier for each configuration that implicitly pointed to the useful information conveyed by each pre-processing pair of parameters.

For this reason, each data set was split into training and validation set using 75% of the subjects in the training set and the other 25% in the validation set. Since we are working with human subjects, the splitting is performed taking care that a subject that is included in the training set cannot be include in the validation set. For this reason and in order to learn more robust meta-classifiers, each data set was split 30 times into training and validation set, which results with 30 different meta-classifiers for each configuration.

Because for each configuration we have 30 different meta-classifiers that are evaluated using the ensemble of 17 performance measures and the decision matrix used for the evaluation methodology requires only one per configuration, we preformed the experiments in two scenarios:

- Best split for each configuration;
- Average of all splits for each configuration.

In the first scenario, the evaluation methodology was first applied within each configuration in order to find the best meta-classifier (i.e. best split). After that, the best meta-classifiers for each configuration were evaluated again using the evaluation methodology in order to select the most promising meta-classifier, that indicated to the most promising pre-processing parameters.

In the second scenario, the results from 30 splits for each configuration were aggregated by averaging the results for each performance measure separately. This was made with the purpose to obtain more robust results, following the cross-fold validation idea.

Since for the evaluation methodology the selection of the generalized preference function is also crucial, for each scenario, we tested two different generalized preference functions: the usual and the V-shape. This was made with the purpose to see if it influenced the end result. In the case of the V-shape generalized preference function, the threshold of strict preference is set to the maximum difference that exists for each preference measure from all pairwise comparisons according to that performance measure.

At the end, we provided sensitivity analysis, in order to see the influence of the included performance measures by removing the correlated measures with regard to some thresholds using the Pearson [4] and Spearman [34] correlation, separately. The Pearson correlation coefficient assesses linear relationships, while the Spearman's correlation assesses monotonic relationships (whether linear or not). The value of both coefficients can be between -1 and 1.

Best Split for Each Configuration. In the case of the usual preference function, the best meta-classifiers within each configuration, which are results when the PROMOTHEE method is used within each configuration, are presented in

Table 4. The first column presents the pre-processing parameters used for the segment length and cut-off frequency for baseline removal. The last column provides the ranking for each combination. These rankings come form the PROMOTHEE method when the best meta-classifiers from all configurations are compared.

Using the Table 4, the best results are obtained using the meta-classifier for the configuration with the segment length of 10 s and cut-off frequency for baseline removal 0.30 Hz, the second best is obtained for the segment length of 20 s and the cut-off frequency of 0.45 Hz, and the third with the segment length of 30 s and the cut-off frequency of 0.15 Hz.

Table 4. Performance results for best meta-classifier trained for each configuration using the Usual generalized preference function.

Comb.	ACC	KAPPA	PRC	ROC	F	COR	PR	RC	RAE	RRSE	RMSE	INF	MAR	MF	LL	MI	PRS	Ranking
10/0.05	55.16	0.33	0.54	0.71	0.53	0.32	0.54	0.55	68.23	108.14	0.51	0.31	0.37	0.55	56.59	0.18	96.75	14
10/0.10	46.99	0.24	0.53	0.68	0.45	0.25	0.54	0.47	77.09	109.25	0.54	0.27	0.29	0.47	32.67	0.12	58.12	26
10/0.15	55.30	0.30	0.53	0.70	0.55	0.33	0.56	0.55	66.71	104.72	0.50	0.32	0.34	0.55	40.72	0.19	61.14	15
10/0.20	49.82	0.24	0.48	0.64	0.50	0.24	0.51	0.50	78.10	113.74	0.54	0.24	0.23	0.50	24.91	0.09	42.61	30
10/0.25	54.01	0.31	0.52	0.69	0.54	0.31	0.55	0.54	71.47	110.71	0.52	0.32	0.30	0.54	33.26	0.14	57.64	21
10/0.30	**63.14**	**0.44**	**0.62**	**0.78**	**0.64**	**0.47**	**0.68**	**0.63**	**58.84**	**95.76**	**0.46**	**0.47**	**0.45**	**0.63**	**52.12**	**0.22**	**93.10**	**1**
10/0.35	56.38	0.28	0.60	0.72	0.56	0.32	0.56	0.56	67.75	101.45	0.49	0.32	0.32	0.56	25.18	0.13	40.82	18
10/0.40	50.19	0.24	0.48	0.64	0.50	0.24	0.51	0.50	80.58	116.81	0.55	0.23	0.27	0.50	26.72	0.10	45.47	29
10/0.45	52.68	0.30	0.48	0.66	0.51	0.28	0.52	0.53	75.96	112.93	0.53	0.27	0.34	0.53	32.58	0.15	54.57	22
10/0.50	52.68	0.29	0.49	0.67	0.50	0.28	0.50	0.53	73.16	112.33	0.53	0.27	0.34	0.53	29.21	0.13	49.54	23
20/0.05	56.88	0.35	0.55	0.73	0.54	0.34	0.53	0.57	63.21	106.86	0.51	0.33	0.42	0.57	45.39	0.21	73.83	11
20/0.10	54.39	0.32	0.53	0.67	0.54	0.34	0.62	0.54	69.39	109.42	0.52	0.37	0.32	0.54	58.17	0.16	102.90	16
20/0.15	50.58	0.26	0.53	0.66	0.52	0.28	0.55	0.51	79.19	109.17	0.53	0.29	0.25	0.51	25.55	0.10	47.01	25
20/0.20	57.14	0.32	0.55	0.70	0.57	0.33	0.57	0.57	67.37	104.82	0.50	0.34	0.34	0.57	29.84	0.15	47.90	12
20/0.25	51.64	0.25	0.51	0.66	0.51	0.25	0.52	0.52	75.33	109.22	0.51	0.26	0.23	0.52	26.49	0.11	44.91	24
20/0.30	50.71	0.24	0.49	0.63	0.51	0.25	0.54	0.51	77.12	110.01	0.52	0.26	0.22	0.51	32.03	0.11	58.00	27
20/0.35	65.56	0.37	0.63	0.73	0.65	0.39	0.65	0.66	56.85	94.44	0.46	0.39	0.39	0.66	19.70	0.13	34.84	6
20/0.40	51.03	0.24	0.45	0.61	0.51	0.23	0.51	0.51	78.26	115.49	0.55	0.24	0.22	0.51	39.74	0.10	68.30	28
20/0.45	61.03	0.41	0.58	0.76	0.59	0.41	0.59	0.61	65.11	93.24	0.44	0.41	0.45	0.61	53.41	0.25	86.30	2
20/0.50	54.87	0.33	0.51	0.67	0.55	0.33	0.56	0.55	77.03	103.46	0.49	0.34	0.35	0.55	35.22	0.16	60.30	20
30/0.05	58.64	0.36	0.58	0.75	0.57	0.37	0.56	0.59	61.19	101.95	0.49	0.36	0.40	0.59	70.00	0.21	115.57	5
30/0.10	54.15	0.32	0.53	0.68	0.55	0.34	0.59	0.54	72.85	109.31	0.52	0.35	0.30	0.54	68.93	0.23	115.65	13
30/0.15	60.96	0.41	0.60	0.75	0.62	0.43	0.64	0.61	62.35	97.53	0.47	0.43	0.42	0.61	45.74	0.20	80.81	3
30/0.20	58.48	0.38	0.53	0.69	0.57	0.37	0.58	0.58	67.72	105.90	0.50	0.37	0.41	0.58	47.47	0.21	77.22	10
30/0.25	52.73	0.30	0.54	0.69	0.53	0.34	0.59	0.53	74.38	108.59	0.52	0.36	0.32	0.53	52.02	0.19	88.54	19
30/0.30	56.07	0.33	0.52	0.68	0.56	0.33	0.56	0.56	70.54	105.38	0.50	0.32	0.33	0.56	43.67	0.16	79.52	17
30/0.35	58.37	0.37	0.58	0.74	0.57	0.37	0.57	0.58	64.60	101.66	0.48	0.37	0.40	0.58	49.26	0.22	79.46	8
30/0.40	57.04	0.36	0.58	0.74	0.57	0.38	0.62	0.57	67.69	103.16	0.51	0.38	0.39	0.57	62.47	0.22	102.85	9
30/0.45	59.41	0.38	0.59	0.73	0.59	0.38	0.59	0.59	68.63	100.51	0.47	0.39	0.38	0.59	45.21	0.15	88.38	7
30/0.50	60.48	0.40	0.59	0.74	0.60	0.41	0.60	0.60	68.74	95.42	0.45	0.41	0.41	0.60	37.36	0.18	67.44	4

In the case of V-shape function, the best meta-classifiers within each configuration together with their rankings are presented in Table 5. Using it, we can see that the three best configurations are the same as in the case when the usual generalized preference function is used.

However, if we look at the rankings, there are several configurations with different rankings. For example, the rankings obtained with the usual preference function are: 14, 26, 15, 30, 21, 1, 18, 29, 22, 23, 11, 16, 25, 12, 24, 27, 6, 28, 2, 20, 5, 13, 3, 10, 19, 17, 8, 9, 7, and 4, while the rankings obtained using the V-shape generalized preference function are: 14, 27, 16, 28, 22, 1, 18, 30, 24, 25, 11, 12, 23, 15, 26, 21, 5, 29, 2, 20, 7, 13, 3, 10, 19, 17, 9, 4, 8, and 6. Comparing these rankings, there is no big deviations between the rankings, the biggest one is the configuration where the signal length is 30 s and the cut-off frequency is 0.40 Hz, when the rankings change from 9 to 4, going from usual to V-shape

Table 5. Performance results for best meta-classifier trained for each configuration using the V-shape generalized preference function [47].

Comb.	ACC	KAPPA	PRC	ROC	F	COR	PR	RC	RAE	RRSE	RMSE	INF	MAR	MF	LL	MI	PRS	Ranking
10/0.05	55.16	0.33	0.54	0.71	0.53	0.32	0.54	0.55	68.23	108.14	0.51	0.31	0.37	0.55	56.59	0.18	96.75	14
10/0.10	46.99	0.24	0.53	0.68	0.45	0.25	0.54	0.47	77.09	109.25	0.54	0.27	0.29	0.47	32.67	0.12	58.12	27
10/0.15	55.30	0.30	0.53	0.70	0.55	0.33	0.56	0.55	66.71	104.72	0.50	0.32	0.34	0.55	40.72	0.19	61.14	16
10/0.20	51.46	0.22	0.51	0.67	0.49	0.23	0.50	0.51	73.99	110.49	0.52	0.24	0.28	0.51	19.38	0.09	29.71	28
10/0.25	54.01	0.31	0.52	0.69	0.54	0.31	0.55	0.54	71.47	110.71	0.52	0.32	0.30	0.54	33.26	0.14	57.64	22
10/0.30	**63.14**	**0.44**	**0.62**	**0.78**	**0.64**	**0.47**	**0.68**	**0.63**	**58.84**	**95.76**	**0.46**	**0.47**	**0.45**	**0.63**	**52.12**	**0.22**	**93.10**	**1**
10/0.35	56.38	0.28	0.60	0.72	0.56	0.32	0.56	0.56	67.75	101.45	0.49	0.32	0.32	0.56	25.18	0.13	40.82	18
10/0.40	50.19	0.24	0.48	0.64	0.50	0.24	0.51	0.50	80.58	116.81	0.55	0.23	0.27	0.50	26.72	0.10	45.47	30
10/0.45	52.68	0.30	0.48	0.66	0.51	0.28	0.52	0.53	75.96	112.93	0.53	0.27	0.34	0.53	32.58	0.15	54.57	24
10/0.50	52.68	0.29	0.49	0.67	0.50	0.28	0.50	0.53	73.16	112.33	0.53	0.27	0.34	0.53	29.21	0.13	49.54	25
20/0.05	56.88	0.35	0.55	0.73	0.54	0.34	0.53	0.57	63.21	106.86	0.51	0.33	0.42	0.57	45.39	0.21	73.83	11
20/0.10	56.07	0.34	0.55	0.72	0.52	0.33	0.53	0.56	69.25	106.40	0.50	0.33	0.42	0.56	48.09	0.20	77.33	12
20/0.15	57.24	0.24	0.57	0.65	0.57	0.23	0.58	0.57	66.19	103.87	0.50	0.23	0.24	0.57	11.33	0.07	20.14	23
20/0.20	57.14	0.32	0.55	0.70	0.57	0.33	0.57	0.57	67.37	104.82	0.50	0.34	0.34	0.57	29.84	0.15	47.90	15
20/0.25	51.64	0.25	0.51	0.66	0.51	0.25	0.52	0.52	75.33	109.22	0.51	0.26	0.23	0.52	26.49	0.11	44.91	26
20/0.30	55.56	0.28	0.58	0.70	0.56	0.30	0.57	0.56	66.80	101.72	0.48	0.30	0.29	0.56	12.89	0.08	20.42	21
20/0.35	65.56	0.37	0.63	0.73	0.65	0.39	0.65	0.66	56.85	94.44	0.46	0.39	0.39	0.66	19.70	0.13	34.84	5
20/0.40	51.03	0.24	0.45	0.61	0.51	0.23	0.51	0.51	78.26	115.49	0.55	0.24	0.22	0.51	39.74	0.10	68.30	29
20/0.45	61.03	0.41	0.58	0.76	0.59	0.41	0.59	0.61	65.11	93.24	0.44	0.41	0.45	0.61	53.41	0.25	86.30	2
20/0.50	54.87	0.33	0.51	0.67	0.55	0.33	0.56	0.55	77.03	103.46	0.49	0.34	0.35	0.55	35.22	0.16	60.30	20
30/0.05	58.64	0.36	0.58	0.75	0.57	0.37	0.56	0.59	61.19	101.95	0.49	0.36	0.40	0.59	70.00	0.24	115.57	7
30/0.10	54.15	0.32	0.53	0.68	0.55	0.34	0.59	0.54	72.85	109.31	0.52	0.35	0.30	0.54	68.93	0.23	115.65	13
30/0.15	60.96	0.41	0.60	0.75	0.62	0.43	0.64	0.61	62.35	97.53	0.47	0.43	0.42	0.61	45.74	0.20	80.81	3
30/0.20	58.48	0.38	0.53	0.69	0.57	0.37	0.58	0.58	67.72	105.90	0.50	0.37	0.41	0.58	47.47	0.21	77.22	10
30/0.25	52.73	0.30	0.54	0.69	0.52	0.34	0.59	0.53	74.38	108.59	0.52	0.36	0.32	0.53	52.02	0.19	88.54	19
30/0.30	56.07	0.33	0.52	0.68	0.56	0.33	0.56	0.56	70.54	105.38	0.50	0.32	0.33	0.56	43.67	0.16	79.52	17
30/0.35	58.37	0.37	0.58	0.74	0.57	0.37	0.57	0.58	64.60	101.66	0.48	0.37	0.40	0.58	49.26	0.22	79.46	9
30/0.40	62.73	0.36	0.59	0.74	0.60	0.43	0.65	0.63	58.09	100.81	0.48	0.48	0.42	0.63	27.00	0.25	40.09	4
30/0.45	59.41	0.38	0.59	0.73	0.59	0.38	0.59	0.59	68.63	100.51	0.47	0.39	0.38	0.59	45.21	0.15	88.38	8
30/0.50	60.48	0.40	0.59	0.74	0.60	0.41	0.60	0.60	68.74	95.42	0.45	0.41	0.41	0.60	37.36	0.18	67.44	6

generalized function. We can also see that changing the generalized preference function from usual to V-shape, the configuration that provides the best meta-classifier can be different. This comes from the reason that the PROMOTHEE method is used within each configuration to find the best split. One such example is the configuration where the segment length is 20 s and the cut-off frequency is 0.30 Hz.

In general, the selection of different preference function does not change the end results. There is no big deviations between the rankings that can be obtained. The only difference is that in the case of the usual generalized preference function, the function only count wins and loses, without taking the amount of difference. While the V-shape function takes into account also how big the win or lose is.

Using the best split experiment, there is no general conclusion which configuration provides most promising results. We can see that the top 10 configuration are spread to all segment lengths. This leads to a question of how robust are the results, or if the selection of the best meta-classifier for each configuration corresponds to a real-life application.

Average of All Splits for Each Configuration. In the case of the usual generalized preference function the averaged performance for each configuration is presented in Table 6. The last column reported the ranking for each configuration that are obtained by the PROMOTHEE method when all configurations are compared using the averaged results.

In the case of V-shape function, the averaged performance for each configuration and their rankings are presented in Table 7.

Using Tables 6 and 7, it follows that the best meta-classifier points to the segment length of 30 s and cut-off frequency of 0.10 Hz, the second best for the segment length of 30 s and the cut-off frequency of 0.15 Hz, and the third with the segment length of 30 s and the cut-off frequency of 0.20 Hz. The top 10 best configurations are when the segment length is 30 s, so this indicates that segment length of 30 s provides the most useful information.

The rankings obtained using the usual generalized preference function are: 16, 20, 21, 14, 12, 15, 18, 26, 17, 27, 19, 11, 30, 22, 28, 23, 29, 25, 13, 24, 4, 1, 2, 3, 7, 10, 8, 6, 5, and 9, while the rankings obtained using the V-shape function are: 16, 21, 19, 14, 12, 15, 18, 26, 17, 29, 20, 11, 28, 22, 30, 23, 27, 25, 13, 24, 5, 1, 2, 3, 7, 10, 8, 6, 4, and 9. Comparing the rankings deviations with the deviations obtained in the case of the best split, we can conclude that this experiment provide more robust rankings with regard to the selection of the generalized preference function.

Table 6. Averaged performance results from all meta-classifiers trained for each configuration using the Usual preference function.

Comb.	ACC	KAPPA	PRC	ROC	F	COR	PR	RC	RAE	RRSE	RMSE	INF	MAR	MF	LL	MI	PRS	Ranking
10/0.05	44.32	0.14	0.45	0.60	0.43	0.14	0.46	0.44	83.80	117.68	0.56	0.14	0.16	0.44	14.64	0.06	24.40	16
10/0.10	43.05	0.12	0.46	0.58	0.43	0.13	0.48	0.43	85.39	119.59	0.57	0.14	0.12	0.43	15.59	0.06	26.19	20
10/0.15	44.02	0.13	0.45	0.59	0.43	0.13	0.46	0.44	84.55	119.00	0.57	0.14	0.14	0.44	14.43	0.06	23.65	21
10/0.20	44.28	0.15	0.44	0.59	0.43	0.15	0.47	0.44	85.16	118.83	0.57	0.16	0.16	0.44	18.22	0.07	30.27	14
10/0.25	45.89	0.15	0.47	0.60	0.45	0.15	0.48	0.46	81.93	116.21	0.55	0.16	0.15	0.46	14.88	0.06	24.46	12
10/0.30	43.78	0.14	0.46	0.60	0.43	0.14	0.47	0.44	83.49	117.40	0.56	0.15	0.14	0.44	15.84	0.06	26.07	15
10/0.35	44.07	0.13	0.46	0.59	0.43	0.14	0.46	0.44	84.54	117.58	0.56	0.13	0.14	0.44	11.94	0.05	18.98	18
10/0.40	42.43	0.11	0.43	0.58	0.41	0.11	0.44	0.42	86.35	120.03	0.57	0.11	0.11	0.42	12.52	0.04	21.03	26
10/0.45	44.51	0.13	0.46	0.59	0.43	0.13	0.45	0.45	83.31	116.29	0.55	0.13	0.15	0.45	10.94	0.05	17.06	17
10/0.50	41.80	0.10	0.44	0.58	0.40	0.10	0.43	0.42	86.91	118.43	0.57	0.10	0.12	0.42	10.41	0.04	16.55	27
20/0.05	42.80	0.13	0.45	0.59	0.42	0.13	0.46	0.43	85.39	118.85	0.57	0.13	0.15	0.43	16.57	0.06	28.14	19
20/0.10	46.08	0.16	0.46	0.59	0.45	0.16	0.49	0.46	81.75	117.28	0.56	0.17	0.17	0.46	18.36	0.06	31.33	11
20/0.15	41.65	0.10	0.44	0.57	0.41	0.11	0.45	0.42	87.05	121.09	0.58	0.12	0.11	0.42	11.59	0.05	18.65	30
20/0.20	42.90	0.12	0.45	0.58	0.42	0.13	0.47	0.43	86.06	118.77	0.57	0.13	0.13	0.43	15.25	0.06	25.31	22
20/0.25	41.97	0.09	0.44	0.57	0.41	0.10	0.45	0.42	86.71	120.46	0.58	0.10	0.10	0.42	11.93	0.05	19.48	28
20/0.30	42.65	0.12	0.44	0.57	0.41	0.11	0.44	0.43	86.93	119.17	0.57	0.12	0.13	0.43	14.81	0.05	24.20	23
20/0.35	41.76	0.10	0.44	0.57	0.40	0.10	0.44	0.42	87.53	120.54	0.58	0.10	0.11	0.42	14.66	0.06	23.60	29
20/0.40	41.76	0.11	0.44	0.57	0.40	0.11	0.45	0.42	87.62	120.57	0.58	0.12	0.12	0.42	15.25	0.06	23.65	25
20/0.45	44.69	0.13	0.47	0.60	0.44	0.14	0.47	0.45	83.58	116.39	0.56	0.15	0.14	0.45	15.72	0.07	24.58	13
20/0.50	42.97	0.10	0.45	0.58	0.42	0.11	0.44	0.43	86.02	118.99	0.57	0.11	0.11	0.43	11.88	0.05	18.69	24
30/0.05	47.96	0.19	0.49	0.62	0.47	0.19	0.50	0.48	78.77	115.69	0.55	0.20	0.21	0.48	23.61	0.09	40.29	4
30/0.01	**49.21**	**0.19**	**0.49**	**0.62**	**0.49**	**0.20**	**0.52**	**0.49**	**78.07**	**114.34**	**0.54**	**0.21**	**0.20**	**0.49**	**21.45**	**0.08**	**36.08**	**1**
30/0.15	47.88	0.20	0.49	0.63	0.47	0.21	0.52	0.48	78.95	114.58	0.55	0.22	0.21	0.48	21.63	0.09	37.32	2
30/0.20	48.21	0.20	0.48	0.62	0.47	0.21	0.51	0.48	79.81	115.27	0.55	0.22	0.22	0.48	24.05	0.10	40.22	3
30/0.25	46.82	0.18	0.48	0.62	0.46	0.18	0.49	0.47	80.50	115.71	0.55	0.19	0.19	0.47	24.06	0.09	40.49	7
30/0.30	45.69	0.16	0.46	0.61	0.44	0.16	0.48	0.46	82.11	116.52	0.56	0.17	0.17	0.46	19.97	0.08	33.25	10
30/0.35	47.53	0.16	0.48	0.60	0.46	0.17	0.50	0.48	79.27	114.75	0.55	0.18	0.16	0.48	19.43	0.08	32.22	8
30/0.40	48.41	0.18	0.48	0.60	0.47	0.18	0.50	0.48	78.94	114.78	0.55	0.19	0.19	0.48	19.29	0.07	32.74	6
30/0.45	48.31	0.18	0.47	0.62	0.47	0.19	0.49	0.48	79.17	114.26	0.54	0.19	0.19	0.48	25.97	0.10	43.66	5
30/0.50	45.79	0.18	0.48	0.63	0.44	0.19	0.50	0.46	82.13	115.70	0.56	0.20	0.21	0.46	19.59	0.07	32.44	9

Sensitivity Analysis. The novelty of the ECGpp framework is in the evaluation methodology, where an ensemble of performance measures is used. However, the selection of the performance measures that will be included in the ensemble can also influence the selection of the most promising configuration. It can happen that the meta-classifier can be good in some performance measures that are correlated, and if their number higher it can influence the results.

For this reason, we continue investigating how the inclusion and exclusion of correlated measures influence the end result. In this case, we used the average of all splits for each configuration with the V-shape generalized preference function. This was done because the average of all splits provides more robust rankings with regard to the selection of the generalized preference function and the V-shape function also takes into account the amount of differences of the wins and loses.

We perform a correlation analysis that uses absolute values of pairwise correlation. So the averaged results for each performance measure for each configuration were first investigated with regard to the correlation analysis, before the ranking was performed. Two types of correlations were explored, the Pearson correlation coefficient [4] and Spearman rank correlation coefficient [34]. While Pearson's correlation assesses linear relationships, Spearman's correlation assesses monotonic relationships (whether linear or not). The value of both coefficients can be between -1 and 1.

After calculating the correlation matrix, we removed the evaluation measures that had the average absolute correlation greater than some threshold. This way, we obtained sets of performance measures that were the least correlated.

We applied commonly-used thresholds 0.80 and 0.90 to remove the highly correlated measures and we come with the following sets of performance measures:

Table 7. Averaged performance results from all meta-classifiers trained for each configuration using the V-shape preference function [47].

Comb.	ACC	KAPPA	PRC	ROC	F	COR	PR	RC	RAE	RRSE	RMSE	INF	MAR	MF	LL	MI	PRS	Ranking
10/0.05	44.32	0.14	0.45	0.60	0.43	0.14	0.46	0.44	83.80	117.68	0.56	0.14	0.16	0.44	14.64	0.06	24.40	16
10/0.10	43.05	0.12	0.46	0.58	0.43	0.13	0.48	0.43	85.39	119.59	0.57	0.14	0.12	0.43	15.59	0.06	26.19	21
10/0.15	44.02	0.13	0.45	0.59	0.43	0.13	0.46	0.44	84.55	119.00	0.57	0.14	0.14	0.44	14.43	0.06	23.65	19
10/0.20	44.28	0.15	0.44	0.59	0.43	0.15	0.47	0.44	85.16	118.83	0.57	0.16	0.16	0.44	18.22	0.07	30.27	14
10/0.25	45.89	0.15	0.47	0.60	0.45	0.15	0.48	0.46	81.93	116.21	0.55	0.16	0.15	0.46	14.88	0.06	24.46	12
10/0.30	43.78	0.14	0.46	0.60	0.43	0.14	0.47	0.44	83.49	117.40	0.56	0.15	0.14	0.44	15.84	0.06	26.07	15
10/0.35	44.07	0.13	0.46	0.59	0.43	0.14	0.46	0.44	84.54	117.58	0.56	0.13	0.14	0.44	11.94	0.05	18.98	18
10/0.40	42.43	0.11	0.43	0.58	0.41	0.11	0.44	0.42	86.35	120.03	0.57	0.11	0.11	0.42	12.52	0.04	21.03	26
10/0.45	44.51	0.13	0.46	0.59	0.43	0.13	0.45	0.45	83.31	116.29	0.55	0.13	0.15	0.45	10.94	0.05	17.06	17
10/0.50	41.80	0.10	0.44	0.58	0.40	0.10	0.43	0.42	86.91	118.43	0.57	0.10	0.12	0.42	10.41	0.04	16.55	29
20/0.05	42.80	0.13	0.45	0.59	0.42	0.13	0.46	0.43	85.39	118.85	0.57	0.13	0.15	0.43	16.57	0.06	28.14	20
20/0.10	46.08	0.16	0.46	0.59	0.45	0.16	0.49	0.46	81.75	117.28	0.56	0.17	0.17	0.46	18.36	0.06	31.33	11
20/0.15	41.65	0.10	0.44	0.57	0.41	0.11	0.45	0.42	87.05	121.09	0.58	0.12	0.11	0.42	11.59	0.05	18.65	28
20/0.20	42.90	0.12	0.45	0.58	0.42	0.13	0.47	0.43	86.06	118.77	0.57	0.13	0.13	0.43	15.25	0.06	25.31	22
20/0.25	41.97	0.09	0.44	0.57	0.41	0.10	0.45	0.42	86.71	120.46	0.58	0.10	0.10	0.42	11.93	0.05	19.48	30
20/0.30	42.65	0.12	0.44	0.57	0.41	0.11	0.44	0.43	86.93	119.17	0.57	0.12	0.13	0.43	14.81	0.06	24.20	23
20/0.35	41.61	0.10	0.44	0.57	0.40	0.10	0.44	0.42	87.53	120.54	0.58	0.10	0.11	0.42	14.66	0.06	23.60	27
20/0.40	41.76	0.11	0.44	0.57	0.40	0.11	0.45	0.42	87.62	120.57	0.58	0.12	0.12	0.42	15.25	0.06	23.65	25
20/0.45	44.69	0.13	0.47	0.60	0.44	0.14	0.47	0.45	83.58	116.39	0.56	0.15	0.14	0.45	15.72	0.07	24.58	13
20/0.50	42.97	0.10	0.45	0.58	0.42	0.11	0.44	0.43	86.02	118.99	0.57	0.11	0.11	0.43	11.88	0.05	18.69	24
30/0.05	47.96	0.19	0.49	0.62	0.47	0.19	0.50	0.48	78.77	115.69	0.55	0.20	0.21	0.48	23.61	0.09	40.29	5
30/0.10	**49.21**	**0.19**	**0.49**	**0.62**	**0.49**	**0.20**	**0.52**	**0.49**	**78.07**	**114.34**	**0.54**	**0.21**	**0.20**	**0.49**	**21.45**	**0.08**	**36.08**	**1**
30/0.15	47.88	0.20	0.49	0.63	0.47	0.21	0.52	0.48	78.95	114.58	0.55	0.22	0.21	0.48	21.63	0.09	37.32	2
30/0.20	48.21	0.20	0.48	0.62	0.47	0.21	0.51	0.48	79.81	115.27	0.55	0.22	0.22	0.48	24.05	0.10	40.22	3
30/0.25	46.82	0.18	0.48	0.62	0.46	0.18	0.49	0.47	80.50	115.71	0.55	0.19	0.19	0.47	24.06	0.09	40.49	7
30/0.30	45.69	0.16	0.46	0.61	0.44	0.16	0.48	0.46	82.11	116.52	0.56	0.17	0.17	0.46	19.97	0.08	33.25	10
30/0.35	47.53	0.16	0.48	0.60	0.46	0.17	0.50	0.48	79.27	114.75	0.55	0.18	0.16	0.48	19.43	0.08	32.22	8
30/0.40	48.41	0.18	0.48	0.60	0.47	0.18	0.50	0.48	78.94	114.78	0.55	0.19	0.19	0.48	19.29	0.07	32.74	6
30/0.45	48.31	0.18	0.47	0.62	0.47	0.19	0.49	0.48	79.17	114.26	0.54	0.19	0.19	0.48	25.97	0.10	43.66	4
30/0.50	45.79	0.18	0.48	0.63	0.44	0.19	0.50	0.46	82.13	115.70	0.56	0.20	0.21	0.46	19.59	0.07	32.44	9

Table 8. Averaged performance results from all meta-classifiers trained for each configuration using the V-shape preference function and Pearson correlation with threshold set at 0.80.

Comb.	PR	LL	Ranking
10/0.05	0.45	14.64	18
10/0.10	0.46	15.59	16
10/0.15	0.45	14.43	22
10/0.20	0.44	18.22	17
10/0.25	0.47	14.88	13
10/0.30	0.46	15.84	14
10/0.35	0.46	11.94	20
10/0.40	0.43	12.52	29
10/0.45	0.46	10.94	21
10/0.50	0.44	10.41	30
20/0.05	0.45	16.57	15
20/0.10	0.46	18.36	11
20/0.15	0.44	11.59	28
20/0.20	0.45	15.25	19
20/0.25	0.44	11.93	27
20/0.30	0.44	14.81	25
20/0.35	0.44	14.66	24
20/0.40	0.44	15.25	23
20/0.45	0.47	15.72	12
20/0.50	0.45	11.88	26
30/0.05	0.49	23.61	3
30/0.10	0.49	21.45	5
30/0.15	**0.49**	**21.63**	**1**
30/0.20	0.48	24.05	2
30/0.25	0.48	24.06	6
30/0.30	0.46	19.97	10
30/0.35	0.48	19.43	7
30/0.40	0.48	19.29	9
30/0.45	0.47	25.97	4
30/0.50	0.48	19.59	8

- 0.80 (Pearson): precision (PR) and log-likelihood (LL);
- 0.90 (Pearson): precision (PR), root mean squared error (RMSE), and log-likelihood (LL),

and

- 0.80 (Spearman): root relative squared error (RRSE) and log-likelihood (LL);

Table 9. Averaged performance results from all meta-classifiers trained for each configuration using the V-shape preference function and Pearson correlation with threshold set at 0.90.

Comb.	PR	RMSE	LL	Ranking
10/0.05	0.45	0.56	14.64	16
10/0.10	0.46	0.57	15.59	19
10/0.15	0.45	0.57	14.43	22
10/0.20	0.44	0.57	18.22	18
10/0.25	0.47	0.55	14.88	12
10/0.30	0.46	0.56	15.84	14
10/0.35	0.46	0.56	11.94	17
10/0.40	0.43	0.57	12.52	28
10/0.45	0.46	0.55	10.94	15
10/0.50	0.44	0.57	10.41	27
20/0.05	0.45	0.57	16.57	20
20/0.10	0.46	0.56	18.36	13
20/0.15	0.44	0.58	11.59	30
20/0.20	0.45	0.57	15.25	21
20/0.25	0.44	0.58	11.93	29
20/0.30	0.44	0.57	14.81	23
20/0.35	0.44	0.58	14.66	26
20/0.40	0.44	0.58	15.25	25
20/0.45	0.47	0.56	15.72	11
20/0.50	0.45	0.57	11.88	24
30/0.05	0.49	0.55	23.61	5
30/0.10	0.49	0.54	21.45	3
30/0.15	0.49	0.55	21.63	2
30/0.20	0.48	0.55	24.05	4
30/0.25	0.48	0.55	24.06	6
30/0.30	0.46	0.56	19.97	10
30/0.35	0.48	0.55	19.43	7
30/0.40	0.48	0.55	19.29	8
30/0.45	**0.47**	**0.54**	**25.97**	**1**
30/0.50	0.48	0.56	19.59	9

– 0.90 (Spearman): root relative squared error (RRSE), markedness (MAR), and log-likelihood (LL).

After determining the set of all performance measures for each threshold and each correlation type, we evaluated the meta-classifiers results in order to select the promising configuration. The rankings obtained using Pearson and

Table 10. Averaged performance results from all meta-classifiers trained for each configuration using the V-shape preference function and Spearman correlation with threshold set at 0.80.

Comb.	RRSE	LL	Ranking
10/0.05	117.68	14.64	16
10/0.10	119.59	15.59	23
10/0.15	119.00	14.43	21
10/0.20	118.83	18.22	15
10/0.25	116.21	14.88	13
10/0.30	117.40	15.84	14
10/0.35	117.58	11.94	20
10/0.40	120.03	12.52	28
10/0.45	116.29	10.94	17
10/0.50	118.43	10.41	25
20/0.05	118.85	16.57	18
20/0.10	117.28	18.36	11
20/0.15	121.09	11.59	30
20/0.20	118.77	15.25	19
20/0.25	120.46	11.93	29
20/0.30	119.17	14.81	22
20/0.35	120.54	14.66	27
20/0.40	120.57	15.25	26
20/0.45	116.39	15.72	12
20/0.50	118.99	11.88	24
30/0.05	115.69	23.61	6
30/0.10	114.34	21.45	3
30/0.15	114.58	21.63	4
30/0.20	115.27	24.05	2
30/0.25	115.71	24.06	5
30/0.30	116.52	19.97	10
30/0.35	114.75	19.43	7
30/0.40	114.78	19.29	8
30/0.45	**114.26**	**25.97**	**1**
30/0.50	115.70	19.59	9

Spearman correlation with 0.80 and 0.90 thresholds are presented in Tables 8, 9, 10, and 11, respectively. Using these tables, we can conclude that the best top 10 configurations are obtained with a segment length 30 s. To see how the best 10 configurations change their rankings when different set of performance measures are included, we present their rankings in Fig. 3.

Table 11. Averaged performance results from all meta-classifiers trained for each configuration using the V-shape preference function and Spearman correlation with threshold set at 0.90.

Comb.	RRSE	MAR	LL	Ranking
10/0.05	117.68	0.16	14.64	16
10/0.10	119.59	0.12	15.59	23
10/0.15	119.00	0.14	14.43	21
10/0.20	118.83	0.16	18.22	14
10/0.25	116.21	0.15	14.88	12
10/0.30	117.40	0.14	15.84	15
10/0.35	117.58	0.14	11.94	19
10/0.40	120.03	0.11	12.52	28
10/0.45	116.29	0.15	10.94	17
10/0.50	118.43	0.12	10.41	25
20/0.05	118.85	0.15	16.57	18
20/0.10	117.28	0.17	18.36	11
20/0.15	121.09	0.11	11.59	30
20/0.20	118.77	0.13	15.25	20
20/0.25	120.46	0.10	11.93	29
20/0.30	119.17	0.13	14.81	22
20/0.35	120.54	0.11	14.66	27
20/0.40	120.57	0.12	15.25	24
20/0.45	116.39	0.14	15.72	13
20/0.50	118.99	0.11	11.88	26
30/0.05	115.69	0.21	23.61	4
30/0.10	114.34	0.20	21.45	5
30/0.15	114.58	0.21	21.63	3
30/0.20	115.27	0.22	24.05	2
30/0.25	115.71	0.19	24.06	6
30/0.30	116.52	0.17	19.97	10
30/0.35	114.75	0.16	19.43	9
30/0.40	114.78	0.19	19.29	8
30/0.45	**114.26**	**0.19**	**25.97**	**1**
30/0.50	115.70	0.21	19.59	7

Using Fig. 3, we can see that there are not large deviations between the rankings of the configurations when different sets of performance measures are involved. The best configuration (30 s, 0.01 Hz) when all measures are used changes its ranking when the highly correlated measures are excluded, but it is still in top 10 best configurations. The configuration with parameters (30 s,

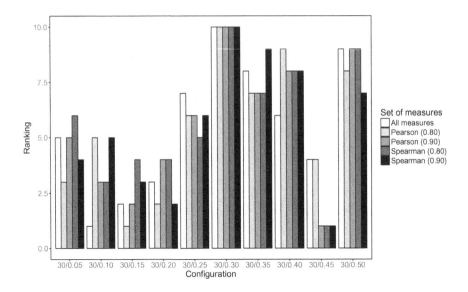

Fig. 3. Top 10 best configurations rankings for different set of performance measures.

0.30 Hz) is the last ranked one in all cases when different sets of performance measures were used. The configuration (30 s, 0.45 Hz) become first one when highly correlated measures were excluded.

In addition, to see the robustness of the obtained rankings, we calculated the absolute differences between the rankings of each configuration with each subset of performance measures and the rankings obtained using all performance measures. Next, we provided the mean value and the standard deviation of the rankings differences that can provide a conclusion about the robustness of the evaluation methodology. The mean values and standard deviations are presented in Table 12.

Using Table 12, we can conclude that the evaluation methodology is robust to inclusion and exclusion of correlated measures that can be seen from the descriptive statistics. We also need to point that there are configurations, such as the configuration with parameters (30 s, 0.45 Hz) that change is rankings from 4 to 1 (see Fig. 3), however if we compare the performance measures from practical point of view there is no significant practical difference. The configurations that are in the best top 10 are always the best, only small deviations between their rankings can be observed when different sets of performance measures are used. However, the best way of using the evaluation approach is to use as many as possible performance measures that are least correlated.

Table 12. Descriptive statistics for robustness of the rankings.

Difference	Mean	Standard deviation
(Pearson (0.80) − All measures)	1.40	1.26
(Pearson (0.90) − All measures)	1.00	1.05
(Spearman (0.80) − All measures)	1.40	0.96
(Spearman (0.90) − All measures)	1.60	1.17

5 Conclusions

We presented a new framework, the ECGpp, which can be used for selecting the most promising parameters for pre-processing of ECG signals that will be further involved in some predictive analysis. It consists of four levels: i) defining the pairs of pre-processing parameters that should be tested, ii) learning signal representation for each configuration of parameters, iii) predictive analysis, and iv) evaluation of the results that leads to selecting the most promising configurations of parameters.

To present how the framework works, we explored different configurations of parameters that can be used for pre-processing of ECG signals that are further used for blood pressure classification. Two parameters were investigated: the signal (i.e. segment) length and the cut-off frequency that is used for baseline removal. We tested 30 different configurations, each one a combination of a signal length that can be one from 10 s, 20 s, or 30 s, and a cut-off frequency starting from 0.05 Hz till 0.50 Hz, with a step of 0.05 Hz.

Evaluation results obtained using a data set of five commercially available sensors showed that by using a signal length of 30 s, it follows that it carries the most valuable information. This is compliant with the optimal ECG sample lengths needed for building predictive models available from state-of-the-art literature [45, 48]. Evaluation also demonstrated that good performance can be achieved even for the lower cut-off frequencies where the ECG components overlap with the baseline wander noise [55].

The main benefit of the ECGpp framework is in the evaluation methodology. It is made using an ensemble of performance measures in order to make more general conclusion and not being biased only to specific performance measures. We used 17 different performance measures that can be used for multi-class classification. The performance measures were manually selected. However, we additionally investigated how the selection of the performance measures influence the final result. For this reason, the framework was tested for the inclusion and exclusion of correlated measures considering linear and monotonic correlations. Evaluations showed that robust rankings are obtained and there are not large deviations between the rankings with regard to the set of performance measures.

Further such kind of analysis can even provide more information, by not using only the best configuration for predictive analysis, but to use several best of them for information fusion approaches.

Acknowledgements. The authors acknowledge the financial support from the Slovenian Research Agency (research core funding No. P2-0098, and project Z2-1867).

References

1. AHA: Understanding blood pressure readings (2016). http://www.heart. org/HEARTORG/Conditions/HighBloodPressure/AboutHighBloodPressure/Und erstanding-Blood-Pressure-Readings_UCM_301764_Article.jsp
2. Ahmad, S., et al.: Electrocardiogram-assisted blood pressure estimation. IEEE Trans. Biomed. Eng. **59**(3), 608–618 (2012)
3. Ahonen, L., Cowley, B., Torniainen, J., Ukkonen, A., Vihavainen, A., Puolamäki, K.: Cognitive collaboration found in cardiac physiology: study in classroom environment. PLoS One **11**(7), e0159178 (2016)
4. Benesty, J., Chen, J., Huang, Y., Cohen, I. (Eds.): Pearson correlation coefficient. In: Benesty, J., Chen, J., Huang, Y., Cohen, I. (eds.) Noise Reduction in Speech Processing. Springer Topics in Signal Processing, vol. 2, pp. 1–4. Springer, Heidelberg (2009). https://doi.org/10.1007/978-3-642-00296-0_5
5. Biosignals, B.: Emotion faros (2016)
6. Brans, J.-P., Mareschal, B.: Promethee methodsos. In: Figueira, J., Greco, S., Ehrogot, M. (eds.) Multiple Criteria Decision Analysis: State of the Art Surveys. ISORMS, vol. 78, pp. 163–186. Springer, New York (2005). https://doi.org/10. 1007/0-387-23081-5_5
7. Brans, J.P., Vincke, P.: Note—a preference ranking organisation method: (the PROMETHEE method for multiple criteria decision-making). Manage. Sci. **31**(6), 647–656 (1985)
8. Breiman, L.: Bagging predictors. Mach. Learn. **24**(2), 123–140 (1996)
9. Canning, J., et al.: Noninvasive and continuous blood pressure measurement via superficial temporal artery tonometry. In: 2016 IEEE 38th Annual International Conference of the Engineering in Medicine and Biology Society (EMBC), pp. 3382–3385. IEEE (2016)
10. i Carós, J.M.S.: Continuous non-invasive blood pressure estimation. Ph.D. thesis, ETH (2011)
11. Chan, K., Hung, K., Zhang, Y.: Noninvasive and cuffless measurements of blood pressure for telemedicine. In: Proceedings of the 23rd Annual International Conference of the IEEE Engineering in Medicine and Biology Society, 2001, vol. 4, pp. 3592–3593. IEEE (2001)
12. Choi, Y., Zhang, Q., Ko, S.: Noninvasive cuffless blood pressure estimation using pulse transit time and Hilbert-Huang transform. Comput. Electr. Eng. **39**(1), 103–111 (2013)
13. Cosoli, G., Casacanditella, L., Pietroni, F., Calvaresi, A., Revel, G.M., Scalise, L.: A novel approach for features extraction in physiological signals. In: 2015 IEEE International Symposium on Medical Measurements and Applications (MeMeA), pp. 380–385. IEEE (2015)
14. Eftimov, T., Korošec, P., Koroušić Seljak, B.: Data-driven preference-based deep statistical ranking for comparing multi-objective optimization algorithms. In: Korošec, P., Melab, N., Talbi, E.-G. (eds.) BIOMA 2018. LNCS, vol. 10835, pp. 138–150. Springer, Cham (2018). https://doi.org/10.1007/978-3-319-91641-5_12
15. Eke, A., Herman, P., Kocsis, L., Kozak, L.: Fractal characterization of complexity in temporal physiological signals. Physiol. Meas. **23**(1), R1 (2002)

16. Freund, Y., Schapire, R.E., et al.: Experiments with a new boosting algorithm. In: ICML, vol. 96, pp. 148–156. Citeseer (1996)
17. Goldberger, A.L., et al.: PhysioBank, PhysioToolkit, and PhysioNet. Circulation **101**(23), e215–e220 (2000)
18. Goli, S., Jayanthi, T.: Cuff less continuous non-invasive blood pressure measurement using pulse transit time measurement. Int. J. Rec. Dev. Eng. Technol. **2**(1), 87 (2014)
19. Hacks, C.: e-health sensor platform v2. 0 for arduino and raspberry pi (2015)
20. Hassan, M.K.B.A., Mashor, M.Y., Mohd Nasir, N.F., Mohamed, S.: Measuring of systolic blood pressure based on heart rate. In: Abu Osman, N.A., Ibrahim, F., Wan Abas, W.A.B., Abdul Rahman, H.S., Ting, H.N. (eds.) 4th Kuala Lumpur International Conference on Biomedical Engineering 2008. IFMBE Proceedings, vol. 21, pp. 595–598. Springer, Heidelberg (2008). https://doi.org/10.1007/978-3-540-69139-6_149
21. Hearst, M.A., Dumais, S.T., Osuna, E., Platt, J., Scholkopf, B.: Support vector machines. IEEE Intell. Syst. Appl. **13**(4), 18–28 (1998)
22. Ilango, S., Sridhar, P.: A non-invasive blood pressure measurement using android smart phones. IOSR J. Dent. Med. Sci. **13**(1), 28–31 (2014)
23. Johnstone, J.A., Ford, P.A., Hughes, G., Watson, T., Garrett, A.T.: Bioharness™ multivariable monitoring device: part. I: validity. J. Sports Sci. Med. **11**(3), 400 (2012)
24. Kim, N., et al.: Trending autoregulatory indices during treatment for traumatic brain injury. J. Clin. Monit. Comput. **30**(6), 821–831 (2016)
25. Kugiumtzis, D., Tsimpiris, A.: Measures of analysis of time series (MATS): a MAT-LAB toolkit for computation of multiple measures on time series data bases. arXiv preprint arXiv:1002.1940 (2010)
26. Li, Y., Gao, Y., Deng, N.: Mechanism of cuff-less blood pressure measurement using MMSB. Engineering **5**(10), 123 (2013)
27. Liao, Y., Vemuri, V.R.: Use of k-nearest neighbor classifier for intrusion detection. Comput. Secur. **21**(5), 439–448 (2002)
28. Liaw, A., Wiener, M., et al.: Classification and regression by randomForest. R news **2**(3), 18–22 (2002)
29. Marani, R., Perri, A.G.: An intelligent system for continuous blood pressure monitoring on remote multi-patients in real time. arXiv preprint arXiv:1212.0651 (2012)
30. McBride, J.C., et al.: Spectral and complexity analysis of scalp EEG characteristics for mild cognitive impairment and early Alzheimer's disease. Comput. Methods Programs Biomed. **114**(2), 153–163 (2014)
31. Monge-Álvarez, J.: Higuchi and Katz fractal dimension measures (2015). https://www.mathworks.com/matlabcentral/fileexchange/50290-higuchi-and-katz-fractal-dimension-measures/content/Fractaldimensionmeasures/HiguchiFD.m
32. Morabito, F.C., Labate, D., La Foresta, F., Bramanti, A., Morabito, G., Palamara, I.: Multivariate multi-scale permutation entropy for complexity analysis of Alzheimer's disease EEG. Entropy **14**(7), 1186–1202 (2012)
33. Mouradian, V., Poghosyan, A., Hovhannisyan, L.: Noninvasive continuous mobile blood pressure monitoring using novel PPG optical sensor. In: 2015 IEEE Topical Conference on Biomedical Wireless Technologies, Networks, and Sensing Systems (BioWireleSS), pp. 1–3. IEEE (2015)
34. Myers, L., Sirois, M.J.: Spearman correlation coefficients, differences between. In: Encyclopedia of Statistical Sciences, vol. 12 (2004)

35. Nye, R., Zhang, Z., Fang, Q.: Continuous non-invasive blood pressure monitoring using photoplethysmography: a review. In: 2015 International Symposium on Bioelectronics and Bioinformatics (ISBB), pp. 176–179. IEEE (2015)

36. Patil, T.R., Sherekar, S.: Performance analysis of Naive Bayes and J48 classification algorithm for data classification. Int. J. Comput. Sci. Appl. **6**(2), 256–261 (2013)

37. Payne, R., Symeonides, C., Webb, D., Maxwell, S.: Pulse transit time measured from the ECG: an unreliable marker of beat-to-beat blood pressure. J. Appl. Physiol. **100**(1), 136–141 (2006)

38. Program, N.H.B.P.E., et al.: The seventh report of the joint national committee on prevention, detection, evaluation, and treatment of high blood pressure (2004)

39. Rish, I., et al.: An empirical study of the Naive Bayes classifier. In: IJCAI 2001 Workshop on Empirical Methods in Artificial Intelligence, vol. 3, pp. 41–46. IBM, New York (2001)

40. Sackl-Pietsch, E.: Continuous non-invasive arterial pressure shows high accuracy in comparison to invasive intra-arterial blood pressure measurement. Unpublished manuscript (2010)

41. Sahani, A.K., Ravi, V., Sivaprakasam, M.: Automatic estimation of carotid arterial pressure in ARTSENS. In: 2014 Annual IEEE India Conference (INDICON), pp. 1–6. IEEE (2014)

42. Sahoo, A., Manimegalai, P., Thanushkodi, K.: Wavelet based pulse rate and blood pressure estimation system from ECG and PPG signals. In: 2011 International Conference on Computer, Communication and Electrical Technology (ICCCET), pp. 285–289. IEEE (2011)

43. Schroeder, E.B., Liao, D., Chambless, L.E., Prineas, R.J., Evans, G.W., Heiss, G.: Hypertension, blood pressure, and heart rate variability. Hypertension **42**(6), 1106–1111 (2003)

44. Seo, J., Pietrangelo, S.J., Lee, H.S., Sodini, C.G.: Noninvasive arterial blood pressure waveform monitoring using two-element ultrasound system. IEEE Trans. Ultrason. Ferroelectr. Freq. Control **62**(4), 776–784 (2015)

45. Shdefat, A.Y., Joo, M.I., Choi, S.H., Kim, H.C.: Utilizing ECG waveform features as new biometric authentication method. Int. J. Electr. Comput. Eng. (IJECE) **8**(2), 658 (2018)

46. Simjanoska, M., Gjoreski, M., Gams, M., Madevska Bogdanova, A.: Non-invasive blood pressure estimation from ECG using machine learning techniques. Sensors **18**(4), 1160 (2018)

47. Simjanoska., M., Papa., G., Seljak., B.K., Eftimov., T.: Comparing different settings of parameters needed for pre-processing of ECG signals used for blood pressure classification. In: Proceedings of the 12th International Joint Conference on Biomedical Engineering Systems and Technologies - Volume 4: BIOSIGNALS, pp. 62–72. INSTICC, SciTePress (2019). https://doi.org/10.5220/0007390100620072

48. Takahashi, N., Kuriyama, A., Kanazawa, H., Takahashi, Y., Nakayama, T.: Validity of spectral analysis based on heart rate variability from 1-minute or less ECG recordings. Pacing Clin. Electrophysiol. **40**, 1004–1009 (2017)

49. Tanaka, S., Nogawa, M., Yamakoshi, T., Yamakoshi, K.I.: Accuracy assessment of a noninvasive device for monitoring beat-by-beat blood pressure in the radial artery using the volume-compensation method. IEEE Trans. Biomed. Eng. **54**(10), 1892–1895 (2007)

50. Technology, Z.: Zephyr bioharness 3.0 user manual (2017). https://www.zephyranywhere.com/media/download/bioharness3-user-manual.pdf

51. Thomas, S.S., Nathan, V., Zong, C., Soundarapandian, K., Shi, X., Jafari, R.: BioWatch: a noninvasive wrist-based blood pressure monitor that incorporates training techniques for posture and subject variability. IEEE J. Biomed. Health Inform. **20**(5), 1291–1300 (2016)

52. Trobec, R., Tomašić, I., Rashkovska, A., Depolli, M., Avbelj, V. (eds.): Commercial ECG systems. In: Body Sensors and Electrocardiography. SAST, pp. 101–114. Springer, Cham (2018). https://doi.org/10.1007/978-3-319-59340-1_6

53. Winderbank-Scott, P., Barnaghi, P.: A non-invasive wireless monitoring device for children and infants in pre-hospital and acute hospital environments (2017)

54. Wong, M.Y.M., Poon, C.C.Y., Zhang, Y.T.: An evaluation of the cuffless blood pressure estimation based on pulse transit time technique: a half year study on normotensive subjects. Cardiovasc. Eng. **9**(1), 32–38 (2009)

55. Xu, Y., Luo, M., Li, T., Song, G.: ECG signal de-noising and baseline wander correction based on ceemdan and wavelet threshold. Sensors **17**(12), 2754 (2017)

Health Informatics

Investigating User's Preference for Anthropomorphism of a Social Robot Trainer in Physical Rehabilitation

Baisong Liu, Panos Markopoulos[✉], and Daniel Tetteroo[✉]

Department of Industrial Design, Eindhoven University of Technology, De Zaale, Eindhoven, The Netherlands
{b.liu2,p.markopoulos,d.tetteroo}@tue.nl

Abstract. Developments in social robotics raise the prospect of robots coaching and interacting with patient during rehabilitation training assuming a role of a trainer. This raises questions regarding the acceptance of robots in this role and more specifically, to what extent the robot should be anthropomorphic. This paper presents the results of an online experiment designed to evaluate the user acceptance of Socially Assistive Robots (SARs) as rehabilitation trainers, and the effect of anthropomorphism on this matter. User attitudes were surveyed with regards to variations of the robot's anthropomorphism as a rehabilitation trainer. The results show that 1) participants are accepting towards SAR-assisted rehabilitation therapies, 2) higher anthropomorphism is generally preferred but does not affect patient's acceptance towards such therapy and technology. Qualitative data brings insight to patient technology acceptance, needs for rehabilitation training and the effect of anthropomorphism.

Keywords: Socially Assistive Robot · Anthropomorphism · Rehabilitation user-centered design · Acceptance

1 Introduction

The application of robotic technology in the domain of physical rehabilitation is an area of ongoing research [17]. Projects have developed robotic technology to support physically impaired patients, such as mobility aids for aging and motor function impaired users, assisting users in loaded walking [5] and supporting rehabilitation training exercises [11, 21]. Such projects have shown that robots can help to improve the quality and quantity of rehabilitation training. However, the current trend mostly concerns with physically supporting (parts of) the patients [2, 25].

Apart from above-mentioned researches, SAR recently has also been proposed as a promising solution to issues with rehabilitation exercises. Socially Assistive Robotics (SAR) provides assistance through social interaction [9]. The use of SAR in rehabilitation training has been demonstrated as promising [7], due to its potential benefits of enhancing patient training compliance, cost reduction, privacy, improving engagement, and flexibility in training scenarios [26]. A feasibility study has proven the potential

© Springer Nature Switzerland AG 2020
A. Roque et al. (Eds.): BIOSTEC 2019, CCIS 1211, pp. 381–394, 2020.
https://doi.org/10.1007/978-3-030-46970-2_18

of such application [16]. A further study has suggested that even very simple robot behavior might benefit compliance in stroke rehabilitation exercises [13]. A more recent study looks further into the strategies of such application domain, it underlined the link between personalized robot behavior and user task performance in rehabilitation training [24].

Within social robot research domain, taxonomies of components concerning socially interactive robots [9, 12] shows that human-oriented perception is an important focus in SAR interaction design. However, as the above-mentioned studies investigated possible engagement strategies with SAR in rehabilitation, there hasn't been a study that looks into the general acceptance for such application by its target user. On a grand scale, general robot acceptance studies have investigated the effects on acceptance of specific robotic traits, such as gender of the voice [8], facial expressions [19] and gestures [27]. Regarding SAR, [12] have identified the following factors to be of influence on acceptance: 1) the user's attitude towards the robot, 2) the robot's field performance, 3) robot-displayed emotions, 4) appearance and dialog, and 5) personality. These studies explore robot acceptance regardless of a specific context, and thus provide general conclusions and directions for further research. On the other hand, a branch of social robot acceptance study focuses on specific contexts and user groups, typically children, elderly and autism patients. For example, the Almere Model has been proposed for testing and predicting elderly users' acceptance of assistive social agent technologies, suggesting 12 factors to be of influence [14]. Another study employed a zoomorphic companion robot (Nabaztag) into an elderly user's home to gain insights on social robot acceptance, focusing on users building a long-term relationship with a social robot in domestic settings [15]. Even though current study has not made any direct comparison among acceptance in different context, but current results already imply that robot's acceptance has a strong association with its tasks. Different tasks could require the robot to take on different genders and different role and associated behavior.

Anthropomorphism of social robots is a powerful factor influencing the user's experience, including empathy [19], enjoyment, and other social emotions [1]. Anthropomorphism is proposed to be expressed in appearance and behavior [3]. So far studies have explored different factors of anthropomorphic appearance embodied in the design of robots, for example through facial expressions [19], voice [23] and gesture [22]. As it has been suggested that user responses to anthropomorphic robotics are context based [6], it is important to explore the effects of anthropomorphism for specific contexts and use cases, such as that of physical rehabilitation.

2 Research Questions

As above- mentioned, the acceptance for application of SAR is an important issue for later design and deploy of this technology in the context of rehabilitation training, and the preferred anthropomorphic level can affect user's perception and in turn reflect in the effectiveness of such application. The studies took a user-centered approach to explore above questions. The initial research included one study for exploring these issues, then according to the results and feedback for the study, we planned an iteration as study 2, to further verify the results and to clear up the ambiguity of user's preference for different anthropomorphic appearance. In this research, we are interested in:

RQ1) What is the patient's accepting attitude towards having a robot trainer for their rehabilitation training?

RQ2) How does the level of anthropomorphism in SAR form-design influence patients' acceptance in the context of rehabilitation training?

RQ3) What are patients' preferences and concerns regarding SAR within the context of rehabilitation training?

3 Study 1

For Study 1 [18], we used an illustration of a fictional scenario with a patient performing her rehabilitation exercise with the help of a robot trainer (see Fig. 1). To answer RQ1 and 2, we designed a between-subject study 1-1 with three levels of anthropomorphic appearances. Study 1-2 aimed at answering RQ3, the robot in the scenario is left blank and participants were asked to pick one to fill the blank from the three options based on their own rehabilitation experience and preferences.

3.1 Material

Study 1 utilized illustrated scenarios describing a designed interaction between a patient and a robot trainer. As the nature of SAR is to provide assistance through social measures, the robot trainers in the scenarios take the role of a training coach that provides the patient with information related to the therapy, instructions for the exercise and verbal motivational prompts. The story of the scenario is based on observations of clinical treatment and was further improved by consulting experienced physical therapists. The scenarios featured three versions of the robot trainer, differing in their level of anthropomorphic appearances. In the studies discussed above, robotic anthropomorphism is expressed mainly through facial expressions and gestures. Therefore, the three versions of the robot trainer included one with human-like body structure and expressions, one with only expressions, and one with none of the two, to represent high, medium and low levels of anthropomorphism in robot form design (See Table 1 and 2). A small survey was conducted as a manipulation check, the concepts are proven to express the desired anthropomorphic level.

3.2 Measurements and Procedure

Negative Attitude towards Robot Scale (NARS) questionnaire [20] was used before the scenarios in both Study 1-1 and 1-2, as a check to make sure that participants hold similar opinions about robot across all conditions. Credibility/Expectancy questionnaire [4] and the TAM (Technology Acceptance Model) questionnaire were used to evaluate the participants' acceptance of the robot assisted therapy and the robot trainer. As manipulation check, we asked the user to rate the look of the robot trainer on a 10-point Machine-like to Human-like scale. Besides quantitative measurements, we also used open questions to collect qualitative data to help with interpreting the results. The structure of the survey for study 1-1 and 1-2 are listed in Table 1 and 2.

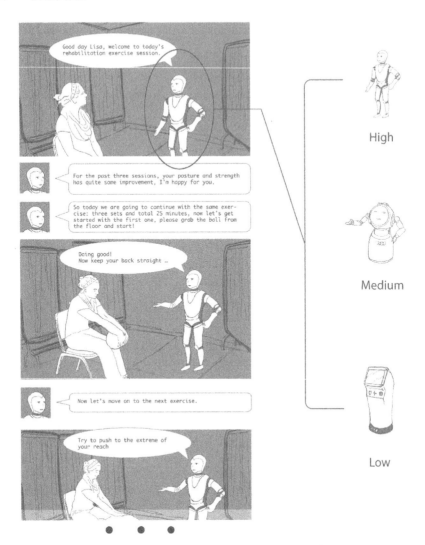

Fig. 1. Scenario and robot anthropomorphic design.

3.3 Participants

Participants were recruited through a crowdsourcing platform. Participants were expected to be or formerly involved in physical rehabilitation training. The study took four groups of participants (N = 103, after screening, average age 37). Detailed numbers of participants and group allocations are listed in Table 3. Study 1 were published on Amazon Mechanical Turk on July 12, 2018 and lasted 14 days. Each participant spent around 10 min on the study. Based on the minimum hourly wage, the reward was set at 1.5 USD.

To ensure the quality of the answers collected, we set a three-step screening scheme. First, workers on Amazon Mechanical Turk had to answer three questions, proving

Table 1. Structure of Study 1-1 [18].

Screening questions
General attitude towards social robots
NARS questionnaire Open question regarding attitude towards working with social robots
Scenario "Lisa's Rehabilitation Training Session with Robot Trainer"
Attitude towards robot-assisted Rehabilitation therapy
Credibility/Expectancy questionnaire Open question regarding attitude towards robot–assisted rehabilitation therapy
Attitude towards robot trainer in rehabilitation therapy
TAM questionnaire Open question regarding attitude towards robot trainer in rehabilitation therapy
Manipulation check
Rate Robot Trainer's look on a scale from Machine-like to Human-like Open question regarding attitude towards robot–assisted rehabilitation therapy

that they had experience in physical rehabilitation, to access the survey. Secondly, four reverse questions (changing positive statements into negative ones, e.g. "*I found the robot trainer easy to interact with*" into "*I found the robot trainer difficult to interact with*") were also planted within the survey to check for satisficing behavior in answering the survey. Lastly, we put an eight-digit password at the end of the survey for claiming the reward, only visible to participants who finished the survey. We set the survey to be only available to workers with approval rate higher than 97% percent and job experience less than 5000 to further ensure the quality of the answer.

Table 2. Structure of Study 1-2 [18].

Screening Questions
Scenario "Lisa's Rehabilitation Training Session with Robot Trainer" with the trainer left blank
User preference for the given concept
Choose the desired robot trainer from the three given concepts Open questions regarding the choice Open questions about further improvements for the therapy and the robot trainer
Manipulation check
Rate three Robot Trainers' look on a scale from Machine-like to Human-like respectively

Table 3. Study participants [18].

Study	Conditions	Participants
Study 1-1	HA (High Anthropomorphism)	28 (HA1 - HA28)
	MA (Medium Anthropomorphism)	24 (MA1 - HA24)
	LA (Low Anthropomorphism)	20 (LA1 - LA20)
Study 1-2	–	31 (ST1 - ST31)

3.4 Results

Manipulation check in study one shows that the different level of anthropomorphic looks were perceived as intended, a one-way ANOVA analysis showed significant difference in study 1-1 (F (2-70) = 22.79, p < .001) and study 1-2 (F (2, 89) = 121.34, p < .001).

A one-way ANOVA analysis showed no significant difference on NARS and Credibility/Expectancy questionnaires. Such result on NARS shows that the participants from all groups have similar accepting attitude for robots, and results of Credibility/Expectancy questionnaires show that anthropomorphic appearances does not have effect on participants' acceptance for the robot trainer therapy. ANOVA analysis on TAM questionnaire found a significant preference for the low anthropomorphic concept (M = 5.34, SD = 1.2), over the high anthropomorphic (M = 4.43, SD = 1.71) and the medium anthropomorphic concept (M = 4.02, SD = 1.7) on the factor Self-Efficacy (SE), F (2, 68) = 3.8, p < .05. No significant effects of anthropomorphism were found for the rest of the factors, namely Perceived Ease of, Perceived Usefulness, Behavioral Intention, Attitude and Subjective Norm.

In study 1, we collected qualitative data regarding patient's acceptance, needs and their preference for the appearances. Above results will be discussed in the findings section. Among the results, qualitative analysis shows participant's preference for a higher anthropomorphic robot trainer; however, TAM questionnaire discovered a high self-efficacy in the low anthropomorphic concept. Such results brought unclear answer for RQ2. Therefore, to bring clarity to this issue, we conducted a study 2 as an iteration to 2) clarify the answer for RQ2, and 2) verify the results for study 1.

4 Study 2

4.1 Methods

Study 2 took the two preferred concepts from study 1, namely the high and low anthropomorphic concepts, and developed the same scenarios with actual picture showing a patient doing the same rehabilitation training with actual commercialized robots (See Fig. 2). Concept high anthropomorphism is represented by robot Pepper by SoftBank, and concept low anthropomorphic with HSR by TOYOTA. And similar as study 1, this study is also divided into two parts (Study 2-1 and 2-2) with the same structure. Study 2 took the same measures and sampling methods as in study 1, and took three groups of participants (N = 29(HA) + 32(LA) + 28(Study 2-2) = 89, average age 36) (See Table 4).

Table 4. Study participants.

Study	Conditions	Participants
Study 2-1	HA (High Anthropomorphism)	29 (HA29 – HA58)
	LA (Low Anthropomorphism)	32 (LA21 – LA53)
Study 2-2	–	28 (ST32 – ST60)

4.2 Results

One-way ANOVA analysis did not find any significant difference on all measures except the manipulation check question (F (1, 59) = 17.14, p = 0.000). Such result on NARS shows that the participants from all groups have similar accepting attitude for robots, and on Credibility/Expectancy and TAM questionnaires, it shows that anthropomorphic appearances does not have effect on participants' acceptance for the robot trainer therapy and robot trainer technology.

5 Findings

The two studies above provided insights on: 1) general attitude towards SARs, 2) Acceptance of SAR assisted rehabilitation therapy and robot trainer, and 3) effects of anthropomorphism on the acceptance of SAR assisted rehabilitation therapy and robot trainer.

5.1 General Attitude Towards Socially Assistive Robots

With the NARS questionnaire, we tested participants' negative attitude towards situations of interaction with robots, social influence of robots and emotional interaction with robots. The three factors from both studies scored lower or around average (average scored is 3), since NARS is a negative attitude questionnaire, these lower scores suggest a positive attitude towards the factors.

An open coding analysis on the answers for the questions following the NARS questionnaire specified that robotic technology is desired for its precision, being objective, convenience, efficiency, opening up possibilities for more privacy and eliminating negative social encounters. Negative opinions clustered around technological possibilities, and cultural and ethical concerns. Below are the two factors concerning acceptance for SARs.

Public Perception of Robot Technology

"I think it has the potential to be very interesting and constructive, but hasn't been fully developed" (HA7)

"I might feel alone working with robot as robots don't have cognitive behavior" (MA12)

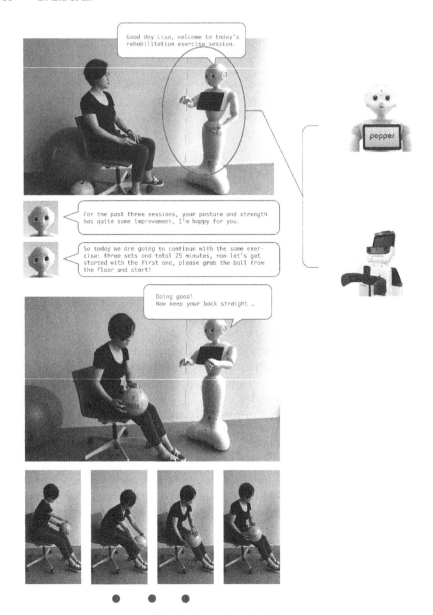

Fig. 2. Scenario in Study 2.

The capability of a robot is questioned based on participants' general knowledge for current technological advancement. 7 quotes suggested robots are best suited for the kind of jobs that are simple, repetitive and do not need complicated judgment. In the participants' opinions, current robotic-related technologies still lack flexibility to handle emergencies and cannot make proper judgement for complex situations. Such technological perception proposed a limitation for participants in terms of the tasks assumed possible for robots to take on, and the possible lack of confidence working with a robot that takes on complex tasks.

Technology-Related Attitude and Beliefs

> *"Not comfortable. Humans are losing the ability to think and react without assistance." (HA21)*
>
> *"Not a fan, I can see the appeal, but I'm sure if there is a living person who needs the money." (LA6)*

Based on the references people use in the comments, it was heavily implied that the related movies, TV shows and news broadcast plays a role in people's opinions for robot technology. Societal and ethical concerns are expressed in the comments. Correspondingly, a recent study suggested that the anthropomorphic appearances of a social robot can pose a threat to human distinctiveness [10]. Designs of SAR application should take this factor into consideration.

5.2 Acceptance of SAR in Rehabilitation Therapy and as Robot Trainer

The Credibility/Expectancy questionnaire was used in to evaluate how much patients believe and how much they feel that the social robot can be an effective aid during rehabilitation training. In Study 1-1, The mean scores for the three groups show that participants for conditions HA and LA have positive opinions on the credibility (HA: $M = 18.82$, $SD = 5.18$, LA: $M = 17.26$, $SD = 7.4$) and expectancy (HA: $M = 17.95$, $SD = 4.26$, LA: $M = 17.16$, $SD = 6.64$) of the training (average score is 14), and participants for condition MA have neutral scores for credibility ($M = 15.30$, $SD = 7.21$) and expectancy ($M = 14.87$, $SD = 6.18$). Study 2-1 agreed with the results from Study 1 with both factors scored above average (Credibility (HA: $M = 16.66$, $SD = 6.13$, LA: $M = 18.07$, $SD = 4.89$), Expectancy (HA:$M = 16.45$, $SD = 4.85$, LA: $M = 17.84$, $SD = 4.16$)).

The TAM questionnaire was used to measure the acceptance of the robot trainer. Mean scores from both studies suggest that participants perceive the robot trainer as easy-to-use (PEU & SE), have a neutral attitude towards the concept (A) and are neutral with regards to its perceived usefulness (PU). Finally, participants have a below average mean score for the factors behavioral intention (BI) and subjective norm (SN).

All the qualitative data regarding the therapy and the robot trainer from study 1 and 2 were included in an open coding analysis, the results are discussed in the three following topics.

Patients' Needs for SAR-Assisted Rehabilitation Training. Based on the contents of the scenario provided, participants expressed the services they considered important in their own rehabilitation therapies, also with confirmation of what was shown in the scenarios. Over 100 quotes were collected and summarized into 9 categories of needs presented in Table 5.

Perceived Benefits of SAR-Assisted Rehabilitation Training

"My own rehabilitation therapy was with a human, but it accomplished the same purpose." (HA17)

Table 5. Patient needs for SAR-assisted rehabilitation therapy [18].

Pre-session		
Plan making		Planning for short/long term rehabilitative training plan
Therapy informing		Information about the session including exercises, time, sporting facilities, goal, key points etc.
During session		
Exercise guidance	Demonstration	Step by step instruction about the exercise being practiced, with sufficient information for self-evaluation for the quality of the exercise
	Guiding information	Counts of the movements, breathing techniques, breaks, next exercise etc.
Performance evaluation and correction		Therapist need to have an on-going evaluation of patients physical and mental state, exercise performance, then provide them with correction information, reminder of key considerations of the exercise, motivational prompts as they deem as needed
Hands-on assistance and therapies	Posture correction	Hands-on correction for posture when the correction information is not well understood
	Hands-on therapies	Massages etc.
Safety supports	Case of emergencies	Possible situations might occur during the session like broken sporting facilities, physical instabilities and other factors that can potentially interfere with the session
	Sports injuries	Dealing with spots injuries with physical and informational support
Emotional interaction	Social interaction	Patients suggest that social interactions with the therapist can help them to be calm and relax, mentally getting ready for the exercises
	Motivational support	Providing timely motivational support when the patient is experiencing physical difficulties
After session		
Progress summary		Summarizing the session, helping the patient to reflect on his/her progress
Plan for next session		Information about short/long-term sessions later

Mean scores of Credibility/Expectancy questionnaire show that participants have above average expectations from the rehabilitation therapy provided by a robot trainer.

Self-directed practice is considered to be an important component in rehabilitation therapy [25]. Quotes from the questionnaire confirmed that the process is mostly done by the patient him/herself and demands consistency and certain quantity. To this end, participants have confidence in having a robot trainer providing guidance, feedback and motivational prompts. The following additional benefits is also expected of a robot trainer to provide:

– Providing stable and basic services while eliminating human errors and interference

Some participants mentioned their rehabilitation experience, during which, there were moments that they felt neglected, misdiagnosed or given the wrong instructions and being interrupted by inappropriate social interactions. These participants believed a robot trainer to be more goal-oriented, therefore enabling them to better focus on the training exercise and eliminating possible human errors.

– Financial benefits and cost effectiveness

Cost efficiency and flexibility were expected by the participants, tele-rehabilitation is one of the most promising usage cases that can be developed for robot trainer.

Concerns about SAR-Assisted Rehabilitation Therapy. Concerns primarily focused on the loss of human factors. Participants questioned how the robot will make up for the loss of human specific values in rehabilitation therapy e.g. empathy, perceptions on the patients and the overall rehabilitation training based on experience and expertise, capability of dealing with emergencies, evaluating patients' training performance and providing emotional support. The lack of humanness also related to participants' lack of trust in the robot trainer. On top of this, patients doubted whether the motivational prompts would be perceived as sincere, instead of "programmed".

5.3 Patients' Preference for Anthropomorphic Appearance

Regarding the preferred anthropomorphic level, we discover that higher anthropomorphic concepts in both studies are clearly the better fit for rehabilitation training. However, the reason for such preference does not lie in the acceptance for the therapy or the technology, but in the subjective perception of the functional and aesthetic design of the concepts. A friendly and aesthetically pleasing design that fits the tasks of the robot trainer is found to be an ideal appearance for robot trainer. Anthropomorphic is found to help with using emotional expressions in the interaction by SAR.

In both studies, participants were asked to choose their preferred version of the robot trainer. Participants preferred the high anthropomorphic concept (17 out of 31), followed by the medium anthropomorphic concept (9/31) and low anthropomorphic concept (5/31). Similar question in study 2 got 24 votes out of 28 for high anthropomorphic look. TAM questionnaire found a significant difference in study 1-1 in self-efficacy, with

392 B. Liu et al.

the low anthropomorphic concept scored the highest, however study 2 did not replicate such results. According to the comments, the high anthropomorphic concept in study 1 looks very futuristic, which could seem to be intimidating or challenging to get familiar with. Comparatively, the materials in study 2 is realistic and less advanced, which could lower the perceived challenge for self-efficacy. Based on the currents results, it is clear that a higher anthropomorphic look is preferred by patients in rehabilitation trainings. However, such preference is not expressed through users' acceptance for the therapy and the technology, because study 2 did not replicate the results in self-efficacy in study 1.

Open coding analysis on the reasons for participants choice specified that the human-like look seems to convey more emotions and more "relatable". But looking human isn't always ideal. Some participants also like the concept better because it does not look too human-like. Human-likeness also brought disapproval because that "the line on pepper' head looks like his head is cracked open" and that "the neutral facial expression looks a little disturbing". A few comments suggested that Pepper should have more facial expression. Thus far even we find out that higher anthropomorphic appearance is more preferred, but the exact preferred level of anthropomorphic appearance for a robot trainer has not been specified. This is a necessary question to discuss since it is likely that anthropomorphism in robot trainer appearances is a double edge sword, and it is not "the more the better". Also, a unique group of quotes appeared for the high anthropomorphism concept. These 15 quotes inquired whether the robot would provide hands-on training assistance. This highlights a potential link between the robot's appearance and users' expectations about its functionality.

Apart from anthropomorphism, the design also effects participants preference. Qualitative analysis points out that the high anthropomorphic concept design in both studies 1) look warm, friendly, cute and personal, 2) seems most able to provide a better and more varied service, especially in study 2-2, people commented that pepper's screen can be very helpful with interaction. The aesthetic design is often mentioned in participants' reasons for their choice. According to the data, people generally prefer friendly and aesthetically-pleasing look of the robot, the design should also fit the task of the robot trainer, and stereotypes of the profession should also be properly expressed in the design. In this study set-up, the aesthetic is inseparable from anthropomorphism, so will be the same case for a real field application of a robot, therefore we suggest any further exploration regarding robot appearances should also consider the importance of aesthetics.

Reason for participants who chose one of the other two concepts were 1) participants feel safe around them, 2) participants are unfamiliar with the high anthropomorphic concept, not knowing what to expect, and 3) a robot trainer with high anthropomorphic appearance, but only voice interaction, is considered unintelligent. Some comments point out that the high anthropomorphic concepts look childish, which could imply that people expect the look of the robot trainer to convey a certain level of professionalism.

6 Conclusion

This work explores patients' acceptance for socially assistive robot in rehabilitation settings, and the effect of anthropomorphic form factor in robotic design in this context.

We discovered that participants have a neutral to positive attitude towards SARs and it's use in rehabilitation therapy as trainer. The SAR technology in therapies is regarded easy to use but participants generally lack intention for using the system, which is possibly due to unfamiliarity with SAR technology.

Participants have a clear preference for high anthropomorphic concept for a robot trainer, but the effect of anthropomorphic appearances does not lie in technology acceptance or the attitude for the therapy. However, such preference is also linked to the design elements of the concept, especially aesthetic design. For a robot trainer to be well accepted, the anthropomorphic level and the design should fit the tasks that was demanded by patients, such process should consider patients' expectation, aesthetic preference and task-related stereotypes. Based on the insights, further work should be done in clarifying patient's demands for the therapy, dealing with patient's concerns, and facilitating trust for the robot trainer.

References

1. Bartneck, C., Bleeker, T., Bun, J., Fens, P., Riet, L.: The influence of robot anthropomorphism on the feelings of embarrassment when interacting with robots. Paladyn. J. Behav. Robot. **1**, 109–115 (2010). https://doi.org/10.2478/s13230-010-0011-3
2. Cardona, M., Destarac, M.A., Garcia, C.E.: Exoskeleton robots for rehabilitation: state of the art and future trends. In: 2017 IEEE 37th Central America and Panama Convention (CONCAPAN XXXVII), pp. 1–6. IEEE, Managua (2017)
3. Choi, J., Kim, M.: The usage and evaluation of anthropomorphic form in robot design, p. 15 (2008)
4. Devilly, G.J., Borkovec, T.D.: Psychometric properties of the credibility/expectancy questionnaire, p. 14 (2000)
5. Ding, Y., et al.: Biomechanical and physiological evaluation of multi-joint assistance with soft exosuits. IEEE Trans. Neural Syst. Rehabil. Eng. **25**, 119–130 (2017). https://doi.org/10.1109/TNSRE.2016.2523250
6. Epley, N., Waytz, A., Cacioppo, J.T.: On seeing human: a three-factor theory of anthropomorphism. Psychol. Rev. **114**, 864–886 (2007). https://doi.org/10.1037/0033-295X.114.4.864
7. Eriksson, J., Mataric, M.J., Winstein, C.J.: Hands-off assistive robotics for post-stroke arm rehabilitation. In: 9th International Conference on Rehabilitation Robotics, ICORR 2005, pp. 21–24. IEEE, Chicago (2005)
8. Eyssel, F., Kuchenbrandt, D., Bobinger, S.: 'If you sound like me, you must be more human': on the interplay of robot and user features on human-robot acceptance and anthropomorphism, p. 2 (2012)
9. Feil-Seifer, D., Mataric, M.J.: Socially assistive robotics. In: 9th International Conference on Rehabilitation Robotics, ICORR 2005, pp. 465–468. IEEE, Chicago (2005)
10. Ferrari, F., Paladino, M.P., Jetten, J.: Blurring human-machine distinctions: anthropomorphic appearance in social robots as a threat to human distinctiveness. Int. J. Soc. Robot. **8**, 287–302 (2016). https://doi.org/10.1007/s12369-016-0338-y
11. Feys, P., et al.: Robot-supported upper limb training in a virtual learning environment: a pilot randomized controlled trial in persons with MS. J. NeuroEng. Rehabil. **12** (2015). https://doi.org/10.1186/s12984-015-0043-3
12. Fong, T., Nourbakhsh, I., Dautenhahn, K.: A survey of socially interactive robots. Robot. Auton. Syst. **42**, 143–166 (2003). https://doi.org/10.1016/S0921-8890(02)00372-X

13. Gockley, R., Matarić, M.J.: Encouraging physical therapy compliance with a hands-off mobile robot. In: Proceeding of the 1st ACM SIGCHI/SIGART Conference on Human-Robot Interaction - HRI 2006, p. 150. ACM Press, Salt Lake City (2006)

14. Heerink, M., Kröse, B., Evers, V., Wielinga, B.: Assessing acceptance of assistive social agent technology by older adults: the almere model. Int. J. Soc. Robot. **2**, 361–375 (2010). https://doi.org/10.1007/s12369-010-0068-5

15. Klamer, T., Allouch, S.B.: Acceptance and use of a social robot by elderly users in a domestic environment. IEEE (2010)

16. Kang, K.I., Freedman, S., Mataric, M.J., Cunningham, M.J., Lopez, B.: A hands-off physical therapy assistance robot for cardiac patients. In: 9th International Conference on Rehabilitation Robotics, ICORR 2005, pp. 337–340. IEEE, Chicago (2005)

17. Laut, J., Porfiri, M., Raghavan, P.: The present and future of robotic technology in rehabilitation. Curr. Phys. Med. Rehabil. Rep. **4**, 312–319 (2016). https://doi.org/10.1007/s40141-016-0139-0

18. Liu, B., Markopoulos, P., Tetteroo, D.: How anthropomorphism affects user acceptance of a robot trainer in physical rehabilitation. In: HEALTHINF 2019 - 12th International Conference on Health Informatics, Proceedings; Part of 12th International Joint Conference on Biomedical Engineering Systems and Technologies, BIOSTEC 2019, Pp. 30–40 (2019)

19. Moosaei, M., Das, S.K., Popa, D.O., Riek, L.D.: Using facially expressive robots to calibrate clinical pain perception. In: Proceedings of the 2017 ACM/IEEE International Conference on Human-Robot Interaction - HRI 2017, pp. 32–41. ACM Press, Vienna (2017)

20. Nomura, T., Kanda, T., Suzuki, T., Kato, K.: Psychology in human-robot communication: an attempt through investigation of negative attitudes and anxiety toward robots, pp. 35–40. IEEE (2004)

21. Popescu, N., Popescu, D., Ivǎnescu, M.: Intelligent robotic approach for after-stroke hand rehabilitation. In: Proceedings of the 9th International Joint Conference on Biomedical Engineering Systems and Technologies, pp. 49–57. SCITEPRESS - Science and Technology Publications, Rome (2016)

22. Salem, M., Eyssel, F., Rohlfing, K., Kopp, S., Joublin, F.: To err is human(-like): effects of robot gesture on perceived anthropomorphism and likability. Int. J. Soc. Robot. **5**, 313–323 (2013). https://doi.org/10.1007/s12369-013-0196-9

23. Siegel, M., Breazeal, C., Norton, M.I.: Persuasive robotics: the influence of robot gender on human behavior. In: 2009 IEEE/RSJ International Conference on Intelligent Robots and Systems, pp. 2563–2568. IEEE, St. Louis (2009)

24. Tapus, A., Mataric, M.J.: Socially assistive robots: the link between personality, empathy, physiological signals, and task performance. In: AAAI Spring Symposium: Emotion, Personality, and Social Behavior, pp. 133–140 (2008)

25. Vitiello, N., Mohammed, S., Moreno, J.C.: Guest editorial wearable robotics for motion assistance and rehabilitation. IEEE Trans. Neural Syst. Rehabil. Eng. **25**, 103–106 (2017). https://doi.org/10.1109/TNSRE.2017.2665279

26. Winkle, K., Caleb-Solly, P., Turton, A., Bremner, P.: Social robots for engagement in rehabilitative therapies: design implications from a study with therapists. In: Proceedings of the 2018 ACM/IEEE International Conference on Human-Robot Interaction - HRI 2018, pp. 289–297. ACM Press, Chicago (2018)

27. Zaga, C., de Vries, R.A.J., Li, J., Truong, K.P., Evers, V.: A simple nod of the head: the effect of minimal robot movements on children's perception of a low-anthropomorphic robot. In: Proceedings of the 2017 CHI Conference on Human Factors in Computing Systems - CHI 2017, pp. 336–341. ACM Press, Denver (2017)

Dementia and mHealth: On the Way to GDPR Compliance

Joana Muchagata[1]([✉]) [iD], Soraia Teles[1,2] [iD], Pedro Vieira-Marques[1] [iD],
Diogo Abrantes[1] [iD], and Ana Ferreira[1] [iD]

[1] CINTESIS - Centro de Investigação em Tecnologias e Serviços de Saúde,
Faculty of Medicine, University of Porto, Porto, Portugal
{joanamuchagata,pmarques,djm,amlaf}@med.up.pt
[2] Institute of Biomedical Sciences Abel Salazar, University of Porto, Porto, Portugal
stsousa@icbas.up.pt

Abstract. Innovative technological solutions for people with some kind of mental or cognitive health issues, have the potential to keep the brain active and help them to be as independent as possible in their daily lives. Therefore, those solutions can improve the overall older adult's quality of life and, particularly, of those with dementia or Mild Cognitive Impairment (MCI). In a previous paper, the authors discussed the potential of mobile apps for people with dementia and their compliance with the GDPR (General Data Protection Regulation). However, and despite all the advantages, a lack of security standards or guidelines and low GDPR compliance was noticed on the analysed MCI mobile apps. This may raise serious concerns, as older adults living with this condition, may be particularly susceptible and vulnerable to risk of privacy breaches. This paper extends that work by using lessons learned and extracted requirements (e.g., GDPR and visual security requirements), together with an adaptable access control model (e.g., SoTRAACE), to build mHealth mockups for people with MCI based on a use-case of a persona, an older adult with a slight decline in cognitive abilities who uses a computer-assisted/mobile cognitive training application to delay his cognitive decline. The authors also aim to bring awareness to researchers, designers, developers and health professionals for the improvement of security and privacy of mHealth for dementia.

Keywords: Mild Cognitive Impairment (MCI) · Dementia Ambient Assisted Living (AAL) · Cognitive training · Security and privacy access control · General Data Protection Regulation (GDPR) · SoTRAACE mHealth applications

1 Introduction

The increase of life expectancy and low birth rates are at the heart of the demographic changes occurring in the world [1]. People are living longer, and demographic, and social trends, have led to an increased number of older adults in industrialized countries, affecting the provision of public and private health and care services [2].

Population ageing is contributing to a greater prevalence of chronic diseases, and countries with higher shares of older people typically have a greater proportion of people

© Springer Nature Switzerland AG 2020
A. Roque et al. (Eds.): BIOSTEC 2019, CCIS 1211, pp. 395–411, 2020.
https://doi.org/10.1007/978-3-030-46970-2_19

with dementia (PWD) [3]. Due to dementia's high prevalence and its economic and social impact on families, caregivers and communities, the condition was established as a public health priority [4–6]. Among older adults, this group of disorders is one of the major causes of disability and dependency, thus frequently requiring long term or permanent care [7]. Long term care can include home nursing, community care and assisted living [1]. With the high demand for healthcare equipment, infrastructures and institutions to ensure the elderly population well-being, additional pressure is placed on the economy and social systems, causing healthcare costs to escalate [3].

Ambient Assisted Living (AAL) solutions have come into the spotlight by their potential cost-effectiveness, as those can support dependent older adults to live longer in their preferred environment (e.g., at home) improving their well-being, autonomy, independence, security and safety, while reducing costs for society and public health systems [2, 8]. When an older adult suffering from dementia or Mild Cognitive Impairment (MCI) is required, and still able to actively use such technological solutions - which is not always the case as AAL solutions can be embedded in the environment and used in a passive way - there are additional challenges to consider. Several security and privacy concerns are at stake because older adults living with such conditions might be particularly susceptible and vulnerable to the risk of privacy breaches. As people living with MCI and dementia might show a poor judgment of situations [9], they can be at greater risk of malicious or unintended acts. MCI and dementia can reduce an individuals' ability to consider the implications of sharing personal information (e.g., sensitive information or geolocation data), recognize scams such as phishing emails or websites, follow recommended password guidelines, among others [10].

In a previous paper, Muchagata et al. [11] discussed the potential of mobile apps to improve the overall patients and caregivers' quality of life and, particularly, of those with dementia. Some apps are aimed at stimulating cognitive functions, keeping the brain active, and, by this way, helping people to be as independent as possible in their daily lives. However, a lack of security standards and guidelines on those mobile apps was noticed. After analyzing 18 apps aimed at stimulating cognitive functions of people with dementia, for GDPR (General Data Protection Regulation) compliance, the results showed that the mandated requirements are still not implemented in most of them, in order to ensure privacy and security in the interactions between users and mobile apps [11].

This paper extends previous research on GDPR compliance by applying lessons learned in this field as well as knowledge on adaptable access control models, to AAL environments for people with dementia. That paper builds on SoTRAACE (Socio-Technical Risk-Adaptable Access Control), an access control model proposed by Moura et al. [7], which has the potential to better adapt users' access control needs to each security reality and context.

This work presents a use-case of a persona described as an older adult with MCI, who shows a slight decline in cognitive abilities and uses a computer-assisted/mobile cognitive training application aimed at delaying cognitive decline. The paper shows how SoTRAACE, by integrating GDPR key requirements, can help defining mHealth mockups for such a scenario. This work intends to bring awareness to researchers, designers, developers and health professionals for the improvement of security and privacy of mHealth for dementia.

2 Related Work

2.1 Ageing, Cognitive Decline and Mild Cognitive Impairment

Mild Cognitive Impairment (MCI) is a term used to describe the progressive decline in cognitive function beyond expectation from normal ageing, due to damage or disease in the brain [12], causing a slight but noticeable decline in cognitive abilities, including memory and thinking skills [12]. When affecting memory, it can lead the person to forget important information such as appointments, paying bills, conversations or recent events. As MCI is also related with thinking skills, this can influence the person's attention, the ability to make the right decisions and the capability to easily and quickly complete a sequence of steps required to complete a complex task [13].

Approximately 15 to 20% of people aged 65, or older, have MCI [13], and are at an increased risk of developing Alzheimer's or another type of dementia. However, not everyone with MCI develops dementia, and in some individuals, it can revert to normal cognition or remain stable [13].

A decline of cognitive abilities is a part of normal ageing. However, in cases when there is a greater risk for the development of dementia, strategies to prevent or slow a decline in cognitive abilities can be very relevant [14].

A healthy lifestyle including mental and social activities as well as healthy eating habits, affect cognitive functions and are associated with less cognitive decline in old age [15]. Therefore, the Alzheimer's Association [13] suggests coping strategies that may help to slow the decline of cognitive skills, including (i) Practice regular exercise; (ii) Control cardiovascular risk factors, e.g., stop smoking; (iii) Choose a healthy diet that includes fresh fruits and vegetables, whole grains and lean proteins; and (iv) Participate in mentally and socially stimulating activities. Hence, the field is prolific in interventions and initiatives aimed at promoting the adoption of such strategies, including health education projects, physical activity programs and interventions aimed at stimulating cognitive functions.

2.2 Computer-Assisted Cognitive Training for Older Adults with MCI

Efforts have been devoted at preventing or slowing the cognitive decline both in normal ageing and on clinically diagnosed cognitive impairment. In the last decade, adding to the traditional, paper-based, cognitive training programs, a plethora of computer-assisted cognitive training programs have been developed with this purpose.

Cognitive interventions aim to improve cognitive problems experienced by older adults, with the goal of maximizing their current function and reducing the risk of, or slowing, cognitive decline. Cognitive training is among those interventions, which involves guided practice on a set of standardized tasks addressing specific aspects of cognition (memory, language, attention or executive functions). It also involves teaching strategies (visual imagery, spaced retrieval and memory strategies) [16].

Computer-assisted cognitive training has the advantage of being flexible and comprehensive enough to allow a systematic training of specific cognitive functions (e.g., memory, executive functions). Moreover, the computer is able to automatically measure success/failure, provide immediate feedback and quickly adapt the program to the person's rhythm and goals/needs [17]. When a computer-assisted cognitive training program is available to be used outside the institutional context (e.g., hospital or private clinic), in a personal computer with internet connection, additional gains include the ubiquity and convenience of such resources, which can be used in any place, at any time, and monitored aloof by a healthcare professional.

Promising evidence has been collected with regards to the safeness and efficacy of Computer-assisted cognitive training programs for cognition in older adults, even though mixed findings have been reported on efficacy, depending on the population and cognitive domains under analysis [18]. Regarding MCI, a recent systematic review and meta-analysis concluded that Computer-assisted cognitive training is effective on global cognition, specific cognitive domains (attention, working memory, learning, and memory), and psychosocial functioning, with limited to moderate effects being found in those domains [18].

Popular examples of computer-assisted cognitive training programs include the brain-training game "Brain Age", which comprises elements of reading aloud and simple arithmetic calculations. This program shows that brain-training games have beneficial effects in terms of cognitive abilities [15]. In another experience, Günther et al. [17] tested a computer-assisted cognitive training (CAT) program with 19 elderly aged between 75 and 91 years old identified with age-associated memory impairment. The CAT program included tasks designed to increase attention, visual and motor performance, reaction time, vigilance, attentiveness, memory, verbal performance and general knowledge. Several of these exercises were identical to real-life tasks and helped increase the motivation to use them. Significant improvements were observed in the majority of cognitive functions [17].

2.3 Online Security and Privacy

Despite the potentials of solutions such as the ones previously described, human-computer interactions can raise several security and privacy challenges.

Access control is one of the first interactions between users and systems and it can help providing a more adapted and adequate access to the environment, being particularly important for people with special requirements. It also has the potential to early detect and prevent security problems thereby helping to avoid more serious harm [19]. Various access control models exist to provide such features but currently, mHealth applications require more adaptable means to provide security and privacy decisions at the interactional level [20]. The SoTRAACE model (Fig. 1) [7] takes Role Based Access Control (RBAC) entities [21], together with contextual (e.g., work, home, public places), technological (e.g., type of device, network connection) and user's interaction profiling, to perform a quantitative and qualitative risk assessment analysis to support a smart decision-making on the most secure and usable way to access and display information. SoTRAACE also integrates an Adaptable Visualization Module (AVM) module to improve availability, security and privacy of visualized data [22], for each request situation. If users have specific interaction needs, such is the case of patients with MCI, AVM can also take that into account and integrate those needs (recurrent alarms and messages to remind or notify users about the activities they need to perform) within the context of how, when and where data are being displayed [20].

For other specific requirements, Break the Glass (BTG) [21], a solution for access provision in emergency or unanticipated situations, is also available, and Delegation can be provided for an unauthorized professional to temporarily access patient data, on behalf of an authorized user.

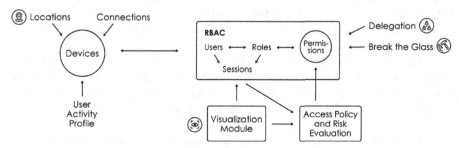

Fig. 1. SoTRAACE - Socio-Technical Risk-Adaptable Access Control Model [7].

2.4 Design and Security Requirements

The authors searched the literature to look for specific validated interface design requirements of the target population (e.g., patients with MCI), as well as, security and privacy needs. Overall, literature produced on this particular topic is scarce and only a few interesting records were identified. Regarding design issues, Onoda et al. [23] emphasize that the touch accuracy for MCI users might cause a difficulty and therefore technical aspects of the devices should be considered, e.g., the layout of buttons and taskbar. Another study stresses that the function of buttons within apps was not always clear because symbols used for the buttons were not recognizable [24]. Sometimes navigation buttons were not big enough or missing. For example, a clear home key was not always available, which they want to have in the app. Also, too many links, screens and clicks within apps compromises the comfort of navigation. This can lead to persons with dementia having difficulty understanding the operation of some apps and getting lost in the navigation menu. MCI users also referred to minimize the need for scrolling, present clear instructions on a step-by-step basis and use recognizable buttons supported by pictograms and text, readable letter types and sizes, a calm interface and background, and contrast between text and background [24]. The use of short clear sentences and the use of easy words were preferred features of the language used by the apps.

On the other hand, regarding the requirements on security and privacy issues, Boulos et al. [25] list the key ingredients necessary for a successful app. These include content quality, usability, need to match the app to consumer's general and health literacy levels, device connectivity standards, security and user's privacy. Peek et al. [26] and Perumal et al. [27] add up to this by stating that improving awareness, the sense of trust and security when using the mobile app, improves its acceptability, which is also described in other works. This is obtained with risk analysis and visual security and privacy adaptations, which ends in higher privacy support and transparency (e.g., by using SoTRAACE with the AVM module).

2.5 General Data Protection Regulation (GDPR) Guidelines

Innovative technological solutions for people with mental or cognitive health issues have conquered a great interest of the scientific community and practitioners in the last years. However, the progression of the mHealth market comes with a growing concern for security and privacy [28] as many tools/systems do not follow design principles and privacy guidelines [11, 29].

In order to respond to the lack of security standards or guidelines to follow as well as to the low or non-existent protection of user's personal data, the European Commission adopted, in 2016, a new stricter legislation for protecting and controlling the processing of individuals' personal data in European member states: the General Data Protection Regulation (GDPR) [30].

In a previous work [11], the authors analyzed whether apps aiming at training cognitive skills such as memory, attention, concentration, language and executive functions comply with the GDPR guidelines and requirements. Eighteen Android apps from Google's Play Store available in English and Portuguese were included in the analysis. The results have shown that most of the key requirements mandated by the GDPR are still not implemented in the available apps and so they do not comply with regulations to ensure privacy and security in the interactions between users and mobile apps. For instance, the majority of the analyzed apps do not have an available privacy policy or terms and conditions (78%; n = 14) at all, suggesting little to no user control of their personal data once entered into the app. In those apps where a privacy policy (22%; n = 4) is available, the information provided is long and vague. Moreover, 7 (39%) apps do not inform the user about what type of data and features they will be accessing when running, and 8 (44%) apps need to access personal data such as location, contacts and photos [11]. This study showed that most apps aiming at training cognitive skills in this sample are not in compliance with the GDPR requirements. This research can be used as a guideline to support further work in defining what a mHealth application for dementia should include to better comply with GDPR. This is the work done and presented in the following sections.

3 Methods

As conclusions from the previous work [11], which this paper extends, the authors gave some recommendations for future research and development in the mHealth field, including: (i) structured guidelines or principles to be used in the process of creating an app should be made available online for all mobile app designers and developers; (ii) a simple, clear, transparent and understandable Privacy Policy should always be available through a button in the main menu or even in another visible part of the app; (iii) explicit consent must be mandatory, being done through a consent screen at the app launch. Hence, when a user is registering on a mobile app, s/he should be asked to opt-in to have their data collected or receive communications (emails or notifications). This screen should also show information about what kind of users' data will be collected and how they are going to be processed; (iv) a functionality must be available where users can ask for their data to be removed or can request their data to be deleted, and have an opt-out of communications/notifications; (v) must have strong encryption algorithms of personal data by default; (vi) every mobile app must include contact information of the business or app developer, allowing users to contact them for support, and, most importantly; (vii) the existence of app regulations made by credible entities related to the app content specially those created for sensitive and vulnerable groups of people.

On the other hand, the SoTRAACE model can exercise further the security and privacy requirements adoption concerning patients' personal data, by improving decision making based on risk assessment of each interaction and associated contextual variables. The model can help define scenarios in different locations and adapt visualization needs to them.

In order to demonstrate and discuss the application of all the interface design requirements, as well as, security and privacy needs described above (Sect. 2.4), which were not considered in the previously analysed applications, a use-case is described in Sect. 4.

The process of defining working mockups starts with the definition of a persona (Sect. 4.1), who represents the main character of the created use-case (a patient living with MCI who uses an online cognitive training tool to improve his cognitive abilities). GDPR requirements and SoTRAACE functionalities are then applied in two scenarios where their adaptation is performed for when the MCI user accesses the app, taking into consideration different contexts and security risks (Sect. 4.2).

A discussion follows this proposal in order to generate and consider various issues that still need to be improved, what can or cannot be adopted from GDPR and SoTRAACE model, and how this research should proceed (Sects. 5 and 6).

4 Use-Case

4.1 Persona Description

Figure 2 describes a persona, who represents the target population (e.g., a person living with MCI and who uses a mobile cognitive training application). His personality, demographics and other attributes are described, as this helps to better conceive what features and functionalities are required to provide usable and useful information when using a mobile cognitive training application.

John (the persona) began to notice some decline in his memory and thinking skills and was recently diagnosed with MCI. He has always been a very active and independent person and he values being able to make his own decisions. Therefore, he hopes his condition does not get worse, to be able to keep his self-confidence and emotional well-being. John is ICT savvy and uses his smartphone and internet daily. Besides having a calendar and reminders application, he is also very enthusiastic about the cognitive training application installed on his smartphone, developed by the local hospital and recommended by his neurologist as a complementary intervention measure. With a personalized training program that can be used at any place with internet connection, he hopes to improve his cognitive skills. Despite the advantage of being able to access the cognitive training program application anywhere, John is concerned about the security and privacy of his personal data.

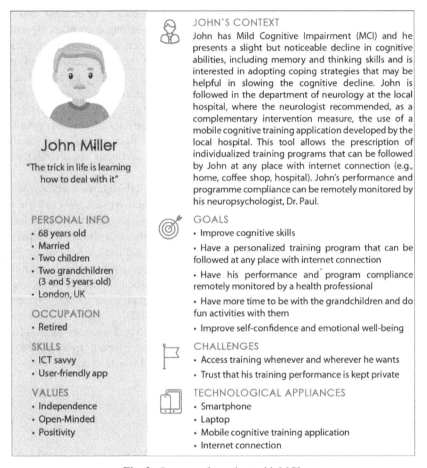

Fig. 2. Persona of a patient with MCI.

4.2 Proposal of SoTRAACE and GDPR Compliant Mobile Application Mockups

As this paper extends a previous research on GDPR compliance as well as the integration of SoTRAACE, in this section, the authors present a use-case of a persona described as an older adult with MCI (Fig. 2). Through mHealth mockups, in Sect. 4.2.1 is presented a scenario with some of the key GDPR requirements applied to a fictitious mHealth app named "Cognicare", while in Sect. 4.2.2 the functionalities of SoTRAACE are integrated with an AAL context.

"Cognicare" is a mobile cognitive training app developed by a local hospital with the aim to be a complementary intervention measure for patients with MCI. This tool allows the prescription of individualized training programs that can be followed by the patient at any place with an internet connection (e.g., home, coffee shop, hospital) (Fig. 3).

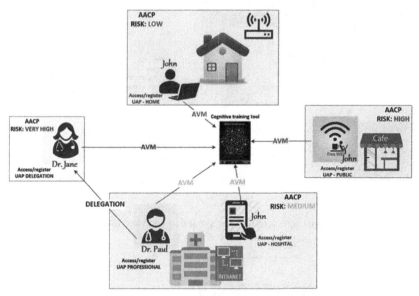

Fig. 3. SoTRAACE model applied to the various online cognitive training context scenarios [19].

4.2.1 Scenario 1: GDPR Guidelines

Regardless of the type of application and the target audience, when a user starts with the app installation s/he must be informed which type of access the mobile app will have in the user's mobile phone in order to be installed [11]. Figure 4 represents the first screen of the "Cognicare" application. This first screen presents information about the features that the mobile app is going to access. And before proceeding with the installation, there is a button for "Privacy Policy".

Unlike the majority of the analysed applications, where the user is confronted with a very extensive text full of jargon, the authors propose a simple, clear and understandable way for users to visualize the most important points related with the Privacy Policy content [30, 31]. Therefore, the relevant items related with the Privacy Policy, which are rendered to the user through icons, have a short and clear explanation (Fig. 5 and Fig. 6). These two figures show information about the kind of users' data that will be collected, and how data will be processed and protected. The full Privacy Policy is linked so users can verify it and see exactly what they are consenting to, regarding their personal information and privacy [32]. The navigation between both screens (Fig. 5 and Fig. 6) is done by clicking on the screen and drag to the side.

Figure 6 also presents an icon for privacy settings management [32]. And, in its turn, Fig. 7 provides, in detail, the available options.

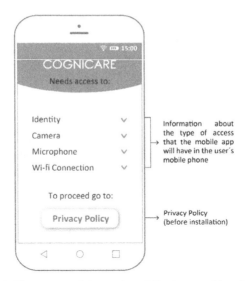

Fig. 4. First screen of the user's mobile phone and installation.

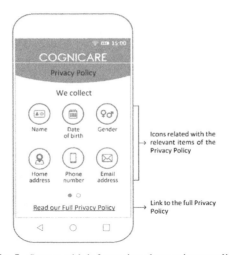

Fig. 5. Screen with information about privacy policy.

Permissions should be customizable in the beginning, and the permissions' icon should always be visible during the entire app and users must be allowed to edit them (Fig. 8 - left) [33]. In this section, the user (John) can edit his profile as well as delete it [30–32]. On "Preferences", he can control whether or not he wants to receive notifications, activate the location and share the results obtained in the training application. Information related with support, contacts, the full privacy policy, and terms and conditions are also available in this menu.

A home button should also be available to allow him to return to the main menu (Fig. 8 - right).

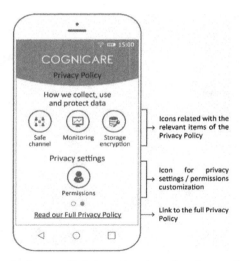

Fig. 6. Screen with information about the privacy policy.

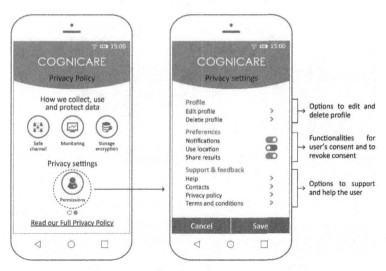

Fig. 7. Customization of user's permissions.

Another important point of the GDPR regulation is about the explicit consent that should be freely expressed by the user through a button or a ticking box complemented with clear, specific and targeted information [30, 31, 34] (Fig. 9). In this case, John may give consent to whomever he considers can have access to his diagnosis.

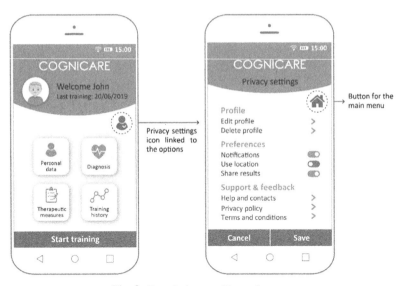

Fig. 8. Permissions and home buttons.

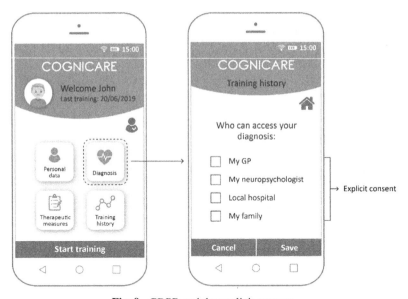

Fig. 9. GDPR and the explicit consent.

4.2.2 Scenario 2: SoTRAACE Model

In this scenario, John is the patient with MCI who uses "Cognicare" a mobile cognitive training app. His performance and program compliance can be remotely monitored by his doctor, or other healthcare professionals, if necessary.

With most existing access control models, privacy of visualized information would be the same independently of the situation, technical measures or user's interaction profile. This way, John would be able to see all the content without any restrictions regardless of his location, time, type of device/network connection, and history of previous interactions. On the other hand, with SoTRAACE, every interactive experience is unique [19].

If John accesses the cognitive training tool at home, the Wi-Fi network is private and protected. Also, it is unlikely the presence of unknown people around, therefore it is improbable the risk of shoulder surfing. Due to these aspects, in this scenario, when accessing the app, the associated risk level is identified as low, thus the AVM component would show all data associated with the tool (Fig. 10). So, after login, the first screen has the name of the user, a photograph and the date of the last training. This screen has also all data associated with the tool, including John's personal data, diagnosis, therapeutic measures, performance history, and, at the bottom, the "Start training" button for accessing training features (Fig. 10).

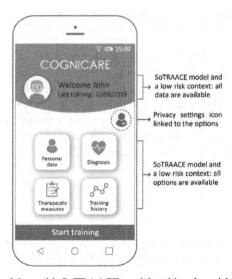

Fig. 10. Visualization of data with SoTRAACE model and in a low risk context (e.g., at home).

However, when John is in a public place, for instance, the hospital (usually a more crowded location), privacy restrictions must be applied (Fig. 11). In this scenario, there is no need to display personal data such as date of birth, complete name or address, and in situations with even higher risk (e.g., in public places with unsecure connections) a more strict policy is enforced and only strictly fundamental data regarding the current training session is available. Consequently, John's name and his photograph are not displayed and only the options related with the training are available ("Start training" and "Training history").

Despite the restrictions in accessing personal information due to a high risk connection, in case of an emergency situation, there is a button" Activate" (Fig. 11) which allows access to all information and options.

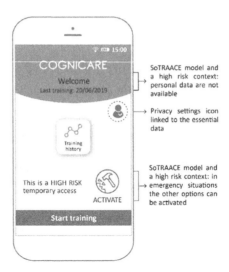

Fig. 11. Visualization of data with SoTRAACE model and in a high risk context.

The same situation also occurs when it comes to third parties accessing data, for instance the professionals monitoring John's evolution. SoTRAACE integrates modules for delegation where unauthorized professionals can temporarily access John's evolution to help assessing his progress. In this situation, SoTRAACE applies even more restrictions as this professional does not need to know any personal information regarding the trainee but only the strictly fundamental information to provide a recommendation (e.g., John's training history). Once accomplished the purpose of this specific access authorization, access is revoked.

5 Discussion

Following the main conclusions of previous research, which this work extends, this paper presents the first step on using the previous lessons learned, for the definition of a preliminary set of mobile mockups for people with MCI, when using an online cognitive training tool. These are directed to the general needs of GDPR, but also to the more specific needs of security and access control decisions (also a GDPR goal) adapted to the contextual requirements of each user's interaction. Furthermore, the requirements are refined to the necessities of the target population, clearly represented by a persona, who can reflect many elderly patients with the same condition all over the world.

In the proposed mockups, GDPR key requirements are taken into account, without compromising MCI needs regarding design specificities. Privacy policy, as well as, data collection content, are simply translated into images and related small and clear expressions, to communicate to the user, mandatory information such as: what data are collected, for what purposes, and how to obtain more information. The same is part of previous research requirements for MCI patients when using mobile apps, e.g., "use recognizable buttons supported by pictograms and text...short clear sentences and the use of easy words were preferred features of the language used by the apps" (similar requirements are described in the GDPR).

There are, however, requirements that cannot be easily translated into the mobile apps. For instance, requirement (vii) on Sect. 3, demands for a standardization and certification infrastructure that can provide available apps with a degree of testing and higher trust, when they pass both standardization and certification requirements. Until now, only generic measures are in place to verify online apps available in both online stores. Attestation and certification are needed to better improve content, privacy and usability/user experience quality, not only in healthcare (which is a very critical domain able to interfere with users' psychological and physical health), but in all domains.

Moreover, beyond generic measures, specific privacy and security features should not be hindering application's use, but need, nevertheless, to be present to instill in the users' mind a feeling of trust. For this matter, data regarding security measures is displayed similarly to the privacy policy, and means to clearly advise the user to know that risk assessment made by the app can provide extra security features to protect their privacy, and not put personal data at a higher risk, unnecessarily, for specific contextual and interactional conditions. Again, for this work, it is clear that access control models need to be more dynamic and adaptable to also provide better transparency, improve user's awareness, trust and perform better informed decisions. The authors believe that SoTRAACE is such a model and currently, work is being done on the development and implementation of the model within an mHealth prototype.

Finally, so that the proposed mockups could be closer to the MCI population, the authors made sure to verify specific design needs so to include them already within the described mockups, in order to avoid the main problems related with usability and accessibility issues, which have already been studied and ascertained by previous research.

Limitations of this work include the fact that no similar work has been done and there is no clear way to compare or improve from that stage. So, a new ground base needs to be started and this implies that mockups are the first step to propose and, obviously, need then to be tested. This has not yet been done, mainly due to time constraints, since this work is part of an extended work, with a limited timeframe. All icons, images and colors are just a representation example and can be altered accordingly to tastes and better usability requirements, after testing. However, the authors tried to follow the design requirements in the literature, e.g., "a calm interface and background, and contrast between text and background".

6 Conclusion

Dementia has high prevalence and high social impact on families, caregivers and communities, all over the world, which makes it a priority for public health and for the continuous search of better and more adaptable solutions. These can help, not only prevent, but minimize its evolution, especially at earlier stages of the condition. However, better care for the privacy and security of dementia patients personal and health data is mandatory. European personal data regulations enforce the requirements to take into account when dealing with those data. This work brings awareness to this issue by applying objective suggestions, not only from the legislation, but also from the technical and design requirements, focused on the target population, to make the proposed mHealth mockups a starting point on the way to make dementia mHealth solutions GDPR, as well as, security and privacy compliant.

Future work includes the refinement and quick testing of the proposed mockups with MCI patients to rapidly modify and adapt more secure and transparent mockups to their real needs.

Acknowledgments. This article was supported by FCT through the Project TagUBig - Taming Your Big Data (IF/00693/2015) from Researcher FCT Program funded by National Funds through FCT - Fundação para a Ciência e a Tecnologia. The author Soraia Teles holds a grant from the Portuguese Foundation for Science and Technology (FCT) (D/BD/135496/2018; PhD Program in Clinical and Health Services Research).

References

1. World Health Organization: Global Health and Aging (2011)
2. Kleinberger, T., Becker, M., Ras, E., Holzinger, A., Müller, P.: Ambient intelligence in assisted living: enable elderly people to handle future interfaces. In: Stephanidis, C. (ed.) UAHCI 2007. LNCS, vol. 4555, pp. 103–112. Springer, Heidelberg (2007). https://doi.org/10.1007/978-3-540-73281-5_11
3. Alzheimer's Disease International: The Global Impact of Dementia: An analysis of prevalence, incidence, cost and trends. World Alzheimer Report 2015 (2015)
4. Prince, M., Wimo, A., Guerchet, M., Ali, G.-C., Wu, Y.-T., Prina, M.: World Alzheimer Report 2015. Alzheimer's Disease International, pp. 1–84 (2015)
5. Winblad, B., et al.: Defeating Alzheimer's disease and other dementias: a priority for European science and society. Lancet Neurol. **15**, 455–532 (2016)
6. World Health Organization: Dementia: a public health priority (2012)
7. Moura, P., Fazendeiro, P., Vieira-Marques, P., Ferreira, A.: SoTRAACE - socio-technical risk-adaptable access control model. In: 2017 International Carnahan Conference on Security Technology (ICCST), Madrid (2017)
8. Bechtold, U., Sotoudeh, M.: Assistive technologies: their development from a technology assessment perspective. Gerontechnology **11**(4), 521–533 (2013)
9. Capucho, P., Brucki, S.M.D.: Judgment in mild cognitive impairment and Alzheimer's disease. Dement. Neuropsychol. **5**, 297–302 (2011)
10. Mentis, H.M., Madjaroff, G., Massey, A.K.: Upside and downside risk in online security for older adults with mild cognitive impairment. In: Conference on Human Factors in Computing Systems - Proceedings (2019)
11. Muchagata, J., Ferreira, A.: Mobile apps for people with dementia: are they compliant with the general data protection regulation (GDPR)? In: HEALTHINF 2019 - 12th International Conference on Health Informatics, pp. 68–77. SCITEPRESS Digital Library, Prague (2019)
12. Petersen, R.: Mild cognitive impairment as a diagnostic entity. J. Intern. Med. **256**(3), 183–194 (2004)
13. Alzheimer's Association: Alzheimer's & Dementia - What Is Dementia? (2018)
14. Zhang, R., Li, F., Li, Y.: Design of a rehabilitation training system for older adults with mild cognitive impairment. In: 2018 11th International Symposium on Computational Intelligence and Design (ISCID), vol. 02, pp. 107–110 (2018)

15. Nouchi, R., Kawashima, R.: Benefits of "smart ageing" interventions using cognitive training, brain training games, exercise, and nutrition intake for aged memory functions in healthy elderly people. In: Tsukiura, T., Umeda, S. (eds.) Memory in a Social Context, pp. 269–280. Springer, Tokyo (2017). https://doi.org/10.1007/978-4-431-56591-8_15

16. Faucounau, V., Wu, Y.-H., Boulay, M., De Rotrou, J., Rigaud, A.-S.: Cognitive intervention programmes on patients affected by Mild Cognitive Impairment: a promising intervention tool for MCI? J. Nutr. Health Aging **14**, 31–35 (2010)

17. Gunther, V.K., Schafer, P., Holzner, B.J., Kemmler, G.W.: Long-term improvements in cognitive performance through computer-assisted cognitive training: a pilot study in a residential home for older people. Aging Mental Health **7**, 200–206 (2003)

18. Hill, N.T., Mowszowski, L., Naismith, S.L., Chadwick, V.L., Valenzuela, M., Lampit, A.: Computerized cognitive training in older adults with mild cognitive impairment or dementia: a systematic review and meta-analysis. Am. J. Psychiatry **174**, 329–340 (2017)

19. Ferreira, A., Teles, S., Vieira-Marques, P.: SoTRAAce for smart security in ambient assisted living. J. Ambient Intell. Smart Environ. **11**(4), 323–334 (2019)

20. Thorpe, J.R., Rønn-Andersen, K.V.H., Bień, P., Özkil, A.G., Forchhammer, B.H., Maier, A.M.: Pervasive assistive technology for people with dementia: a UCD case. Healthc. Technol. Lett. **3**, 297–302 (2016)

21. Ferreira, A., et al.: How to securely break into RBAC: the BTG-RBAC model. In: 2009 Annual Computer Security Applications Conference, pp. 23–31 (2009)

22. Muchagata, J., Ferreira, A.: How can visualization affect security? In: ICEIS 2018 - 20th International Conference on Enterprise Information Systems. SCITEPRESS Digital Library, Poster Presentation in Funchal, Madeira (2018)

23. Onoda, K., et al.: Validation of a new mass screening tool for cognitive impairment: Cognitive Assessment for Dementia, iPad version. Clin. Interv. Aging **8**, 353–360 (2013)

24. Yjf, K., Bergsma, A., Graff, M., Dröes, R.-M.: Selecting apps for people with mild dementia: Identifying user requirements for apps enabling meaningful activities and self-management. J. Rehabil. Assist. Technol. Eng. **4**, 205566831771059 (2017)

25. Boulos, M.N.K., Brewer, A.C., Karimkhani, C., Buller, D.B., Dellavalle, R.P.: Mobile medical and health apps: state of the art, concerns, regulatory control and certification. Online J. Public Health Inform. **5**, 229 (2014)

26. Peek, S.T., Wouters, E.J., van Hoof, J., Luijkx, K.G., Boeije, H.R., Vrijhoef, H.J.: Factors influencing acceptance of technology for aging in place: a systematic review. Int. J. Med. Inform. **83**, 235–248 (2014)

27. Perumal, T., Ramli, A.R., Leong, C.Y.: Interoperability framework for smart home systems. IEEE Trans. Consum. Electron. **57**, 1607–1611 (2011)

28. Papageorgiou, A., Strigkos, M., Politou, E., Alepis, E., Solanas, A., Patsakis, C.: Security and privacy analysis of mobile health applications: the alarming state of practice. IEEE Access **6**, 9390–9403 (2018)

29. Bakker, D., Kazantzis, N., Rickwood, D., Rickard, N.: Mental health smartphone apps: review and evidence-based recommendations for future developments. JMIR Mental Health **3**, e7 (2016)

30. European Union: Regulation (EU) 2016/679 of the European Parliament and of the Council L 119. Official Journal of the European Union (2016)

31. GDPR. https://www.eugdpr.org/the-regulation.html. Accessed 06 Nov 2017

32. OAIC: Mobile privacy: a better practice guide for mobile app developers (2014)

33. Pires, R.J.T.R.: mHealth: o impacto da nova diretiva Europeia de proteção de dados, caso de uso e avaliação. vol. Mestrado em informática médica. FCUP - University of Porto (2016)

34. EDPS: Guidelines on the protection of personal data processed by mobile applications (2016)

Comparison of Texture Features and Color Characteristics of Digital Drawings in Cognitive Healthy Subjects and Patients with Amnestic Mild Cognitive Impairment or Early Alzheimer's Dementia

Sibylle Robens[1], Thomas Ostermann[1]($^{(\boxtimes)}$), Petra Heymann[2], Stephan Müller[3], Christoph Laske[3], and Ulrich Elbing[2]

[1] Witten/Herdecke University, Witten, Germany
{sibylle.robens,thomas.ostermann}@uni-wh.de
[2] Institute of Research and Development in Art Therapies (HKT), University of Applied Science Nürtingen-Geislingen, Nürtingen, Germany
petra.heymann@gmx.de, ulrichelbing@arcor.de
[3] Department of Psychiatry and Psychotherapy, Eberhard Karls University, Tübingen, Germany
{stephan.mueller,christoph.laske}@med.uni-tuebingen.de

Abstract. Color characteristics in combination with gray level co-occurrence matrix (GLCM) texture features of digital drawings were compared between cognitive healthy subjects (Control, n = 67) and individuals clinically diagnosed with amnestic mild cognitive impairment (aMCI, n = 32) or early Alzheimer's dementia (AD, n = 56). It was hypothesized that these variables contribute to the detection of cognitive impairments. Between subject groups comparisons of texture entropy, homogeneity, correlation and image size were conducted were performed with Chi-Square and Kruskal-Wallis tests. The diagnostic power of combining all texture features as explanatory variables was analyzed with a logistic regression model and the area under curve (AUC) of the corresponding receiver operating control (ROC) curve was calculated to discriminate best between healthy and cognitive impaired subjects. Texture and color features differed significantly between subject groups. The AUC for discriminating the control group from patients with early AD was equal 0.86 (95% CI [0.80, 0.93], sensitivity = .80, specificity = .79), and the AUC for discriminating between healthy subjects and all cognitive impaired equal 0.82. (95% CI [0.75; 0.89], sensitivity = .76, specificity = .79) for discriminating healthy controls from MCI patients. Although the study results are very promising, further validation is needed, especially with a larger sample size.

Keywords: Gray level co-occurrence matrix · Color use · Digital device Alzheimer's disease screening

A. Roque et al. (Eds.): BIOSTEC 2019, CCIS 1211, pp. 412–428, 2020.
https://doi.org/10.1007/978-3-030-46970-2_20

1 Introduction

Alzheimer's Disease (AD) is the most common form of dementia and its prevalence and incidence increase with the demographic aging of western countries [1]. It is characterized by a progressive decline of cognitive functions, which affects the ability of carrying out everyday activities. Although the degenerative process of the disease cannot be stopped yet, an early diagnose allows for application of symptomatic therapies which can temporally reduce symptoms and maintain the patient's level of life quality and functioning [1]. People with mild cognitive impairment (MCI) and memory impairment as a hallmark (amnestic MCI, abbreviated aMCI) have a high risk of developing Alzheimer's disease and therefore it is of main interest to identify them in screening tasks.

Early stage symptoms affecting the daily life of the patients include deficits in short-term memory, difficulties in following a conversation and in completing ordinary everyday life tasks. Besides these symptoms, deficits in the handling of spatial relationships and visual images occur as well. This results in difficulties in perception, e.g. in reading and in processing, e.g. drawing or writing [1, 2].

As the process of drawing an object relies on a combination of different cognitive functions, such as fine motor skills, visual perception, memory and creativity, different drawing tasks, often included in neurological test-batteries, are used for early diagnosis and initial assessment of cognitive impairment.

One of the most popular drawing tasks is the clock drawing test [3], which exist in different scoring versions. It has a high sensitivity and specificity in identifying patients with early dementia, but a low sensitivity in detecting persons with mild cognitive deficits [4].

In common drawing tasks, patients draw an object on a sheet of paper and specialists analyze and score the resulting picture. A new approach is the computer aided image analysis of data from digital pens used for drawing. Actual studies suggest that the assessment of the complete drawing process, including kinematic variables, changes in colors, pauses and on-air-movements, can improve the identification of early demented subjects [5–7].

The current analysis is based on a newly developed tree-drawing task, which has been introduced in [7]. Sixty-seven healthy subjects, 32 patients with aMCI and 56 persons diagnosed with early AD were asked to draw a tree by memory with a digital stylus on a device. They could choose between three linewidths and 12 colors. An integrated new software program calculated several characteristics of the drawing process. In the focus of the current study was the analysis of the number of color changes, the painting times with a specific color, the image size in relation to the screen and several texture characteristics based on Haralick's gray-level co-occurrence matrix (GLCM) [8].

The digital texture analysis with the GLCM is a statistical procedure based on the spatial relationship of image pixel. In the medical context, digital texture analysis can be used to analyze pictures of imaging procedures in diagnosis, for example for the differentiation of pathological tissue from healthy one in mammography [9], the identification of bone leasures in images of micro-computer tomography to assess the risk of osteoporotic fractures [10] or the analysis of skin texture images to detect dermatitis and other skin diseases [11].

In the present analysis, which extends the approach of [7], it was hypothesized that the GLCM texture features entropy, correlation, homogeneity in combination with color features and the image size contribute to the differentiation between cognitive healthy and cognitive impaired (aMCI and early AD) subjects.

2   Methods

2.1   Study Subjects

The study included 155 individuals (78 women, 77 men, mean age $= 69.5 \pm 9.9$ years) who were recruited from the Memory Clinic at the University Clinic for Psychiatry and Psychotherapy of Tübingen, Germany. The study was approved by the ethical committee of the University Clinic of Tübingen and all participants signed an informed consent for participation. Subjects were fully physically able to perform the drawings on the tablet and had normal or corrected to normal eyesight and a sufficient hearing ability. Participants were clinically interviewed and tested neuropsychologically with the German version of the modified CERAD (Consortium to Establish a Registry for Alzheimer's Disease) test-battery [12]. If there were signs of not age-related cognitive impairments, further examinations as special laboratory tests and neuroimaging were performed.

Thirty-two persons (13 women, 19 men) were diagnosed with amnestic MCI, according to the criteria of Petersen et al. [13]. Fifty-six individuals (40 women, 16 men) were clinically diagnosed with early AD according to criteria provided by the National Institute of Neurological and Communicative Disorders and Stroke - Alzheimer's Disease and Related Disorders Association (NINCDS-ADRDA) [14].

The control group consisted of sixty-seven persons (25 women, 42 men) without any cognitive abnormalities confirmed by the clinical interview and neuropsychological tests performed at the memory clinic. Descriptive characteristics of age and education level of each subject group are given in Table 1.

2.2   Digital Test Procedure and Device

All subjects performed a digital drawing task, which was introduced by in [5]. They were told to draw a tree from memory without any restrictions to time and structure of the tree. The drawing was performed with a digital pen on a Microsoft Surface-Pro 3 tablet (Fig. 1).

Windows 8.1 Pro software was implemented on this multi-touch digital device with an Intel Core i7-4650U processor (1.7–3.3 GHz). The size of the display area was 25.4 times 16.9 cm with a resolution of 2160 × 1440. The participant could hold the display upright or crosswise by drawing and was able to choose between 3 lines widths and 12 different colors. The participants could become familiar with the device in drawing one sample-tree before the actual test started.

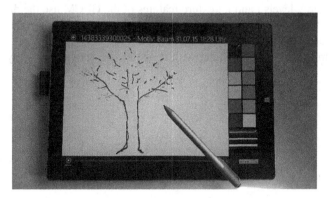

Fig. 1. Digital device and drawing program (Source: [7]).

In the study of Heymann et al. [5] dementia-specialized art therapist examined the drawings and categorized them in pictures of cognitive impaired or unimpaired subjects. In the current study a new software was implemented by attentra GmbH, Tübingen which allowed to objectively record drawing characteristics of the drawing process.

2.3 Image Characteristics

The use of different colors, the number of color changes and different texture characteristics based on the GLCM [8], were analysed in the current study with regard to the ability of discriminating between healthy and cognitive impaired subjects.

Color Variables
The drawing program offered 12 different colors: black, blue, light blue, brown, yellow, orange, light orange, red, pink, light pink, green and light green. The following color variables were analysed:

- **Color Count:** The number of different colors used.
- **Color Changes:** The number of color changes during the total drawing process.
- **% Time Painting** *"color name"*: The percentage of painting time (i.e., the time the digital pen is moved on the device surface) using the color *"color name"*. For this variable similar colors were grouped: (1) light blue and blue into "both blues", (2) light green and green into "both greens", (3) yellow, light orange and orange into "yellow/orange", (4) red, pink and light pink into "yellow/pink".

Gray Level Co-occurrence Texture Characteristics

Texture features calculated from the GLCM [8] provide informations about visual image patterns taking into account the structural arrangement of the image surface. The number of rows and columns of the squared GLCM are equal to the number of different grey-levels of the analysed image. For a specified distance d and an angle θ, the matrix element (i, j) of the GLCM is the frequency a pixel with gray level value i is adjacent to a pixel with grey-level value j. The angle θ indicates the direction of the spatial relationship between both grey levels i and j. Texture features of the GLCM use the distance d $= 1$ (nearest neighbor) and the four angles $\theta = 0°$ (horizontal), $\theta = 45°$ (right-diagonal), $\theta = 90°$ (vertical), and $\theta = 135°$ (left-diagonal).

For example, we look at an image with window size four and four gray levels:

0	1	1	3
0	0	2	3
1	2	3	0
2	3	2	4
0	3	4	2

The resulting GLCM at angle $\theta = 0°$ and distance d $= 1$ is:

	j=0	1	2	3	4
i=0	1	1	1	1	0
1	0	1	1	1	0
2	0	0	0	3	1
3	1	0	1	0	1
4	0	0	1	0	0

If each matrix element is divided by the sum of all matrix elements (in our example $= 15$) the resulting element P(i, j) of the "normalized" GLCM is the probability that this spatial relationship occurs. Several texture measures, which were extracted from this normalized matrix, were proposed in [8]. According to [7] four characteristics were calculated.

With

P(i, j) = Element ij of the normalized GLCM

N = Number of gray levels in the image

$$\mu = \sum_{i,j=0}^{N-1} i P(i, j)$$

$$\sigma^2 = \sum_{i,j=0}^{N-1} P(i, j)(i - \mu)^2$$

the following texture features were calculated:

- **Entropy** [7]: A measure of local variations in the GLCM. It has small values for texturally uniform images.

$$Entropy = \sum_{i,j=0}^{N-1} -\ln P(i,j) P(i,j) \tag{1}$$

- **Correlation** [7]: Measure of the gray level linear association between the pixels at the specified positions relative to each other.

$$correlation = \sum_{i,j=0}^{N-1} P(i,j) \frac{(i-\mu)(j-\mu)}{\sigma^2} \tag{2}$$

- **Homogeneity** [7]: Measure of image uniformity. It has large values if the image has only few gray levels.

$$homgeneity = \sum_{i,j=0}^{N-1} \frac{P(i,j)}{1+(i-j)^2} \tag{3}$$

- **Format Full Frame** [7]: Measure of the area which is covered by image pixels in relation to the total screen area of the digital device.

2.4 Statistical Analysis

Descriptive statistics including boxplots and frequency polygon charts were calculated for image characteristics. Group comparisons were performed with Chi-Square tests, Kruskal-Wallis tests (comparisons between healthy control, aMCI and early AD) and Wilcoxon rank-sum tests (pairwise comparisons). Logistic regression models with corresponding receiver operating characteristic curves were calculated to discriminate best between healthy and cognitive impaired subjects. Based on Youden-index calculation sensitivity and specificity were determined. All statistical calculations were done using SAS (Version 9.4) and p-values $< .05$ were considered significant.

3 Results

Statistical characteristics of demographic data and drawing results are listed separately for each subject group in Table 1.

Table 1. Means (standard deviations), medians and interquartile ranges (IQR) of demografic and drawing variables by subject group (healthy control, aMCI, early AD).

	N	Mean (Std Dev)	Median	IQR [1st, 3rd quartile]
Healthy Control				
Gender (female/male)	25/42			
Age (yrs)	67	65.85 (10.30)	65	[59, 74]
Education (yrs)	66	14.08 (3.03)	15	[12, 17]
Color Count	67	4.64 (1.77)	4	[3, 6]
Color Changes	67	7.07 (4.66)	6	[4, 9]
% Time painting black	67	4.60 (10.49)	0	[0, 0.53]
% Time painting brown	67	25.87 (19.33)	27.28	[7.02, 37.85]
% Time painting blue	67	0.87 (3.76)	0	[0, 0]
% Time painting yellow/orange	67	9.93 (13.93)	2.82	[0, 15]
% Time painting red/pink	67	5.48 (9.04)	0	[0, 12.5]
% Time painting green	67	53.25 (21.79)	53.4	[38.33, 67.01]
Texture Entropie	67	0.85 (0.51)	0.74	[0.44, 1.15]
Texture Homogenity	67	0.97 (0.02)	0.97	[0.96, 0.98]
Texture Correlation	67	0.94 (0.03)	0.95	[0.92, 0.97]
Format Full Frame	67	0.83 (0.16)	0.88	[0.72, 0.99]
aMCI				
Gender (female/male)	13/19			
Age (yrs)	32	71.31 (7.99)	72	[66, 77.5]
Education (yrs)	32	12.34 (3.25)	12	[11, 15]
Color Count	32	3.84 (1.72)	4	[3, 5]
Color Changes	32	5.56 (4.26)	5	[5.5, 7.5]
% Time painting black	32	13.46 (28.40)	0	[0, 8.51]
% Time painting brown	32	37 (28.78)	35.89	[11.21, 55.85]
% Time painting blue	32	0.41 (1.63)	0	[0, 0]
% Time painting yellow/orange	32	5.02 (10.19)	0	[0, 4.24]
% Time painting red/pink	32	7.53 (12.41)	0	[0, 12.7]
% Time painting green	32	36.57 (24.01)	39.93	[19.91, 52.47]

(*continued*)

Table 1. (*continued*)

	N	Mean (Std Dev)	Median	IQR [1st, 3rd quartile]
Texture Entropie	32	0.57 (0.30)	0.49	[0.38, 0.76]
Texture Homogenity	32	0.98 (0.01)	0.98	[0.97, 0.98]
Texture Correlation	32	0.93 (0.05)	0.93	[0.9, 0.96]
Format Full Frame	32	0.75 (0.17)	0.78	[0.63, 0.87]
early AD				
Gender (female/male)	40/16			
Age (yrs)	56	72.71 (9.16)	74	[67, 80]
Education (yrs)	56	11.11 (2.86)	11	[8, 13]
Color Count	56	3.25 (1.63)	3	[2.5, 4]
Color Changes	56	4.30 (4.51)	2.5	[1.5, 6.5]
% Time painting black	56	11.72 (27.92)	0	[0, 8.64]
% Time painting brown	56	25.81 (29.88)	14.97	[0, 44.11]
% Time painting blue	56	1.06 (3.60)	0	[0, 0]
% Time painting yellow/orange	56	12.68 (24.32)	0	[0, 15.69]
% Time painting red/pink	56	5.09 (13.65)	0	[0, 0]
% Time painting green	56	43.64 (31.06)	45.67	[13.72, 64.9]
Texture Entropie	56	0.45 (0.34)	0.31	[0.21, 0.63]
Texture Homogenity	56	0.98 (0.01)	0.99	[0.98, 0.99]
Texture Correlation	56	0.92 (0.05)	0.93	[0.9, 0.95]
Format Full Frame	56	0.65 (0.21)	0.65	[0.5, 0.82]

The education level was high in all three subject groups with mean education years ranging between 11 and 14 years. Mean ages ranged between 66 and 73. The percentage of females was highest in the group of early AD (71%) and lowest in the control group (37%). These demographic differences indicate the importance of an adjustment for the logistic model analysis in Sect. 3.3 concerning age, gender and education.

Examples of drawings of cognitive healthy persons, persons diagnosed with aMCI and persons with early AD are displayed in Fig. 2.

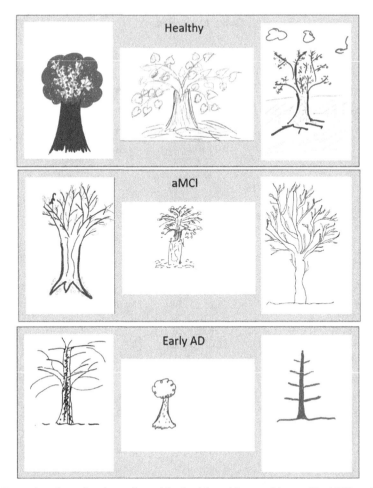

Fig. 2. Examples of tree drawings of cognitive healthy subjects, subjects with aMCI, and subjects with early AD.

3.1 Analysis of Color Variables

In the task of painting a tree, not surprisingly, healthy subjects as well as patients with aMCI or early AD most often used brown and green color. But examining the percentage of painting time with a specific color (see Table 1), there were significant difference between the subject groups for "green" ($p = .002$) which was used in control subjects 53%, in aMCI 37% and in early AD 44% of the painting time.

There were also significant differences between subject groups in the percentages of subjects using a specific color, indicating less color variation in cognitive impaired individuals (Fig. 3). Green and yellow/orange were used significantly more in the healthy control group compared to the aMCI and early AD group (all p-values $< .05$). Brown was also significantly used by more persons in the control group compared to the early AD group (chi-square test, $p = .001$).

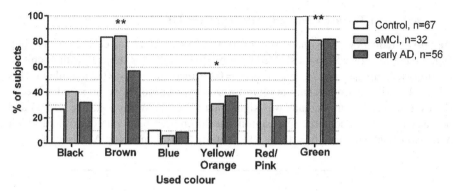

Fig. 3. Percentage of subjects using a specific color, grouped by healthy control, aMCI and early AD. P-values of chi-square test of overall group comparisons: *p < .05, **p < .01. (Color figure online)

Furthermore, there were significant differences in the number of colour changes during the painting process (Fig. 4) between the subject groups (p < .0001) with less color changes in cognitive impaired patients compared to healthy subjects. The variation of colors was most reduced in early demented subjects where 50% changed the color less than twice compared to 10% in the control group and 22% in the aMCI group.

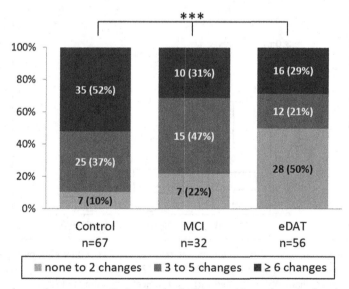

Fig. 4. Number and percentages (in brackets) of subjects with number of color changes during the drawing process. P-value of chi-square test: ***p < .001. (Color figure online)

3.2   Analysis of Texture Characteristics from the GLCM

Entropy. Frequency polygon charts and boxplots separately for each subject group (Fig. 5a and b) showed a right skewed entropy distribution for subjects with cognitive deficits (Median$_{Healthy}$ = 0.74, median$_{aMCI}$ = 0.49, median$_{early\ AD}$ = 0.31, Table 1). This indicated smaller entropies and more uniform images for cognitive impaired subjects. The overall decrease in medians was significant (Kruskal-Wallis test, p < .0001) and the pairwise comparisons revealed significant differences between control and aMCI (Wilcoxon-Rank sum test, p = .007), and between control and early AD (p < .0001).

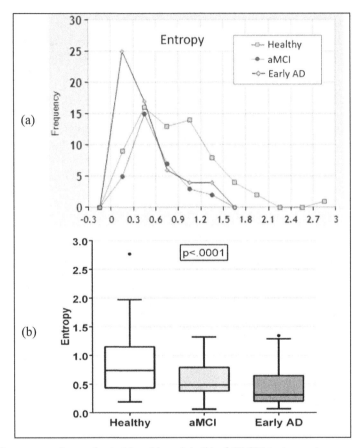

Fig. 5. Frequency polygon charts (a) and boxplots (b) of GLCM texture entropy separately for healthy subjects (n = 67), patients with aMCI (n = 32) and patients with early AD (n = 56). Frequency polygon charts of healthy and early AD subjects according to [7].

Texture Correlation. The three distributions of texture correlation were all left skewed but had smaller peak-values for the aMCI and early AD group (Median$_{Healthy}$ = 0.95, median$_{aMCI}$ = 0.93, median$_{early\ AD}$ = 0.93, Table 1), revealing smaller texture correlations for cognitive impaired subjects (Fig. 6). Median comparisons showed overall significant differences between all groups (p = .017) and significant differences between healthy subjects and patients with early AD (p = .007).

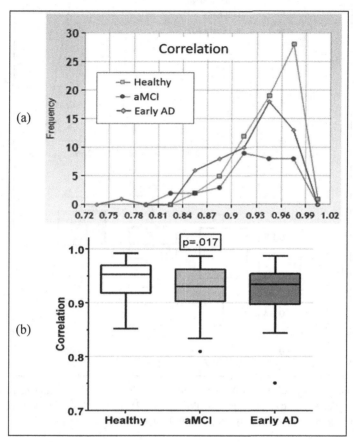

Fig. 6. Frequency polygon charts (a) and boxplots (b) of GLCM texture correlation separately for healthy subjects (n = 67), patients with aMCI (n = 32) and patients with early AD (n = 56). Frequency polygon charts of healthy and early AD subjects according to [7].

Homogeneity. Frequency polygon charts of the three subject groups (Fig. 7a) showed a right shifted distribution especially for the demented group and the boxplots (Fig. 6b) indicated an increase in homogeneity with cognitive impairment. Median comparisons revealed significantly more homogenous images for the demented group compared to the control group (Table 1, Fig. 7b, median$_{Healthy}$ = 0.97, median$_{aMCI}$ = 0.98, median$_{early\ AD}$ = 0.99, p < .0001).

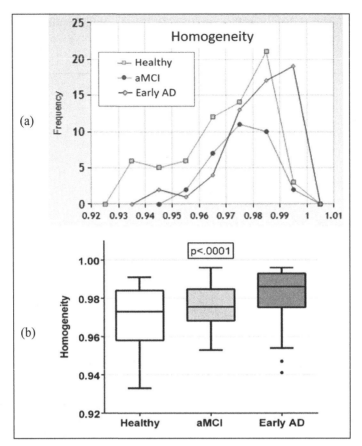

Fig. 7. Frequency polygon charts (a) and boxplots (b) of GLCM texture homogeneity separately for healthy subjects (n = 67), patients with aMCI (n = 32) and patients with early AD (n = 56). Frequency polygon charts of healthy and early AD subjects according to [7].

Format Full Frame. The distribution of the healthy subjects was much more right skewed than the distributions of patients with cognitive deficits, indicating that healthy subjects use more space for their images than cognitive impaired individuals (Fig. 8a). Median values significantly decrease from healthy to early AD (Table 1, Fig. 8b, $median_{Healthy} = 0.88$, $median_{aMCI} = 0.75$, $median_{early\ AD} = 0.65$, p < .0001).

3.3 ROC-Curve Analysis

To analyse the performance of color and GLCM texture features in discriminating between healthy and cognitive impaired subjects, a ROC-curve analysis based on a logistic regression model was carried out. Texture homogeneity, texture entropy, texture correlation, format full frame, and number of color changes were included as factors. The model was adjusted for gender, age and education.

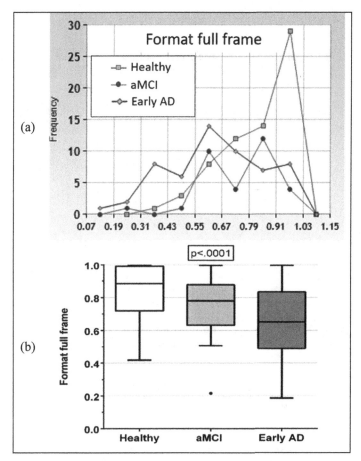

Fig. 8. Frequency polygon charts (a) and boxplots (b) of image size relative to screen size (format full frame) separately for healthy subjects (n = 67), patients with aMCI (n = 32) and patients with early AD (n = 56). Frequency polygon charts of healthy and early AD subjects according to [7].

In the first analysis (Fig. 9a) the group of cognitive impaired persons consisted of aMCI and early AD subjects and was compared with the control group. The AUC of the ROC-curve was equal 0.819 (95% confidence interval CI [0.753; 0.885]. A sensitivity of 76% and a specificity of 78% was calculated with the Youden-Index.

In the second ROC-analysis only patients with early AD built up the group with cognitive deficits (Fig. 9b). The AUC for discriminating healthy from early AD was 0.864 with a sensitivity of 80% and a specificity of 79%.

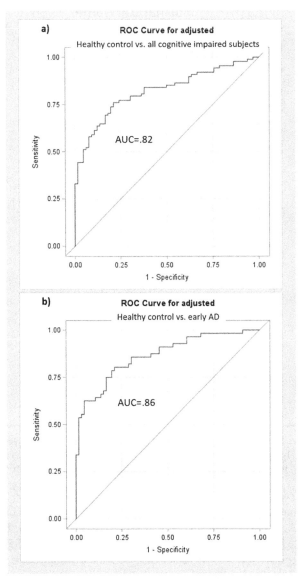

Fig. 9. ROC curve for discrimination of healthy subjects (n = 67) from (a) patients with cognitive impairments (aMCI or early AD, n = 88) and from (b) patients with early AD (n = 56). Texture homogeneity, texture entropy, texture correlation, format full frame, and number of color changes were included as factors and the model was adjusted for gender, age and education.

4 Conclusions

This paper analysed digital image data from a tree-drawing task [5, 7] to investigate if texture features derived from the grey-level co-occurrence matrix and color characteristics of the image can contribute to the detection of patients with mild cognitive impairment and early dementia of Alzheimer's type.

Several drawing deficits have been reported with early stages of AD, e.g. image simplifications, reduced image sizes and disorders of spatial relations and perspectives [2, 15, 16]. In line with these studies we found that images of cognitive impaired subjects had less contrasts, were more homogeneous, and smaller compared to images of healthy subjects.

The use of colors in paintings of AD patients has been described as a reduction in color variations with a preference to yellow-red in early stages and a tendency to darker colors in later stages [17, 18].

In our analysis we did not discover this preference. In contrary, the patients with early AD did use less yellow, orange, red and pink colors than the control subjects. This might be explained by the task of drawing a tree, where all subject groups preferred the colors brown and green. An important aspect we found was a significant reduction in color variation in aMCI and early AD patients.

The ROC-Curve, with all texture characteristics and the number of color changes as explanatory factors, separated cognitive healthy and early demented subjects quite good with an AUC of 0.86. The corresponding sensitivity was 80% and the specificity 79%.

Although our results indicate that the analysis of texture and color features might be a reasonable approach to discriminate between healthy and early demented subjects, considering the severity of the disease and the enormous stress of a wrong diagnosis, a specificity of 79% is too small and further investigations including other drawing characteristics have to be made.

The creative procedure of drawing is assumed to be less stressful than for example memory tests, where the patient is confronted with his cognitive deficits. Using a digital device instead of paper allows for an objective evaluation of drawing features and the images don't have to be rated by a trained specialist.

Although the study results are very promising, further analysis and validation is needed, especially with a larger sample size.

Our future aim is to automatically calculate a decision-value from the linear combination of digital drawing features adjusted for age, gender and education and to support the decision of physicians whether the patient needs further clinical examinations or not.

References

1. Alzheimer's Association: Alzheimer's disease facts and figures. Alzheimer's Dement. **13**, 325–373 (2017)
2. Trojano, L., Gainotti, G.: Drawing disorders in Alzheimer's disease and other forms of dementia. J. Alzheimers Dis. **53**, 31–52 (2016)
3. Shulman, K.I., Gold, D.P., Cohen, C.A., Zucchero, C.A.: Clock-drawing and dementia in the community: a longitudinal study. Int. J. Geriatr. Psychiatry **8**, 487–496 (1993)

4. Ehreke, L., Luck, T., Luppa, M., Konig, H.H., Villringer, A., Riedel-Heller, S.G.: Clock draw-ing test - screening utility for mild cognitive impairment according to different scoring sys-tems: results of the Leipzig Longitudinal Study of the Aged (LEILA 75+). Int. Psychogeriatr. **23**, 1592–1601 (2011)

5. Heymann, P., et al.: Early detection of Alzheimer's disease based on the patient's creative drawing process: first results with a novel neuropsychological testing method. J. Alzheimers Dis. **63**, 675–687 (2018)

6. Muller, S., Preische, O., Heymann, P., Elbing, U., Laske, C.: Diagnostic value of a tablet-based drawing task for discrimination of patients in the early course of Alzheimer's disease from healthy individuals. J. Alzheimers Dis. **55**, 1463–1469 (2017)

7. Robens, S., et al.: Digital picture co-occurrence texture characteristics discriminate between patients with early dementia of Alzheimer's type and cognitive healthy subjects. In: Pro-ceedings of the 12th International Joint Conference on Biomedical Engineering Systems and Technologies, vol. 5, pp. 88–93 (2019)

8. Haralick, R.M., Shanmugam, K., Dinstein, I.: Textural features of image classification. IEEE Trans. Syst. Man Cybern. **3**, 610–621 (1973)

9. Pratiwi, M., Alexander, Harefa, J., Nanda, S.: Mammograms classification using gray-level co-occurrence matrix and radial basis function neural network. Procedia Comput. Sci. **59**, 83–91 (2015)

10. Shirvaikar, M., Huang, N., Dong, X.N.: The measurement of bone quality using gray level co-occurrence matrix textural features. J. Med. Imaging Health Inform. **6**, 1357–1362 (2016)

11. Parekh, R., Mittra, A.K.: Automated detection of skin diseases using texture features. Int. J. Eng. Sci. Technol. **3**(6), 4801–4808 (2011)

12. Morris, J.C., et al.: The consortium to establish a registry for Alzheimer's disease (CERAD). Part I. Clinical and neuropsychological assessment of Alzheimer's disease. Neurology **39**, 1159–1165 (1989)

13. Petersen, R.C.: Mild cognitive impairment as a diagnostic entity. J. Int. Med. **256**, 183–194 (2004)

14. McKhann, G., Drachman, D., Folstein, M., Katzman, R., Price, D., Stadlan, E.M.: Clinical diagnosis of Alzheimer's disease. Report of the NINCDS-ADRDA Work Group* under the Auspices of Department of Health and Human Services Task Force on Alzheimer's Disease, vol. 34, pp. 939–939 (1984)

15. Gragnaniello, D., Kessler, J., Bley, M., Mielke, R.: Copying and free drawing by patients with Alzheimer disease of different dementia stages. Nervenarzt **69**, 991–998 (1998)

16. Kirk, A., Kertesz, A.: On drawing impairment in Alzheimer's disease. Arch. Neurol. **48**, 73–77 (1991)

17. Maurer, K., Prvulovic, D.: Paintings of an artist with Alzheimer's disease: visuoconstructural deficits during dementia. J. Neural Transm. **111**(3), 235–245 (2004)

18. Lee, Y.T., Tsai, Y.C., Chen, L.K.: Progressive changes in artistic performance of a Chinese master with Alzheimer's disease. Cortex **69**, 282–283 (2015)

Standardising Clinical Caremaps: *Model, Method* and *Graphical Notation* for Caremap Specification

Scott McLachlan[1]([⊠]) [iD], Evangelia Kyrimi[1], Kudakwashe Dube[2] [iD], and Norman Fenton[1] [iD]

[1] Queen Mary, University of London, London, UK
s.mclachlan@qmul.ac.uk
[2] Massey University, Palmerston North, New Zealand

Abstract. Standardising care can improve patient safety and outcomes, and reduce the cost of providing healthcare services. Caremaps were developed to standardise care, but contemporary caremaps are not standardised. Confusion persists in terms of terminology, structure, content and development process. Unlike existing methods in the literature, the approach, model and notation presented in this chapter pays special attention to incorporation of clinical decision points as first-class citizens within the modelling process. The resulting caremap with decision points is evaluated through creation of a caremap for women with gestational diabetes mellitus. The proposed method was found to be an effective way for comprehensively specifying all features of caremaps in a standardised way that can be easily understood by clinicians. This chapter contributes a new standardised method, model and notation for caremap content, structure and development.

Keywords: Caremap · Clinical documentation · Flow diagrams

1 Introduction

Florence Nightingale introduced formal and descriptive documentation that would transform healthcare and become a vital component of effective care delivery [1]. *Clinical care process specification* (CCPS), or care modelling, which allows clinicians to create, amongst other things, caremaps that specify the workflow to be followed in caring for a patient suffering from a specific health condition [2] were developed from Nightingale's notation and reporting methods. While some CCPS present as templates to guide evidence-based care, others provide templates for charting individual patient needs, metrics or treatments. CCPS ensure continuity and quality of care for the patient [1, 3]. Most contemporary clinical documents were developed and refined during the 1980's and 1990's in response to a number of key needs, including: (i) the need to control costs; and, (ii) to improve the quality of patient care [4, 5]. Drawing on project management (PM) and total quality management (TQM) tools that were more common to industry,

© Springer Nature Switzerland AG 2020
A. Roque et al. (Eds.): BIOSTEC 2019, CCIS 1211, pp. 429–452, 2020.
https://doi.org/10.1007/978-3-030-46970-2_21

hospital managers attempted to reengineer hospital care processes with the aim of reducing clinical resource use and error rates, and improving patient outcomes [6, 7]. In spite of the potential for those reductions, clinical costs have continued to increase, and error rates continue to occur with distressing frequency [8].

Although the British Medical Association and Royal College of Nursing developed a joint guidance stating that use of standardised forms are beneficial in reducing variation in healthcare practice [9], a wide range of terms exist for CCPS, including:

- *Clinical practice guidelines* (CPG) [10] which are sometimes also known as:

  - *Consensus-based guidelines* (CBG) [11]; and,
  - *Local operating procedures* (LOP) [12, 13];

- *Clinical decision rules* (CDR) [14];
- *Clinical pathways* [15];
- *Care plans* [16];
- *Treatment protocols* [17]; and
- *Caremaps* [2, 18].

The key issue limiting the effectiveness of these terms is that authors do not agree on whether some of them represent distinct clinical documents [19–21], or are synonymous [22–24]. There is a clear lack of *standardisation of definitions, presentations and development processes for most types of clinical documentation*. While, for some of these terms, standardisation has been attempted, these attempts have either been incomplete or only further added to the confusion [18, 25, 26]. The use of different terms and versions of the same clinical care specification in different units within the same care facility, and between different care facilities, is becoming a serious problem. In the modern, increasingly digital, healthcare environment greater amounts of data are generated and captured daily, including from diagnostic devices used, or sensors worn by the patient while in the community. Any differences in the documentation approach or data recording method results in fragmented data, complicates the integration of data about the same patient from different sources, and inhibits health information exchange (HIE) [27, 28].

Researchers have proposed different approaches to develop CCPS and different ways of specifying them [18, 25]. These approaches vary greatly in their complexity level, design approach, content and representational structures [18, 25]. These variances lead to substantial and ubiquitous differences in communication and information transfer between clinicians providing care for the same patient. This affects the quality of care and introduces additional risk of harm for as many as 25% of all patients [28, 29]. Error reporting documentation is another area that also suffers from lack of standardisation. While clinicians and clinical researchers are professionally obliged and assumed to be honest and transparent in reporting identified errors, it is unlikely that current error statistics are representative of the entire scope of the problem [30–32].

Standardised CCPS ensures sufficiently high-quality information is recorded, enabling documents to be read quicker and content within to be better retained, all with the effect of improving overall patient safety and outcomes [18, 29, 33–35]. Standardised approaches to CCPS, ensure that each time a healthcare provider approaches each type of CCPS, the format and content are consistent with expectations [18].

Standardisation of CCPS brings many other benefits than purely operational or clinical. For example, a common problem with most clinical data is that they lack one or more of the elements of *integrity, integration and interoperability* (III). This has been described as the *data triple-I issue* [36] and is presently seen as one of the biggest single barriers to Learning Health Systems (LHS) [36, 37]. Standardisation of CCPS make possible the support to mitigate the data triple-I issue, particularly *computer interpretability*, which in turn supports data standardisation and increases the chances for successful EHR and LHS implementation [37].

Unfortunately, there has been little research into the standardisation of caremaps and other results of clinical care process modelling [25, 38, 39]. *The objective of this chapter is to address this challenge by exploring a model and graphical notation that makes it easy for clinicians to understand and allow clinicians to comprehensively specify caremaps.*

Supporters perceive care processes standardisation as an effective approach for dropping healthcare service variations and delivery cost, while at the same time maintaining or even increasing efficacy, quality and safety, improving patient experience and quality of life [40, 41]. However, healthcare is still one of the slowest sectors to accept and implement process standardisation, and to prove the positive impact on patient outcomes [41, 42]. This is due to clinician resistance as care standardisation is considered by many as 'cookbook' or 'cookie cutter medicine' that can only be effective after they have ruled out the unique needs of each individual [41, 43–45]. Given the overconsumption and financial crisis common to healthcare service delivery globally, standardisation of care processes can help clinicians provide managed care that is thought to decrease resource consumption and overall healthcare cost, and the incidence of inappropriate or ineffective care [46, 47].

Standardisation vs Innovation

Standardisation is ubiquitous in our daily lives [48]. Examples might include the USA's CAFÉ and similar international fuel economy standards used to govern efficiency and emissions of new motor vehicles offered for sale [49]; standards instituted for terminology and language, especially for mission-critical applications like satellite and aeronautical navigation systems [50] and air traffic control [51]; and standards used to ensure safe development, testing, production, prescription and administration of medicines [52, 53]. Standardisation has been described as the activity of establishing and recording a limited set of solutions to actual or potential matching problems directed at benefits for the party or parties involved in balancing their needs and intending and expecting that these solutions will be repeatedly or continuously used during a certain period by a substantial number of the parties for whom they are meant [54]. Standards generally consist of rules, guidelines, templates or characteristics for activities, or their results, that are provided for common and repeated use [55].

Innovation involves the development and implementation of a new or significantly improved product, service or process, and includes all scientific, technological, organisational, financial and commercial steps which are, or are intended to lead to the implementation of the innovation [56, 57]. Innovation in technology and strategy is both a catalyst for modern economic growth [56, 58], and standardisation [59, 60]. Yet standardisation, especially that which is unofficial or voluntary, is believed to be something that innately inhibits innovation [56, 61]. Growing insight into the role standardisation plays in enabling innovation is forcing reconsideration of this belief [48, 56, 62].

Several approaches have demonstrated the beneficial role standards can have in supporting innovation. Interoperability standards describe how different components in an ecosystem work together, for example, the hardware and software in ICT systems [63]. Anticipatory standards describe the operation and interoperation of components of future systems not yet in operation [64]. Formal standards are high-quality but have a considerable development lead time as they are carefully deliberated by standards-writing organisations, such as the International Standards Organisation (ISO) and International Engineering Task Force (IETF) [65]. De facto standards autonomously stem from processes and interactions within the ecosystem, such as the dominance of Microsoft's operating system in personal computing or resilience of the QWERTY keyboard layout which while being originally designed to mitigate adjacent keys jamming on early mechanical typewriters, is still seen on devices like touch screens which have no moving parts [63, 65]. Standards can also be described in terms of their particularisation or extent to which they are standardised: whether the organisation, service or approach is, for example, wholly, or largely, standardised [66].

Motor vehicle production and use is restrained by a great many standards: directing safety, materials application, pollution, operation and maintenance. The same standards governing fuel efficiency and emissions discussed earlier, and which have removed many vehicles with inefficient large-bore engines from sale, actually stimulated innovation. This innovation includes the recently released homogenous charge gasoline compression engines using a system described as Spark Controlled Compression Ignition (SCCI). SCCI is claimed to reduce fuel consumption by as much as 20% [67, 68]. The standards also produced competition in innovation with another major vehicle manufacturer also releasing new technology this year, the Variable Compression Turbocharged (VC-T) engine [69]. There were also innovations that delivered the fully electric vehicle (fEV) by Tesla: a product that sits in a market space that can only continue to innovate in order to meet anticipated standards requiring all passenger/commuter vehicles to become electric [70, 71]. While the standards discussed operate to ensure that motor vehicles marketed today cause less pollution, they do not, for example, act inhibit a manufacturers choice of colour, luxury options or the model name that might adorn your next vehicle. And as we have seen, far from inhibiting innovation, standards can beneficially support novel innovations.

When it comes to the practice of medicine, a large array of standards applies to almost every action a clinician may seek to undertake. Built on a base of clinical practice guidelines, evidence-based medicine is perhaps the most broadly applied and well-known standardisation in medicine [26, 72]. This work investigates standardisation in the context of health informatics, finding current efforts often focus on some element of how the clinician interacts with the system, data entry, composition or presentation. In this review, no example was located that was investigating the potential for fundamental underlying issues to have arisen when non-standardised clinical documentation was digitised by a variety of hospitals and health sectors in the creation of EHR platforms. The clinical documentation that HIS and the now ubiquitous EHR were engaged to replace should be investigated as one potential source giving rise to the barriers that inhibited HIS and EHR adoption, and which currently restrain integration of LHS in clinical practice.

2   Literature Review and Related Works

Caremaps Background

The term caremap refers to a graphical representation of the sequence of patient care activities to be performed for a specific medical condition suffered by either a patient or a cohort [73–75]. Caremaps have been in use, in one form or another, for around forty years [6, 7, 76]. Caremaps aim to standardise health care practice by organising and sequencing care workflow, ensuring standard of care, timely interventions and uniform outcomes using an appropriate level of resources [25, 73, 76, 77]. Caremaps also help track variance in clinical practice, as they provide a simple and effective visual method for identifying when care practice has deviated from the routine evidence-based pathway [73, 78].

The literature presents three different descriptions for the origin of caremaps, with distinct points of intersection between each that make it difficult to assess which may be the true history:

1. Caremaps were an output of the Centre for Case Management (CCM) in 1991 [79]. CCM's CareMaps were similar in form and function to existing clinical pathways and were applied to specific patient populations that were commonly treated in many hospitals [79]. CCM went on to trademark the double-capitalised version CareMap but had not within the first decade undertaken any research to demonstrate the effectiveness of the concept whose invention they claimed [80].
2. Caremaps naturally evolved as an expansion of earlier case management and care plans [7].
3. Caremaps were developed during the 1980's at the New England Medical Centre (NEMC) [75, 81].

Caremaps arose in nursing where they incorporate and extend the critical pathways and bring established project management methodologies into healthcare delivery [24, 57, 62]. Indeed, from the early 1980's nurses were the primary users of caremaps [44, 68].

Caremap Terminology

Definitions from literature of the early- to mid 1990's in principle agreed that the caremap presents as a graph or schedule of care activities described *on a timeline* and *performed as part of the patient's treatment* by *a multidisciplinary team* to produce *identified health outcomes* [2, 7, 73–77]. Even though the structure and content of caremaps has changed markedly during the last three decades, this general definition still applies.

Caremaps can be observed under three similar but different titles: (i) caremaps; (ii) CareMaps; and (iii) care maps. The first, *caremaps*, appears to have been the original title prior to the CCM trademarking the second, *CareMaps*, in the early 1990's [77, 79]. In literature published after 1994 that uses the first, *caremaps*, it is not uncommon to also see some mention of CCM or their trademark [82] although this is not always the case [83, 84]. The use of *care maps* has also been seen, possibly as a defence to potential issues that might arise from confusion with the CCM trademark, as no author used this third type in context or with reference to the CCM [73, 85].

There is disagreement on whether caremaps are a separate format of clinical tool [19–21], or simply another term for care pathways, clinical pathways, critical pathways and care plans [22–24]. This disagreement is exemplified by flow diagrams that are internally describe as a "care map", yet are captioned 'clinical pathway' by the author (e.g. in Fig. 1 of Thompson et al. [86] and Fig. 5 on page 45 of Yazbeck [87]). Yazbeck (ibid) further presents a number of similar flow diagrams for care management, describing them using a range of terms including 'care map', 'care pathway', and 'algorithm'.

Caremap Evolution and Current Context

Starting in the early 1990's, Nursing caremaps were more textual than their contemporary counterparts, and had a structure made up of two components: (1) *Problem and Outcomes Specification*: identifying patient problems and necessary outcomes within a time-frame; and (2) *Task and Activity Specification*: a breakdown and description of day-by-day tasks and activities on a critical path [73, 74]. Later approaches specified the care map in three components: (1) *the flow chart diagram*; (2) the transitional text-based *care map of activities* broken down day-to-day, and; (3) the *evidence* base relied upon in their construction [78]. These methods of specifying and presenting the caremap may have resulted in the terminology confusion that still persists today. More recent caremaps are specified as a flow diagram made up of clinical options for a particular condition. Thus, modern caremaps contain multiple possible paths based on: (i) symptomatology; (ii) diagnostic results, and; (iii) how the patient responds to treatment [88, 89].

Traditional caremaps considered elements such as anxiety, rehabilitation, education, prevention and coping strategies and were intended to restore the patient as close to a normal quality of life as was possible given their diagnosis [73–75]. Starting from 1999 there began to be examples of *transitional caremaps*: while still being text-based, these were limited to interventions necessary to treat the primary diagnosis [25, 82]. As caremaps evolved into graphical representations we observe *contemporary caremaps* presented as separate but complementary components to the clinical pathway or CPG [79, 84]. A summary of the relevant elements of each caremap type is presented in Table 1.

Table 1. Summary and comparison of caremap evolution stages (from [18]).

	Traditional (1980's to mid-1990's) *	Transitional (Mid-1990's to mid 2000's) *	Contemporary (2004 onwards) *
Primary author	Nurses	Nurses and doctors	Doctors
Context	Holistic	Primary condition	Single diagnostic, screening and/or intervention event
Foci	Restoring the patient to normal life	Outcomes, cost and resource consumption	Efficiency of care delivery and outcomes, reduction of practice variation, bridge the gap between evidence and practice
Presentation	Text-based	Text-based with some early flow examples	Flow diagram or graph
Status	Independent document	Independent or sometimes incorporated with CP document	Self-contained but often found appended to/contained in CPG

Caremaps are found in many healthcare domains, including: *paediatric surgery* [88], *nursing* [89], *oncology* [90], *diagnostic imaging* [91], *obstetrics* [4] and *cardiology* [76]. Even within these examples, there exists significant variance in complexity level, design approach, content and the representational structures used.

Related Works: Efforts to Standardise Caremaps
Numerous contemporary caremap examples were found annexed to hospital-based clinical CPGs. Contemporary caremap literature tended to focus on establishing the clinical condition justifying creation of the caremap, such as: determination of incidence, risk factors and patient outcomes [88]; diagnosis and stabilisation of patients with an acute presentation [89]; and, protocolising of ongoing treatment [85]. Presentation or discussion of a development process or the elements used in construction were rare, and more often had to be inferred from a thorough reading of each paper.

We found a single article written by a veterinarian and a lawyer which attempted a systematic description of the process for contemporary caremap development [92]. This article primarily focused on standardisation for the purpose of cost containment, and provides an example of mapping for a surgical procedure [92]. Given their focus and particular caremap construction model which, through their own exemplar application, only includes a temporally-ordered single-path representation of the gross steps of patient care, their paper was at best, merely formative. By their own admission, they deliberately limited relevant data analysed during the input design phase to what they felt was truly critical for identifying and understanding outliers. This results in a model lacking clinical applicability and a distinct lack of detail surrounding each care process. Their method requires significant work to adequately support true standardised clinical caremap development.

Hospital management and clinical literature opinions changed during the early 2000's, with a distinct focus shift towards the theme of standardisation [6, 7, 93, 94]. Researchers, politicians, those engaged in hospital governance, and some clinicians recognised standardisation should be considered of paramount importance to the future of healthcare delivery [94]. Standardisation of such things as clinical decisions, diagnostic and therapeutic methods, evidence-based guidelines, care approaches, practice standards and clinical information was sought [5, 8, 94, 95]. Standardisation in the name of quality care and outcomes would become the single-minded national focus of healthcare service delivery for entire countries [5, 95]. Promoted with great passion, this type of standardisation has seen multiple teams within the same country, or even within the same organisation, expending effort on developing standardisation frameworks with some degree of similarity and overlap [96–98]. However, this drive towards standardisation has had little effect on the definition, development and structure of much of the current clinical documentation, because as we approached the end of the first full decade of standardisation, calls for standardised clinical care documents continue to increase [18, 38, 39, 95, 99, 100]. An unmet need can also be seen in calls to resolve poorly standardised taxonomy and nomenclatures currently used in developing and cataloguing clinical documentation [101].

3   Research Process and Methodology

Literature Review. A search was conducted across a range of databases using the terms 'caremap', 'CareMap', and 'care map'. A citation search drawn from all included papers was also performed. This search identified 1,747 papers. Once duplicates, papers not based in the nursing, medical or healthcare domains, and those using the term "care map" in other contexts were removed a core pool of 115 papers remained.

Development of Review Framework Using Thematic Analysis. Initially, each paper was reviewed using content and thematic analysis [102] and concept analysis [103] to identify and classify terminology, construction and content elements and to infer the caremap development processes.

Methodology for Standardisation of Caremaps. Literature reviews have a ground-level consensus forming function that allows for identification of implementation techniques and the degree of accord between authors within a domain [104, 105]. The literature pool was used to identify common definition, structure and content elements for caremaps. In addition, process steps that were consistently described led us to a standardised caremap development process.

Methodology for Evaluation of Proposed Standard for Caremaps. Case Studies are a grounded comparative research methodology with a well-developed history, robust qualitative procedures and process validation [106]. The case study approach provides a real-life perspective on observed interactions and is regularly used in information sciences [107, 108]. Case studies are considered as developed and validated as any other scientific method and are an accepted method where more rigid approaches to experimental research cannot or do not apply [109, 110]. The standardised development process and resulting caremap are both evaluated using case studies of examples from the authors' other works.

4   Standardisation of Caremaps: *Exemplar for Standardising CCPS*

Clinical Decisions in Caremaps

Graphically modelling patient care for a given medical condition is not new. Several approaches and presentation styles have been proposed, including: *UML process modelling* to represent the ongoing clinical management of a chronic condition [111]; *business process modelling notation* (BPMN) to visually map the treatment flow captured in clinical pathways [112]; and, *influence diagrams* to model the structure of complex clinical problems, identifying **decisions** to be made, *the sequence in which those decisions may arise*, the *information available to make the decision* and the *probability of uncertain events* [113]. Caremaps presentation style and content has changed significantly since their conception in the 1980's. Currently, contemporary caremaps used in clinical medicine present as an immature information visualisation approach [18]. Apart from lacking standardisation, existing caremaps lack also a comprehensive representation of clinical ***decision points*** (DP).

Until recently, caremaps lacked standardisation in structure, content and development [18]. The authors proposed and presented what is stated here as TaSC (*Towards a Standard for Caremaps*): a model for standardising the development and presentation of clinical caremaps [18]. Based on TaSC, each node within the caremap represents activities related to patient care. In addition, nodes are often seen to represent one or more latent clinical decisions, such as selecting the appropriate treatment path for each patient. Our prior work has pointed out the presence of these latent DPs within caremaps as well as the absence of a way to identify and represent them [18]. This chapter explores these issues and proposes an extension to TaSC for identifying and representing DPs with decision criterion.

There are several clinical decisions that might be embedded within a caremap node. For instance, a treatment activity may require the clinician to consider whether aseptic technique is required, which dressing to use or which clinical resource to assist during treatment. The majority of these decisions have no direct impact on the flow of care or the pathway of the patient within the caremap. Thus, only decisions that have an impact on the path to be taken by the patient should be considered as separate DPs within the caremap.

Clinical decisions that may lead to DPs in a caremap result from six aspects of clinical activities identified by Richardson et al. [114] as follows:

Clinical Evidence: The identification and selection of clinical evidence from clinical trials and clinical practice guidelines for use in creating tools like caremaps necessitates decisions regarding how to gather the right clinical findings properly and interpret them soundly.

Diagnosis: During diagnosis decisions are made regarding the selection and interpretation of diagnostic tests.

Prognosis: Prognosis requires decisions of how to anticipate a given patient's likely course.

Therapy: Therapy decisions consider how to select treatments that do more good than harm.

Prevention: Screening and reducing a patient's risk for disease prevention decisions.

Education: Consideration of how to teach the clinician, patient or patient's family what is needed fall within the remit of education decisions.

5   Approach and Method for Standardising the Model and Notation for Caremap Specifications

This section describes the current state, and potential starting point for any standard for caremaps, as resolved from the review of the literature.

Caremap Development Process with Consensus Formation

The literature was used initially to establish consensus on common structure, content and development processes that had previously been used in the creation of caremaps, and which may be relevant in defining standard caremap and development processes. The case studies were used to evaluate and refine the elements of each.

To address the stated aim of this research, we focused our research on tertiary care (hospital-borne) caremaps and specifically the following three components whose characteristics came out of the thematic analysis, and make up the review framework.

Structure	What is the representational structure and notation for expressing contemporary caremaps?
Content	What content types are consistently seen in contemporary caremaps?
Development	What are the process steps followed for developing contemporary caremaps?

Standardising the Caremap Structure

Each caremap flow diagram identified from the literature had its own visual element and notation style. The most common observed was a rectangle for representing the process step, which are usually called an activity. Contemporary caremaps contain a set of nodes that represent patient care activities. However, the literature shows there is no consistency in the way an activity may be represented. Different shapes including rectangular boxes with rounded [86] or squared corners [85, 93, 115], plain text [79], or even arrows [116] have been used. In some cases, activities that diverge to different and mutually exclusive pathways may be represented by a diamond [23, 115]. The flow from one activity to another has been illustrated with arrows [78, 88, 115], or simple lines [23, 79]. The literature also lacks clarity as to whether a caremap should have entry and exit points. In some cases, neither is present [78, 86], while in others these points are an implicit [23] or explicit part of the diagram [115]. Finally, most caremaps contained multiple pathways and were sometimes presented as multi-level flow charts [93, 115].

Standardising the Caremap Content

An activity in the caremap represents a specific medical process. Three broad medical activities that are regularly observed are; diagnosis, treatment and ongoing monitoring/management [86, 117]. A set of desired outcomes is a common caremap component [85, 88, 93, 115]. Time, presented either as a duration or a dynamic care process, is often included in the caremap [84]. Finally, an explanation related to the activities and/or the arrows might also be part of the caremap [78, 84, 86, 88]. The former helps to better describe an activity, while the latter to justify the flow transition from one activity to another and/or the path to be taken based on the clinical decision being made.

Standardising the Caremap Development Process

The process of developing a contemporary caremap is a research topic that has been frequently neglected. Only one in every six papers gives any information concerning the development process. Unfortunately, very few papers provide any clear description of the development process [44, 86, 117]. For the remaining, the caremap development process can only be inferred [79, 85, 115].

6 TaSC: Proposed Standard for Caremaps

This section presents a solution for standardising caremap structure and content, and an approach for caremap development distilled directly from analysis of the CCPS literature. During the course of refining and evaluating TaSC the presence of previously undescribed DPs that would be assistive in identifying the appropriate treatment path for patients was realised. As a result, TaSC also incorporates a standard approach to describing DPs relevant to path selection, and based around the six aspects of clinical work from which clinical decisions arise listed earlier.

Standardising Caremap Structure

The TaSC entity relationship model shown in Fig. 1 describes the relationships among the caremap's structural elements. All elements and their notation are presented in Table 2. The standardised structural model for the caremap is then demonstrated in the content model shown in Fig. 2.

Figure 1 presents the model for the caremap specification that we believe has the key features necessary to comprehensively specify a clinical caremap by using a minimal set of representational constructs or elements. The representational elements of the caremap in this model lead to a representation notation that is simple and easy for clinicians to understand and use in authoring caremaps. In the caremap model, which is presented by using the UML class diagram, the caremap can either nest or link to another caremap. A caremap contains Pathways such that each present as a sequence of Elements. These include the Activity nodes within which clinical efforts occur, as well as the functional EntryPoint, ExitPoint, ExclusionPoint and DecisionPoint (DP) elements. Each DP represents some clinical decision to be made based on one or more Criterion, which can

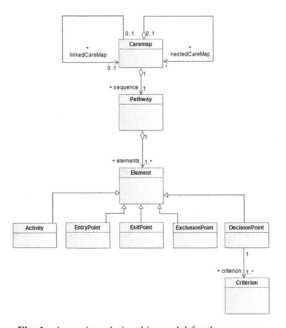

Fig. 1. An entity relationship model for the caremap.

include such things as the patient's risk factors, symptomatology and response to treatment, and often as identified from the results of clinical tests. The Pathway describes both: (i) the timing of necessary activities, that is, when activities should occur and how long to wait before performing the next activity; and, (ii) the route or selected order of events identified as a result of the impact of DP Criterion.

Table 2. The TaSC content type, activities and decisions (adapted from [18]).

	Element	Description	Notation
1	*Entry point*	Beginning of the caremap	
2	*Exit point*	End of the caremap	
3	*Exclusion point*	Exclusion from the caremap, as the patient does not belong to the targeted population	
4	*Activity*	A care or medical intervention that is associated with a medical content type *(see Table X in next section)*	
5	*Nested Activity*	An activity that has an underlying caremap	
6	*Decision*	A cognitive process of selecting a course of action that is associated with a medical content type *(see Table X in next section)*	
7	*Nested Decision*	A decision that has an underlying caremap	
8	*Flow*	Transition from one activity to another along the pathway	
9	*Multiple pathways*	Flow from an antecedent activity to a number of successors from which a decision point arises	
10	*Decision Criterion*	Conditional values used to identify the path to be taken based on the clinical decision being made	Xxx
11	*Nested caremap connection*	Connection between an activity and its nested caremap	
12	*Multi-level caremap connection*	Connection between a series of linked caremaps	

Corresponding to each representational construct presented in the caremap model in Fig. 1, a set of notational elements have been designed to allow caremaps to be specified according to the model. Table 2 presents the notation to represent each caremap element in the model. The notation is inspired by the standardised pictorial approach of UML. The application and use for each element is described within Table 2.

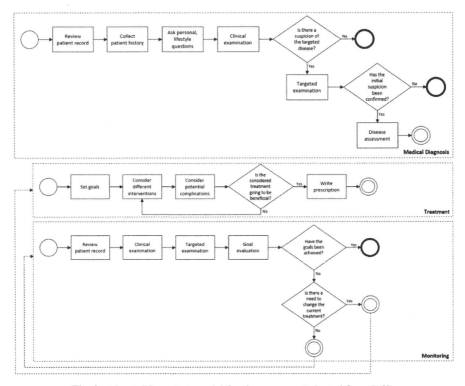

Fig. 2. The TaSC content model for the caremap (adapted from [18]).

Standardising Caremap Content

Diagnosis, treatment and ongoing management/monitoring are the three main content types captured in TaSC. As shown in Table 3, these three broad content types are related to a set of specific medical activities, the information captured, and relevant DPs. Finally, referring back to the content model presented previously in Fig. 2 we see that each content type represents a different caremap level, and that the activities and decisions are components of the caremap.

Table 3. Caremap content type, activities, data and decisions (adapted from [18]).

Content type	Activity (associated with Content Type)	Data/information captured	Decision (associated with Content Type)
Diagnosis	Review patient records	Demographics Medical history	Is there a suspicion of the targeted disease?
	Collect patient history	Family history Comorbidities	
	Ask personal, lifestyle questions	Habits (risk factors)	
	Clinical examination	Signs/symptoms	
	Targeted examination	Diagnostic test results	Has the initial suspicion been confirmed?
	Disease assessment	Diagnosis	
Treatment	Set goals	Expected outcomes	Is the considered treatment going to be beneficial?
	Consider different interventions	Possible treatments	
	Consider potential complications	Variances from expected outcomes	
	Write prescription	Selected treatment Treatment details	
Monitoring	Review patient records	Previous test results Previous symptoms	Have the goals been achieved? Is there a need to change the current treatment?
	Clinical examination	Signs/symptoms	
	Targeted examination	Diagnostic test results	
	Evaluate goals	Progression	

Standardising the Caremap Development Process

TaSC development process is divided into 6 phases, as shown in Fig. 3. The development steps have been clustered into three primary groups: (a) those undertaken before caremap development commenced; (b) those undertaken during development and refinement of the caremap, and; (c) those that come after the caremap has been refined and approved for implementation. At first, the conceptual framework should be decided and a multi-disciplinary team should be assembled. In the next phase it is important to clarify and challenge current practice. The knowledge and current data should be studied and potential variations from the current practice should be anticipated. Reviewing and evaluating the available evidence is the last phase before caremap development. Figure 3 illustrates that as new knowledge becomes available and more lessons are learned through caremap evaluation and implementation, the caremap should be revised [117].

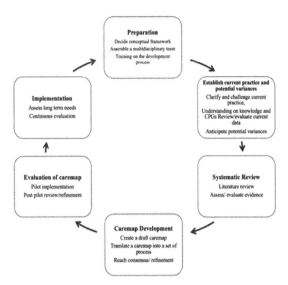

Fig. 3. Caremap development lifecycle [18].

7 Evaluation: A Study Using TaSC to Develop and Specify Caremaps in a Standardised Way

As part of a project to design and build LHS intended to reducing clinical overuse while empowering patients to actively participate in their own healthcare, the EPSRC-funded PAMBAYESIAN project (www.pambayesian.org) is creating Bayesian Network (BN) models to predict treatment needs for individual mothers with gestational diabetes mellitus (GDM). The process initially required us to create three caremaps for: (1) diagnosis; (2) management, and; (3) postnatal follow up.

Inputs: Inputs were: (a) clinical practice guidelines for the care of women with diabetes in pregnancy; and, (b) review and consensus from midwives and diabetologists.

Development: An iterative development process was used wherein the decision scientist and midwifery fellow worked together to deliver an initial version of the caremap based on the CPG and clinical experience. This initial caremap was revised and refined during a number of sessions with clinicians. Figure 4a presents the resulting clinical management caremap for GDM.

Extending the Caremaps: While using the caremaps to develop BNs for supporting diagnostic and treatment decisions for GDM we found the process was significantly simpler and more efficient when latent decisions relevant to selecting the appropriate treatment path for patients, and embedded in each caremap, were identified and included in the caremap. The GDM caremaps were redeveloped as caremaps with DPs.

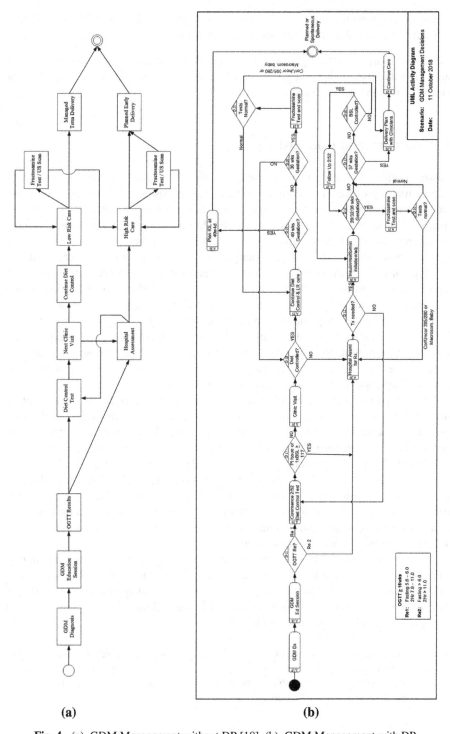

Fig. 4. (a). GDM Management without DP [18]. (b). GDM Management with DP.

Figure 4b shows the same clinical management caremap, however the DP have now been expounded in place of the previous activity node.

Validation: Validation was performed through consultation seeking consensus from three diabetologists with tertiary care experience of obstetric patients managed using the CPGs used in the caremaps' creation.

8   Summary and Conclusions

Standardisation of care through the means of guidelines and caremaps is sometimes seen as limiting clinicians' ability to make decisions based on the patient presenting before them, seemingly giving rise to *cookie-cutter medicine*. A range of clinical care process specification (CCPS) documents exist. The disagreement that persists within the domain regarding their name, form and function shows that they are not standardised. This lack of standardisation can put patients at risk, and has in some cases, caused harm. One type of CCPS, *caremaps*, are a form of standardised clinical documentation that can improve patient safety and outcomes while prompting clinicians with information and visual cues necessary to clinical decisions regarding the appropriate treatment path for their patients. Caremaps have evolved during the last three decades from primarily text-based presentations developed by nurses, to flow-based visual aids prepared by doctors to be representative of diagnostic and treatment processes. These contemporary caremaps have been presented in a variety of ways and with vastly different levels of content. Contemporary caremaps lacked standardisation.

This chapter presented one solution for standardising caremap structure, content and clinical decisions, and an approach for caremap development distilled directly from analysis of the collected pool of academic literature. The development process was evaluated and refined during the development of caremaps for management of patients with GDM. The resulting caremaps were validated by expert consensus.

If used consistently, the methods presented in this chapter could bring standardisation to caremaps and ensure that as clinical staff move between busy units in a tertiary care setting, they are not distracted from the patient in an effort to understand the care flow model. Every caremap would be familiar and time can be given over to treating their patient, not trying to understand the document.

Future work should address a standard approach for digital development and imputation of the caremap by clinicians, and representation of caremap logic in other computer-aware and algorithmic forms including BNs and Influence Diagrams (Fenton and Neil 2018). These can form part of an LHS and aid in the making of population-to-patient level predictions about treatment and health outcomes.

Acknowledgements. SM, EK and NF acknowledge support from the EPSRC under project EP/P009964/1: PAMBAYESIAN: Patient Managed decision-support using Bayes Networks. KD acknowledges funding and sponsorship for his research sabbatical at QMUL from the School of Fundamental Sciences, Massey University.

References

1. Iyer, P., Camp, N.: Nursing Documentation: A Nursing Process Approach, 2nd edn. Mosby Year-book, St Louis (1995)
2. Gordon, D.: Critical pathways: a road to institutionalizing pain management. J. Pain Symptom Manag. **11**(4), 252–259 (1996)
3. Fischbach, F.: Documenting Care Communication, the Nursing Process and Documentation Standards. F.A. Davis, Philadelphia (1991)
4. Comreid, L.: Cost analysis: initiation of HBMC and first CareMap. Nurs. Econ. **14**(1), 34–39 (1996)
5. Trowbridge, R., Weingarten, S.: Clinical pathways. In: Shojania, K., Duncan, B., McDonald, K., Wachter, R. (eds.) Making Health Care Safer: A Critical Analysis of Patient Safety Practices. Evidence Report/Technology Assessment, vol. 43. AHRQ, Rockville (2001). AHRQ Publication No. 01-E058
6. Gemmel, P., Vandaele, D., Tambeur, W.: Hospital process orientation (HPO): the development of a measurement tool. Total Qual. Manag. Bus. Excellence **19**(12), 1207–1217 (2008)
7. Zander, K.: Integrated care pathways: eleven international trends. J. Integr. Care Pathways **6**, 101–107 (2002)
8. Morris, A.: Decision support and safety of clinical environments. BMJ Qual. Saf. Healthcare **11**, 69–75 (2002)
9. Freeman, K., Field, R., Perkins, G.: Variations in local trust do not attempt cardiopulmonary resuscitation (DNACPR) policies: a review of 48 English healthcare trusts. BMJ Open **5**, e006517 (2015)
10. Seidman, M., et al.: Clinical practice guideline: Allergic rhinitis. Otolaryngology - Head Neck Surg. **152**, s1–s43 (2015)
11. Beskow, L., Dombeck, C., Thompson, C., Watson-Ormond, J., Weinfurt, K.: Informed consent for bio-banking: consensus-based guidelines for adequate comprehension. Genet. Med. **17**(3), 226–233 (2015)
12. Hennaut, E., et al.: Prospective cohort study investigating the safety and efficacy of ambulatory treatment with oral cefuroxime-axetil in febrile children with urinary tract infection. Front. Pediatr. **6**, 237 (2018)
13. RHW. Local Operating Procedures: A-Z Links (2019). https://www.seslhd.health.nsw.gov.au/royal-hospital-for-women/policies-and-publications
14. Holmes, J., Sokolove, P., Brant, W., Kuppermann, N.: A clinical decision rule for identifying children with thoracic injuries after blunt torso trauma. Ann. Emerg. Med. **39**(5), 492–499 (2002)
15. Downey, L., Cluzeau, F., Chalkidou, K., Morton, M., Sadanandan, R., Bauhoff, S.: Clinical pathways, claims data and measuring quality/measuring quality of care: the authors reply. Health Aff. **36**(2), 382a (2017)
16. Handelsman, Y., et al.: American association of endocrinologists and American College of Endocrinology: clinical practice guidelines for developing a diabetes mellitus comprehensive care plan - 2015. Endocrine Practice **21**, 1–87 (2015)
17. Salmonson, H., Sjoberg, G., Brogren, J.: The standard treatment protocol for paracetamol poisoning may be inadequate following overdose with modified release formulation: a pharmacokinetic and clinical analysis of 53 cases. Clin. Toxicol. **56**(1), 63–68 (2018)
18. McLachlan, S., Kyrimi, E., Dube, K., Fenton, N.: Clinical caremap development: how can caremaps standardise care when they are not standardised? Paper presented at the 12th International Joint Conference on Biomedical Systems and Technologies (BIOSTEC 2019), vol. 5. HEALTHINF, Prague (2019)

19. Kehlet, H.: Fast-track surgery: an update on physiological care principles to enhance recovery. Langenbeck's Arch. Surg. **396**(5), 585–590 (2011)
20. Solsky, I., et al.: Perioperative care map improves compliance with best practices for the morbidly obese. Surgery **160**(6), 1682–1688 (2016)
21. Zander, K.: Quantifying, managing and improving quality Part 1: How CareMaps link C.Q.I. to the patient. New Defn. **7**(4), 1–4 (1992)
22. Holocek, R., Sellards, S.: Use of detailed clinical pathway for bone marrow transplant patients. J. Pediatr. Oncol. Nurs. **14**(4), 252–257 (1997)
23. Li, W., Liu, K., Yang, H., Yu, C.: Integrated clinical pathway management for medical quality improvement based on a semiotically inspired systems architecture. Eur. J. Inf. Syst. **23**(4), 400–471 (2014)
24. O'Neill, E., Dluhy, N.: Utility of structured caer approaches in education and clinical practice. Nurs. Outlook **48**(3), 132–135 (2000)
25. Bumgarner, S., Evans, M.: Clinical Care Map for the ambulatory lapropscopic cholecystectomy patient. J. PeriAnaesthesia Nurs. **14**(1), 12–16 (1999)
26. Shiffman, R., Shekelle, P., Overhage, J., Slutsky, J., Grimshaw, J., Deshpande, A.: Standardised reporting of clinical practice guidelines: a proposal from the Conference on Guideline Standardisation. Ann. Internal Med. **139**(6), 493–498 (2003)
27. De Pietro, C., Francetic, I.: E-Health in Switzerland: the laborious adoption of the federal law on electronic health records (EHR) and health information exchange (HIE) networks. Health Policy **122**(2), 69–74 (2018)
28. Piwek, L., Andrews, S., Joinson, A.: The rise of consumer health wearables: promises and barriers. PloS Med. **13**(2), e1001953 (2016)
29. Brennan, P., et al.: Surgical specimin handover from the operating theatre to laboratory: can we improve patient safety by learning from aviation and other high-risk organisations? J. Oral Pathol. Med. **47**(2), 117–120 (2018)
30. Leape, I.: The preventability of medical injury Trans. In: Bogner, M. (ed.) Human Error in Medicine, pp. 13–25. CRC Press (2018)
31. Naveh, E., Katz-Navon, T., Stern, Z.: Readiness to report medical treatment errors: the effects of safety procedures, safety information and priority of safety. Med. Care **44**(2), 117–123 (2006)
32. Yelland, I., et al.: Prevalence and reporting of recruitment, randomisation and treatment errors in clinical trials: a systematic review. Clin. Trials **15**(3), 278–285 (2018)
33. Christian, C., et al.: A prospective study of patient safety in the operating room. Surgery **139**(2), 159–173 (2006)
34. Gu, X., Liu, H., Itoh, K.: Inter-department patient handoff quality and its contributing factors in Chinese hospitals. Cogn. Technol. Work **1**(11), 133–143 (2018)
35. Valenstein, P.: Formatting pathology reports: applying four design principles to improve communication and patient safety. Arch. Pathol. Lab. Med. **132**(1), 84–94 (2008)
36. McLachlan, S.: The largest single barrier to Learning Health Systems. A presentation at the 2nd Annual Pambayesian Workshop Event. Queen Mary University of London, London (2019)
37. McLachlan, S., et al.: A framework for analysing learning health systems: are we removing the most impactful barriers? Learn. Health Syst. (2019). https://doi.org/10.1002/lrh2.10189
38. McDonald, A., Frazer, K., Cowley, D.: Caseload management: an approach to making community needs visible. Br. J. Commun. Nurs. **18**(3), 140–147 (2013)
39. Mitchell, S., Plunkett, A., Dale, J.: Use of formal advance care planning documents: a national survey of UK Paediatric Intensive Care units. Arch. Disease Childhood **99**(4), 327–330 (2014)
40. Appleby, J., Raleigh, V., Frosini, F., Bevan, G., Gao, H., Slay, J.: Variations in healthcare: the good, the bad and the inexplicable (2011)

41. Zarzuela, S., Ruttan-Sims, N., Nagatakiya, L., DeMerchant, K.: Defining standardisation in healthcare. Mohawk Shared Serv. **15** (2015)
42. Leotsakos, A., et al.: Standardisation in patient safety: the WHO High 5's project. Int. J. Qual. Health Care **26**(2), 109–116 (2014)
43. Corbett, E.: Standardised care vs. personalisation: can they coexist? Quality and process improvement. Health Catalyst (2016). https://www.healthcatalyst.com/standardized-care-vs-personalization-can-they-coexist
44. Giffin, M., Giffin, R.: Market memo: critical pathways produce tangible results. Health Care Strategy Manag. **12**(7), 1–17 (1994)
45. Rotter, T., et al.: A systematic review and meta-analysis of the effects of clinical pathways on length of stay, hospital costs and patient outcomes. BMC Health Serv. Res. **8**, 265 (2008)
46. Keyhani, S., Falk, R., Howell, E., Bishop, T., Korenstein, D.: Overuse and systems of care: a systematic review. Med. Care **51**(6) (2014)
47. Martin, E.: Eliminating waste in healthcare. ASQ Healthcare Update **14** (2014)
48. Blind, K.: The impact of standardisation and standards on innovation (2013)
49. Crandall, R., Graham, J.: The effect of fuel economy standards on automobile safety. J. Law Econ. **32**(1), 97–118 (1989)
50. Curey, R., Ash, M., Thielman, L., Barker, C.: Proposed IEEE inertial systems terminology standard and other inertial sensor standards. Paper presented at the PLANS 2004. Position Location and Navigation Symposium, Monterey, CA (2004)
51. Jones, A.: Perceptions on the development of a care pathway for people diagnosed with schizophrenia on acute psychiatric units. J. Psychiatric Mental Health Nurs. **10**(6), 669–677 (2003)
52. Hoag, S., Ramachandruni, H., Shangraw, R.: Failure of Prescription Prenatal Vitamin Products to Meet USP Standards for Folic Acid Dissolution: six of nine vitamin products tested failed to meet USP standards for folic acid dissolution. J. Am. Pharm. Assoc. **37**(4), 397–400 (1997)
53. Milstien, J., Costa, A., Jadhav, S., Dhere, R.: Reaching international GMP standards for vaccine production: challenges for developing countries. Expert Rev. Vaccines **8**(5), 559–566 (2009)
54. de Vries, H.: Standardisation - what's in a name? Terminolog **4**(1), 55–83 (1997)
55. ISO/IEC. Standardisation and Related Activities - General Vocabulary (2004). Retrieved from: Geneva
56. Blind, K.: Standardisation: A catalyst for innovation. Retrieved from: Rotterdam, Netherlands (2009)
57. OECD. Oslo Manual: Guidelines for collecting and interpreting innovation data (2005). Retrieved from: Paris
58. Baumol, W.: Entrepreneurship, innovation and growth: the David-Goliath symbiosis. J. Entrepreneurial Finance **7**(2), 1–10 (2002)
59. Allen, R., Sriram, R.: The role of standards in innovation. Technol. Forecasting Soc. Change **64**(2–3), 171–181 (2000)
60. Egyedi, T., Sherif, M.: Standards' dynamics through an innovation lens: next generation ethernet networks. Paper presented at the First ITU-T Kaleidoscope Academic Conference-Innovations in NGN: Future Network and Services (2008)
61. Reddy, N., Cort, S., Lambert, D.: Industrywide technical product standards. R & D Manag. **19**(1), 13–25 (1989)
62. Williams, K., Ford, R., Bishop, I., Loiterton, D., Hickey, J.: Realism and selectivity in data-driven visualisations: a process for developing viewer-oriented landscape surrogates. Landscape Urban Plan. **81**, 213–224 (2007)
63. Williams, R., Graham, I., Jakobs, K., Lyytinen, K.: China and Global ICT standardisation and innovation. Technol. Anal. Strategic Manag. **23**(7), 715–724 (2011)

64. Cargill, C.: A five-segment model for standardization Trans. In: Kahin, B., Abbate, J. (eds.) Standards Policy for Information Infrastructure. MIT Press, Cambridge (1995)

65. Belleflamme, P.: Coordination on formal vs. de facto standards: a dynamic approach. Eur. J. Polit. Econ. **18**(1), 153–176 (2002)

66. Tether, B., Hipp, C., Miles, I.: Standardisation and particularisation in services: evidence from Germany. Res. Policy **30**, 1115–1138 (2001)

67. Kosawatz, J.: Rekindling the spark. Mech. Eng. Mag. Sel. Art. **139**(11), 28–33 (2017)

68. Mazda. Performance: Skyactiv-X (2019). https://www.mazda.com.au/imagination-drives-us/performance—skyactiv-x/

69. Mizuno, H.: Nissan gasoline engine strategy for higher thermal efficiency. Combust. Engines **169**(2), 141–145 (2017)

70. Chrisafis, A., Vaughan, A.: France to ban sales of petrol and diesel cars by 2040. Guardian (2017). https://www.theguardian.com/business/2017/jul/06/france-ban-petrol-diesel-cars-2040-emmanuel-macron-volvo

71. Coren, M.: Nine countries say they'll ban internal combustion engines. So far, it's just words (2018). https://qz.com/1341155/nine-countries-say-they-will-ban-internal-combustion-engines-none-have-a-law-to-do-so/

72. Timmermans, S., Angell, A.: Evidence-based medicine, clinical uncertainty, and learning to doctor. J. Health Soc. Behav. **42**, 342–359 (2001)

73. Marr, J., Reid, B.: Implementing managed care and case management: the neuroscience experience. J. Neurosci. Nurs. **24**(5), 281–285 (1992)

74. Ogilvie-Harris, D., Botsford, D., Hawker, R.: Elderly patients with hip fractures: improving outcomes with the use of care maps with high-quality medical and nursing protocols. J. Orthopaedic Trauma **7**(5), 428–437 (1993)

75. WIlson, D.: Effect of managed care on selected outcomes of hospitalised surgical patients. (Master of Nursing), University of Alberta, Alberta, Canada (1995)

76. Hampton, D.: Implementing a managed care framework through care maps. J. Nurs. Adm. **23**(5), 21–27 (1993)

77. Blegen, M., Reiter, R., Goode, C., Murphy, R.: Outcomes of hospital-based managed care: a multivariate analysis of cost and quality. Manag. Care: Obstetrics Gynaecol. **86**(5), 809–814 (1995)

78. Houltram, B., Scanlan, M.: Care maps: atypical antipsychotics. Nurs. Standard **18**(36), 42–44 (2004)

79. Dickinson, C., Noud, M., Triggs, R., Turner, L., Wilson, S.: The antenatal ward care delivery map: a team model approach. Aust. Health Rev. **23**(3), 68–77 (2000)

80. Jones, A., Norman, I.: Managed mental health care: problems and possibilities. J. Psychiatric Mental Health Nurs. **5**, 21–31 (1998)

81. Schwoebel, A.: Care mapping: a common sense approach. Indian J. Pediatr. **65**(2), 257–264 (1998)

82. Philie, P.: Management of blood-borne fluid exposures with a rapid treatment prophylactic caremap: one hospital's four-year experience. J. Emergency Nurs. **27**(5), 440–449 (2001)

83. Griffith, D., Hampton, D., Switzer, M., Daniels, J.: Facilitating the recovery of open-heart surgery patients through quality improvement efforts and CareMAP implementation. Am. J. Critical Care **5**(5), 346–352 (1996)

84. Saint-Jacques, H., Burroughs, V., Watkowska, J., Valcarcel, M., Moreno, P., Maw, M.: Acute coronary syndrome critical pathway: chest PAIN caremap. A qualitative research study provider-level intervention. Critical Pathways Cardiol. **4**(3), 145–604 (2005)

85. Royall, D., et al.: Development of a dietary management care map for metabolic syndrome. Can. J. Dietetic Practice Res. **75**(3), 132–139 (2014)

86. Thompson, G., deForest, E., Eccles, R.: Ensuring diagnostic accuracy in pediatric emergency medicine. Clin. Pediatric Emergency Med. **12**(2), 121–132 (2011)

87. Yazbeck, A.: Reengineering of business functions of the hospital when implementing care pathways. Ph.D. University of Ljubljana (2014)

88. Chan, E., Russell, J., Williams, W., Van Arsdell, G., Coles, J., McCrindle, B.: Postoperative chylothorax after cardiothoracic surgery in children. Ann. Thoracic Surg. **80**(5), 1864–1870 (2005)

89. deForest, E., Thompson, G.: Advanced nursing directives: integrating validated clinical scoring systems into nursing care in the pediatric emergency department. Nurs. Res. Practice (2012)

90. BCCancer. Gallbladder: 3 Primary Surgical Therapy. http://www.bccancer.bc.ca/books/gallbladder

91. WAHealth. Diagnostic Imaging Pathways: Bleeding (First Trimester)

92. Sackman, J., Citrin, L.: Cracking down on the cost outliers. Healthcare Finance Manag. **68**(3), 58–63 (2014)

93. Chu, S., Cesnik, B.: Improving clinical pathway design: lessons learned from a computerised prototype. Int. J. Med. Inform. **51**, 1–11 (1998)

94. Panz, V., Raal, F., Paiker, J., Immelman, R., Miles, H.: Performance of the CardioChek (TM) PA and Cholestech LDX (R) point-of-care analysers compared to clinical diagnostic laboratory methods for measurement of lipids: cardiovascular topic. Cardiovascular J. South Africa **16**(2), 112–116 (2005)

95. Hubner, U., et al.: The need for standardised documents in continuity of care: results of standardising the eNurse summary. Stud. Health Technol. Inform. **160**(2), 1169–1173 (2010)

96. NHS. Quality and Outcomes Framework (QOF), enhanced services and core contract extraction specifications (2018). https://digital.nhs.uk/data-and-information/data-collections-and-data-sets/data-collections/quality-and-outcomes-framework-qof

97. NHS. Commission for Quality and Innovation (2019). https://www.england.nhs.uk/nhs-standard-contract/cquin/

98. NICE. Standards and Indicators (2018). https://www.nice.org.uk/standards-and-indicators

99. Ilott, I., Booth, A., Rick, J., Patterson, M.: How do nurses, midwives and health visitors contribute to protocol-based care? A synthesis of the UK literature. Int. J. Nurs. Stud. **47**(6), 770–780 (2010)

100. Wilson, M.: Making nursing visible? Gender, technology and the care plan as script. Inf. Technol. People **15**(2), 139–158 (2002)

101. Harrison, J., Young, J., Price, M., Butow, P., Solomon, M.: What are the unmet supportive care needs of people with cancer? A systematic review. Supportive Care Cancer **17**(8), 1117–1128 (2009)

102. Vaismoradi, M., Jones, J., Turunen, H., Snelgrove, S.: Theme development in qualitative content analysis and thematic analysis. J. Nurs. Educ. Practice **6**(5), 100–110 (2016)

103. Stumme, G.: Formal concept analysis. In: Staab, S., Studer, R. (eds.) Handbook on Ontologies. Springer, Berlin (2009)

104. Bero, L., Grilli, R., Grimshaw, J., Harvey, E., Oxman, A., Thomson, M.: Closing the gap between research and practice: an overview of systematic reviews of interventions to promote the implementation of research findings. The cochrane effective practice and organization of care review group. BMJ (Clin. Res.) **317**(7156), 465–468 (1998)

105. Cook, J., et al.: Quantifying the consensus on anthropogenic global warming in the scientific literature. Environ. Res. Lett. **8**(2), 024024 (2013)

106. McLachlan, S.: Realism in Synthetic Data Generation. (Master of Philosophy in Science MPhil), Massey University, Palmerston North, New Zealand (2017)

107. Cable, G.: Integrating case study and survey research methods: an example in information systems. Eur. J. Inf. Syst. **3**(2), 112–126 (1994)

108. Lee, A.: A scientific method for MIS case studies. MIS Q. 33–50 (1989)

109. Eisenhardt, K.: Building theories from case study research. Acad. Manag. Rev. **14**(4), 532–550 (1989)
110. Yin, R.: Applications of Case Study Research. SAGE (2011)
111. Knape, T., Herderman, L., Wade, V., Gargan, M., Harris, C., Rahman, Y.: A UML approach to process modelling of clinical practice guidelines for enactment. Stud. Health Technol. Inform. 635–640 (2003)
112. Scheuelein, H., et al.: New methods for clinical pathways—business process modeling notation (BPMN) and tangible business process modeling (t. BPM). Langenbeck's Arch. Surg. **397**(5), 755–761 (2012)
113. Gomez, M., Bielza, C., Fernandez del Pozo, J., Rios-Insua, S.: A graphical decision-theoretic model for neonatal jaundice. Med. Decis. Making **27**(3), 250–265 (2007)
114. Richardson, W., Wilson, M., Nishikawa, J., Hayward, R.: The well-built clinical question: a key to evidence-based decisions. ACP J. Club **123**(3), A12–A13 (1995)
115. Panzarasa, S., Madde, S., Quaglini, S., Pistarini, C., Stefanelli, M.: Evidence-based careflow management systems: the case of post-stroke rehabilitation. J. Biomed. Inform. **35**(2), 123–139 (2002)
116. Gopalakrishna, G., Langendam, M., Scholten, R., Bussuyt, P., Leeflang, M.: Defining the clinical pathway in cochrane diagnostic test accuracy reviews. BMC Med. Res. Methodol. **16**(153) (2016)
117. Huang, B., Zhu, P., Wu, C.: Customer-centered careflow modeling based on guidelines. J. Med. Syst. 36, 3307–3319 (2012)

Towards a More Reproducible Biomedical Research Environment: Endorsement and Adoption of the FAIR Principles

Alina Trifan(✉) and José Luís Oliveira

DETI/IEETA, University of Aveiro, Aveiro, Portugal
{alina.trifan,jlo}@ua.pt

Abstract. The FAIR guiding Principles for scientific data management and stewardship are a fundamental enabler for digital transformation and transparent research. They were designed with the purpose of improving data quality, by making it Findable, Accessible, Interoperable and Reusable. While these principles have been endorsed by both data owners and regulators as key data management techniques, their translation into practice in quite novel. The recent publication of FAIR metrics that allow for the evaluation of the degree of FAIRness of a data source, platform or system is a further booster towards their adoption and practical implementation. We present in this paper an overview of the adoption and impact of the FAIR principles in the area of biomedical and life-science research. Moreover, we consider the use case of biomedical data discovery platforms and assess the degree of FAIR compatibility of three such platforms. This assessment is guided by the FAIR metrics.

Keywords: Biomedical and life-science research · Data discovery platforms FAIR principles · Reproducible research · FAIR metrics

1 Introduction

The FAIR guiding principles - FAIR stands for Findable, Accessible, Interoperable and Reusable - were proposed with the ultimate goal of reusing valuable research objects [41]. They represent a set of guidelines for turning data more meaningful and reusable. They emphasize on the necessity to make data discoverable and interoperable not just by humans, but by machines as well. These principles do not provide strict rules or standards to comply with, but rather focus on conventions that enable data interoperability, stewardship and compliance against data and metadata standards, policies and practices. They are not standards to be rigorously followed, but rather permissive guidelines.

The principles are aspirational, in that they do not strictly define how to achieve a state of FAIRness. Depending on the needs or constraints of different research communities, they can be open to interpretation. Independently of this openness, they were designed to assist the interaction between those who want to

© Springer Nature Switzerland AG 2020
A. Roque et al. (Eds.): BIOSTEC 2019, CCIS 1211, pp. 453–470, 2020.
https://doi.org/10.1007/978-3-030-46970-2_22

use community resources and those who provide them. When followed, they are beneficial for both data and system owners and users that seek access to these data and systems. These principles have rapidly been adopted by publishers, funders, and pan-disciplinary infrastructure programmes as key data management issues to be taken into consideration. This can be explained as data management closely relates to interoperability and reproducibility [10].

Generic and research-specific initiatives, such as the European Open Science Cloud[1], the European Elixir infrastructure[2] and the USA National Institutes of Health's Big Data to Knowledge Initiative[3] are some of the current initiatives that endorse the FAIR principles and are committed to provide FAIR ecosystems across multi-disciplinary research areas. Moreover, the European Commission has recently made available a set of recommendations and demands for open data research that are explicitly written in the context of FAIR data[4]. Besides these, several European infrastructures aimed at large scale populational and healthcare research, such as the European Health Data Network[5] and Big Data for Better Outcomes[6] promote these principles as the underlying guide for delivering transparent, reproducible and qualitative research.

Straightforward FAIR-dedicated initiatives such as GOFAIR[7], FAIRsFAIR[8] or FAIRSharing[9] work towards building connected infrastructures of FAIR resources, improve their interoperability and reusability and generally adding value to data by capitalizing on the FAIR principles. They make use of infrastructures that already exist in European countries to create a federated approach for turning the FAIR principles a working standard in science. FAIRDOM[10] alike, a web platform uilt for collecting, managing, storing, and publishing dat alika, models, and operating procedures endorses the FAIR guiding principles as improvements to existing research management practices.

With regard to biomedical and life-science data sources, data interoperability and reusability has been a hot topic over the last decade, strongly correlated with the evolution of the so called Big Data in Healthcare. Despite the incremental increase of the use and storage of electronic health records, research communities still tends to use these data in isolation. Unfortunately more than 80% of the datasets in current practice are effectively unavailable for reuse [18]. This is just one of the factors behind the reproducibility crisis that is manifesting in the biomedical arena [24]. Apart from data still being gathered in silos unavailable outside of the owning institution or country, data privacy concerns and unclear

---

[1] http://eoscpilot.org.

[2] http://www.elixir-europe.org.

[3] http://commonfound.nih.gov/bd2k/.

[4] http://ec.europa.eu/research/participants/data/ref/h2020/grants_manual/hi/oa_pilot/h2020-hi-oa-data-mgt_en.pdf.

[5] www.ehden.eu.

[6] http://bd4bo.eu/.

[7] https://www.go-fair.org.

[8] fairsfair.eu.

[9] https://fairsharing.org/.

[10] https://fair-dom.org/about-fairdom/.

data management approaches are critical barriers for sharing and reusing data. The FAIR principles have been enabling the global debate about better data stewardship in data-driven and open science, and they have triggered funding bodies to discuss their application to biomedical and life-sciences systems. A wide adoption of these principles by the data sources and systems that handle biomedical data has the ability to solve this reproducibility crisis, by ensuring secure interoperability among heterogeneous data sources.

In this paper we propose an overview of the adoption of these principles by the biomedical, life-science and in a more bread sense, health related research communities. We review current approaches of FAIR ecosystems and while such system already perform self-assessments of their methodologies for following the FAIR principles, our exhaustive literature search revealed only a handful of such assessments. We therefore overview FAIR practices that have been thoroughly documented. The FAIR principles are identified as system requirements by several data discovery platforms and biomedical infrastructures, although many of them fall short in really exposing a deep evaluation of their adoption. As such, we dive deeper into the challenges of translating these principles into practice. We chose three biomedical data discovery platforms, as a use case for identifying the methodologies through which they follow the FAIR guidelines.

The present manuscript is an extension of the article presented by the same authors at HealthInf 2019, the 12th International Conference on Health Informatics, held in Prague, Czech Republic [34]. In the current manuscript the Introduction includes further insight into the importance and endorsement of the FAIR Principles within the biomedical and healthcare research communities. In this paper we broaden the scope of the research question behind it and we not only proposes an open assessment of three biomedical data discovery platforms, but we complement it with an overview of FAIR self-assessments that have been recently published. Moreover, the assessment done is extended with more insights into how the FAIR metrics were applied. The Discussion takes into consideration the scientific advances that the FAIR principles have enabled so far and argues on possible challenges that are still to be overcome from the practical point of view of their implementation.

This paper is structured in 5 more sections. A detailed presentation of the FAIR principles is covered in Sect. 2, followed by an overview of biomedical and healthcare FAIR-endorsing initiatives in Sect. 3. The adoption of the FAIR principles by these platforms is analyzed in Sect. 4. We then review self-assessing publications and we propose an open FAIR evaluation of 3 biomedical platforms. We discuss the importance of this adoption for the biomedical and life-science research communities and the current challenges in Sect. 5. We draw our final remarks in Sect. 6.

2   FAIR Guiding Principles

The FAIR principles were intended as a set of guidelines to be followed in order to enhance the reusability of any type of data. They put specific emphasis on enhancing the ability of machines to automatically find and (re)use the data, in addition to supporting its (re)use by individuals. The goal is that, through the pursuit of these principles, the quality of a data source becomes a function of its ability to be accurately found and reused. Although they are currently not a strict requirement, nor a standard in biomedical data handling systems, these principles maximize their added-value, by acting as a guidebook for safeguarding transparency, reproducibility, and reusability.

The FAIR principles as initially proposed by [41] are detailed in Table 1. In a nutshell, if a data source is intended to be FAIR, sufficient metadata must be provided to automatically identify its structure, provenance, licensing and potential uses, without having the need to use specialized tools. Moreover, any access protocols should be declared where they do or do not exist. The use of vocabularies and standard ontologies further benefit to the degree of FAIRness of a data set.

Table 1. The FAIR Guiding Principles as originally proposed in [41].

Findable	**F1**. (meta)data are assigned a globally unique and persistent identifier
	F2. data are described with rich metadata (defined by R1 below)
	F3. metadata clearly and explicitly include the identifier of the data it describes
	F4. (meta)data are registered or indexed in a searchable resource
Accessible	**A1**. (meta)data are retrievable by their identifier using a standardized communications protocol
	A1.1 the protocol is open, free, and universally implementable
	A1.2 the protocol allows for an authentication and authorization procedure, where necessary
	A2. metadata are accessible, even when the data are no longer available
Interoperable	**I1**. (meta)data use a formal, accessible, shared, and broadly applicable language for knowledge representation
	I2. (meta)data use vocabularies that follow FAIR principles
	I3. (meta)data include qualified references to other (meta)data
Reusable	**R1**. (meta)data are richly described with a plurality of accurate and relevant attributes
	R1.1 (meta)data are released with a clear and accessible data usage license
	R1.2 (meta)data are associated with detailed provenance
	R1.3 (meta)data meet domain-relevant community standards

The way these principles should manifest in reality was largely open to interpretation and more recently some of the original authors revisited the principles, in an attempt to clarify what FAIRness is [18]. They addressed the principles as a community-acceptable set of rules of engagement and a common denominator between those who want to use a community's resources and those who provide them. An important clarification was that FAIR is not a standard and it is not equal to open. The initial release of the FAIR principles were somehow misleading in the sense that accessibility was associated with open access. Instead, in the recent extended explanation of what these principles really mean, the A in FAIR was redefined as "Accessible under well defined conditions". This means that data do not have to be open, but the data access protocol should be open and clearly defined. In fact, data itself should be "as open as possible, as closed as needed".

The recognition that computers must be capable of accessing a data object autonomously was the core to the FAIR principles since the beginning. The recent re-interpretation of these principles maintains their focus on the importance of data being accessible to autonomous machines and further clarifies on the possible degrees of FAIRness. While there is no such notion as unFAIR, the authors discuss the different levels of FAIRness that can be achieved. As such, the addition of rich, FAIR metadata is the most important step towards becoming maximally FAIR. When data objects themselves can be made FAIR and open for reuse, the highest degree of FAIRness can be achieved. When all of these are linked with other FAIR data, the Internet of FAIR data is reached. Ultimately, when a large number of applications and services can link and process FAIR data, the Internet of FAIR Data and Services is attained.

3   Biomedical and Life-Science FAIRness

Massive amounts of data are currently available and being produced at an unprecedented rate in all domains of life sciences worldwide. The large volume and heterogeneity of data demand rigorous data standards and effective data management. This includes modular data processing pipelines, APIs and end-user interfaces to facilitate accurate and reliable data exchange, standardization, integration, and end user access [31]. Along with biomedical and life sciences research, the biopharmaceutical industry R&D is becoming increasingly data-driven and can significantly improve its efficiency and effectiveness by implementing the FAIR guiding principles. Recent powerful analytical tools such as artificial intelligence, data mining and knowledge extraction would be able to access the data required in the learning process. The implementation of FAIR is a differentiating factor to exploit data so that they can be used more effectively but also for catalysing external collaborations and for leveraging public datasets. FAIR data support such collaborations and enable insight generation by facilitating the linking of data sources and enriching them with metadata [42].

In the healthcare context, similarly to the biopharma industry, current practices are highly data-driven. Machine learning algorithms capable of securely learning from massive volumes of patients' deidentified clinical data is an appealing and noninvasive approach toward personalization. Health personalization is expected to revolutionize current health outcomes. To reach this goal, a scalable big data architecture for the biomedical domain becomes essential, based on data standardization to transform clinical, biomedical and life science data into FAIR data [33]. With a new perspective on the FAIR principles applied to healthcare, Holub et al. [8] argue that biological material and data should be viewed as a unified resource. This approach would facilitate access to complete provenance information, which they consider a prerequisite for reproducibility and meaningful integration of the data. They even proposed an extension of the FAIR Principles for healthcare, to include additional components such as quality aspects and meaningful reuse of the data, incentives to stimulate effective enrichment of data sets and biological material collections, and privacy-respecting approaches for working with the human material and data.

The NIH Big Data to Knowledge (BD2K) initiative aims to facilitate digitally enabled biomedical research. Within the BD2K framework, the Commons initiative is intended to establish a virtual environment that will facilitate the use, interoperability, and discoverability of digital research objects. It seeks to promote the widespread use of biomedical digital resources by ensuring that they are FAIR. There are four established working subgroups with the aim of bringing some of the high level concepts established by the BD2K Commons into practice, one of them being solely dedicated to the development of FAIRness metrics [9]. In Europe, the German Network for Bioinformatics Infrastructure collects, curates, and shares life-science data. The work of the center is guided by the FAIR principles. This research initiative developed several different tools as contributions to FAIR data, models, and experimental methods storage and exchange [43]. Similarly, FAICE (FAIR Collaboration and Experiments) allow for comprehensive machine-readable description of an experiment that enables replication as well as modification to reuse other input data or a different execution environment [10].

On the genomics spectrum, publicly available gene expression datasets are growing at an accelerating rate. Such datasets hold value for knowledge discovery, particularly when integrated. Although numerous software platforms and tools have been developed to enable reanalysis and integration of genomics datasets, large-scale reuse is harden by minimal requirements for standardized metadata that are ofthen not met. The ultimate goal of initiatives as the Gene Expression Omnibus is to make such repositories more FAIR [39]. Likewise, to unlock the full potential of genome data and to enhance data interoperability and reusability of genome annotations, the Semantic Annotation Platform with Provenance (SAPP) was developed [12]. As an infrastructure supporting FAIR computational genomics, it can be used to process and analyze existing genome annotations. Because managing FAIR genome annotation data requires a considerable administrative load, SAPP stores the results and their provenance in a Linked Data format, thus enabling the deployment of mining capabilities of the Semantic Web.

Access to consistent, high-quality metadata is critical to finding, understanding, and reusing scientific data. The W3C Semantic Web for Health Care and the

Life Sciences Interest Group identified Resource Description Framework (RDF) vocabularies that could be used to specify common metadata elements and their value sets, thereby enabling the publication of FAIR data [4]. The usage of ontologies adds to transforming data from database schemas into FAIR data. An ontology, combined with Semantic Web technologies, are a strong contributor to the FAIRness of a system by facilitating their reproducibility. One such example is the Radiation Oncology Ontology, a platform that contains classes and properties between classes to represent clinical data and their relationships in the radiation oncology domain following the FAIR principles. The ontology along with Semantic Web technologies show how to efficiently integrate and query data from different sources without a priori knowledge of their structures. When clinical FAIR data sources are combined using the mentioned technologies, new relationships between entities are created and discovered, representing a dynamic body of knowledge that is continuously accessible and increasing [33].

4   FAIRness into Practice

While the FAIR principles have been both identified as key requirements of data management systems and endorsed by multiple research infrastructures and funding bodies over the last years, there are only a handful of scientific publications that address the assessment of the FAIR degree of biomedical, life-science or health related platforms or systems. Dataverse [15], for instance, is an open-source data repository software designed to support public community or institutional research repositories. Open PHACTS[11], a data integration platform for drug discovery, UniProt [25], an online resource for protein sequence and annotation data and the EMIF Catalogue [35], are some of the few FAIR self-assessed data discovery and integration platforms.

Another example is Datasets2Tools, a repository indexing bioinformatics analyses applied to datasets and bioinformatics software tools. It provides a platform for not only the discovery of these resources, but to their compliance with the FAIR principles. Users are enabled to grade digital objects according to their compliance with the FAIR principles. When a user submits a FAIR evaluation, its scores are stored in the database, aggregated with the feedback from all other users, and displayed on the corresponding landing pages. The FAIRness evaluation information is also incorporated within the search ranking system, where users can prioritize and identify resources based on their overall FAIRness score [32].

A detailed FAIR assessment is proposed by Rodriguez et al. [27], who describe the process of migrating the Pathogen-Host Interaction Database (PHI-base) to a form that conforms to each of the FAIR Principles. They detail the technical and architectural decisions, including observations of the difficulty of each step. They examine how multiple FAIR principles can be addressed simultaneously through careful design decisions, including making data FAIR for both humans and machines with minimal duplication of effort. They argue that FAIR data

---

[11] http://www.openphactsfoundation.org/.

publishing involves more than data reformatting and that the sole use of Semantic Web or Linked Data resources is not sufficient for reaching a high level of FAIRness. They explore the value-added by the FAIR data transformation by testing out the result through integrative questions that could not easily be asked over traditional Web-based data resources [27].

Several other examples on how the FAIR principles are translated into practice come from research areas that are either limited by the amount of data available or by the rareness of study events. As such, the Immune Epitope Database (IEDB) has the mission to make published experimental data relating to the recognition of immune epitopes easily available to the scientific public. Vita et al. [38] examine how IEDB complies with the FAIR principles and identify broad areas of success, but also areas for improvement, through a systematic inspection. The IEDB does comply with a number of the FAIR principles to a high standard, but at the same time, several areas for improvement were identified [38]. Another example is the area of pharmacovigillance. OpenPVSignal is an ontology aiming to support the semantic enrichment and rigorous communication of pharmacovigilance signal information in a systematic way. It focuses on publishing signal information according to the FAIR data principles, and exploiting automatic reasoning capabilities upon the interlinked signal report data. OpenPVSignal is developed as a reusable, extendable and machine-understandable model based on Semantic Web standards. An evaluation of the model against the FAIR data principles was performed by Natsiavas et al. [19]. Project Tycho, an open-access database comprising million counts of infectious disease cases and deaths reported for over a century by public health surveillance in the United States was recently upgraded to version 2.0. The main changes reflected in this new version were the use of standard vocabularies to encode data, improving thus compliance with FAIR [21].

In the rare diseases spectrum, the Open Source Registry for Rare Diseases (OSSE) provides a software for the management of patient registries. In this area, networking and data exchange for research purposes remains challenging due to interoperability issues and due to the fact that small data chunks are stored locally. A pioneer in this area, the OSSE architecture was adapted so as to follow the FAIR Data Principles. The so called FAIR Data Point [30] was integrated in order to provide a description of metadata in a FAIR manner. This is an important first step towards unified documentation across multiple registries and the implementation of the FAIR Data Principles in the rare disease area [28].

A metadata model, along with a data sharing framework designed to improve findability and reproducibility of experimental data inspired by FAIR principles were proposed by Karim et al. [11]. The developed system is evaluated against competency questions collected from data consumers, and thereby proven to help to interpret and compare data across studies. The authors follow an incremental approach to achieve optimal FAIRness of the data sets and report on the initial degree of FAIRness that was achieved. Their implementation is not complete in terms of coverage of all FAIR principles, but provides a starting point and a good example of practical applications of Semantic Web technologies for FAIR data sharing.

Table 2. The template for creating FAIR Metrics retrieved from https://github.com/FAIRMetrics.

Field	Description
Metric Identifier	FAIR Metrics should, themselves, be FAIR objects, and thus should have globally unique identifiers
Metric Name	A human-readable name for the metric
To which principle does it apply	Metrics should address only one sub-principle, since each FAIR principle is particular to one feature of a digital resource; metrics that address multiple principles are likely to be measuring multiple features, and those should be separated whenever possible
What is being measured	A precise description of the aspect of that digital resource that is going to be evaluated
Why should we measure it	Describe why it is relevant to measure this aspect
What must be provided	What information is required to make this measurement?
How do we measure it	In what way will that information be evaluated?
What is a valid result	What outcome represents "success" versus "failure"?
For which digital resource(s) is this relevant	If possible, a metric should apply to all digital resources; however, some metrics may be applicable only to a subset. In this case, it is necessary to specify the range of resources to which the metric is reasonably applicable
Example of their application across types of digital resource	Whenever possible, provide an existing example of success, and an example of failure

4.1 FAIR Metrics

Along with the narrative analysis of FAIR principles and their adoption, we propose an assessment following the FAIR metrics recently proposed by some of the original authors of the FAIR guiding principles (Table 2).

The increasing ambiguity behind the initially published principles, along with the need of data providers and regulatory bodies to evaluate their translation into practice led to the establishment of the FAIR metrics group[12], with the purpose of defining universal measures of data FAIRness. Nevertheless, these universal metrics can be complemented by resource-specific ones that can reflect the expectations of one or multiple communities.

---

[12] http://fairmetrics.org.

4.2 FAIR Use Case: Biomedical Discovery Platforms

The integration and reuse of huge amounts of biomedical data currently available in digital format has the ability to impact clinical decisions, pharmaceutical discoveries, disease monitoring and the way population healthcare is provided globally. Storing data for future reuse and reference has been a critical factor in the success of modern biomedical sciences [26]. In order for data to be reused, first it has to be discovered. Finding a dataset for a study can be burdensome due to the need to search individual repositories, read numerous publications and ultimately contact data owners or publication authors on an individual basis. Recent research shows that the time spent by researchers in searching for and identifying multiple useful data sources can take up to 80% of their time dedicated to the project or research question itself [23].

Biomedical data exists in multiple scales, from molecular to patient data. Health systems, genetics and genomics, population and public health are all areas that may benefit from big data integration and its associated technologies [16]. The secondary reuse of citizens' health data and investigation of the real evidence of therapeutics may lead to the achievement of personalized, predictive and preventive medicine [22]. However, in order for researchers to be able to reuse data and conduct integrative studies, they first have to find the right data for their research. Data discovery platforms are one-stop shops that enable clinical researchers to identify datasets of interest without having to perform individual, extensive searches over distributed, heterogeneous health centers.

There are currently many data discovery platforms, developed either as warehouses or simply aggregators of metadata that link to the original data sources. A warehouse platform, the Vanderbilt approach [3] contains both fully de-identified research data and fully identified research that is made available taking into consideration access protocols and governance rules. A cataloguing toolkit is proposed by Maelstrom Research, built upon two main components: a metadata model and a suite of open-source software applications [1]. When combined, the model and software support implementation of study and variable catalogues and provide a powerful search engine to facilitate data discovery. Disease oriented platforms, such as The Ontario Brain Institute's (Brain-CODE) [37] are designed with a very explicit, yet not limited, purpose of supporting researchers in better understanding a specific disease. Brain-CODE addresses the high dimensionality of clinical, neuroimaging and molecular data related with various brain conditions. The platform makes available integrated datasets that can be queried and linked to provincial, national and international databases. Similarly, the breast cancer (B-CAN) platform [40] was designed as a private cancer data center that enables the discovery of cancer-related data and drives research collaborations aimed at better understanding this disease. Still in the spectrum of cancer discovery, the Project Data Sphere was built to voluntarily share, integrate, and analyze historical cancer clinical trial data sets with the final goal of advancing cancer research [6]. In the rare disease spectrum, RD-Connect [5] links genomic data with patient registries, biobanks, and clinical bioinformatics tools in an attempt to provide a FAIR rare disease complete ecosystem.

Among most established initiatives, Cafe Variome [13] provides a general-purpose, web-based, data discovery tool that can be quickly installed by any genotype–phenotype data owner and turn data discoverable. MONTRA [29], another full-fledged open-source discovery solution, is a rapid-application development framework designed to facilitate the integration and discovery of heterogeneous objects. Both solutions rely on a catalogue for data discovery and include extensive search functionalities and query capabilities.

Linked Data is also explored in discovery platforms, such as YummyData [44] which was designed to improve the findability and reusability of life science datasets provided as Linked Data. It consists of two components, one that periodically polls a curated list of SPARQL endpoints and a second one that monitors them and presents the information measured. Similarly, the Open PHACTS Discovery Platform [7] leverages Linked Data to provide integrated access to pharmacology databases. Still in the spectrum of Linked Data, FAIRSharing is a manually curated searchable portal of three linked registries [17] that cover standards, databases and data policies in the life sciences.

Further contributors to the degree of FAIRness of such systems are APIs that enable machines to discover and interact with FAIR research objects. One such example is the smartAPI[13] [45], which was developed with the aim to make APIs FAIR. It leverages the use of semantic technologies such as ontologies and Linked Data for the annotation, discovery, and reuse of APIs. Considering the diversity, complexity and increasing volume of biomedical research data, Navale et al. argue that cloud based platforms can be leveraged to support several different ingest modes (e.g. machine, software or human entry modes) to make data more FAIR [20].

All these platforms address data discovery from different perspectives, integrating or linking to different types of biomedical data. Another aspect that they share is that they identify the FAIR principles as requirements of their architectures, as well as enablers of data discovery. Although the high majority of these platforms emphasize the importance of providing a way for machines to discover and access the data sets, they are heterogeneous in the way they address the FAIR guidelines. A recent systematic review on biomedical discovery platforms [36] argues that 45% (9 out of 20) of the studies included in the review indicate the FAIR principles as requirements, without providing details on their implementation. For the evaluation that we propose in this paper, we have chosen three of the previously overviewed data discovery platforms that identify the FAIR principles as guidelines for their development. We are keen on understanding their approaches in following the guiding principles. We first overview the scope and methods of these platforms and we present in a narrative form their partial or total compliance with the FAIR principles.

Among the three platforms we chose for this assessment, the Maelstrom Research cataloguing toolkit presented by [1] is built upon two main components: a metadata model and a suite of open-source software applications. The model sets out specific fields to describe study profiles, characteristics of the

---

[13] www.smart-api.info.

subpopulations of participants, timing and design of data collection events and variables collected at each data collection event. The model and software support implementation of study and variable catalogues and provide a powerful search engine to facilitate data discovery. Developed as an open source and generic tool to be used by a broad range of initiatives, the Maelstrom Research cataloguing toolkit serves several national and international initiatives. The FAIR principles have been identified from early on as a requirement of its architecture. With respect to Findability, each dataset is complemented by rich metadata. To ensure quality and standardization of the metadata documented across networks, standard operating procedures were implemented. In what concerns Accessibility, when completed, study and variable-specific metadata are made publicly available on the Maelstrom Research website. Using information found in peer-reviewed journals or on institutional websites, the study outline is documented and validated by study investigators. Thus, the linkage with other FAIR metadata is achieved. Where possible, data dictionaries or codebooks are obtained, which contributes to the data interoperability.

Many life science datasets are nowadays represented via Linked Data technologies in a common format (the Resource Description Framework). This makes them accessible via standard APIs (SPARQL endpoints), which can be understood as one of the FAIR requirements. While this is an important step toward developing an interoperable bioinformatics data landscape it also creates a new set of obstacles as it is often difficult for researchers to find the datasets they need. YummyData provides researchers the ability to discover and assess datasets from different providers [44]. This assessment can be done in terms of metrics such as service stability or metadata richness. YummyData consists of two components: one that periodically polls a curated list of SPARQL endpoints monitoring the states of their Linked Data implementations and content and another one that presents the information measured for the endpoints and provides a forum for discussion and feedback. It was designed with the purpose to improve the findability and reusability of life science datasets provided as Linked Data and to foster its adoption. Apart from making data available to software agents via an API, the adoption of Linked Data principles has the potential to make data FAIR.

FAIRSharing, originally named Biosharing, is a manually curated searchable portal of three linked registries [17]. These resources cover standards, databases and data policies in the life sciences broadly encompassing the biological environmental and biomedical sciences. The manifest of the initiative is that FAIRSharing makes these resources findable and accessible - the core of the FAIR principle. Every record is designed to be interlinked providing a detailed description not only on the resource itself but also on its relations with other life science infrastructures. FAIRSharing is working with an increasing number of journals and other registries and its focus is to ensures that data standards, biological databases and data policies are registered, informative and discoverable. Thus, it is considered a pivotal resource for the implementation of the ELIXIR-supported FAIR principles.

Our biomedical discovery use-case assessment follows the previously identified FAIRness metrics, applied to each of the 13 items of the FAIR guiding principles. For each of the principles, we outline next the questions that we tried to answer in the evaluation and the name of the metric, within brackets. The following information is a summary of the FAIR metrics description proposed by some of the original authors of the guiding principles[14]:

- F1 (Identifier uniqueness) Whether there is a scheme to uniquely identify the digital resource.
- F1 (Identifier persistence) Whether there is a policy that describes what the provider will do in the event an identifier scheme becomes deprecated.
- F2 (Machine-readability of metadata) The availability of machine-readable metadata that describes a digital resource.
- F3 (Resource identifier in metadata) Whether the metadata document contains the globally unique and persistent identifier for the digital resource.
- F4 (Indexed in a searchable resource) The degree to which the digital resource can be found using web-based search engines.
- A1.1 (Access Protocol) The nature and use limitations of the access protocol.
- A1.2 (Access authorization) Specification of a protocol to access restricted content.
- A2 (Metadata longevity) The existence of metadata even in the absence/ removal of data.
- I1 (Use a knowledge representation language) The use of a formal, accessible, shared, and broadly applicable language for knowledge representation.
- I2 (Use FAIR Vocabularies) The metadata values and qualified relations should themselves be FAIR, for example, terms from open, community-accepted vocabularies published in an appropriate knowledge-exchange format.
- I3 (Use qualified references) Relationships within (meta)data, and between local and third-party data, have explicit and 'useful' semantic meaning.
- R1.1 (Accessible Usage License) The existence of a license document, for both (independently) the data and its associated metadata, and the ability to retrieve those documents.
- R1.2 (Detailed Provenance) That there is provenance information associated with the data, covering at least two primary types of provenance information: who/what/when produced the data (i.e. for citation) and why/how was the data produced (i.e. to understand context and relevance of the data).
- R1.3 (Meets Community Standards) Certification, from a recognized body, of the resource meeting community standards.

This evaluation allowed us to identify the FAIR requirements already satisfied and the ones that are not undressed, or unclear. Our findings show a high level of FAIRness achieved by the three platforms, mainly favored by the rich metadata with which each of these platform complement the actual data sources. In all cases the metadata can be accessed both by humans and machines through a

---

[14] https://github.com/FAIRMetrics/Metrics/blob/master/ALL.pdf.

unique and persistent identifier, mostly in the form of an URI. Moreover, the use of FAIR standards and vocabularies contributes to their degree of FAIRness. This is complemented in two of the platforms by the ability to link to other FAIR metadata, which speaks for the data interoperability and reusability. Still related to reusability, the use of Linked Data by two of the platforms is one of its strong enablers. Last but not least, all of the platforms support machine discoverability and access, by providing dedicated APIs. The main unclear aspect was the access protocol, which was not trivial to identify. Another weak point was the lack of quantifiable certification that the resources meet community standards. We present our summarized assessment in Table 3.

With respect to Findability, we can argue that FAIRsharing exposes a higher quality of FAIRness as all resources are identified by truly globally and unique identifiers, following a schema similar to the Digital Object Identifiers used in the case of scientific publications. All three portals have clearly defined and easily findable data description sections, that link to the origin of the data in question. They all support search capabilities for the identification of the resources they hold. Additionally, Google Dataset Search engine indexes FAIRsharing resources. Regarding Accessibility, the only requirement that we were not able to retrieve based on the publications behind these platforms is the one related to the prevalence of the metadata when original date is no longer available. Interoperability wise, apart from using FAIR compliant vocabularies, both FAIRSharing and the Maelstrom Catalogue link to Pubmed publications, when existing. YummyData uses LinkedData technologies, which contributes to its higher interoperability.

Table 3. Assessment of the FAIRness of each of the three discovery platforms based on the FAIRness metrics. X represents a satisfied requirement and - means that no proof to support the requirement was found. This table was originally published in [35].

Platform	F1	F2	F3	F4	A1.1	A1.2	A2	I1	I2	I3	R1.1	R1.2	R1.3
Maelstrom catalogue	X	X	X	X	X	–	–	X	X	X	–	X	–
YummyData	X	X	X	X	X	X	–	X	X	–	X	X	–
FAIRsharing	X	X	X	X	X	X	–	X	X	X	X	X	–

These open applications have benefitted from strong alignment with the FAIR principles, which have facilitated their adoption by many different research bodies. As an example, YummyData and FAIRSharing have been identified by Wise et al. [42] as important FAIR tools, that enable other research projects to transition towards a more FAIR development and data re(use).

5   Discussion

Researchers need tools and support to manage, search and reuse data as part of their research work. In the biomedical area, data discovery platforms, either in the shape of data warehouses or metadata integrators that link to original data silos support the researcher in the process of finding the right data for a given research topic. However, finding the right data is not sufficient for conducting a study. Data should be not only qualitative and accessible under clear and well-defined protocols, but it should also be interoperable and reusable in order to maximize the research outcomes. The FAIR guiding principles are recommendations on the steps to follow in order to increase the meaningfulness and impact of data and are strongly related to data management. FAIR compliant biomedical data discovery platforms have the ability to support biomedical researchers throughout all the steps from finding the right data source to reusing it for secondary research. This can ultimately lead to better health and healthcare outcomes. Ultimately, these principles give an important contribution to the reproducibility of research.

Big biomedical data creates exciting opportunities for discovery, but are often seen as make difficult for capturing analyses and outputs in forms that are FAIR [14]. The FAIR guiding principles have been widely endorsed by publishers, funders, data owners and innovation networks across multiple research areas. However, up until recently, they did not strictly define how to achieve a state of FAIRness and this ambiguity led to some qualitatively different self-assessments of FAIRness. A new template for evaluating the FAIRness of a data set or a data handling system, recently proposed by some of the original authors of the principles, offers a benchmark for a standardized evaluation of such self-assessments. In this paper we have applied them to three different biomedical data discovery platforms in order to estimate their FAIRness. Moreover, we sought to understand the impact that the adoption of these guidelines has in the quality of the output produced by these platforms and to what degree ensuring data reusability and interoperability turns data more prone to be reused for secondary research.

This analysis revealed that the adoption of the FAIR principles is an ongoing process within the biomedical community. However, the FAIR-compliance of a resource or system can be distinct from its impact. The platforms discussed exposed a high level of FAIRness and an increased concern for enabling data discovery by machines. While FAIR is not equal to Linked Data, Semantic Web technologies along with formal ontologies fulfill the FAIR requirements and can contribute to the FAIRness of a discovery platform.

With digital patient data increasing at an exponential rate and having understood the importance of reusing these data for secondary research purposes, it is highly important to ensure its interoperability and reusability. Recently developed data search engines such as DataMed [2] and Google DataSet Search[15] are powered by machine readable metadata and are a powerful stimulus into turning datasets more FAIR. The assessment of data FAIRness is a key element for providing a common ground for data quality to be understood by both data owners and data users. If up until recently the open interpretation of the FAIR guiding principles could lead to assessment biases, the recently published FAIR metrics support more than ever the implementation of the common ground. For this, the biomedical research community should continue to challenge and refine

---

[15] https://toolbox.google.com/datasetsearch.

their implementation choices in order to achieve a desirable Internet of FAIR Data and Services.

6   Conclusions

The FAIR principles demand well-defined qualities and properties from data resources but at the same time they allow a great deal of freedom with respect to how they should be implemented. In this work we reviewed current approaches taken in the areas of biomedical and life-science research for putting them into practice and, as a use case, we further evaluated the approaches followed by three different biomedical data discovery platforms in providing FAIR data and services by following the recently published FAIR metrics. These fresh examples highlighted the increasing impact of the FAIR principles among the biomedical and life-science research community. By acting in accordance with the FAIR metrics we, as a community, can reach an agreed basis for the assessment of data quality and not only add value to data, but ensure reproducibility, transparency and ultimately facilitate research collaborations.

Acknowledgements. This work has received support from the Innovative Medicines Initiative 2 Joint Undertaking (JU) under grant agreement No 806968 and from the Integrated Programme of SR&TD SOCA (Ref. CENTRO-01-0145-FEDER-000010). The JU receives support from the European Union's Horizon 2020 research and innovation programme and EFPIA.

References

1. Bergeron, J., Doiron, D., Marcon, Y., Ferretti, V., Fortier, I.: Fostering population-based cohort data discovery: the Maelstrom research cataloguing toolkit. PLoS ONE **13**(7), e0200926 (2018)
2. Chen, X., et al.: Datamed-an open source discovery index for finding biomedical datasets. J. Am. Med. Inform. Assoc. **25**(3), 300–308 (2018)
3. Danciu, I., et al.: Secondary use of clinical data: the Vanderbilt approach. J. Biomed. Inform. **52**, 28–35 (2014)
4. Dumontier, M., et al.: The health care and life sciences community profile for dataset descriptions. PeerJ **4**, e2331 (2016)
5. Gainotti, S., et al.: The RD-Connect Registry & Biobank Finder: a tool for sharing aggregated data and metadata among rare disease researchers. Eur. J. Hum. Genet. **26**(5), 631 (2018)
6. Green, A.K., et al.: The project data sphere initiative: accelerating cancer research by sharing data. Oncologist **20**(5), 464–e20 (2015)
7. Groth, P., Loizou, A., Gray, A.J., Goble, C., Harland, L., Pettifer, S.: API-centric linked data integration: the open PHACTS discovery platform case study. Web Semant.: Sci. Serv. Agents World Wide Web **29**, 12–18 (2014)
8. Holub, P., et al.: Enhancing reuse of data and biological material in medical research: from FAIR to FAIR-health. Biopreserv. Biobank. **16**(2), 97–105 (2018)
9. Jagodnik, K.M., et al.: Developing a framework for digital objects in the big data to knowledge (BD2K) commons: report from the commons framework pilots workshop. J. Biomed. Inform. **71**, 49–57 (2017)

10. Jansen, C., Beier, M., Witt, M., Frey, S., Krefting, D.: Towards reproducible research in a biomedical collaboration platform following the FAIR guiding principles. In: Companion Proceedings of the 10th International Conference on Utility and Cloud Computing, pp. 3–8. ACM (2017)
11. Karim, M.R., et al.: Towards a FAIR sharing of scientific experiments: improving discoverability and reusability of dielectric measurements of biological tissues. In: SWAT4LS (2017)
12. Koehorst, J.J., van Dam, J.C., Saccenti, E., Martins dos Santos, V.A., Suarez-Diez, M., Schaap, P.J.: SAPP: functional genome annotation and analysis through a semantic framework using FAIR principles. Bioinformatics 34(8), 1401–1403 (2017)
13. Lancaster, O., et al.: Cafe Variome: general-purpose software for making genotype-phenotype data discoverable in restricted or open access contexts. Hum. Mutat. 36(10), 957–964 (2015)
14. Madduri, R., et al.: Reproducible big data science: a case study in continuous FAIRness. PLoS ONE 14(4), e0213013 (2019)
15. Magazine, D.L.: The dataverse network®: an open-source application for sharing, discovering and preserving data. D-lib Mag. 17(1), 2 (2011)
16. Martin-Sanchez, F., Verspoor, K.: Big data in medicine is driving big changes. Yearb. Med. Inform. 9(1), 14 (2014)
17. McQuilton, P., et al.: BioSharing: curated and crowd-sourced metadata standards, databases and data policies in the life sciences. Database 2016 (2016)
18. Mons, B., Neylon, C., Velterop, J., Dumontier, M., da Silva Santos, L.O.B., Wilkinson, M.D.: Cloudy, increasingly FAIR; revisiting the FAIR data guiding principles for the European Open Science Cloud. Inf. Serv. 37(1), 49–56 (2017)
19. Natsiavas, P., Boyce, R.D., Jaulent, M.C., Koutkias, V.: OpenPVSignal: advancing information search, sharing and reuse on pharmacovigilance signals via FAIR principles and semantic web technologies. Front. Pharmacol. 9, 609 (2018)
20. Navale, V., McAuliffe, M.: Long-term preservation of biomedical research data. F1000Research 7 (2018)
21. van Panhuis, W.G., Cross, A., Burke, D.S.: Project Tycho 2.0: a repository to improve the integration and reuse of data for global population health. J. Am. Med. Inform. Assoc. 25(12), 1608–1617 (2018)
22. Phan, J.H., Quo, C.F., Cheng, C., Wang, M.D.: Multiscale integration of -omic, imaging, and clinical data in biomedical informatics. IEEE Rev. Biomed. Eng. 5, 74–87 (2012)
23. Press, G.: Cleaning big data: most time-consuming, least enjoyable data science task, survey says. Forbes, 23 March 2016
24. Prinz, F., Schlange, T., Asadullah, K.: Believe it or not: how much can we rely on published data on potential drug targets? Nat. Rev. Drug Discov. 10(9), 712 (2011)
25. Pundir, S., Martin, M.J., O'Donovan, C.: UniProt protein knowledgebase. In: Wu, C.H., Arighi, C.N., Ross, K.E. (eds.) Protein Bioinformatics. MMB, vol. 1558, pp. 41–55. Springer, New York (2017). https://doi.org/10.1007/978-1-4939-6783-4_2
26. Razick, S., Močnik, R., Thomas, L.F., Ryeng, E., Drabløs, F., Sætrom, P.: The eGenVar data management system-cataloguing and sharing sensitive data and metadata for the life sciences. Database 2014 (2014)
27. Rodríguez-Iglesias, A., et al.: Publishing FAIR data: an exemplar methodology utilizing PHI-base. Front. Plant Sci. 7, 641 (2016)
28. Schaaf, J., et al.: OSSE goes FAIR-implementation of the FAIR data principles for an open-source registry for rare diseases. Stud. Health Technol. Inform. 253, 209–213 (2018)

29. Silva, L.B., Trifan, A., Oliveira, J.L.: Montra: an agile architecture for data publishing and discovery. Comput. Methods Programs Biomed. **160**, 33–42 (2018)
30. da Silva Santos, L., et al.: FAIR data points supporting big data interoperability. In: Enterprise Interoperability in the Digitized and Networked Factory of the Future. ISTE, London pp. 270–279 (2016)
31. Stathias, V., et al.: Sustainable data and metadata management at the BD2K-lincs data coordination and integration center. Sci. Data **5**, 180117 (2018)
32. Torre, D., et al.: Datasets2Tools, repository and search engine for bioinformatics datasets, tools and canned analyses. Sci. Data **5**, 180023 (2018)
33. Traverso, A., van Soest, J., Wee, L., Dekker, A.: The radiation oncology ontology (ROO): publishing linked data in radiation oncology using semantic web and ontology techniques. Med. Phys. **45**(10), e854–e862 (2018)
34. Trifan, A., Oliveira, J.: FAIRness in biomedical data discovery, pp. 159–166, January 2019. https://doi.org/10.5220/0007576401590166
35. Trifan, A., Oliveira, J.L.: A FAIR marketplace for biomedical data custodians and clinical researchers. In: 2018 IEEE 31st International Symposium on Computer-Based Medical Systems (CBMS), pp. 188–193. IEEE (2018)
36. Trifan, A., Oliveira, J.L.: Patient data discovery platforms as enablers of biomedical and translational research: a systematic review. J. Biomed. Inform. **93**, 103154 (2019)
37. Vaccarino, A.L., et al.: Brain-CODE: a secure neuroinformatics platform for management, federation, sharing and analysis of multi-dimensional neuroscience data. Front. Neuroinform. **12**, 28 (2018)
38. Vita, R., Overton, J.A., Mungall, C.J., Sette, A., Peters, B.: FAIR principles and the IEDB: short-term improvements and a long-term vision of obo-foundry mediated machine-actionable interoperability. Database **2018** (2018)
39. Wang, Z., Lachmann, A., Ma'ayan, A.: Mining data and metadata from the gene expression omnibus. Biophys. Rev. **11**(1), 103–110 (2018). https://doi.org/10.1007/s12551-018-0490-8
40. Wen, C.H., et al.: B-CAN: a resource sharing platform to improve the operation, visualization and integrated analysis of TCGA breast cancer data. Oncotarget **8**(65), 108778 (2017)
41. Wilkinson, M.D., et al.: The FAIR guiding principles for scientific data management and stewardship. Sci. Data **3** (2016)
42. Wise, J., et al.: Implementation and relevance of FAIR data principles in biopharmaceutical R&D. Drug Discov. Today **24**(4), 933–938 (2019)
43. Wittig, U., Rey, M., Weidemann, A., Mueller, W.: Data management and data enrichment for systems biology projects. J. Biotechnol. **261**, 229–237 (2017)
44. Yamamoto, Y., Yamaguchi, A., Splendiani, A.: YummyData: providing high-quality open life science data. Database **2018** (2018)
45. Zaveri, A., et al.: smartAPI: towards a more intelligent network of web APIs. In: Blomqvist, E., Maynard, D., Gangemi, A., Hoekstra, R., Hitzler, P., Hartig, O. (eds.) ESWC 2017. LNCS, vol. 10250, pp. 154–169. Springer, Cham (2017). https://doi.org/10.1007/978-3-319-58451-5_11

Author Index

Printed in the United States
By Bookmasters